"The Physics of Resistance Exercise *is a welcome addition to the fitness*
*other book has addressed. I wish I had this information years ago. I would ha*
*time on useless exercises. Great going, Doug!"*

—Richard Baldwin, Ph.D.
Professor of History/Humanities
Gulf Coast State College

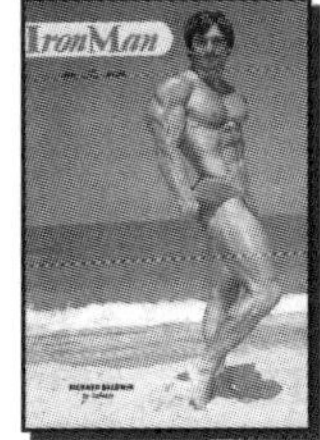


**Richard Baldwin** is Professor Emeritus, Social Sciences Division, Gulf Coast State College. An accomplished former competitive bodybuilder, having won Mr. Texas ('72), Mr. USA ('75), and Mr. Florida ('78), and twice finished 2nd place in Mr. Universe ('79 and '80), he has two master's degrees (one in theology, and one in Greek and Latin), as well as a Ph.D. in literature. Dubbed the "Modern Apollo" of his time by *Iron Man* magazine, Dr. Baldwin has devoted much of his career as an educator to helping people better understand the aging process.

✦ ✦ ✦

*"I've known Doug Brignole since 1979—39 years to date. We met when he was competing for the Teenage Mr. California title, at the age of 19. Throughout my many years involved in the sport, I can honestly say that Doug is one of the most passionate, sincere, and intelligent of all the bodybuilders I have had the pleasure to know. There are very few bodybuilders who have achieved the same degree of physique elegance and artistry as Doug Brignole, and there are probably very few scholars (non-bodybuilders) who have reached his level of knowledge related to exercise mechanics, as Doug Brignole. But Doug has achieved both.* The Physics of Resistance Exercise *is the culmination of Doug's 40+ years in the sport, passionately pursuing the ultimate in physical development, as well as the scientific knowledge about how to best optimize efficient biomechanics. It's an honor to regard Doug Brignole as my friend, and my pleasure to recommend this outstanding book."*

—Samir Bannout
Member, IFBB Hall of Fame

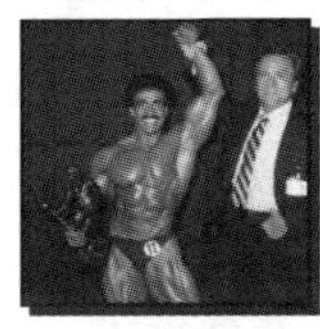

**Samir Bannout** born and raised in Beirut, Lebanon, is widely regarded as one of the best, most aesthetic and most symmetrical bodybuilders of all time. He competed in 58 competitions over a 37-year period of time, winning numerous international titles including the prestigious Mr. Olympia title in 1983—which is considered by many individuals as the highest honor in bodybuilding. Known as the "Lion of Lebanon," he is the last Mr. Olympia to weigh under 200 lbs.

✦ ✦ ✦

*"One of the outstanding features of Doug Brignole's extraordinary exploration of* The Physics of Resistance Exercise *is his appreciation for the importance of addressing psychological factors affecting exercise practices, athleticism definitions, strength building assumptions, and resistance to changing routines used to achieve different fitness goals. Doug not only raises the bar in physical training by his vast experience and expertise in biomechanics, he also raises awareness of the profound roles played by personal biases, historical beliefs, and societal values in our pursuit of athletic prowess and muscular development."*

—Ellen Basian, Ph.D.
Clinical Psychologist
Los Angeles, CA

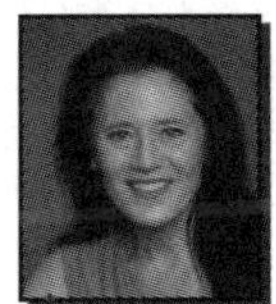

**Ellen Basian** has been in private practice since graduating from the Northwestern University Medical School in 1993. Her diverse experience in clinical psychology emphasizes an integrated treatment approach for mind-body fitness with individuals, couples, and groups.

✦ ✦ ✦

*"In* The Physics of Resistance Exercise, *Doug Brignole uses a rational and systematic approach to answer the question: What are the most efficient movements for building muscle? Drawing from anatomy, physics, exercise science, and extensive experience, Brignole makes a compelling case that a specific set of basic movements should make up the bulk of a person's physical culture practice, while dispelling a number of fitness industry myths in the process."*

—Stephan J. Guyenet, Ph.D.
Obesity Researcher
Author

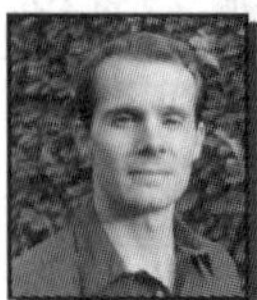

**Stephan J. Guyenet** is a health writer whose work ties together neuroscience, physiology, evolutionary biology, and nutrition to offer explanations and solutions to the global problem with excess body weight. He received a B.S. in biochemistry from the University of Virginia and a Ph.D. in neurobiology at the University of Washington. He is the author of the popular health website Whole Health Source, as well as the well-received book *The Hungry Brain*.

✦ ✦ ✦

*"Through the many years in which I've been involved in weight lifting, power lifting, and physical fitness, I've never read a more intelligent analysis of the biomechanics of resistance exercise, for the purpose of physique/muscular development, than* The Physics of Resistance Exercise. *Doug Brignole has done a remarkable job of explaining the elements that factor into this type of training. This book will likely revolutionize the way 'resistance exercise' is taught from this point forward."*

—Frederick C. Hatfield, Ph.D.
Co-founder and President
ISSA

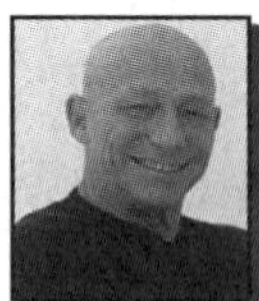

**Frederick C. Hatfield**, nicknamed Dr. Squat, was an American world champion powerlifter. He also co-founded the International Sports Sciences Association, an organization that certifies personal trainers. He earned a B.S. degree in physical education at Southern Connecticut State University, an M.S. degree in social sciences of sport from the University of Illinois at Urbana-Champaign, and a Ph.D. in psychology, sociology, and motor learning from Temple University. (Note: Dr. Hatfield passed away on May 14, 2017—several months after giving this endorsement.)

✦ ✦ ✦

*"Doug Brignole's extensive knowledge of the human musculoskeletal system, as demonstrated in* The Physics of Resistance Exercise, *is very impressive. It is obvious that he has done quite a bit of research and study, and that he clearly understands the mechanics of the body. What's most astounding is his ability to then connect the ideal mechanics of the human body with the physics that makes an exercise more or less efficient (muscle load versus energy cost). It's wonderful to see resistance exercise being approached from the perspective of safe and efficient movement, instead of the contortionist version we often see, or focusing primarily on simply moving a very heavy weight. It makes good sense to exercise in ways that provide a muscle with the most load, while simultaneously reducing the stress on the bones and joints."*

—Ronald S. Kvitne, M.D.
Partner, Kerlan-Jobe Orthopaedic Clinic
Los Angeles, CA

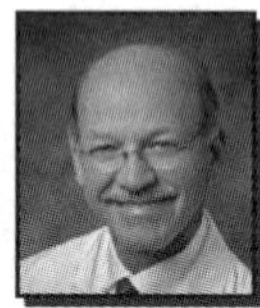

**Ronald S. Kvitne** is a renowned orthopaedic surgeon who has been practicing medicine for almost four decades. A 1982 graduate of the University of California, San Francisco School of Medicine, he is the head team physician for both the Los Angeles Angels of Anaheim (professional baseball team) and the Los Angeles Kings (professional ice hockey team).

✦ ✦ ✦

*"Doug Brignole brings together cutting-edge exercise science and decades of experience as a world-class athlete in* The Physics of Resistance Exercise. *As a former engineer and professional bodybuilder, I appreciate the solid foundation of exercise science, combined with real world applications. The concepts presented are solid, and, once mastered, will take your training to a new level. This book is a MUST-READ, if you're serious about understanding the WHYs and HOWs of all the sets, reps, and training that you do as an athlete!"*

—Lee Labrada
International Professional Bodybuilding Champion
Author

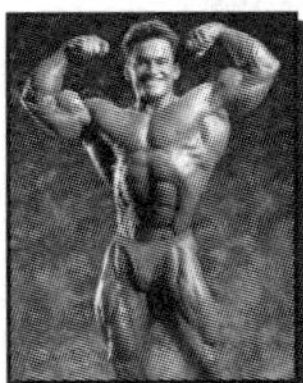

**Lee Labrada** is one of the world's most well-known and celebrated bodybuilding champions. He holds 22 professional bodybuilding titles, including the IFBB Mr. Universe, and is one of few pro bodybuilders in history to consistently place in the top four at the Mr. Olympia competition (the "Super Bowl" of bodybuilding) for seven consecutive years—a feat he shares with Arnold Schwarzenegger. In 2004, Lee was inducted into the IFBB Pro-Bodybuilding Hall of Fame. He has appeared on the covers of more than 100 bodybuilding and fitness magazines and has been featured on CNBC, FOX, NBC, ABC, CBS, CNN, and ESPN as a fitness and nutrition expert.

✦ ✦ ✦

*"I have known Doug Brignole since 1986, when we presented a series of sports and fitness seminars in Pasadena, California. Throughout the years, Doug's theoretical and practical expertise has stood as a national and international reference in the field. His book—*The Physics of Resistance Exercise*—contains a wealth of knowledge regarding proper training procedures and methodology, as viewed from the perspective of a bodybuilding champion, as well as from a person of great maturity and wisdom. I have learned a great deal from Doug, and it is my sincere wish that you will too."*

—Guillermo A. Laich, M.D., Ph.D.
Professor of Medical and Surgical Pathology
University Alfonso X el Sabio (UAX—Madrid)

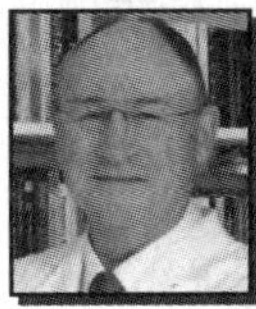

**Guillermo A. Laich** is a world-renowned physician, based in Madrid, Spain. His medical specialties include clinical psychiatry, plastic surgery, sports medicine, internal medicine, and surgical pathology. With an extensive professional history in medicine and sports sciences, he is often invited to speak at professional meetings. In addition, he has had noteworthy involvement with the martial arts community, particularly karate.

✦ ✦ ✦

*"So much of what is considered 'conventional wisdom' about resistance exercise exists as anecdote—'tips' passed down from one person to another. The belief in the effectiveness of certain exercises is often garnered by the appearance of the person promoting that exercise, as if there isn't a better method by which exercises can be evaluated. Ignored in all this is the biomechanical factors that are involved in each exercise. In* The Physics of Resistance Exercise, *Doug Brignole has tackled this problem successfully by presenting, in a precise and easy-to-understand manner, how the musculoskeletal system works, and the role of physics during resistance exercise. The brilliance of this book is Doug's ability to explain and illustrate to the reader how this knowledge can be utilized to get the best results, with the least wasted energy and the least risk of injury."*

—David H. Le, M.D.
Orthopedic Surgeon

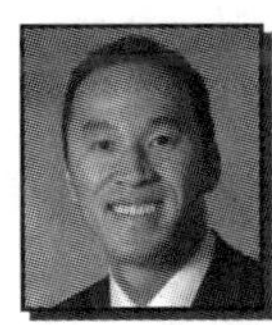

**David H. Le** is an orthopedic surgeon, based in Los Angeles, who has been practicing sports medicine since graduating from Tufts University School of Medicine in 2004. Born in Vietnam and raised in Southern California, he is affiliated with Los Angeles Kaiser Permanente, specializing in knees and hips.

✦ ✦ ✦

*"I found* The Physics of Resistance Exercise *to be absolutely fascinating. Clearly, the human body is made up of levers, which naturally follow the same rules of physics as do all other mechanical systems and structures. I also found it remarkable that Doug Brignole was able to apply these well-established principles to the human anatomy, in the performance of resistance exercise, and then to simplify the myriad of recommendations we are all given by the fitness industry down to those that are most efficient and safe. This is the best book on the subject of resistance exercise I've ever read. In fact, I cannot imagine anyone being in the business of teaching resistance exercise, and NOT understanding the bio-mechanical principles that are presented in this book. After reading Doug's book, I made several changes to my own workout regime and can attest I feel better, and have experienced improved results."*

—Jeffrey R. Mackey, Ph.D.
Physics/Astrophysics
NASA

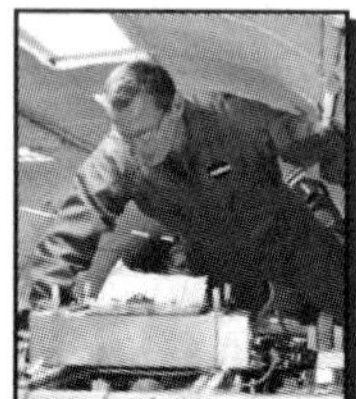

**Jeffrey R. Mackey** has been both a safety engineer and optical research engineer providing support service work under contract at NASA Glenn Research Center since 1990 and has taught part-time in the Physics Department at Cleveland State University since 2007. Dr. Mackey obtained an A.B. in physics from Kenyon College in 1985, an M.S. in optical physics from Cleveland State University in 1994, and his Ph.D. in engineering from the Electrical Engineering and Computer Science Department at the University of Toledo in 2002. During his career, he has authored or co-authored numerous peer-reviewed articles and has been involved in a considerable number of research projects for NASA. He also has presented papers at a variety of professional meetings.

✦ ✦ ✦

*"As an orthopedic surgeon and spine specialist, and also from the perspective of being personally involved in weight lifting for many years, I can honestly say that Doug Brignole's understanding of human mechanics is extraordinary. Doug's knowledge of the anatomy, combined with his grasp of physics, allow him to have a unique and valuable perspective on the safest and most productive way to engage in resistance exercise.* The Physics of Resistance Exercise *is an outstanding book."*

—Hooman Melamed, M.D.
Orthopedic Surgeon/Spine Specialist
Marina Del Rey, CA

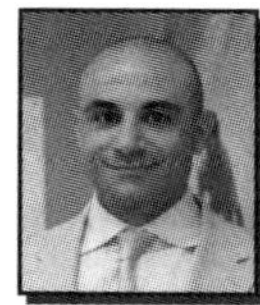

**Hooman Melamed** is a well-respected orthopedic surgeon, based in Marina Del Rey, CA. A pioneer in the field of minimally invasive spine surgery, Dr. Melamed regularly appears as a medical expert on television.

*"As a professor of sociology, my focus is on the cultural behaviors that are adopted by populations—often in the absence of good reasoning. Humans tend to be 'copy cats,' which is evidenced by fashion trends, the use of slang, and also religious, cultural and political views. Therefore, it's easy to see how an obsession with 'physical power' has allowed exercise bias to exist for many decades. This appears to have led many people to favor 'compound' exercises, and eschew 'isolation' exercises, even though physics and anatomical analysis do not support those beliefs. In* The Physics of Resistance Exercise, *Doug Brignole does a great job of breaking down the physics of what determines the load on a muscle, thereby revealing that traditional exercise selections are often based more on bias than on science, or even logic. This book reveals that there are far better ways of achieving one's goal of muscular development—with less wasted effort and less abuse on the joints—than has been used traditionally."*

—Adrian James Tan, Ph.D.
Professor of Sociology
University of North Texas

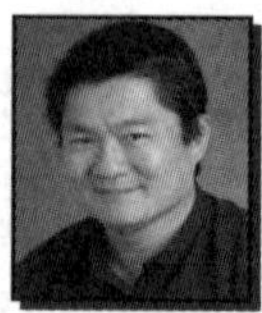

**Adrian James Tan** is a professor of sociology at the University of North Texas, as well as the author or co-author of three books, including "Million Dollar Muscle," which he wrote with Doug Brignole. Dr. Tan obtained a bachelor's degree in English and philosophy, as well as a master's degree in sociology and international affairs—both from Ohio University. He earned his Ph.D. in sociology from the University of North Texas.

✦ ✦ ✦

# THE PHYSICS OF RESISTANCE EXERCISE

## An Analysis and Application of Biomechanical Principles in Resistance Exercise

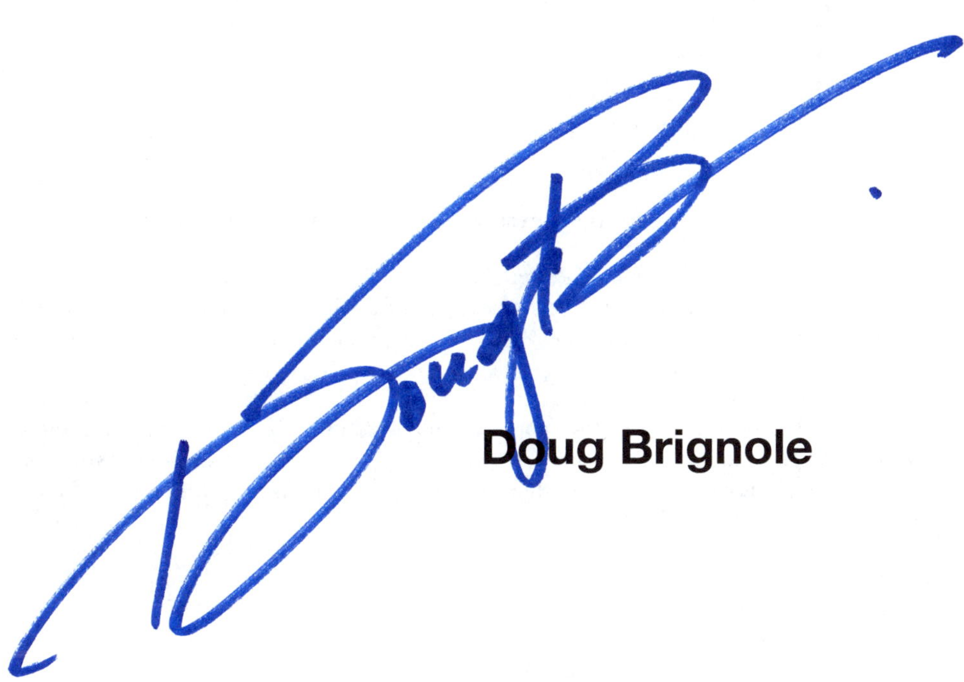

Doug Brignole

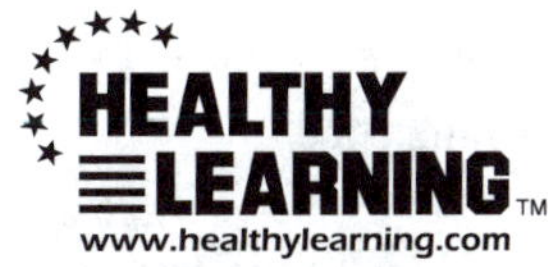

ISBN: 978-1-60679-497-5
Cover design: Cheery Sugabo
Book layout: Cheery Sugabo
Cover images: ScienPro/Shutterstock.com; Duntrune Studios/Shutterstock.com
Back cover author photo: Robert Reiff

Healthy Learning
P.O. Box 1828
Monterey, CA 93942
www.healthylearning.com

# DEDICATION

*Dedicated to the loving memory of my mother,*

*Ines Ortiz Bolocco de Brignole*

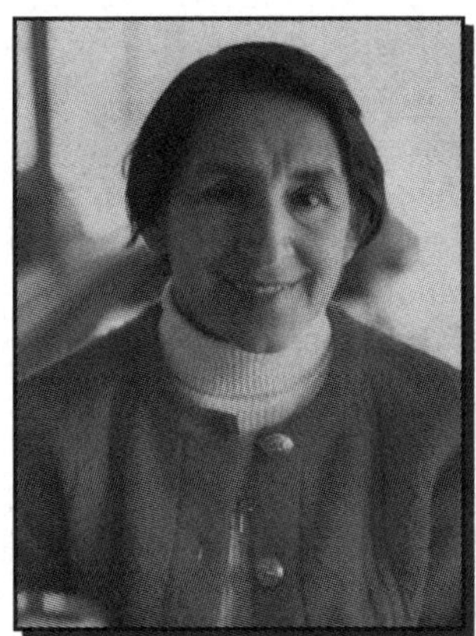

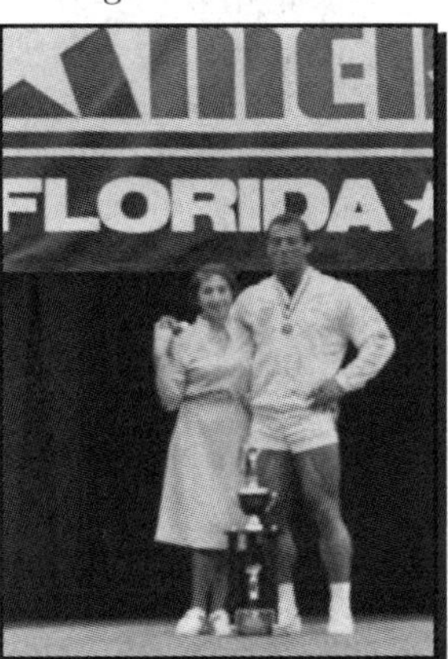

# FOREWORD

Every year, thousands of youth and young adults begin a resistance training program in an attempt to either enlarge their muscle size for enhanced physical appearance or to increase their muscle strength for improved athletic performance. Most of these new fitness enthusiasts perform standard resistance exercises, as recommended by fitness professionals, personal trainers, and friends, or as presented in books, magazines, and websites. These standard resistance exercises are generally effective for the first few months of training, during which time most new participants experience gains in both muscle size and strength. Sooner or later, however, they encounter either an exercise-related injury or a muscle-development plateau. One reason for these unintended occurrences is that many popular resistance exercises present a relatively high risk of injury, a relatively low training stimulus to the target muscles, or both.

When faced with exercise-related injuries, most people discontinue their resistance training program altogether. When faced with muscle-development plateaus, many people increase their training volume by performing more exercises and more sets of each exercise. For those individuals who have less favorable musculoskeletal genetics, high-volume resistance training typically leads to overuse injuries that can become chronic problems. For those exercisers who have more favorable musculoskeletal genetics, high-volume resistance training may be effective for eliciting additional gains in muscle size and strength. Adherence to high-volume resistance training programs, however, is physically demanding, mentally challenging, and time-consuming.

Thankfully, there is a safe and productive alternative to high-volume resistance training, based on more appropriate exercise selection and more effective exercise performance. In this comprehensive resistance training textbook, Doug Brignole presents a physics perspective for maximizing muscle development by *doing the right exercises and doing them right.* Doug applies his extensive knowledge of biomechanics to both the principles of resistance training and the practical applications of exercise performance.

The first 17 book chapters clearly explain the physics principles that are essential for optimal performance of all resistance exercises. Doug demonstrates an unusual ability to simplify complex biomechanical concepts through excellent examples and precise illustrations, so that readers can make appropriate practical applications to their exercise selection and execution.

The next eight book chapters discuss specific resistance exercises for essentially all of the larger and smaller muscles. Doug details the strengths and weaknesses of various exercises, presents the most effective exercises for enhancing muscle development and avoiding injuries, and describes how to properly perform those exercises for best results.

Doug's understanding of physics principles and musculoskeletal biomechanics is exceptionally impressive, as are the physique titles that he has achieved by putting this knowledge into practice throughout his 40-plus years of championship bodybuilding. As a former Mr. California, Mr. America, and Mr. Universe, Doug certainly knows how to train hard in the weight room. Equally important, Doug also knows how to train safely and efficiently (with fewer exercises and sets), by ensuring that each exercise provides maximum stimulus to the target muscle(s).

If you would like to enhance your muscle development with more productive exercises that offer lower injury risk and higher training effect, then you are reading the right book. You will definitely gain greater understanding of how your muscles work, how to work your muscles, and how to think critically about each exercise that you perform.

After reading and contemplating Doug's physics-based analyses of resistance exercises, I made some beneficial changes in my strength training program. I am very confident that the information presented in this cutting-edge text will enable you to also make some advantageous exercise modifications in your strength training program.

—Wayne L. Westcott, Ph.D.
Professor of Exercise Science, Quincy College,
Quincy, Massachusetts
Author of 28 strength training books/textbooks

# CONTENTS

Dedication ........................................................ 7
Foreword by Wayne L. Westcott, Ph.D. ........................................................ 8
Prologue by Bill Pearl ........................................................ 16
Introduction ........................................................ 19

**CHAPTER 1:** The Levers of the Human Body ........................................................ 25

- Determining the Amount of Magnification of Levers
- Types of Levers (Class 1, Class 2, and Class 3)
- Primary Levers and Secondary Levers
- Tilting the Secondary Lever on a Different Plane
- Evaluating the Effect of the Secondary Lever on the Squat
- Comparing Two Versions of the Standing Side Dumbbell Raise
- Summary

**CHAPTER 2:** Active Levers and Neutral Levers ........................................................ 37

- Comparing an Efficient Lever vs. an Inefficient Lever
- Assessing Exercise Efficiency
- Supine Dumbbell Press (as a Pectoral Exercise)
- Hanging Leg Raises (as an Abdominal Exercise)
- Squats (as a Quadriceps Exercise)
- When a "Neutral" Lever Is Made Dangerously "Active"
- Summary

**CHAPTER 3:** Mechanical Disadvantage ........................................................ 51

- Application During a Standing Barbell Curl
- When "Mechanical Disadvantage" Meets an "Active Lever"
- A Mechanical Disadvantage Only Occurs With "Flexion" Joints and Muscles
- List of Muscles That Experience Mechanical "AD-vantage" and "DIS-advantage"
- Higher Risk of Injury When Training the Biceps, Pecs, Hamstrings, and Lats, Due to Mechanical Disadvantage
- Pectoral Injuries
- Latissimus Dorsi Injuries
- Hamstring Injuries
- Summary

**CHAPTER 4:** The Resistance Curve ........................................................ 65

- What Is a Resistance Curve?
- Types (and Directions) of Resistance

- Manipulating the Resistance Curve
- The Ideal Resistance Curve: "Early Phase Loading"
- Comparing the Resistance Curves of Several "Side Raise" Exercise Versions for the Lateral Deltoids
- Summary

**CHAPTER 5:** The Apex and the Base ........................................ 79

- What Defines the Apex and the Base?
- Transference of Load After Crossing the Apex or Base
- The Four Resistance Quadrants
- Application
- Another Example
- How the Apex and/or Base Interact With a Secondary Lever
- Summary

**CHAPTER 6:** Primary and Secondary Resistance Sources and Other Forces ........................................ 91

- What Defines a Secondary Resistance?
- When a Secondary Resistance Pulls a Different Direction Than the Primary Resistance
- Composite Direction of Resistance
- Improperly Adding a Second Resistance Source
- Centrifugal Force and Momentum
- Momentum Meets Ground Reaction Force and Friction Force
- Summary

**CHAPTER 7:** Alignment ........................................ 103

- The Consequence of Misalignment
- Alignment of Movement and of Resistance
- The Viewing Plane of Alignment
- Summary

**CHAPTER 8:** Opposite Position Loading ........................................ 113

- The Load Is Always Greatest Opposite the Direction of Resistance
- Proper Positioning of a Muscle Relative to Resistance
- Summary

**CHAPTER 9:** "Dynamic" vs. "Static" Muscle Contraction and Range of Motion ........................................ 125

- The Difference Between Dynamic and Static Muscle Contraction
- Using Dynamic Tension for Target Muscles and Isometric Tension for Stabilizing Muscles
- How Much Range of Motion Is Enough?
- A Bit of History: The Marketing of Isometric Exercise
- Summary

**CHAPTER 10:** The "All or Nothing" Principle of Muscle Contraction and the Myth of "Shaping" a Muscle .............................. 139

- What Is the "All or Nothing" Principle?
- Folklore Regarding Changing Muscle Shape
- Summary

**CHAPTER 11:** Reciprocal Innervation and Active and Passive Insufficiency............................................................145

- What Is Reciprocal Innervation?
- The Relationship Between Reciprocal Innervation and the Apex/Base
- What Is Active and Passive Insufficiency?
- Using Reciprocal Innervation to Structure Workouts
- A More Sensible Approach
- Creating a Workout Structure
- Intensity, Recovery, and Adaption
- Relieve Muscle Cramping With Reciprocal Innervation
- Summary

**CHAPTER 12:** "Compound" vs. "Isolation"—The Origins of the Debate.......................................................................155

- The Birth of "Physical Culture"
- Comparing "Compound" vs. "Isolation" Exercises for Muscle Loading
- Is a Critical Evaluation of a Compound Exercise "Immoral"?
- Survival and Heroism
- Comic Books and Mythology
- The Folly of Impressing Observers
- Departures From Logic
- Leg Extension "Shearing"
- Summary

**CHAPTER 13:** Peripheral Recruitment—Comparing Compound and Isolation Exercises ..................................................... 169

- Assertions in Favor of Compound Exercise
- Reality Check: Compound Exercise Fallacies
- Comparing Compound Exercise vs. Isolation Exercise
- The Bias in Favor of Compound Exercise
- The Mechanical Inefficiency of Most Compound Exercises and the Folly of Prioritizing the Lifting of "Heavy" Weight
- Summary

**CHAPTER 14:** Momentum and the Use of "Good Form"....................... 183

- The Difference Between Good Form vs. Bad Form: Momentum
- Momentum Example #1
- Momentum Example #2
- Momentum Example #3
- Momentum Example #4

- "Cheating" in Two Ways
- "Bouncing" on a Stability Ball
- Acceptable Applications of Momentum
- Kettlebell Training and Momentum
- Summary

**CHAPTER 15:** Balance/Core Exercises in Physique Development Training........................................................191

- The Origin of "Balance Training"
- What Is Balance and Equilibrium?
- What Is Proprioception?
- Who Needs Proprioceptive Exercise?
- The Folly of Combining Instability With Strength Training
- Bait and Switch: "Balance" Training Being Sold as Fitness Training
- The Compromises of Training While Unstable
- What Is the "Core," and How to Train the Core Correctly?
- Summary

**CHAPTER 16:** "Cross Education" and the Benefits of Unilateral Exercise ...............................................................207

- What Is Cross Education?
- The Benefits of Unilateral Resistance Exercise
- Using Cross Education to Improve Muscular Symmetry
- Redefining "Unilateral" Exercise
- When to Use Isolated Unilateral, Alternating Unilateral, and Simultaneous Unilateral Exercise
- "Unidirectional Focus" and the Avoidance of Moving Limbs in the Opposite Direction During Resistance Exercise
- "Bilateral Deficit" (BLD)
- Summary
- Cited References

**CHAPTER 17:** Assessing and Selecting Exercises, Using "Ideal" Biomechanical Parameters................................................ 221

- Using Biomechanical Factors to Evaluate the Potential Benefits and Risks of Resistance Exercise
- The Role of Evolution in Determining Natural Human Motion
- Determining Which Movements Are Most "Natural," Most Productive, and Most Safe
- Referencing Joint Design in Exercise Evaluation
- Referencing the Direction of a Muscle's Fibers
- Recognizing the Difference Between Bad, Good, Better, and Best Exercises
- Is Changing Exercises Regularly Necessary?
- Does the Body Really Adapt to the Same Exercises?
- Testing the Theory
- Summary

**CHAPTER 18:** Pectorals and the Serratus Anterior ................................ 235

- The Best Anatomical Movement for Pectoral Exercise
- The Myth of Incline Movement for the Upper Pecs
- Evaluating Other Angles for Pectoral Exercise
- Anatomy and Function of the Pectoralis Minor
- Anatomy and Function of the Coracobrachialis
- Anatomy and Function of the Serratus Anterior
- Summary

**CHAPTER 19:** Latissimus Dorsi and "Upper-Back" Muscles ................. 251

- Anatomy of the "Lats"
- Determining the Ideal Anatomical Motion for Exercising the Lats
- Determining the Ideal Direction of Resistance for the Lats
- The Muscles of the "Upper Back": Middle Trapezius, Teres Major, Infraspinatus, and Teres Minor
- The Best Exercise for the "Upper Back"
- What About the Upper Trapezius?

**CHAPTER 20:** Deltoids—Lateral, Anterior, and Posterior ..................... 267

- Anatomy of the Lateral Deltoids
- "Lateral Abduction" Is the Ideal Direction of Anatomical Movement for the Lateral Deltoids
- Identifying the Ideal Direction of Resistance for "Lateral Abduction"
- Exercise Options for the Lateral Deltoids
- Anatomy of the Anterior Deltoids
- Identifying the Ideal Anatomical Motion for the Anterior Deltoids
- Exercise Options for the Anterior Deltoids
- Anatomy of the Posterior Deltoids
- Identifying the Ideal Anatomical Motion for the Posterior Deltoids
- Exercise Options for the Posterior Deltoids

**CHAPTER 21:** Biceps, Triceps, and Forearms ........................................ 285

- Anatomy and Function of the Biceps Brachii
- The Ideal Anatomical Motion of the Biceps
- The Ideal Direction of Resistance for the Biceps
- Vulnerability of the Biceps/Mechanical Disadvantage
- The Effect of Hand/Wrist Position During Biceps Exercises
- Anatomy of the Triceps
- The Ideal Anatomical Movement for the Triceps
- The Ideal Direction of Resistance for the Triceps
- Anatomy and Function of the Forearms
- Exercise Options for the Forearm Flexors and Extensors

**CHAPTER 22:** Quadriceps and Hamstrings ........................................... 311

- Anatomy of the Quadriceps
- Analysis of Common Exercises for the Quadriceps
- Anatomy of the Hamstrings

**CHAPTER 23:** Glutes, Adductors, and Hip Flexors ................................ 339

- Anatomy of the Gluteus Maximus
- The Ideal Anatomical Motion for the Gluteus Maximus
- Exercise Options for the Gluteus Maximus
- Anatomy of the Gluteus Medius and Gluteus Minimus
- Anatomy of the Femural Adductors
- Anatomy of the Hip Flexors
- Should You Work Your Hip Flexors?
- Developing the Hip Flexors for Physique Display
- Exercise Options for the Hip Flexors

**CHAPTER 24:** Calves, Abs, and Lower Back........................................... 357

- Anatomy of the Calves
- The Function of the Gastrocnemius vs. the Soleus
- Impossible to Emphasize "Inner" Calf vs. "Outer" Calf
- Ideal Foot Position, When Training the Calves
- Range of Motion, When Training the Calves
- The Proper Amount of Resistance, When Training the Calves
- Anatomy of the Rectus Abdominis
- Best Number of Reps for Training the Abs
- The Anatomy of the Erector Spinae and the Myth of the "Lower Back"
- Summary
- References

**CHAPTER 25:** Internal and External Obliques, Transverse Abdominis, and Shoulder Rotators .................................................... 385

- Anatomy and Function of the Obliques
- Ideal Direction of Resistance for Training the Obliques
- Range of Motion and Limitations of Spinal Mobility
- Commentary About Other Exercises for the Obliques
- Anatomy of the Transverse Abdominis
- Shoulder Rotators (AKA the Rotator Cuff Muscles)

**CHAPTER 26:** In Conclusion ................................................................. 405

- The Causes of "Bad" Choices Related to Exercise
- The Influence of Fitness Magazines
- Dubious Endorsement by Trusted Authorities
- Misinformed "Experts"
- Knowledge vs. Beliefs
- Psychological Barriers to New (Better) Information

About the Author ........................................................................................ 416

# PROLOGUE

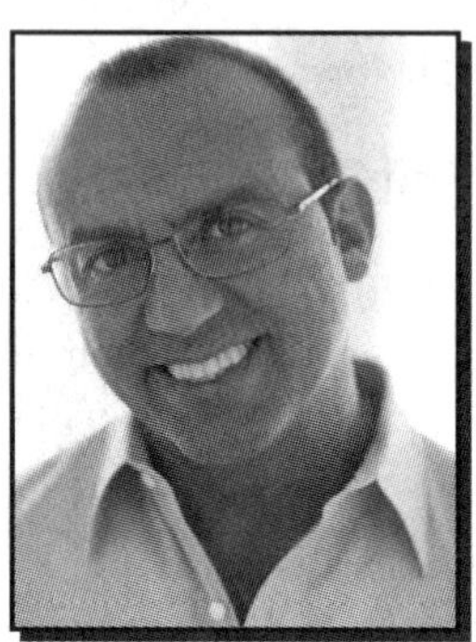

Doug Brignole began weight training when he was 14 years old. His goal was to increase his body weight, because he was very thin, and his Junior High School coach told him it's better to gain muscle weight than fat weight. So, he convinced his mother to buy him a home barbell set, and an adjustable bench. The barbell set came with a "*Weight Training Guide Book.*"

Doug followed the advice and examples in the book, but immediately realized that many exercises did not feel right. In some cases, he felt that certain exercises were very uncomfortable, i.e., the movement felt "unnatural." In other instances, he was not able to feel the "target" muscle working or perceived that the exercise did not have a "logical trajectory." This observation alone is interesting, because most 14-year-old kids don't question the "correctness" of an exercise. If they feel any joint strain, or don't feel the muscle working, they typically assume they're doing it wrong, or assume they just don't know how the exercise is supposed to feel.

On the other hand, Doug noticed that some exercises DID feel "right." He observed that certain other exercises felt very "natural," and that the objective—the trajectory of the movement—was obvious and logical. Those "good" exercises didn't twist or distort a joint. They didn't seem awkward, and they seemed to follow a path that permitted an obvious stretch of the "target muscle," followed by an obvious contraction of that muscle. Doug thought to himself, "*All* exercises *should* feel like that."

From the age of 14, Doug realized there should be some similarity in ALL the "good" exercises. They should all follow similar mechanical patterns, he thought. What's mechanically good for one exercise should be good for all exercises, and what makes another exercise mechanically "'bad," would make *all* exercises "bad." There must be a set of "rules" or principles by which an exercise can be qualified as "good" or "bad," or somewhere in between.

No such reference book existed, however. Indeed, it's prudent and wise for a person who participates in resistance exercise, to be curious about how it works—mechanically speaking—or to insist that their trainer be equipped with that knowledge.

In 1975, at the age of 15, "Dougie" (as I've always called him) joined my gym in Pasadena, California. Actually, we made an agreement, whereby he would help me maintain the gym on the weekends. I paid him, of course, but he would also earn his next week's membership, in advance. He was bright, inquisitive, dedicated, and very focused from the day he walked into my gym. On occasion, he worked out with me, but on other times, he worked out with the other established bodybuilders who also worked out there, including Jim Morris, Clint Beyerle, Dave Johns, Chris Dickerson, Dennis Tinnerino, and Boyer Coe.

Since Doug first began training, however, he was always a free-thinker. He didn't assume the pro bodybuilders he worked out with, knew all there was to know about weight training and building muscle. He was very analytical. Every one of Dougie's workouts was "exploratory." He's tried every single exercise, and noted the key characteristics of each, e.g., the direction of the resistance relative to the target muscle's position, the angle at which resistance pulls on the target muscle's operating lever, etc. He's participated in cadaver dissections, created replica limbs and performed his own tests with them, studied anatomy, and read physics books. He realized that despite there not being a reference book that explains what features characterize an exercise as mechanically good or bad, there are definitely patterns that all "good" exercises follow. Exercises that fail to follow those mechanical patterns are varying degrees of "inferior," depending on how many of the mechanical characteristics are not in compliance.

Dougie began competing in bodybuilding at the age of 16. At 19 years old, he won Teenage Mr. California and Teenage Mr. America. He won the 1982 AAU Mr. California title at the age of 22, and he won his division in the 1986 AAU Mr. America and Mr. Universe competitions, at the age of 26. From 1991 through 2019, he competed in a number of other competitions, ending his competitive career in 2019, at the age of 59—43 years after he began. Doug won first place in his final competition—the 2019 AAU Mr. Universe—at almost 60 years old. It was his second time winning this title, and his condition was significantly better than many others in the competition who were decades younger than him.

Few competitive bodybuilders ever reach a 40-year span of competitions. Fewer still have been able to achieve "as good" or "better" condition when they were over the age of 50, than they achieved at the age of 26—but this is the case with Dougie. His condition at 54 years old was arguably "as good" or "better" than when he won Mr. America (medium-tall division) at the age of 26. I believe this is due entirely to his advanced understanding of biomechanics and his ability to make each workout *much more efficient* than "conventional" workouts. His approach to resistance exercise is focused on less wasted energy, less strain on the spine and the joints, and better (more direct) muscle stimulation.

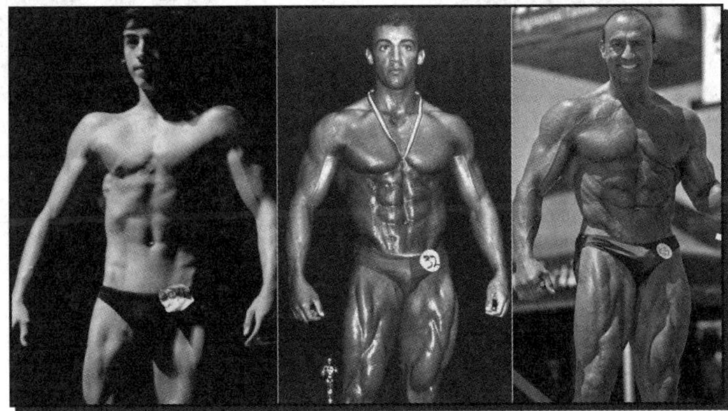

Doug Brignole at the age of 16 (far left), 22 (center), and 54 (far right)

Throughout his competitive career, Doug's physique was regarded as one of the "most aesthetic" of all time. Some bodybuilding observers have even included him in their top 10, although this is subjective, of course. In any case, Doug's physique has been lauded for its balance, symmetry, definition, and elegance. He is one of a handful of bodybuilders who did not compete in "professional" competitions, yet is compared to Frank Zane, Francis Benfatto, and Bob Paris, who are some of the greatest (most aesthetic) professional bodybuilders in the history of the sport.

In 1984—at the age of 24—Dougie opened a beautiful 10,000 square-foot gym in California (which he later expanded to 25,000 square feet), and managed it for 11 years. He has conducted seminars throughout the U.S., as well as overseas. He has written numerous articles for the leading fitness publications—most notably *Iron Man Magazine*—and has provided "continuing education credits" (CECs) to numerous personal trainers, by way of his educational courses. He is also the co-author of *Million Dollar Muscle* (along with Adrian Tan, Ph.D., professor of sociology), which is a university textbook that examines the fitness industry from a sociological perspective.

Dougie's greatest contribution, however, might be the rational and scientifically sound insight he has brought to the field of resistance exercise for physique development, through his teachings of biomechanics. His insights are profound, and will likely change the way resistance exercise is taught, the way machines are designed, the way gyms are equipped, and the way trainers are educated. More importantly, Dougie's teachings will allow consumers to achieve their fitness goals with the utmost level of efficiency and safety.

—Bill Pearl
Mr. California
Mr. America
Four-time Mr. Universe winner
Trainer of numerous bodybuilding champions
Author of six books

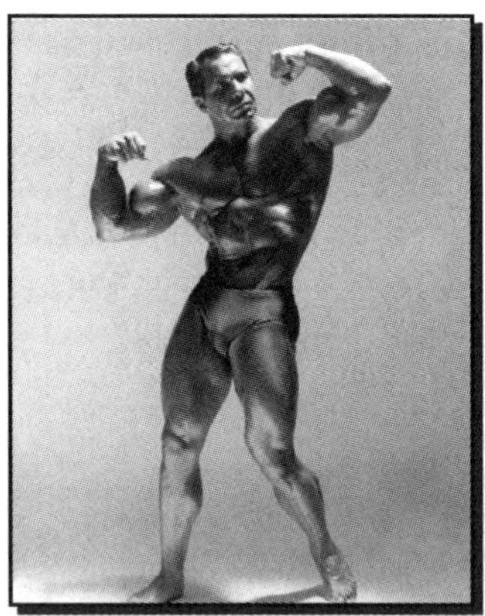

Bill Pearl in 1971

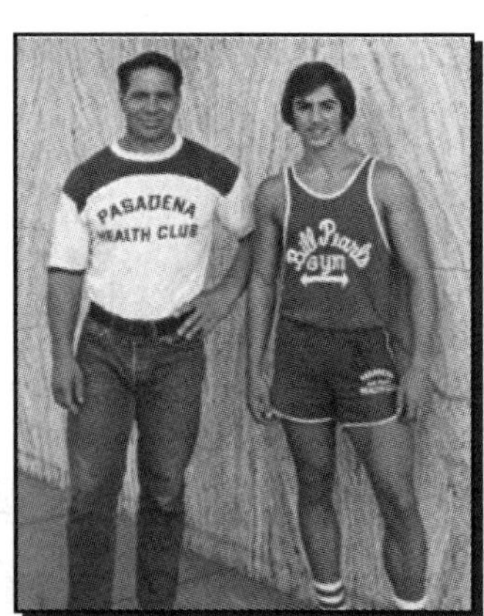


Bill Pearl & Doug Brignole in 1976

# INTRODUCTION

If you have spent any amount of time performing conventional weight training exercises like barbell squats, dead lifts, overhead presses, incline presses, upright rows, bent-over barbell rows, seated low pulley rows, and hanging leg raises—to name just a few—I can say with absolute certainty that you have not exercised efficiently. You have spent more time and energy than is necessary, you have not stimulated your target muscles as well as you could have, and you have exposed your joints and spine to a significant and unnecessary risk of being injured.

I realize these are bold statements to make. I assure you, however, that you will understand exactly what I mean, after you've read this book. The fact is that a very high percentage of what is typically taught about "resistance exercise selection"—for the goal of muscular development—is either entirely incorrect, or simply not the wisest strategy for the intended goal. The reasons for this are clearly explained throughout this book.

What is most important to understand is that the human body is essentially a system of pulleys and levers. Muscles are very much like "pulleys," and our bones (limbs) are essentially "levers." Thus, the universal principles of physics (i.e., "classical mechanics"), which apply to all things that are structural and/or mechanical, also apply to the human body. These principles of physics, combined with some basic precepts regarding the human musculoskeletal system and muscle physiology, allow us to clearly determine which exercises are best for each muscle group.

What has been missing from mainstream fitness instruction is a standardized set of rules—criteria—by which all exercises can be evaluated. There needs to be a checklist of mechanical factors that can be applied across the board—to all resistance exercises—which allows people to determine whether an exercise is mechanical "good" (optimally productive, efficient, and safe), mechanically "bad," or somewhere in between. Somehow, the fitness industry has failed to acknowledge that there are biomechanical factors that determine how "good" (productive, efficient and safe) a resistance exercise is, as well as how "bad" it is. This absence of biomechanical guidelines has resulted in "bad" exercises being unjustly glorified, while "good" exercises have been overlooked.

"Bad" exercises are ones that only deliver a small percentage of the load we're using to the target muscle. "Bad" exercises are the ones that unnecessarily load (and strain) non-target muscles more than they load the target muscles. "Bad" exercises are the ones that unnecessarily strain joints and the spine. "Bad" exercises are the ones that waste time and energy, because they either fail to move the target muscle's operating lever (limb) in the ideal anatomical direction, or they use a direction of resistance that fails to provide alignment, does not provide "early phase loading," does not allow a complete range of motion, and a number of other essential factors.

We have been misled—essentially fooled—by misinformed, misguided, or dishonest self-proclaimed "gurus" and a commercially driven industry, into performing highly *in*efficient exercises that make us think we're "beastly" (because we are able to move lots of weight), yet fail to optimally stimulate the target muscles and expose us to far more risk of injury than is necessary.

Once you understand the biomechanical principles that determine which exercises are "good" or "bad," you will be able to pursue your training with much more efficiency and effectiveness. You will be able to load your target muscles more, while using less weight, wasting less energy, and putting less strain on your bones, joints, and spine.

The biomechanical principles of which you should be aware fall under two general categories:

- The ideal direction of anatomical movement for each muscle
- The ideal direction of resistance for each movement

Every skeletal muscle has an "ideal" *direction of movement*—a motion that moves that muscle's operating lever (limb) though a pathway that most purely represents that muscle's function. When an exercise precisely mimics that motion, it allows that particular muscle to function with the greatest percentage of efficiency. When an exercise fails to mimic that muscle's ideal motion, the muscle participates in whatever "non-specific" motion you have selected, but with progressively less efficiency. The degree of departure from the "ideal" direction of motion—away from that which correctly mimics the muscle's ideal motion—determines the degree to which you will compromise the ability of that muscle to fully benefit from the exercise.

Furthermore, skeletal *joints* also have parameters of "ideal" motion—limits of "natural" movement. The parameters of a given joint's movement typically match the ideal motion produced by the skeletal muscle(s) that operates that joint. In other words, the ideal motion of a particular skeletal muscle allows the joint operated by that muscle to function as "naturally" as possible. Motions (exercises) that are distinctly aberrant (different) from a muscle's ideal movement also tend to strain the joint that is operated by that muscle. Numerous examples of this factor will be detailed in this text.

Separate from the "ideal direction of anatomical motion" is the issue of the "ideal direction of resistance" for the anatomical motion being executed during an exercise. The *direction of resistance* of a given exercise plays a significant role in the effectiveness, efficiency and safety of that exercise. When we perform any "resistance exercise," the resistance being used applies its force on the lever(s) of our body in a specific direction. That direction of resistance is not incidental. In fact, it has profound outcomes.

The direction of an exercise's resistance determines which muscles are loaded, as well as which ones are not. It is not the direction of movement that determines which muscles are loaded. It is the direction of the resistance that determines which muscle(s) is loaded, based on "the line of force" (aka, "opposite position loading")—a universal physics principle. The direction of an exercise's resistance also determines how much (as a percentage) of the load being used is placed on the target muscle.

In addition, the direction of resistance determines the alignment of the exercise, which translates to efficiency—how much of the load is being applied productively or is being misdirected. The alignment of an exercise (whether it's correct or not) also impacts the injury risk potential of that exercise. The direction of resistance also determines the "resistance curve" of the exercise, which could be highly productive (if it matches the strength curve of the target muscle) or very *un*productive (if it fails to match the strength curve of the target muscle).

Without doubt, there are "bad," "good," "better," and "best" ways of selecting the exercises we choose to perform. Some of you may be wondering if this book (i.e., the concepts it discusses) will be too complicated for you to understand. You can be assured, however, that this book has been written in plain language, using plenty of examples, and utilizing over 900 images (photos and illustrations) to help you understand. In addition, there is a synopsis at the end of each chapter that gives you "the bottom line." As such, even if you are not able to fully understand the "why," you will still understand the "what."

Resistance exercises are not all equal, in terms of productivity, efficiency, and safety. Each exercise has a distinct biomechanical profile, which can be clearly identified once you know what to look for. The factors involved in an exercise's biomechanical profile enable you to ascertain whether an exercise can be classified as "good" or "bad". These include the following:

- Which levers (bones) are perpendicular with the given resistance, and which ones are not, during a particular exercise?
- At what point in the range of motion of an exercise is your target muscle's operating lever (your forearm, when you are performing a *biceps curl,* for example) perpendicular with resistance, parallel with resistance, or somewhere in between?
- From what angle is the target muscle pulling on its operating lever? For example, at some points in the range of motion of a *curling* exercise, the biceps pulls on the forearm perpendicularly, while at other times, it pulls on the forearm more from a parallel angle. This factor is significant, because it helps you decide which exercise you should not do, as well as how to perform the exercise you should do.
- Is the operating lever (the limb) of the muscle you intend to target, moving directly toward the origin of that muscle? If "yes," then, it's good. If "no," then, the exercise has varying degrees of non-compliance, which compromises its efficiency and its productivity to the degree of the non-compliance.
- During a particular exercise, is the muscle on which you are most focused (prioritizing) working more than the supporting muscles? Or, are the supporting muscles working harder than your target muscle? This factor is affected by the direction of resistance.
- Have you positioned your target muscle directly opposite the direction of resistance? If "yes," then, it's good. If "no," then, the exercise has varying degrees of being inefficient or unproductive.
- When you do multiple exercises for a given muscle, are you able to clearly identify what makes one exercise different from the other? Are you sure all those exercises are worth doing? In fact, there is quite a bit of redundancy in doing more than one exercise for a muscle group (except for pectorals and trapezius), with some exercises being drastically inferior to others.
- Are you performing an exercise with the misguided belief that it's somehow going to change the shape of the target muscle? If an exercise could do that, the mechanism by which it does do that should be understood and verifiable. In fact, the opposite is true—a muscle does not/cannot change its shape. This is a fact that is verifiable.

All of these questions have very specific and scientifically sound answers. If you invest large amounts of time and energy in the pursuit of physique development, you owe it to yourself to know the answers to these questions. If you are in the business of advising people with regard to resistance exercise—if you are a trainer, a coach, or a physical therapist—it is imprudent and irresponsible for you to not know the answers to these questions.

Have you made the mistake of assuming that the gym lore promoted by fitness magazines and uneducated bodybuilders (i.e., lacking education in exercise science) are providing you with accurate information? Have you passed along this "misinformation," believing it was accurate, but, in fact, you aren't actually sure of its veracity? Isn't it time that you clearly understood the mechanics of resistance exercise, so that you can stop wasting your time and energy, and risking injury, because you're performing exercises inefficiently, or you're doing exercises that are not even worth doing?

Exercise "efficiency" relates to the cost/benefit of an exercise. Exercise efficiency determines how "diluted" and safe an exercise is. Ideally, you want to ensure you're getting the "full potency" of the exercise, without dilution and without joint distortion. An inefficient exercise is one that delivers less than 100% of the available resistance to the target muscle. Thus, an inefficient exercise—for example, one that only delivers 50% of the resistance being used, to the target muscle—requires that twice as much weight be used, in order to deliver the same amount of load to the target muscle, as an efficient exercise would require.

Very often—in conventional weight training—people engage in exercises that require them to use far more weight than is necessary, because it gratifies their ego and fools them into thinking that the target muscle is getting more load. In fact, the length of the limb (which may be influenced in two ways) and the angle of the limb (relative to the direction of resistance) determine the percentage of the load (being used) that is delivered to the target muscle. A muscle does not "know" whether the load it feels is a heavy weight being magnified less (by the length and angle of the limb) or a lighter weight being magnified more. Therefore, it is sensible to focus more on "efficiency" (high load, with less weight), and spare the unnecessary strain on the bones, joints, and spine that occur with the use of very heavy weight. Either way, the muscle is loaded the same amount.

Since the inception of "weight training," people have been debating which exercises are "good" or "bad," based almost entirely on misconceptions and myths. In fact, determining which exercises are good or bad (efficient/productive) is very easy to determine, because the process mostly involves simple math, basic physics, and a bit of anatomical knowledge. Many of the same physics principles are used to determine the structural integrity of a bridge, or the efficiency and stability of a crane. These are universal principles. There is no need to interject opinion, folklore, or mythology in the selection of exercises. It's all perfectly quantifiable.

There are some exercise-related factors that are more biological, than mechanical—for example, understanding the difference between higher reps with less weight versus lower reps with heavier weight. This type of issue involves a different kind of science called "exercise physiology." Exercise *selection*, however, should be based entirely on "biomechanics." Exercise selection should not be ambiguous. It is not dependent on a "mind/muscle connection." Rather, it is based on a simple set of rules that are entirely logical, which apply the same way to every person—man or woman, old or young. Everyone's joints and muscles operate the same way, mechanically speaking.

To be clear, I am not suggesting that "inefficient" (traditional) exercises do not produce positive results. Clearly, there is lots of evidence, where people have achieved a remarkable level of fitness, using traditional exercises. Rather, it's a matter of efficiency—"not so good," "good," "better," and "best." Even an exercise that rates a "2" (on a scale of 1 to 10) is better than sitting on the couch, watching TV, while eating potato chips. The question is, should you use an exercise that rates a "2," instead of an exercise that rates a "10?" In fact, there's no logical reason to use an inefficient exercise—not even in addition to using an efficient exercise. It would be better to do twice as many sets of the better exercise, than it would to do half the sets with the good exercise, and half with the bad exercise.

You can achieve a result that is "as good" or better, using more efficient exercises, as you could achieve with conventional exercises—but with much less skeletal strain, little or no risk of injury, and much less effort. The key is to apply the physics of fitness to your resistance exercises.

The first 17 chapters of this book address concepts that are either mechanical (physics principles) or factors related to basic muscle physiology (e.g., "dynamic muscle tension" versus "isometric muscle tension," "reciprocal innervation," "unilateral exercise" versus "bilateral exercise," etc.). Chapters 18 through 25 discuss the individual muscle groups. These chapters explain what is not quite correct about many traditional exercises that are used for those muscles, and which exercises are better—based on the information presented in the first 17 chapters. The factors that determine what constitutes a good exercise versus a not-so-good exercise are undeniable, as you will soon see.

The final chapter of this book—Chapter 26—addresses the issue of "what or whom you should believe," with regard to information on exercise selection. Unfortunately, a number of the sources we've all come to believe as accurate and trustworthy are actually not very accurate or trustworthy. This realization will likely be "a bitter pill to swallow" for some people. There are bound to be some individuals who will be shocked—possibly even angry or in denial—that the beliefs they've held for so long are incorrect. In reality, there is a long history of people denying truths, simply because previous beliefs are rooted in dogma.

I encourage you to open your mind, use your sense of reason, try the experiments I recommend throughout the book, and allow yourself to explore the alternatives I suggest in this book. Ultimately, I firmly believe that you will be very happy you did.

—Doug Brignole

# CHAPTER 1

# THE LEVERS OF THE HUMAN BODY

- *The human body is made up of levers. Limbs and appendages (a collection of bones acting as a unit) are acted upon by muscles which cross over articulations (joints). Joint movement is thus produced when the muscles that cross those joints, contract (shorten).*
- *All levers magnify resistance and force. The universal laws of physics, as they apply to levers, work the same with regard to the levers of the human body.*
- *Therefore, all resistance exercises you perform are subject to magnification of force, as well as other mechanical principles. Understanding and complying with these principles allows you to work with optimum efficiency in the pursuit of physique development.*

Anatomical movement is caused by muscles pulling on the various "levers" of the body, thereby moving joints, the axis between bones, which are also known as "articulations." Sometimes, those levers are individual bones, like a femur (thigh bone). Other times, they are comprised of two, side-by-side bones, like a forearm or a lower leg. Sometimes, the "lever" is a group of bones, like a hand or a foot. Still other times, it's the entire torso or the head (the skull), acting as a lever. All of these levers are acted upon by muscles, which cause joints to bend, extend, or rotate, thereby creating movement.

The fundamental basis of resistance exercise is the deliberate loading of a lever (a forearm, for example), for the purpose of strengthening and developing the muscle that causes that particular lever to move. The amount of resistance imposed on any muscle is the result of a combination of factors. These include the weight being used (barbell, dumbbells, cables, machines, etc.), as well as the magnification caused by the length of the "levers" (bones/limbs) involved, in addition to factors that include the angle of the lever relative to the direction of resistance, the angle of the muscle pulling on the bone, the position of the target muscle relative to the direction of resistance, etc. All of these factors will be addressed in this book in due time.

During a *standing dumbbell curl*, for example, a 10-pound weight that is placed in the exerciser's hand will impose a challenge on the biceps that is *more* than the 10 pounds. In reality, the weight in the hand is *magnified* by a factor that is directly related to the length of the forearm. In normal, day-to-day resistance training, it is not necessary to know the exact amount of this magnification. It is important, however, to have a sense of the magnification itself, and how a given exercise compares with another exercise, based on the length of the lever being used.

When I conduct seminars, I typically use a lever device (Figure 1-1) to demonstrate the magnification effect of levers. Using this same lever device, I also demonstrate another concept, called "mechanical advantage and disadvantage," which will be discussed in Chapter 3.

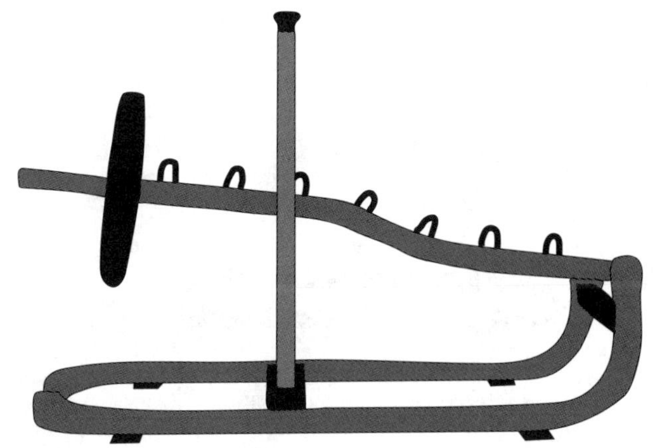

Figure 1-1

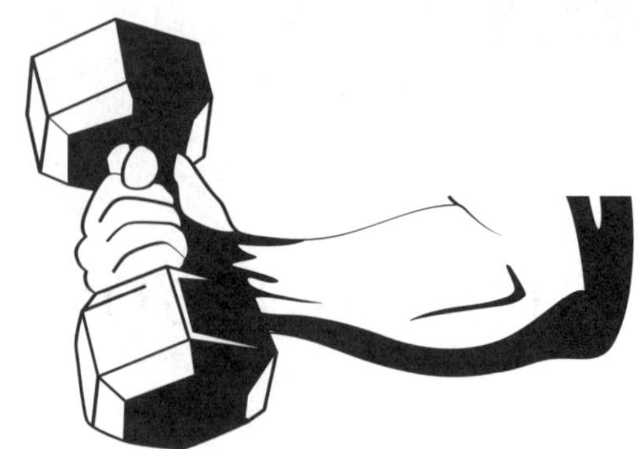

Figure 1-2

I begin my seminars by asking the audience to imagine that this lever device in front of them is their forearm, and that the weight-holder on the end of the lever is their hand. The pivot on the other end of the lever device is their theoretical "elbow."

Initially, I take a 10-pound plate and slide it onto the holder. I then ask the individuals in the audience the following question: "If you held a 10-pound weight in your hand, with your forearm parallel to the ground, how much resistance would your biceps be holding?" To some, the answer may seem to be "10 pounds," which is the answer that some people call out.

I then pick up a fishing scale, which has a hook on it. I connect that hook to the first loop on the lever—the one that is closest to the weight at the end of the lever. Essentially, this is the place where an exerciser's "wrist" would be. Next, I pull straight up on the fishing scale, until the lever lifts slightly off its perch, and ask an audience member to read the measurement on the scale. "10 pounds," the observer calls out. "Fine," I respond.

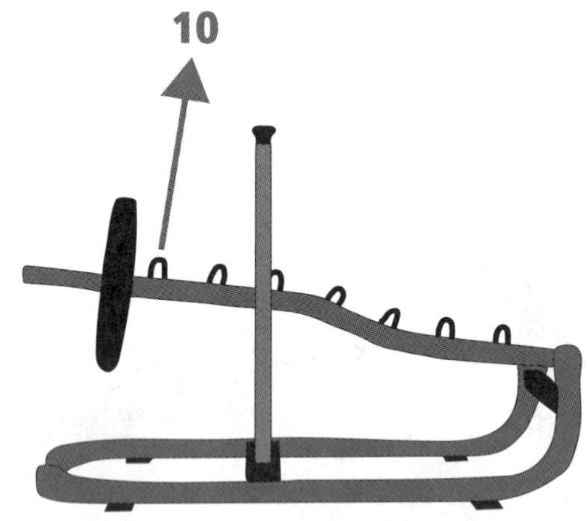


Figure 1-3

I then move the fishing scale to the next hook, moving away from the "hand," in the direction of the "elbow." I pull up on the scale, and ask the audience member to read the measurement. "23 pounds," the observer calls out. I move the fishing scale to the next hook, further away from the hand. I then pull up on the scale, and ask for the reading. "38 pounds," the audience member calls out.

I continue moving the fishing scale down the length of the lever device. Each time I move it, the scale measures a higher amount. Finally, I arrive at the final hook on the lever—the one located approximately an inch away from the pivot. This position is the actual place (approximately), where a person's biceps would attach to the forearm, and from which the biceps would be pulling on that forearm.

Finally, I pull up on the scale, and ask for the reading. "112 pounds," the individual calls out. Of course, by now, the audience has become somewhat restless.

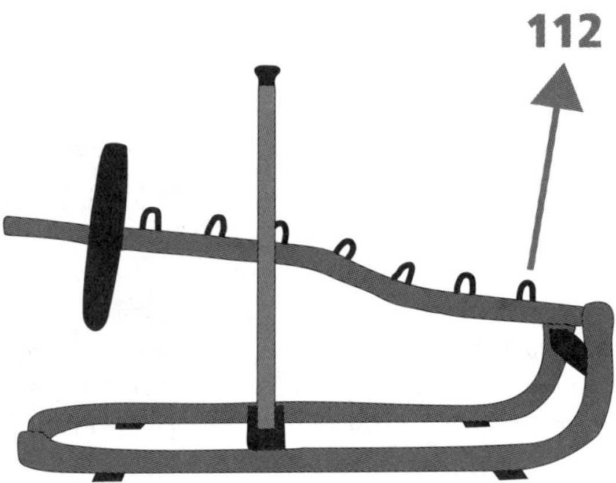


Figure 1-4

At that point, I playfully ask, "Isn't that still a 10-pound weight you're holding in your hand?" I then rhetorically inquire, "Didn't some people say their biceps would be pulling 10 pounds when their hand is holding a 10 pound weight?"

In fact, the biceps *never* pulls directly on the weight that is in your hand. The biceps pulls on the lever (your forearm), which is holding the weight that is in your hand. Furthermore, the biceps is pulling on the forearm from a point that is about 12 inches behind the weight, and about one inch in front of the elbow (the pivot). That would be a 12-to-1 ratio. In other words, the weight is magnified by a factor of 12 (approximately), depending on the length of the exerciser's forearm.

Figure 1-5 illustrates how a lever magnifies resistance. Regardless of the weight that is actually being held, lifted, pushed, or pulled, the operating lever (the limb) *always* magnifies the amount of resistance that the muscle must move.

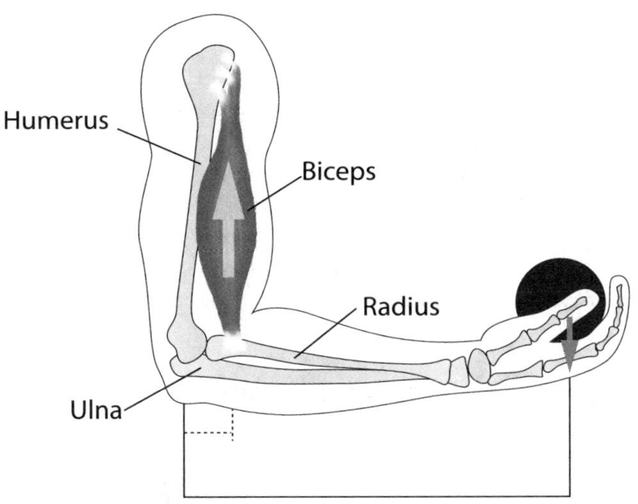


Figure 1-5

There are additional factors that further alter the resistance (increasing or decreasing it), which will be discussed shortly. It's important, however, to understand that muscles never pull directly on the weights. In reality, *they pull on levers* that are holding the weights, an action that occurs in accordance with the laws of physics.

## Determining the Amount of Magnification of Levers

The basic *universal formula* that determines the amount of magnification of levers is *R x RA = F x FA*. *The same formula applies to all types of levers*, even though the three factors change position, depending on which type of lever is being used.

- "R" represents "resistance," which the amount of weight that is placed upon the lever. On occasion, this factor is called FL ("force load") or just load."
- "RA" represents "resistance arm," which is the lever. More specifically, it is the *length* of the lever that is between the "effort" and the "load." In the case of the class 3 lever in Figure 1-6, it is "the forearm," as measured NOT from the hand to the elbow, but from the hand to the connection of the biceps on the forearm—the point at which the upward "effort" is being applied.
- "FA" represents "force arm," which is the distance between the pivot (the elbow) and the point at which the "effort" is applied on the lever (e.g., the insertion point of the biceps onto the forearm).
- "F" represents "force", which is the amount of muscle force required to hold up (or move) the lever, given the other three factors.

To illustrate the math involved in this formula, use a 15-pound weight, and plug this figure (15 pounds of the resistance) into the *"R"* aspect of the equation.

Then, assume that the distance between the "effort" (the biceps attachment on the forearm) and the weight in the hand is 12 inches. As a result, put a "12" in the *"RA"* ("resistance arm") part of the magnification equation. Given that the objective is to calculate *"F"* (the force required of the biceps), you should leave that blank for now.

Finally, assume that the distance between the elbow and the biceps connection on the forearm is one inch. As such, put a "1" in the *"FA"* spot in the equation. At this point, it would look like the following:

*15 pounds x 12 inches = ______ (Force) x 1 inch*

*Resistance* (R is 15) x *Resistance Arm* (RA is 12 inches) = *Force* (?) x *Force Arm* (FA is 1)

Then, just do the math ...

(15 x 12 = 180) = ? x 1

180 divided by 1 = 180

Therefore ...

*F = 180 pounds*

In other words, in this hypothetical scenario, *the biceps needs to generate 180 pounds of force* (approximately), in order to hold a 15-pound weight in the hand, assuming an average length forearm.

> *Note: In this instance, the forearm is in a horizontal position, and the biceps is pulling perpendicularly on the forearm, as would be the case when the elbow is bent at 90 degrees, and the person is standing upright.*

Of course, a forearm that is longer than 12 inches (as measured from the hand to the biceps insertion near the elbow) would require a little more than 180 pounds of force by the biceps. In turn, a forearm that is less than 12 inches long would require a little less than 180 pounds of force.

In any case, the amount of force the biceps needs to generate, when "curling" a 15-pound dumbbell, is much more than just 15 pounds. This factor is reason enough to not concern ourselves with whether we're lifting "heavy enough." In reality, the only thing that matters is that the target muscle must be challenged.

Using this formula, you could calculate how much force your biceps would have to generate if you were curling 25 or 30 pounds. In fact, you could approximate the amount of force any muscle would have to generate, provided you know the length of the resistance arm, the length of the force arm, and the weight being used, as well as a couple of other factors, which will be addressed soon.

## Types of Levers (Class 1, Class 2, and Class 3)

There are three types of levers—class 1, class 2, and class 3. For the moment, I'd like to examine one of these types, and see how it matches one of the levers in the human body. Then, I'd like to apply the formula that is used to calculate the magnification of any lever.

❑ Class 3 Lever:

The first type of lever I would like to address is a class 3 lever. This type matches that of the *forearm/elbow/biceps*. In the example illustrated in Figure 1-6, you will notice that the lever is horizontal. In other words, it is perpendicular to gravity (which is always vertical), a fact that you should keep in the back of your mind. It is important, as you will see in subsequent chapters.

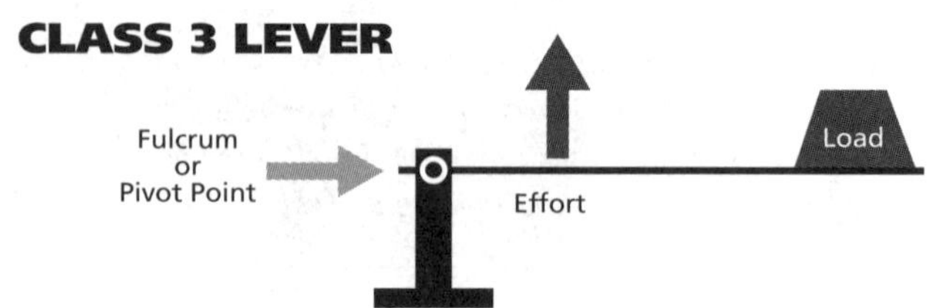


Figure 1-6

In Figure 1-6, the "fulcrum/pivot" would be the *elbow*. The "load" would be the *weight in hand*. The "effort" would be the upward force of the biceps on the lever. Of course, the point from which the "effort" (biceps) is actually applied would be closer to the pivot (i.e., the elbow) than is depicted in Figure 1-6. All-in-all, a class 3 lever simply refers to the fact that the "effort" is *between* the pivot and the load.

❑ Class 2 Lever:

A class 2 lever is one that has the "effort" being applied at the *end* of the lever, rather in between the load and the pivot (illustration below). It requires that the weight ("load") be placed in the *middle* of the lever, with the muscle force being applied at the *end* of the lever. An example of using this type of lever is when you are performing a "*standing calf raise*" (Figure 1-8). This example is rather unique, because class 2 levers are otherwise not commonly found on the human body.

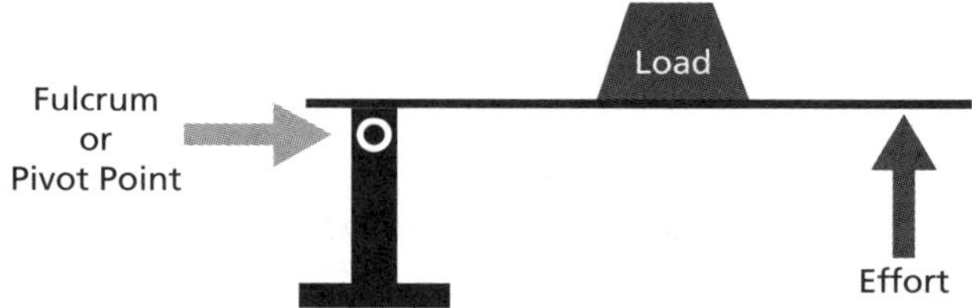


Figure 1-7

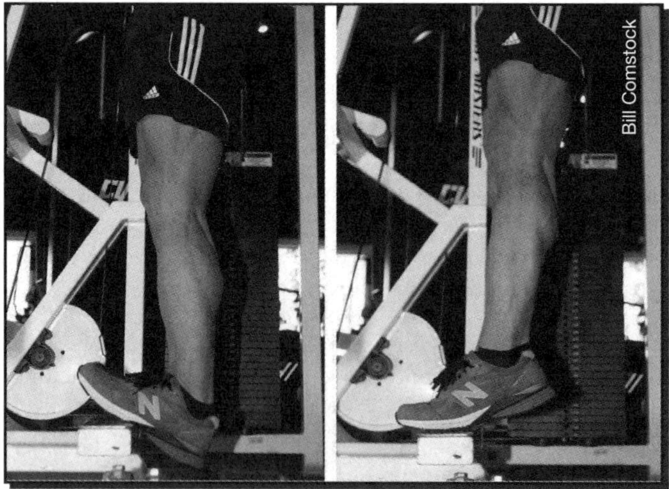


Figure 1-8

During a *standing calf raise*, a person's bodyweight, plus whatever additional weight is placed on the exerciser's shoulders, transfers all the way down to the ankle, and bears *down* on the joint of the foot (Figure 1-9). When the calf muscle contracts, it pulls upward on the heel bone, which elevates the mid-foot carrying the load. The ball of the foot is the pivot, because that's the part of the body that is stationary.

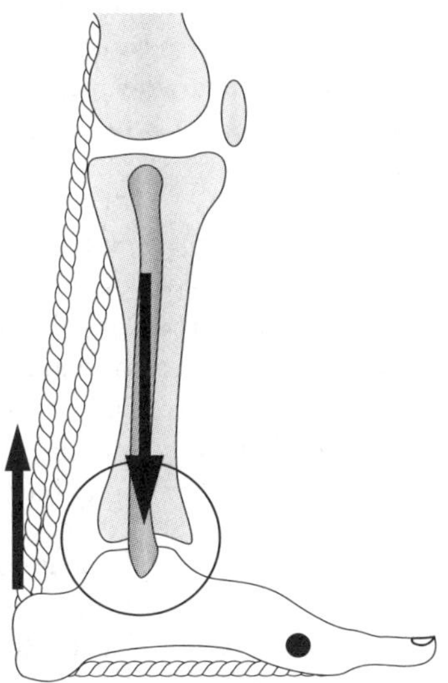

Figure 1-9

In Figure 1-10, you can see how this image is similar to a man using a "wheelbarrow." The force is the man pulling upward on the handles, while the load is whatever is in the wheelbarrow's container, bearing downward with its weight. The wheel is the pivot.

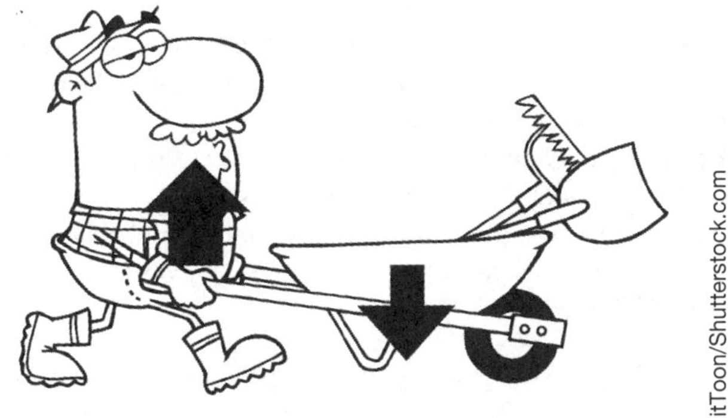


Figure 1-10

Watch what happens, however, when *seated leg press calf extension* is performed. The seat (and therefore the body and the *ankle*) are stationary—not the ball of the foot. The "load" is now the weight (resistance) provided by the machine—not the exerciser's bodyweight. In turn, the pivot is now the ankle, because IT is now stationary.

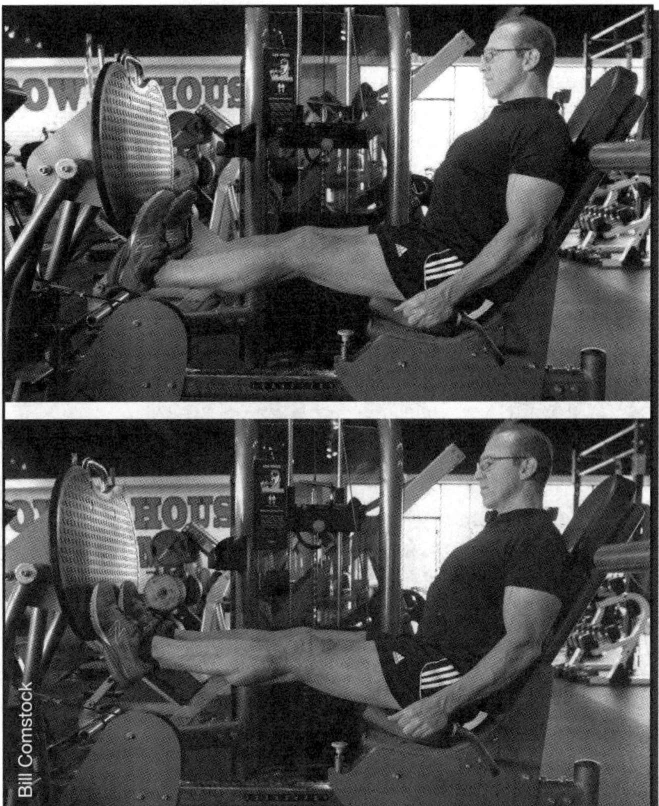


Figure 1-11

❑ Class 1 Lever:

Despite this still being a calf exercise, its characteristics are like that of a class 1 lever—NOT a class 2 lever. The definition of a class 1 lever is having the pivot *between* the load and the force (Figure 1-12).

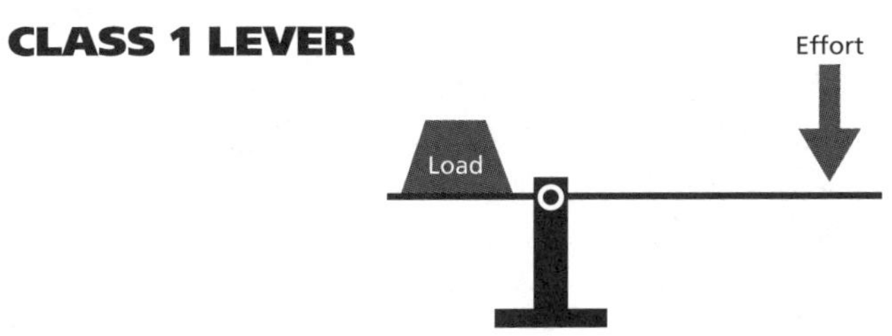


Figure 1-12

Figure 1-13 provides a better view of how a "*leg press calf extension*" sometimes functions as a class 1 lever. The ankle is the pivot, because it's stationary—pivoting between the calf and the forefoot. The load is now the weight bearing downward at the end of the lever (the foot), instead of in the middle of the lever.

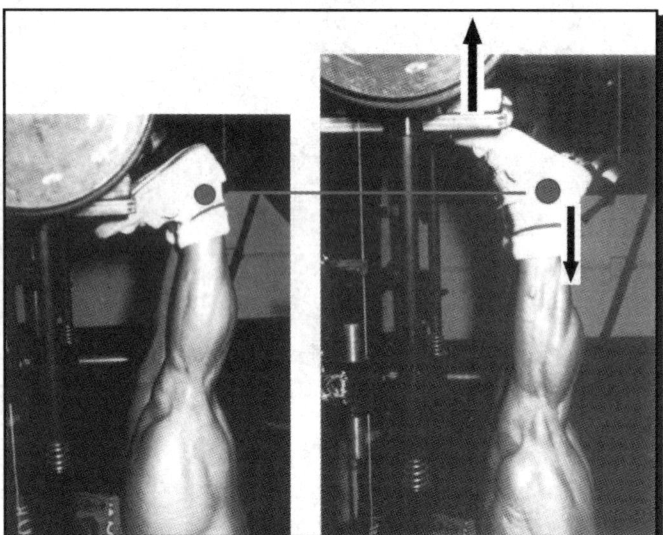

Figure 1-13

Another example of a class 1 lever is shown in Figure 1-14. In this illustration, an arm is viewed from the side. As you can see, the triceps muscle is highlighted, while the elbow (small circle) and the forearm (arrow), are spotlighted. The "up" arrow indicates an upward load, in this instance, provided by a cable, for example. This represents what would happen during a "*triceps cable pushdown*." In Figure 1-14, the forearm is the "resistance arm." The elbow is the "pivot." The triceps is the "effort."

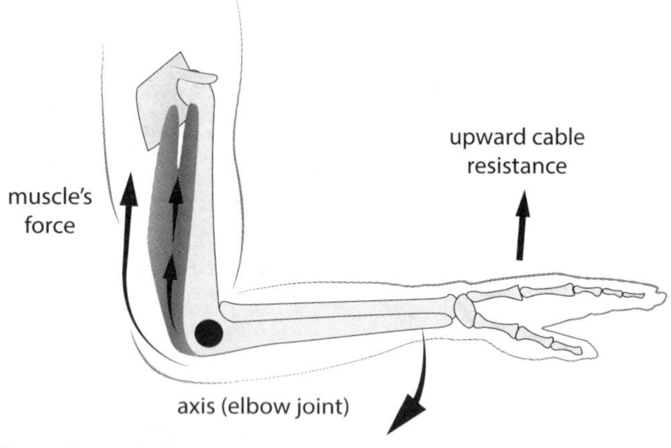


Figure 1-14

When performing a triceps cable pushdown, as the triceps muscle of the arm contracts, it pulls upward on its insertion, on the back of the forearm (similar to the heel bone of the foot, during *calf extensions*). This action causes the pivot (the elbow) to extend/push the forearm downward, against the upward resistance of the cable. The pivot is between the force and the load—a class 1 lever.

Whenever you are lifting a weight (moving resistance), you are using one of the three types of levers—either a class 1, class 2, or class 3. In all cases, the formula for calculating the amount of resistance with which a muscle is loaded, is always the same. On the other hand, quantifying the *exact* amount of resistance that is loaded onto a muscle is not especially important, certainly not on a day-to-day basis.

What does matter is that you understand that your limbs are levers, and whenever you are doing resistance exercise, your body is subject to the laws of physics. In that regard, one of the primary physics principles of physics (as it relates to levers) is that *the weight you are moving is NEVER the resistance your target muscle is getting*. Rather, the resistance that your target muscle is handling is altered (increased or decreased) by the length and position of the operating lever, as well as several other factors.

## Primary Levers and Secondary Levers

In the context of resistance exercise, the bone that is directly connected to your target muscle (by way of muscle insertion), is the "*primary lever*." Whatever other bone is directly attached to the primary lever, but not to the target muscle, is the "*secondary lever*." For example, if your target muscle is your pectorals, then the humerus (the upper arm bone) is the *primary lever*, and the forearm—which is attached to your upper arm bone—is the *secondary lever*.

During the discussion on the biceps, attention was focused exclusively on the *forearm*, as the "operating lever" of the biceps. In that instance, there really is no "secondary lever," other than the hand. Because the hand is very short, relative to the forearm, it's mostly inconsequential.

In situations involving the pectorals, for example (and a few other muscles), the secondary lever could significantly influence the mechanics of the exercise, because of its length. Since the humerus does not have a hand attached directly to its distal end (Figure 1-15), you cannot hold a weight ONLY with the humerus. Because the weight in your hand is attached to the end of the *forearm*, you must consider the effect of the forearm, even though the pectoral muscle does not connect directly to it.

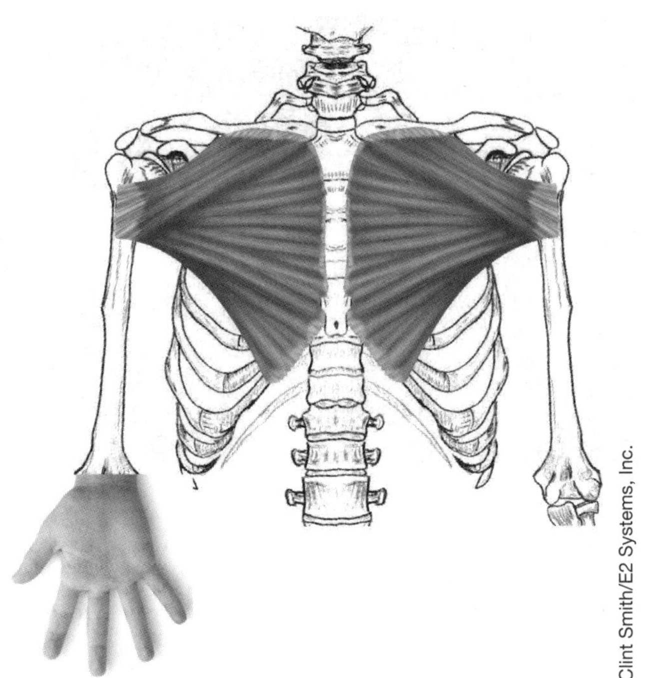


Figure 1-15

If the arm (elbow) is straight, the forearm would only act as an extension of the upper arm. When the elbow is bent, however, depending on the degree of elbow bend, the position of the forearm (relative to gravity) greatly influences the physics of the upper arm, as it relates to the pectorals. Therefore, as the "secondary lever" to the humerus, the position of the forearm, during any pectoral exercise, matters a great deal.

This factor is not only true with regard to exercises involving the pectorals, it's also true any time you load any muscle by way of a secondary or tertiary (third) lever. It applies to exercises for the latissimus dorsi, the teres major, the deltoids, the glutes, the hip flexors, and the shoulder rotators, as well as a few other muscles.

A secondary lever could affect an exercise in several ways. For example, it could act purely as an "extension" of the primary lever—*adding to its length*—which would result in more magnification of the load. A secondary lever could also "double back" over (or under) a primary lever, thereby *reducing the effective length* of the primary lever, which would decrease its magnification of the load. It could also act as "neutral" lever—neither increasing nor decreasing the magnification of the primary lever.

A secondary lever could also ROTATE its primary lever. If the secondary lever is allowed to tilt in a direction that is NOT aligned with the primary lever, it would "torque" (turn) its primary lever. If this is intentional, as would be the case when doing an exercise for the infraspinatus and/or subscapularis (the rotator cuff muscles of the shoulder joint), it's fine. On the other hand, if it's unintentional, as would be the case when improper form is used on pressing motions, it could be potentially injurious.

You should examine some of these possibilities, so that you can fully understand what a secondary lever is, how it interplays with its primary lever, and how it could affect the muscle(s) that connect to the primary lever. For example, in Figure 1-16, you can see a person doing a *supine dumbbell press*, for the pectorals. The humerus is the primary lever, because the pectoral muscle is directly connected to it. The forearm is the secondary lever. In this illustration (Figure 1-16), the forearm is behaving as a *neutral* secondary lever, because it is mostly *parallel* with gravity. As long as the forearm stays perfectly vertical, it will behave as a neutral secondary lever.

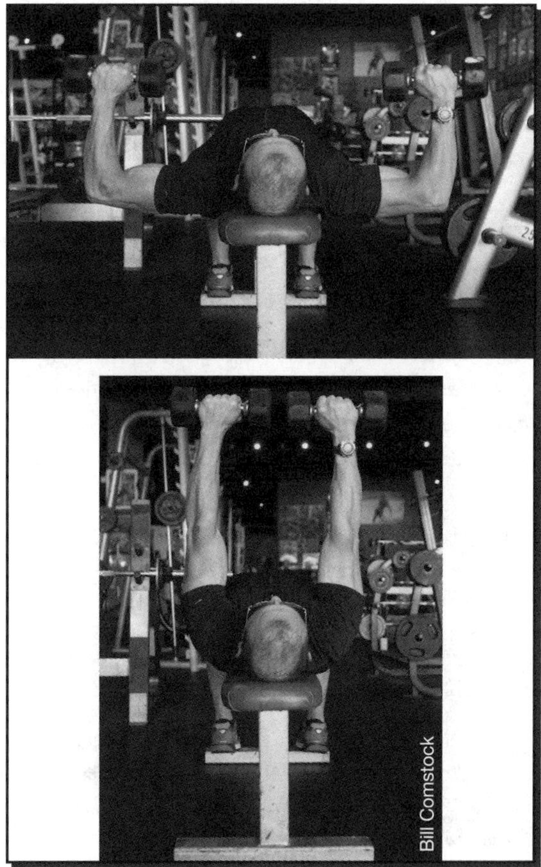


Figure 1-16

Figure 1-17 provides a contrasting example. In this instance, the forearm is *not* staying vertical (parallel with gravity)—at least not in this descended position of the movement. When the forearm breaks from a vertical position—entering various degrees of horizontal, it becomes an "active" secondary lever.

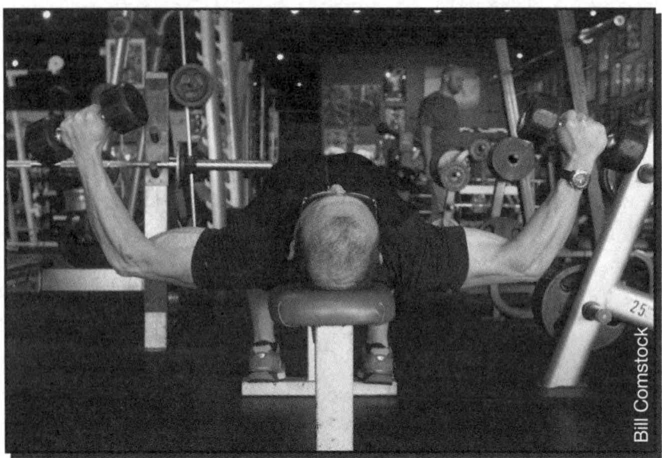


Figure 1-17

Because the forearm is leaning *away* from the where the primary lever pivots (at the shoulder), it essentially "lengthens" the primary lever (the upper arm bone). This factor *increases* the magnification of the weight being used, which further loads the pectorals.

*Note: The forearm is the primary lever of the biceps, so when it leans "outward" (laterally), it actually does two things. Not only does it increase the load to the pectorals, it also engages the biceps. This situation isn't necessarily good or bad. For now, you should just be aware that the bicep engages when the forearm tilts outward, and increases the load to the pectorals.*

In the example illustrated in Figure 1-18, the forearm is tilting *inward*, instead of outward. This factor *decreases* the load to the pectorals, because it effectively "shortens" the upper arm lever, by doubling back over it.

*Note: In this instance, the forearm is also the primary lever of the triceps. As a result, when the forearm leans "inward," it actually does two things. It decreases the load to the pectorals, and it also engages the triceps. As before, this is not necessarily good or bad. For now, you should imply be mindful of the fact that when the forearm tilts inward, it also engages the triceps.*

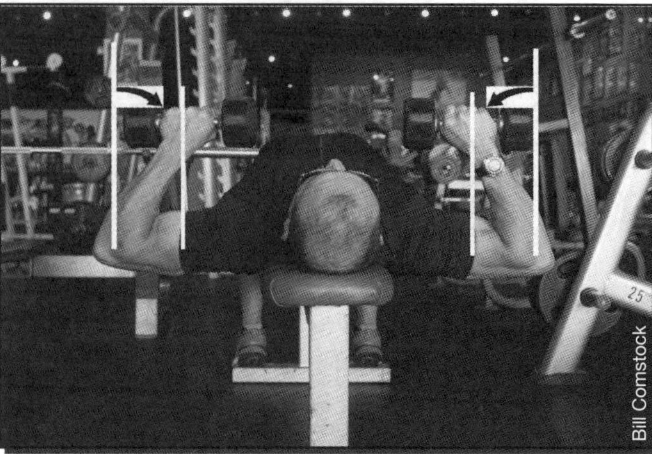


Figure 1-18

Whenever a secondary lever tilts *away* from the pivot of the primary lever, it *increases* the magnification of the primary lever. In turn, whenever a secondary lever tilts *toward* the pivot of the primary lever, it *reduces* the magnification of the primary lever. This outcome is because the secondary lever is either "lengthening" or "shortening" the effective length of the primary lever.

Calculating exactly how much a secondary lever increases or decreases the magnification of the primary lever (due to tilting outward or inward) can be complicated. It's also not necessary. What's important is to have a sense of it, in terms of percentage.

The easiest way to estimate this percentage is to draw an imaginary vertical line straight up through the beginning and the end of the secondary lever, as well as the primary lever, as is done in Figure 1-19. As you can see, the *distance* between the two vertical lines of the forearm is about *half* the distance of the lines of the upper arm. This scenario indicates that the secondary lever has added about 50 percent more "length" (also called the "moment arm") to the primary lever, thereby adding about 50 percent more magnification to it. This same simplified method can be used to approximate the *reduction* of magnification that is caused by a secondary lever "doubling back" over the primary lever.

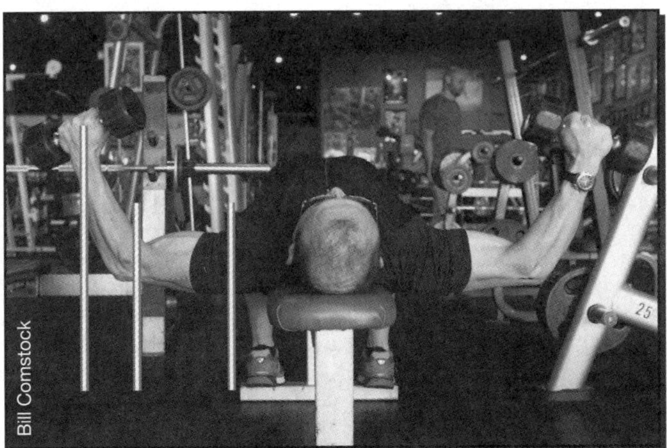

Figure 1-19

In the example illustrated in Figure 1-20, the distance between the line at the hand and the line at the elbow is about half the distance between the line at the shoulder and the line at the elbow. This observation indicates that the secondary lever has reduced the effective length of its primary lever by about HALF, which means the magnification has also been reduced by about half.

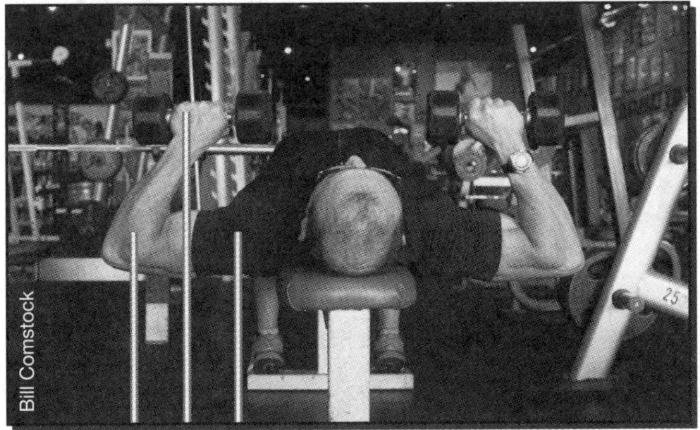

Figure 1-20

It's most effective to use a vertical forearm (neutral lever) when performing this exercise. On the other hand, if you "must" tilt your forearm, it's more sensible to use a slightly lighter weight, tilt the forearm outward, and allow the secondary lever to *increase* the magnification of that weight to the pectorals. It is LESS sensible to use a weight that's heavier than the pecs can handle, and then allow the forearms to tilt inward, which *reduces* the magnification of that weight to the pectorals.

Far too often, a person's ego will try to convince that individual to use the heavier weight (allowing them to believe that they're stronger), but then reducing the load to the pecs, by tilting the forearm inward. That's a bit foolish, because the pecs get the same load either way. The heavier weight simply strains the joints more, and increases the risk of injury.

A muscle does not "know" how much weight is in your hands. It only "senses" how much load it's required to move. Several factors—not the least of which is the position of the secondary lever—determine the actual resistance that is loaded onto the target muscle. It is *never* the actual amount in your hands.

*Note: While it might seem to make sense for you to "open" your elbows quite a bit (on this exercise)—effectively lengthening the primary lever and increasing its magnification to the pectorals—doing so would likely recruit the biceps too much, allowing them to be the "weak link in the chain." In fact, it would be ideal if the weight would be attached directly to the end of the humerus, eliminating the involvement of the forearm. Since that's not possible, however, the next best thing is to simply keep the forearm in the neutral position, throughout the exercise.*

## Tilting the Secondary Lever on a Different Plane

Separate from an "inward" tilt or an "outward" tilt, the forearm could also tilt *backward* or *forward*, when doing a *supine dumbbell press*. This tilting is a potentially dangerous "mistake," in terms of the position of the secondary lever. It would create "external rotation" of the humerus or "internal rotation" of the humerus, respectively (as shown in Figure 1-21) and could result in a serious injury, if the weight being used is substantial.

When the forearm is NOT vertical (as viewed from the side), it means that it has entered a different plain—separate from the one on which the pectorals are working. In either one of these instances, the forearm will begin "falling" either toward the head or toward the feet ("externally" or "internally"), and will require the use of the rotator cuff muscles to prevent the forearm from falling into worse alignment.

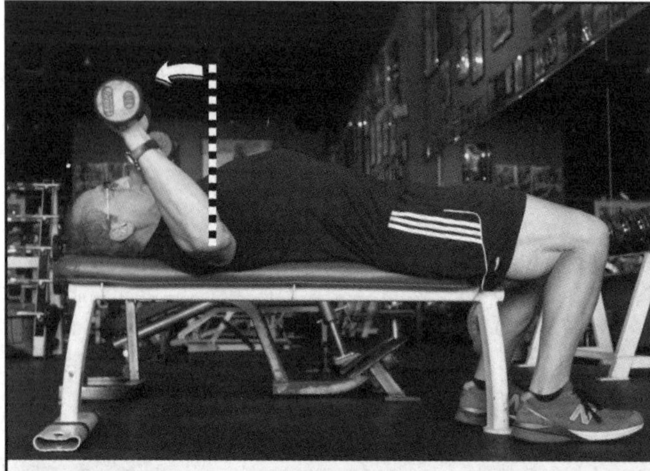

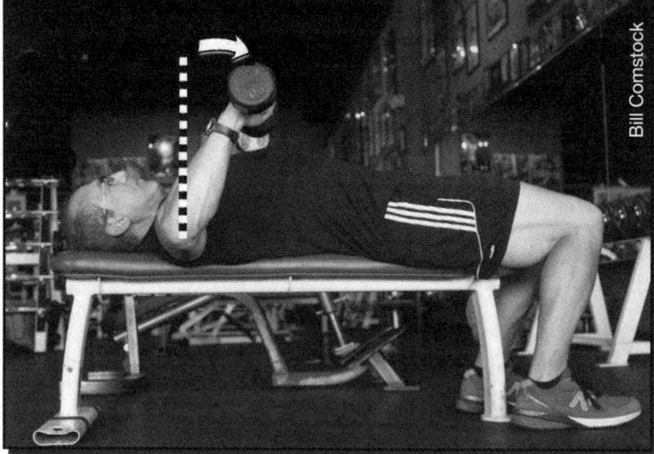


Figure 1-21

Since the weight typically used for pectoral exercises is substantial, this situation could seriously overload the rotator cuff muscles, resulting in an injury. This factor will be discussed in greater detail in Chapter 25. At this point, however, you need to be aware that a secondary lever can greatly influence an exercise, and NOT necessarily in a good way.

## Evaluating the Effect of the Secondary Lever on the Squat

There are a number of characteristics that determine the amount of "load" on a muscle, including the following:

- The *length of the operating lever*, which includes the "addition" or "subtraction" provided by a secondary lever (if applicable)
- The *degree of "perpendicular-ness" of the operating lever*, relative to the direction of resistance
- The angle from which the target muscle is able to pull on its operating lever (mechanical advantage/disadvantage), which will be discussed shortly

An analysis of a squat indicates that the following three primary "levers" are in play:

- The *lower leg* (tibia/fibula—acting as the primary lever of the quads, as well as the secondary lever to the glutes)
- The *upper leg bone* (femur—acting as the primary lever of the glutes)
- The *torso* (acting as the primary lever of the erector spinae)

Because "secondary levers" are addressed in this section, the underlying objective at this point is to evaluate how effectively the glutes are being loaded, as a result of the relationship between the femur and the lower leg, during a *squat*. In that regard, it is important to note that the muscle attachment of the glutes is on the femur. So, the femur is the primary lever of the glutes. During a *squat*, however, the resistance is applied to the glutes by way of the lower leg. The resistance is not being applied directly to the femur. As such, the lower leg is the *secondary lever* of the glutes, and it plays a significant role in this instance.

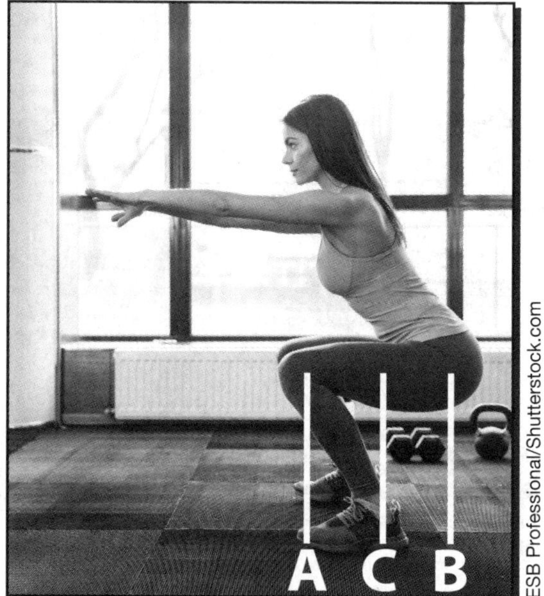


Figure 1-22

Just as was done when evaluating the *supine dumbbell press* (i.e., the forearm tilting either away from or toward the pivot of the primary lever), your attention should be focused in this instance on the lower leg (as the secondary lever) "doubling back" under the femur. As shown in Figure 1-22, the distance from "A" to "B" represents the length of the femur.

The average femur is about 19 inches long. The distance between "A" and "C" is the amount by which the lower leg (as the secondary lever) is reducing the effective length of the femur. As you can see, it's reducing it by about half. As such, the distance between "B" and "C" is all that remains of the "effective" femur length (about 10 inches), after the "reduction." In other words, the glutes are not getting quite as much load as one might think, due to the reduced femur length, during a standard squatting movement.

In addition, this factor also provides a clue concerning "why/how" it is that a person is *able* to squat so much weight. The combination of a reduced femur length (caused by the "doubling back" of the lower leg) *and* the angle of the tibia (shown in Figure 1-22 at about 30 degrees from neutral), means that the quads are only getting about one-third of the "available resistance," while the glutes are getting about 60 percent of the available resistance.

## Comparing Two Versions of the Standing Side Dumbbell Raise

As noted previously, since you cannot hold a dumbbell with only your humerus, you must involve the forearm as a secondary lever in order to load the deltoids. By holding the weights in your hands, you automatically engage the forearm as a secondary lever.

When the exercise is performed with straight arms, as illustrated in Figure 1-23, the forearm acts only as an extension of the upper arm. This factor essentially "lengthens" the primary lever, thereby increasing the magnification of the resistance, which is fine. A longer lever loads the deltoids more than a shorter (bent arm) lever does, even though a lighter weight may be used.

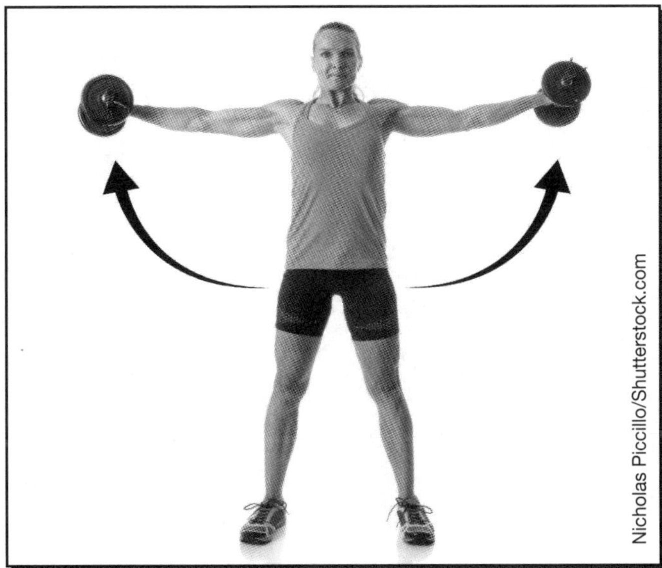

Figure 1-23

The average adult male arm—humerus and forearm combined—is about 30 inches long, from the shoulder to the hand. This means that whatever weight you're using in your hand, while doing "*straight arm side raises*," will be magnified by a factor of (approximately) 28, allowing for a two-inch "force arm." As such, a 10-pound dumbbell would be magnified to approximately 280 pounds (when the arm is perpendicular with the ground), in terms of how much force the deltoid has to produce.

Every once in a while, however, someone is seen in the gym doing the version of this exercise that is shown in Figure 1-24, with their elbows bent. Mechanically speaking, this technique is NOT a better version of a *side raise*. It might seem appealing, because it's "new" or "different." It might also appeal to a person, because a heavier weight can be used. While being able to use a heavier weight might cause some individuals to assume that this version is "better," that is an entirely incorrect assumption.

Yes, you CAN use more weight this way, but that's only because a bent arm magnifies the resistance HALF as much as a straight arm. Whether you use a straight arm with half as much weight, or a bent arm with twice as much weight, the deltoid gets the same load (approximately). Either way, it equals the same NET resistance to the deltoid. In reality, the deltoid does not work any harder, if you're using a heavier weight, with a bent arm.

At this point, you may be thinking that if the deltoids are loaded the same either way—whether using a bent arm with more weight or a straight arm with less weight—"why not do what's more gratifying (i.e., using a heavier weight)?" A very good reason exists, however, why *not* to make that choice.

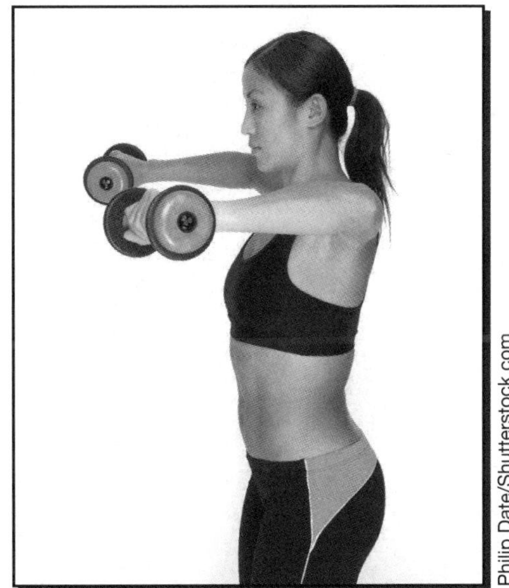

Figure 1-24

When the elbow is straight, the forearm (working as a secondary lever to the humerus) acts ONLY as an *extension* to the humerus. On the other hand, *when the elbow is bent*, the forearm enters into different plane of resistance. Instead of "lengthening" the humerus, the *forearm will now "rotate" (twist) the humerus*. It would be like using the forearm as the handle of a crescent wrench, to TURN the humerus inside the shoulder socket.

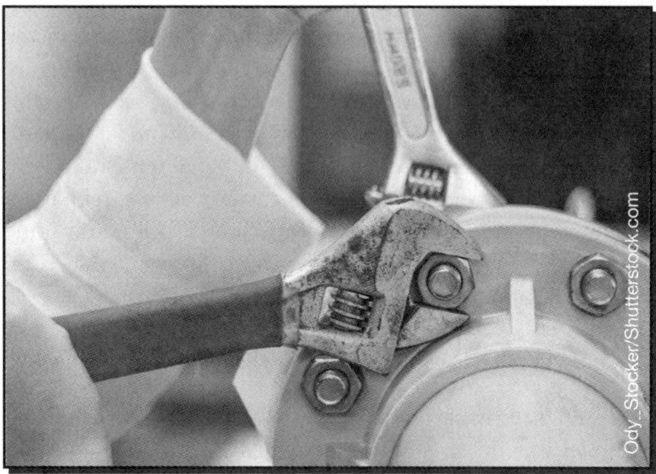


Figure 1-25

In response to this "forward-rotation" of the humerus, the external rotator muscles of the rotator cuff (i.e., the infraspinatus and teres minor) must fight to prevent further forward rotation. This effort could easily strain these muscles, because the weight typically used for deltoids is excessive for these smaller muscles.

As such, the bent-arm version of the *standing side dumbbell raise* would be, at the very least, an *inefficient* way of working the lateral deltoids. You'd be spending more effort, because *you're using a heavier weight*, than if your arms were straight. You would *not, however, be loading the deltoids anymore*. It could also be a risky choice, since the rotator cuff muscles could easily be overloaded.

Some people might try to suggest that working the rotator cuff muscles would be good. In general, I would agree. On the other hand, attempting to do so *while* trying to work the larger, stronger deltoids, would be a risky strategy. It might also compromise the deltoid load. Furthermore, there is a much better way of exercising the external rotators of the shoulders, which will be explained in Chapter 25.

## Summary

The concepts of "lever length" and "secondary levers" are among the most foundational biomechanical factors related to resistance exercise. The issue of the length of the levers is involved in every single resistance exercise you do. Furthermore, the issue of "secondary levers" is involved anytime you try to load a target muscle by applying the resistance to a lever that is NOT directly connected to the target muscle by way of muscle attachment.

It's important to understand how and why a *longer* lever magnifies a load *more*, and a *shorter* lever magnifies a load less. It is also essential to understand how a *secondary lever* can increase or decrease a load placed upon a primary lever, and how a secondary lever can cause strain to muscles unrelated to the target muscle, if the secondary lever moves *out of alignment* with the primary lever.

CHAPTER 2

# ACTIVE LEVERS AND NEUTRAL LEVERS

- *A lever that is perfectly parallel with the direction of resistance is "neutral." It does not require any force to hold it in that position. It is balanced, either over its base or under its pivot.*
- *Conversely, a lever that is perfectly perpendicular with the direction of resistance is fully "active." It is at its "heaviest" at that position, in terms of the effort required to hold it there (all other factors being equal).*
- *Therefore, an exercise for a given target muscle should (ideally speaking) allow that muscle's operating lever to encounter a mostly "active" position, somewhere in its range of motion. This step would allow the target muscle to be loaded with all or most of the available resistance.*
- *Varying degrees of inefficiency occur when an exercise does NOT allow a target muscle's operating lever to interact with resistance in a perpendicular manner.*
- *A lever that is mostly "neutral" only loads its operating muscle with a small percentage of the available resistance. Therefore, you must use much more weight than is necessary, in order to compensate for this reduction, and adequately challenge the muscle that operates that lever.*

As per the *Merriam-Webster Dictionary*, the definition of "efficiency" is: "effective operation as measured by a comparison of productivity versus cost (effort, time and/or money)." In other words, "efficiency"—in the pursuit of muscle growth—means getting the most amount of muscle load, with the least amount of weight used, and the least injury risk. In turn, "inefficiency" would be defined as using more weight, but without more load to the target muscle, which would result in wasted effort.

The previous chapter addressed the fact that the *amount of muscle force* required to move a weight held by a lever is greater than the actual amount of weight being used. The lever "magnifies" the weight that is on the lever, in proportion with the *length* of the lever.

This chapter looks at the fact that the amount of resistance that a weighted lever loads onto its operating muscle also depends on the *position* of that lever, relative to the direction of resistance. For example, in Figure 2-1, the lever is *perpendicular with gravity*, which makes it a fully *"active"* lever. This lever position results in the "heaviest" load to the muscle that holds the lever (i.e., 100 percent of the available resistance).

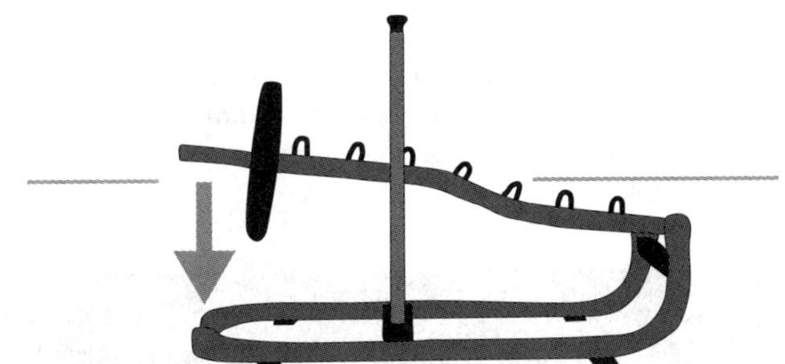

Figure 2-1

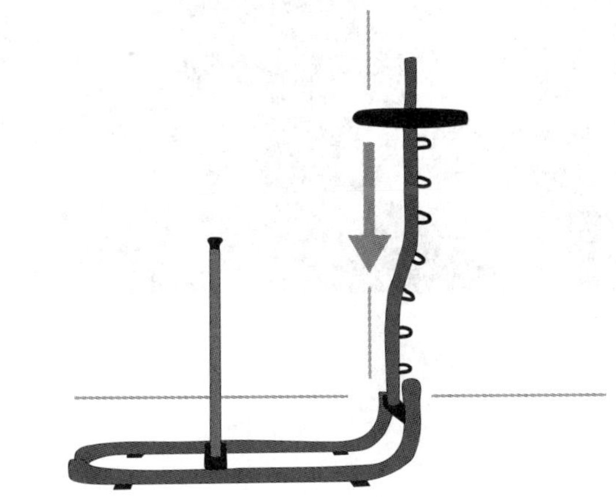

Figure 2-2

In contrast, in Figure 2-2, that same lever is *parallel with gravity*, which makes it a fully *"neutral"* lever. This position results in the "lightest" load to the muscle that holds the lever (i.e., zero resistance). It is important to note that regardless of how much weight is placed on the lever, it will always be NEUTRAL, when that lever is perfectly parallel with gravity (or whatever the direction of resistance happens to be during that exercise). It requires NO force to hold the lever in that position. It is balanced directly over (or under) the pivot.

Accordingly, the *most efficient* exercises are the ones that allow the operating lever of a target muscle (for example, the forearm, as the operating lever of the triceps) to go through a fully or mostly "active" position, somewhere in the range of motion. Exercises that are less efficient do not provide an opportunity for the operating lever to go through a mostly "active" position, somewhere in the range of motion. In fact, some exercises are extremely inefficient, because the operating lever of the target muscle is mostly "neutral" through the *entire* range of motion.

## Comparing an Efficient Lever vs. an Inefficient Lever

In order to address the issue of comparing an efficient lever with an inefficient lever, you might consider developing your TRICEPS muscle, with a standard *"supine dumbbell triceps extension."* In this hypothetical example, you would be exercising with a 20-pound dumbbell in each hand. As you can see in Figures 2-3 and 2-4, the forearm (which is the "operating lever" of the triceps) moves from a position that is just below horizontal (Figure 2-3), up to a position that is almost completely vertical (Figure 2-4).

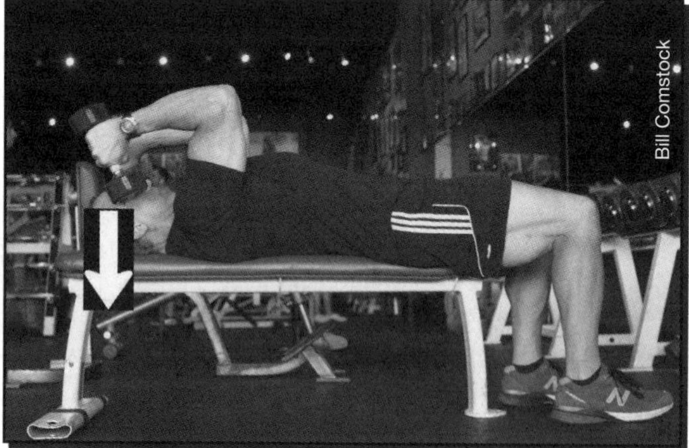


Figure 2-3

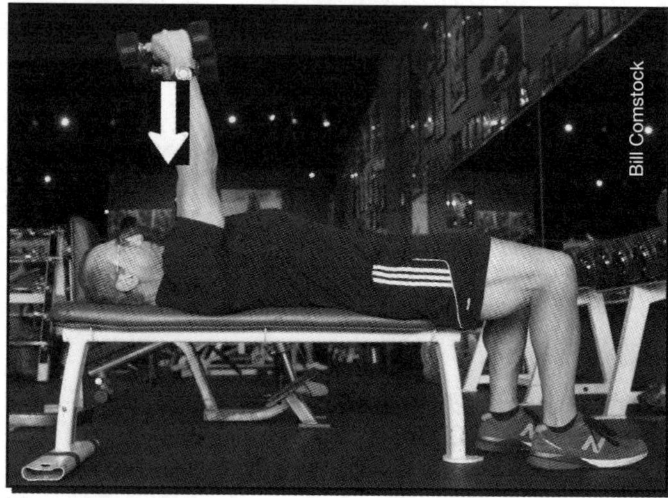


Figure 2-4

Even though *gravity* can't be seen, you are aware that it always pulls straight down. Using a clock for reference, "free weight gravity" always pulls in a 6:00 direction. For clarity's sake, a downward arrow has been included in both Figures 2-3 and 2-4, indicating the direction of gravity. This way, you can compare the angle of the forearm, relative to the "direction of resistance."

> *Note: When using a cable, the "direction of resistance" is toward the pulley, even though gravity pulls the weight stack straight down.*

When the forearm is horizontal, it is PERPENDICULAR with gravity, which would make it fully "active," at that point. A lever that is perpendicular with resistance is a *"100 percent lever."* In other words, all of the "available resistance" is loading the muscle that operates that lever. In this instance, it's the triceps. Then, as the forearm approaches the end of its range of motion, it culminates in a near vertical position. At that point, because it is almost *parallel* with gravity, it is mostly *"neutral."* This factor is important, because a fully neutral lever provides ZERO load to the muscle that operates it.

Doing a bit of math can determine approximately how much resistance each 20-pound dumbbell loads onto each triceps, in the aforementioned example, when the forearm is horizontal (fully "active"). It should be kept in mind that the following calculation is a simplified formula. The exact calculation requires trigonometry, which is not necessary for our purposes. This simplified method is accurate enough to give you a sense of how this particular exercise *compares* to another developmental exercise for the benefit of the triceps.

The average length of an adult male forearm, plus a bit of the hand, is approximately 14 inches. As such, any weight held in the hand would be magnified by a factor of approximately 12 (allowing for a two-inch "force arm"), when the forearm is perpendicular with resistance. Therefore, the 20-pound weight should be multiplied by a factor of 12, which equals 240 pounds. At that point, the load should be multiplied by 100 percent, given that the forearm is acting as a *fully* active lever. Multiplying by 100 percent essentially means that there's no "reduction" of resistance. In other words, 240 pounds is approximately how much is loaded onto each triceps, when a person uses a 20-pound dumbbell to perform a supine dumbbell triceps extension, and the forearm is at the most "active" position, i.e., perpendicular with gravity.

*Note: There is an additional factor that further magnifies resistance—known as "mechanical "disadvantage"—which will be discussed in the next chapter. For the sake of simplicity, however, you should assume, in this instance, that the only magnifier is the length of the forearm.*

For comparative purposes, consider another developmental exercise for the triceps—*parallel bar dips*. In Figure 2-5, you can see that the person's elbow is bent at approximately 90 degrees, which is the same degree of bend that occurs in the descended position of the *supine dumbbell triceps extensions*. During this exercise, however, the forearm is mostly *parallel* with gravity, at the same degree of elbow bend. It only tilts from the vertical (neutral) position by approximately 10 degrees, if that.

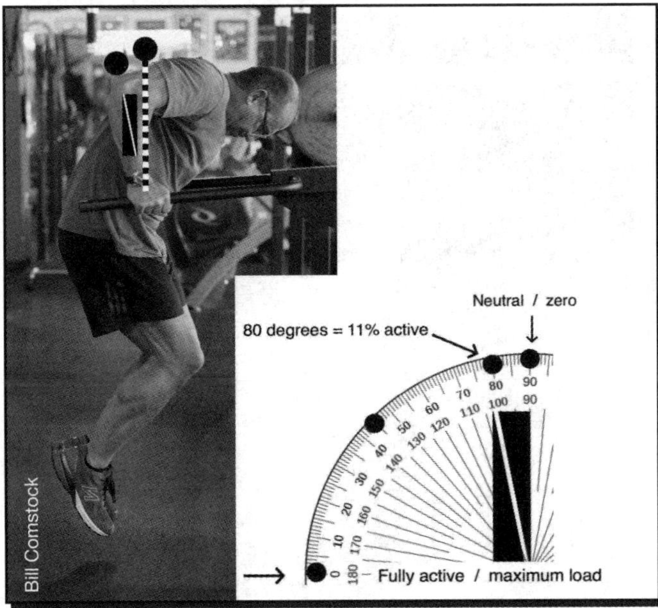


Figure 2-5

As you can see, Figure 2-5 also includes a graph that shows that the *vertical* position (90 degrees from horizontal) is *parallel* with gravity, and is, therefore, "neutral." The next line (on the left) is the 80-degree angle, which is 10 degrees less than vertical. This constitutes 11 percent of the distance between fully vertical and fully horizontal. You should compare that line with the angle of the person's forearm on the left.

Accordingly, if a horizontal lever is 100 percent "active," and a 90-degree lever is completely "neutral," then an 80-degree lever is only 11 percent "active." In other words, during *parallel bar dips*, the percentage of resistance that is loaded onto the triceps is only about 11 percent of that which is "available."

The next step is to do the (simplified) math on these figures. For example, say this exerciser (doing *parallel bar dips*) weighs 180 pounds. The individual has two arms, which translates to 90 pounds per arm. The exerciser's forearm is the same length as the person doing the *supine dumbbell triceps extensions*, which results in a magnification factor of 12. The exerciser is using an 11 percent lever. As such, the following figures need to be added into the equation:

- 180 pounds (bodyweight) divided by 2 (arms) = 90 x 12 (forearm length magnification) x 11 percent = 118.8 pounds.
- Each triceps is being loaded with about 119 pounds of resistance, in the descended position.

At this point, the "efficiency" of each exercise can be compared. In the first exercise, the man was lifting a total weight of 40 pounds (two 20 pound dumbbells), which resulted in each of his triceps being loaded with 240 pounds. In the second exercise, the man was lifting his entire bodyweight of 180 pounds, which resulted in each of his triceps being loaded with 119 pounds.

In reality, *parallel bar dips* require the man to use *4.5 times MORE* resistance (180 pounds) than when he is doing a *supine dumbbell triceps extension* (40 pounds). On the other hand, when performing parallel bar dips, he is loading his triceps with less than *HALF as much* load (119 pounds), as compared with *supine dumbbell triceps extensions* (240 pounds). See the cost/benefit difference?

When you examine the physics of each exercise, it should be *obvious* which is the "better" (more efficient) triceps exercise. The reason parallel bar dips rate so poorly as a triceps exercise, is because the forearm (as the operating lever of the triceps) is barely "active" throughout the entire range of motion. As such, it is only able to deliver 11 percent of the available resistance to the triceps.

If you've ever performed parallel bar dips, you may be thinking that this exercise FEELS like it's providing more load than just 119 pounds. To a point, you are correct. 119

pounds is only what is being loaded onto each of your Triceps. Furthermore, 180 pounds is certainly much heavier than the 40 pounds used when performing supine dumbbell triceps extensions. As such, it is natural that *dips* would feel much more difficult, than would *supine dumbbell triceps extensions.* In fact, just holding your bodyweight at the top of the dipping bars is somewhat challenging, even though neither the forearm nor the upper arm levers are "active" (perpendicular with gravity). As such, there is an enormous amount of vertical pressure on the arm bones, wrists, and hands, even without descending into the movement.

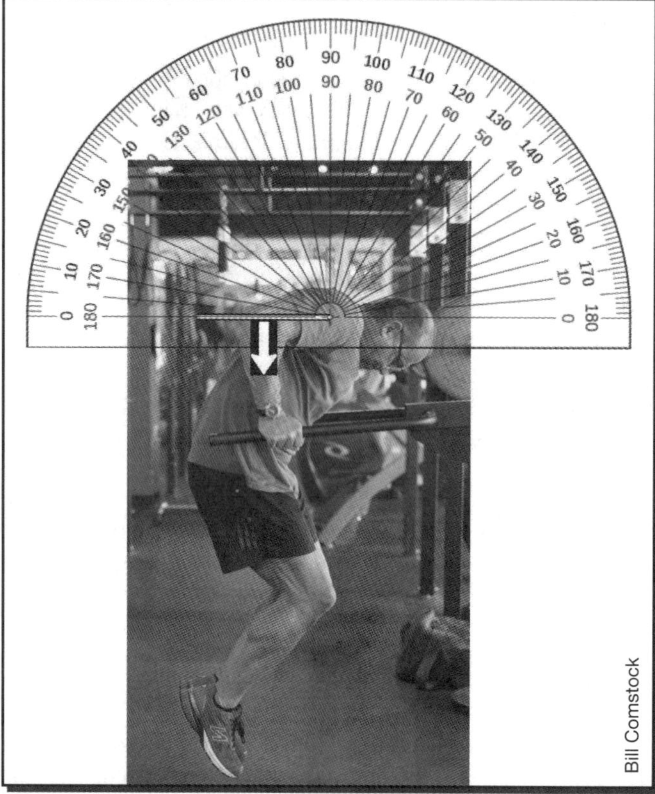


Figure 2-6

In Figure 2-6, a line has been placed that is parallel with the exerciser's humerus (upper arm bone), and an arrow indicating the direction of resistance. These notations show that the humerus is very "active" in the descended position. The humerus mostly loads the pecs, when the elbows are wide. In turn, it mostly loads the *anterior deltoids*, when the elbows are "back," as occurs during parallel bar dips.

At this point, you might be thinking, "great, I could use some anterior deltoid development." Arguably, however, your body weight is "too much" resistance for your anterior deltoids. Furthermore, because the pathway of humeral movement during *parallel bar dips* is *not ideal* for the pectoral fibers, it's compromised as a pectoral exercise. In fact, there are far better pectoral exercises than parallel bar dips, and there are also much better (and safer) anterior deltoid exercises.

As you can see, with regard to *parallel bar dips*, there are several problematic issues. Not only does the exercise involve an inefficient lever loading the triceps, it also entails an efficient lever overloading the anterior deltoids. Furthermore, the exercise has a "less-than-ideal" humeral pathway compromising the potential benefit to the pectorals.

Bench dips (Figure 2-7) are another example of an exercise that is intended as a triceps exercise, but proves to be very *inefficient* in that effort, because the forearm (as the operating lever of the triceps) is mostly in the neutral position throughout the entire range of motion. This exercise also causes the operating lever of the triceps—the forearm—to be mostly parallel with resistance (gravity), rather than mostly perpendicular with it. Furthermore, it induces the upper arm bone/lever (the *humerus*) to be the more active lever. This factor (again) causes the majority of the load to be placed on the anterior deltoids, even though that is not the intended goal of this exercise.

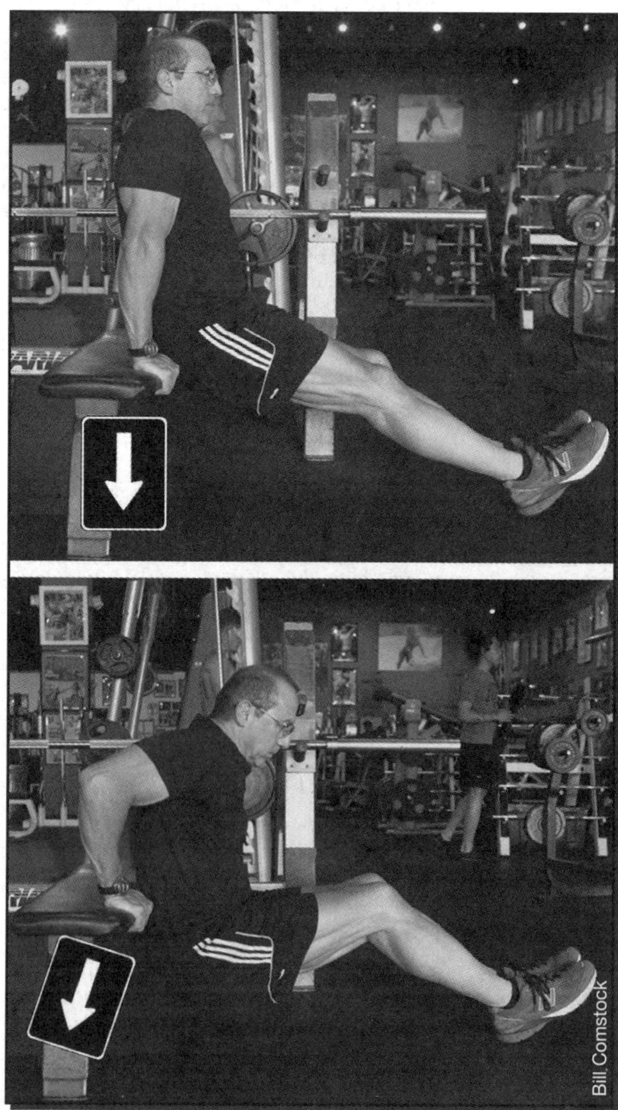


Figure 2-7

In addition, performing bench dips over-stretches the anterior deltoids *even more* than occurs when doing parallel bar dips. All-in-all, this factor should be fairly obvious, based on the fact that the hands are constantly *behind the torso*. At least with parallel bar dips, they are mostly alongside the torso.

Not only are bench dips mostly unproductive for developing the triceps, they could easily strain the anterior deltoids. Once you understand the difference between an *active lever* and a *neutral lever*, the downside of performing bench dips is fairly obvious.

## Assessing Exercise Efficiency

When assessing a resistance exercise, one of the most important factors to identify is which levers are more perpendicular with resistance, and which are less perpendicular, through the range of motion of that exercise. Identifying this feature and putting it into context requires that two other aspects be known:

- The *direction of resistance* ("free weight" gravity, cables, or machine)
- The *muscles* that operate those levers

As a prelude to the discussion of muscular anatomy that appears in Chapters 18 to 25, and to help you fully grasp the concept and application of "*active*" and "*neutral*" levers in exercise assessment, the following list of basic physique muscles and their corresponding operating levers is provided. This list can also be helpful in knowing which muscles are operating the levers that are moving during an exercise.

| Muscle | Operating Lever |
|---|---|
| Pectorals | Humerus (upper-arm bone) |
| Lats | Humerus (upper-arm bone) |
| Deltoids (lateral, posterior, and anterior) | Humerus (upper-arm bone) |
| Trapezius | Scapula/clavicle (shoulder carriage) |
| Biceps | Radius/ulna (forearm) |
| Triceps | Radius/ulna (forearm) |
| Quadriceps | Tibia/fibula (lower leg) |
| Hamstrings | Tibia/fibula (lower leg) |
| Glutes | Femur (upper-leg bone) |
| Hip flexors | Femur (upper-leg bone) |
| Calves | Foot |
| Forearms (flexors/extensors) | Hand |
| Obliques | Spine/torso/pelvis |
| Abdominals | Spine/torso/pelvis |
| Erector spinae | Spine/torso/pelvis |

A limb (e.g., upper arm, forearm, femur, etc.) is usually "operated" by more than one muscle. For example, the humerus (upper-arm lever) is "operated" (moved) by the pecs, the lats, and the deltoids (in three directions), as well as by other smaller muscles. As such, not surprisingly, it's relatively easy to be confused concerning knowing which muscle is actually "working," when the upper arm is moving.

In order to know which muscle is moving a limb (the humerus, for example), you simply need to identify which muscle origin that limb is moving *toward*, when it is moving concentrically. For example, if the humerus is moving toward the sternum, it's the pectorals that are causing that to happen. On the other hand, if the humerus is moving laterally (to your sides), it's the lateral deltoids that are causing that to happen, because the humerus is moving toward the origin of the lateral deltoids. The key point to remember is that muscles always pull their corresponding limbs *toward* their origins.

## Supine Dumbbell Press (as a Pectoral Exercise)

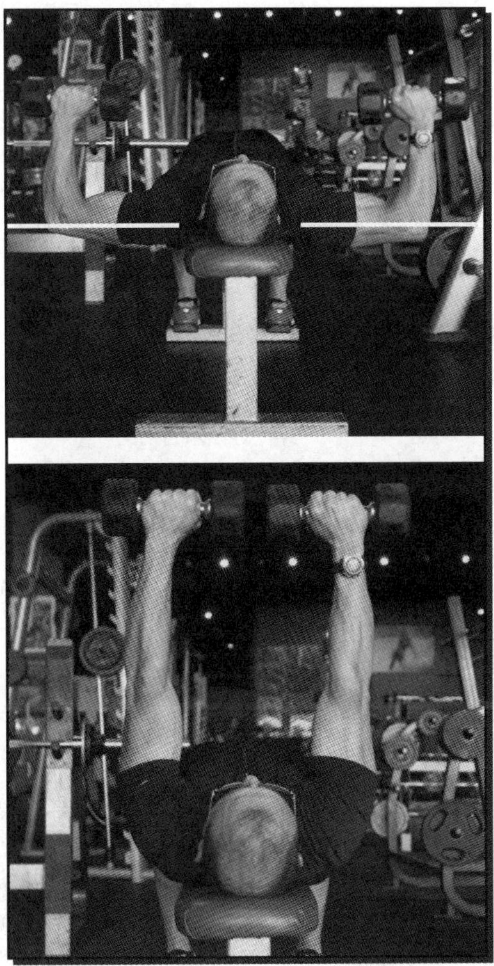


Figure 2-8

As the aforementioned list noted, the "operating lever" of the pectoralis major is the humerus (i.e., the upper-arm bone). The origin of the pectoral fibers is mostly on the sternum (the "sternal fibers"), with some additional fibers originating on the clavicle (the "clavicular fibers"), as well as on the lower ribs (the "costal fibers"). ALL of the pectoral fibers, however, ultimately attach onto the humerus. Therefore, the contraction of any of the pectoral fibers requires the use of the humerus as the *operating lever* of the pectorals.

One of the most important questions to ask, when assessing an exercise involving the pectorals is "Does the operating lever of the pectoralis major (i.e., the humerus) encounter a mostly perpendicular angle with the direction of resistance, during the range of motion?" In the aforementioned exercise (*supine dumbbell press*), the answer is "yes." That "encounter" occurs when the humerus is parallel with the ground, in the descended position, which is why this exercise is a considered a "good" pectoral exercise.

Is there a secondary lever in play in this instance? Yes, the forearm is involved as a secondary lever. Is that lever mostly "active," or mostly "neutral?" It is mostly *neutral*, because it is mostly parallel with resistance, which is also good.

Again, there are other factors that also help determine whether the supine dumbbell press is a "great" exercise or not. The first thing to ascertain, however, is whether or not the operating lever of the pectorals (the humerus) utilizes lever efficiency, somewhere in the exercise's range of motion. It's also important to determine whether another (non-target) muscle's operating lever is more active than that of the target muscle's. If that factor occurs, it would interfere with the loading of the pecs.

## Hanging Leg Raises (as an Abdominal Exercise)

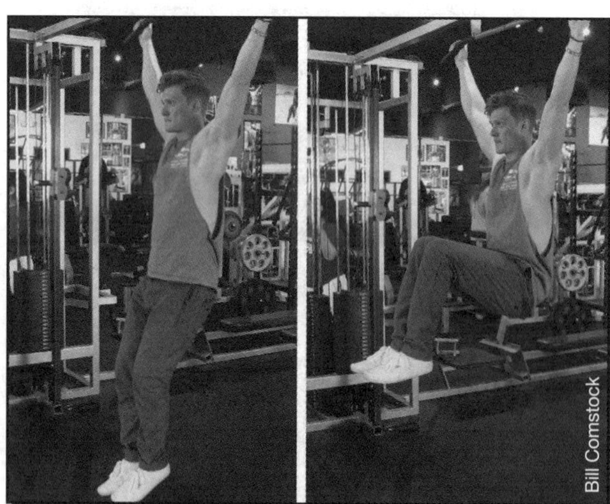

Figure 2-9

The primary objective of performing *hanging leg raises* (Figure 2-9) is to work the abdominal muscles, specifically the rectus abdominis, which is also known as the abs. Is there an "active lever" in this exercise? Yes, the femurs (the upper-leg bones). When they are horizontal, the femur bones cross the point that is perpendicular with gravity. As such, the femurs are fully *active* levers. The femurs, however, are not the operating lever of the abs. This situation is a perfect example of the *wrong lever being active* during an exercise. The femurs are being raised by a different set of muscles, known as the "hip flexors."

As such, what is the operating lever of the abs, as per the aforementioned list? It is the spine/pelvis. However, neither the spine nor the pelvis are in an "active" position during a hanging leg raise. The spine and the pelvis are parallel, or mostly parallel, with gravity, which means that they are neutral or mostly neutral. Therefore, as an abs exercise, this is exercise significantly compromised. There are additional reasons why this exercise is compromised, but this is the first strike against it.

In fact, the rectus abdominis *does not even connect to the legs*, as you can see in Figure 2-10. The abs originate on the *pubic bone of the pelvis*, and attach on the bottom front portion of the ribs. When this muscle contracts, it brings the ribcage toward the pelvis, which requires flexion of the spine. It does NOT, however, require flexion of the hip (as occurs during *hanging leg raises*). While there is a tiny bit of spinal flexion that occurs during *hanging leg raises*, it is not much. More importantly, the spine is NOT interacting perpendicularly with gravity.

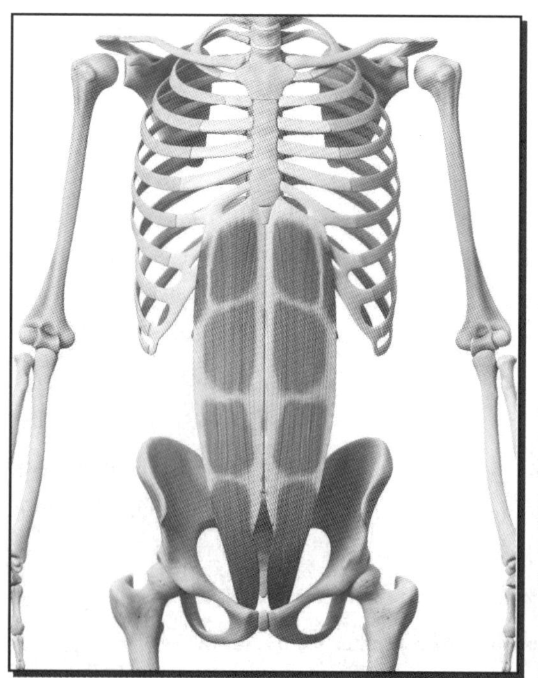

Figure 2-10

As such, the hanging leg raise exercise fails miserably in both of the aforementioned criteria. Instead of the primary lever being most active, it is mostly neutral. Furthermore, instead of the secondary lever being mostly neutral, it's entirely active.

In reality, the *hanging leg raise* is a *very inefficient* exercise. In fact, it could be called "one of the LEAST efficient exercises" commonly performed in a fitness environment. The energy cost is very high, and the benefit to the abs is very low.

## Squats (as a Quadriceps Exercise)

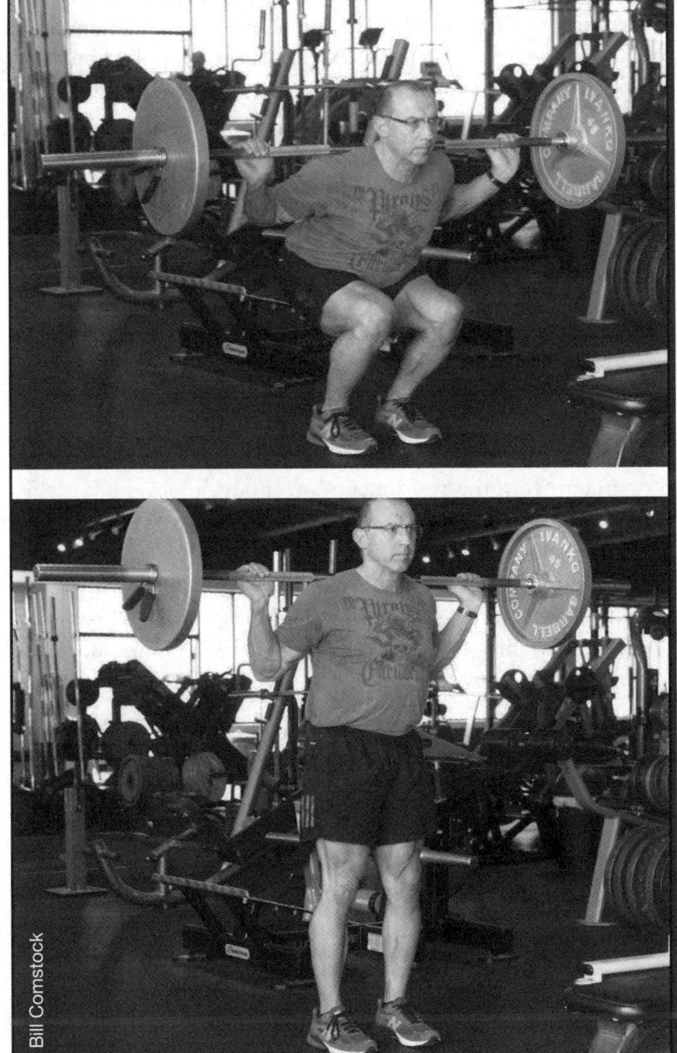

Figure 2-11

The primary objective of performing weighted *squats* is to work the quadriceps, followed closely *behind* (pun intended) by the gluteus. Accordingly, the questions to ask, with regard to performing squats, are, "How active is the lower leg (as the operating lever of the quads) and the upper leg (as the operating lever of the glutes)? Also, is there any other (non-target muscle's) lever that is more "active" than it should be?

Figure 2-12 shows a good perspective of the levers in play. Specifically, Figure 2-12 illustrates the degrees of "perpendicular-ness" of each of these levers. The tibia, for example, is tilting forward about 30 degrees from vertical (60 degrees), which translates to about a 33 percent tilt (30 divided by 90 degrees). Therefore, we could say that the tibia is working with about 33 percent efficiency.

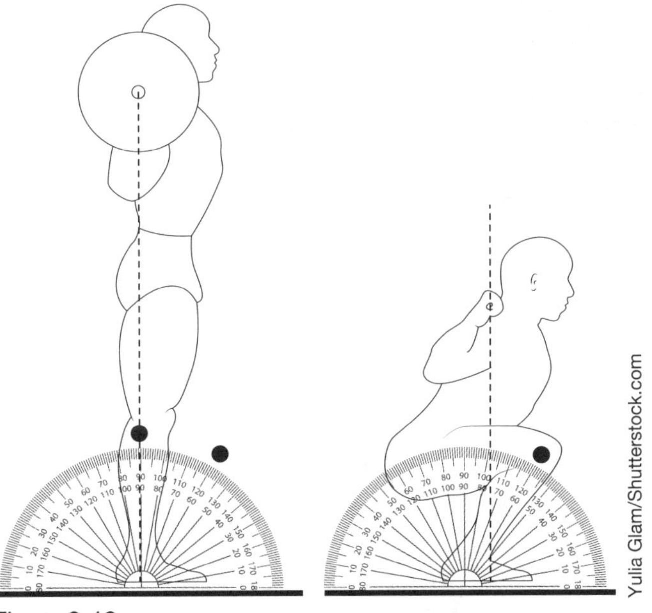

Figure 2-12

The Femur (Figure 2-13) is slightly below horizontal. Since it's a bit beyond perpendicular with gravity, this lever could be called a 100 percent lever. Furthermore, the torso (shown in Figure 2-14) is tilting about 30 degrees from vertical (60 degrees). Therefore, this lever is also about 33 percent active (30 divided by 90).

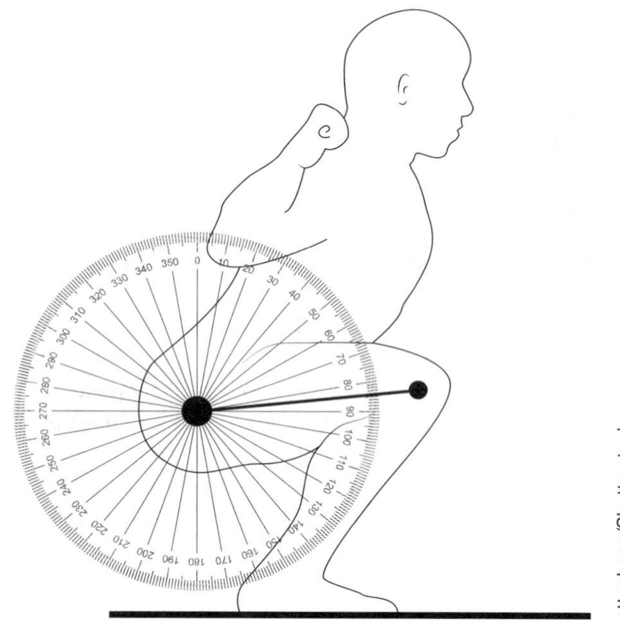

Figure 2-13

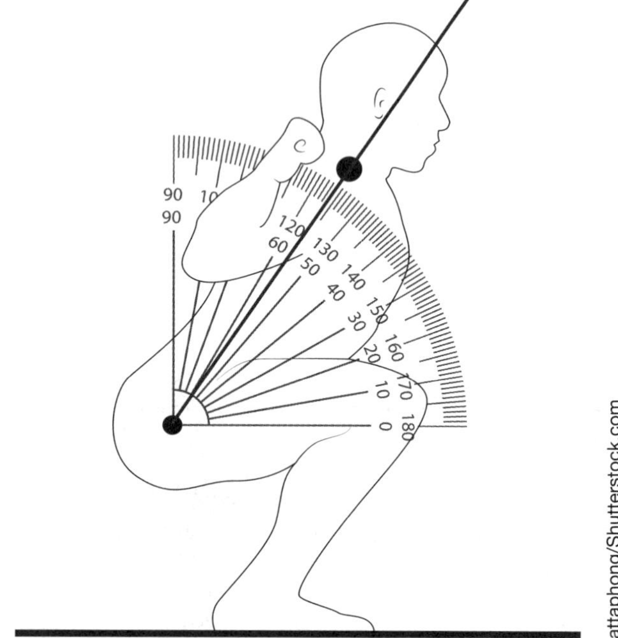

Figure 2-14

The higher the percentage of "active" a lever is, the greater the percentage of the "available resistance" that will be loaded onto the muscle that operates that lever. It should be kept in mind, however, that the "available resistance" is also a factor of the *length* of the lever.

For this reason, the gluteus is not getting quite as much benefit (load) from a squat as it would appear. Even though the femur is 100 percent active (when in the descended position), it is being effectively *shortened* by the "doubling back" of the tibia (*the secondary lever*, as was discussed in the previous chapter). As such, the glutes are working with a femur that is operating with about half its actual length, in this scenario. Therefore, the femur is delivering 100 percent of a *reduced* load, to the glutes. Furthermore, because the tibia is about 33 percent efficient in the descended position of the squat, it's only loading approximately 33 percent of the "available resistance" onto the quadriceps.

Doing a bit of math can help clarify the point. For example, consider a hypothetical situation in which a man is squatting with 225 pounds on his back. His primary goal (ostensibly) is to work his quadriceps. His bodyweight is 200 pounds, but only about 3/4 of that is the weight above his legs. In other words, he is effectively squatting (150 + 225 =) 375 pounds. Since his tibia (length) has a magnification factor of (approximately) 20X, the 375 should be multiplied by 20 (= 7,500 pounds). In turn, that number should be multiplied by his 33 percent lever efficiency factor. That calculation brings it down to 2,475 pounds total, which is then divided by two legs, therefore equaling 1,238 pounds per quadriceps.

That outcome may seem like quite a lot of load on each quadriceps. On the other hand, it's not as much load as it could be (as you'll soon see), and the energy cost of that is also much higher than it could be.

Because the forward tilt of the *torso* is similar to that of the tibia, it is equally "active" as the lever that loads the quads. His torso, however, is a longer lever than is his tibia. As such, it is magnifying the resistance more than the lever that loads the quads. The barbell is resting at the very top of the torso lever, which allows the entire length of the torso to magnify the forward force of the 225 lb. barbell. In other words, his erector spinae (the muscle operating the torso lever) is loaded *more* than are his quads, even though this exercise is not meant as an erector spinae exercise.

At this point, you might ask, "Isn't there a way of getting a *greater percentage* of the available resistance to load onto the quads, and less onto the erector spinae and the spine?" The answer is "yes." You can accomplish this simply by changing the direction of resistance, so that the tibia (the lower leg) interacts more perpendicularly with resistance, than it normally does during barbell squats, and the spine interacts less perpendicularly with resistance, than occurs during barbell squats.

Figure 2-15 shows a "*cable squat.*" You should note that the added resistance is now coming from the cables, which are pulling in a *frontward*/downward direction. Of course, your own bodyweight is still being pulled straight downward. For the sake of simplicity, however, consider that all of the resistance is coming from the cables. As you can see in Figure 2-15 (bottom), the tibia is completely *perpendicular* with the cable. At that point, the tibia is acting with 100 percent efficiency.

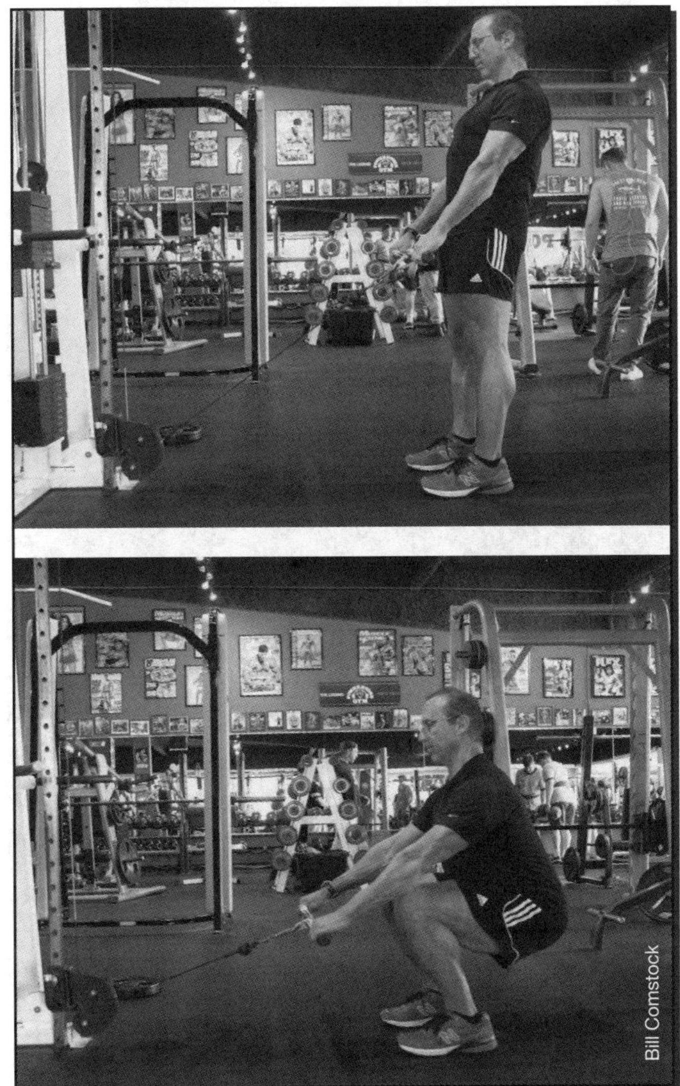

Figure 2-15

In addition to the quadriceps getting 100 percent of the available resistance, there is very little downward loading on the spine. Certainly, there is no metal barbell pushing downward, directly on the vertebrae. Furthermore, because the cable handles are held low, the effective lever length of the torso is lessened, thereby causing less load on the erector spinae, a factor that is also good.

The squat exercise will be covered more in Chapter 22, in the section that discusses the quadriceps. At this point, it can be helpful to consider some other examples that utilize a fully active lever (for the quads), rather than a 33 percent active lever.

For example, a *leg extension* (on a leg extension machine) applies its resistance 100 percent perpendicularly against the lower leg, making the lower leg a 100 percent active lever. Accordingly, if you were using 150 pounds of resistance (75 pounds per ankle), it would load each quadriceps with 1,500 pounds (approximately). Compare that to the 1,238 pounds that each quadriceps would be getting, if you were squatting 225 pounds, and consider the difference in "cost" between the two. As such, leg extensions are much more efficient at delivering a load to the quads, because less weight used still equals more load on the quads.

Figure 2-16 shows a couple of photos of a man doing an exercise called "*sissy squats*." He's holding no additional weight (beyond his bodyweight), compared to the 225 pounds used in the previous examples of a squat. Yet, he's loading his quadriceps *more* with THIS exercise, than he would during a standard barbell squat holding a 225-pound barbell.

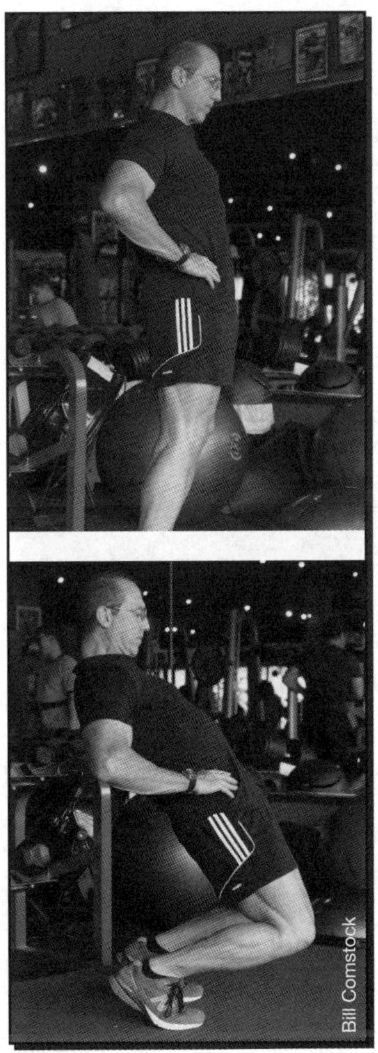

Figure 2-16

His lower leg levers almost reach a fully horizontal angle (almost *fully* "active"), when in the descended position. As you can see, they're about 10 degrees short of being perfectly horizontal. In other words, the tibia reaches about a 90 percent efficiency.

Using the same formula as in the previous exercise (a bodyweight of about 200 lbs.), you should use 150 (200 minus 25 percent), as his "bodyweight" number. He's not using any additional resistance, so the "resistance" amount is still 150 pounds. You should then factor in the magnifier "x20" (for the tibia length), and then factor in the efficiency of 90 percent (150 x 20 x .90 =). The total comes to 2,700 pounds, which is then divided by two legs, which equals 1,350 pounds per quadriceps.

That total is 112 pounds more than the previous squat example. The energy cost in this exercise ("sissy squats") is obviously significantly less. While 375 pounds was used with the *barbell squats*, only 150 pounds was used with the sissy squats. That's *60 percent less* weight, which is 60 percent less energy cost.

As such, the reason why a person is ABLE to squat with so much weight (sometimes as much as 500 pounds, or more) is PRECISELY because of the *inefficiency* of the Tibia angle (33 percent), combined with the shortened femur length (caused by the doubling-back of the lower leg).

If your goal is simply "to move the most amount of weight," even though it doesn't load any of the muscles involved as efficiently as possible, than doing heavy *squats* is fine. On the other hand, for the purpose of building muscle, it would be much wiser to do an exercise with better mechanics. If you do, you can load the target muscles MORE with less weight, while putting LESS stress on your bones, joints, and non-target muscles.

## When a "Neutral" Lever Is Made Dangerously "Active"

You can use this concept (i.e., *active* lever versus *neutral* lever) to determine whether an exercise is efficient, as well as ascertain whether an exercise has a potential risk of injury. For example, Chapter 1 reviewed the issue of the secondary lever, with regard to the supine dumbbell press. It also briefly discussed the internal and external rotation of the humerus that is caused by allowing the forearm to tilt either toward the head or toward the feet. Both were examples of "neutral levers made dangerously active." As such, during a supine dumbbell press, the ideal position for the forearm is to have it be perfectly vertical (neutral), when viewed from the side.

Tilting the forearm *toward the feet* causes the humerus to rotate "internally," and forces the "external shoulder rotators" (infraspinatus and teres minor) to become loaded, in order to prevent further forward rotation. This situation could easily strain the smaller rotator muscles, given the amount of weight that is typically used during a *supine dumbbell press* for the pectorals.

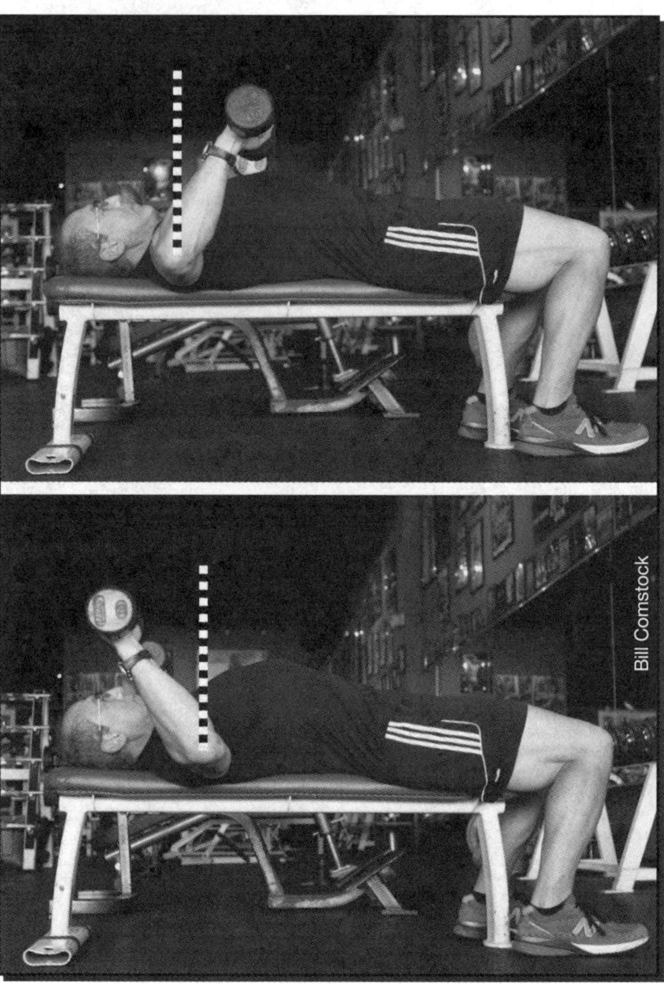


Figure 2-17

The same factor is also true for allowing the forearm to tilt *toward the head*, thereby causing the humerus to rotate "externally." This action would force the internal shoulder rotator (subscapularis) to prevent further backward rotation of the humerus, which could strain the smaller forward rotation muscle.

Figure 2-18 provides a photo of an exerciser doing a "behind-the-neck press" with a barbell. You should note that his right forearm (actually both of his forearms although you can see the right forearm more clearly) is tilting "externally"—toward the rear. This tilt is causing the forearm to be "active," with an external rotational force. Externally rotating the humerus this much (even without weight), inside the shoulder socket, is already very strenuous to the joint. Adding a heavy load further exacerbates the problem.

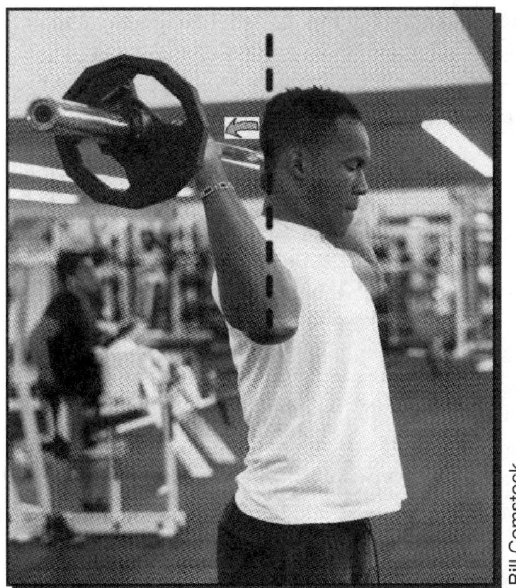

Figure 2-18

Figure 2-19 illustrates an example of the forearm tilting toward the front, instead of toward the rear. Since the humerus attaches to the torso alongside the head (not in front of, nor behind the head), using a *barbell* automatically requires either a backward tilt of the forearms (which behind-the-neck presses require) or a forward tilt of the forearms (which in-front-of-the-neck presses require, in order to allow exercisers to avoid hitting themselves on the head with the barbell. Tilting the forearms either way (forward or backward)—during any kind of pressing movement—strains the muscles of the "rotator cuff." A backward tilt strains the internal rotators, while a forward tilt strains the external rotators.

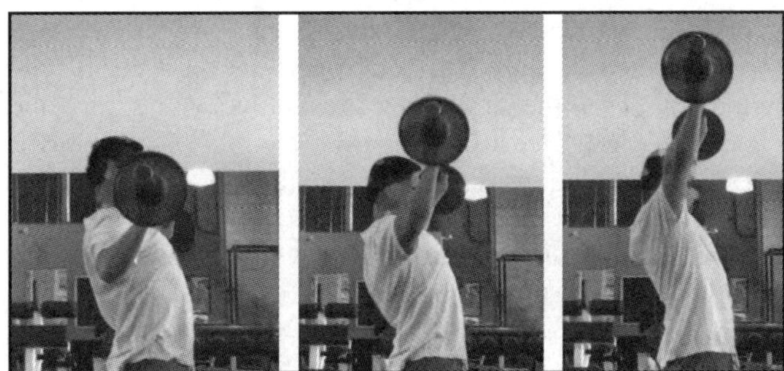
Figure 2-19

Figure 2-19 shows a man forward-tilting his forearm the most in the far left photo, in order to avoid hitting himself in the head. Even after the bar has passed his head, however, he still does not fully "correct" this forward tilt. As discussed previously, part of this situation is due to the fact that most people do not have enough mobility in their shoulder joint to rotate their humerus externally enough to cause their forearm to be perfectly vertical (during an overhead press). Either way, the result in the same. It strains the limits of the smaller, shoulder rotation muscles.

The overhead press would be "less bad," if the forearms could be kept perfectly vertical during the exercise (neutral, as seen from the side)—tilting neither backward nor forward. Theoretically, this step could be accomplished by using dumbbells, instead of a barbell if an exerciser had the shoulder mobility to achieve a perfectly vertical forearm position. In reality, the majority of people do not have that degree of shoulder mobility. The overhead press has several other mechanical problems as well, which will be discussed in Chapter 20 ("Deltoids").

## Summary

A lever that is perfectly parallel with resistance (gravity, a cable, or a machine, etc.) is NEUTRAL, in the sense that it requires no effort from the muscles that operate that lever (i.e., limb) to be held in that position. Knowing when a lever should be neutral, and when it should be active, is very important for maximizing benefit and minimizing injury risk when exercising.

A lever that is perfectly neutral (parallel with resistance) could be defined as having one end either directly over, or directly under, its other end, relative to resistance. For example, a lamp post (Figure 2-20) has its top *directly over* its base. It is not tilting in any direction whatsoever. In contrast, a plumb line has its weight *directly under* its pivot (Figure 2-21). In reality, the reason a plumb line is used in construction, is to identify the neutral position. Buildings are built in a way that requires the least amount of lateral support. Hence, they are constructed "parallel with gravity," using vertical columns, etc.

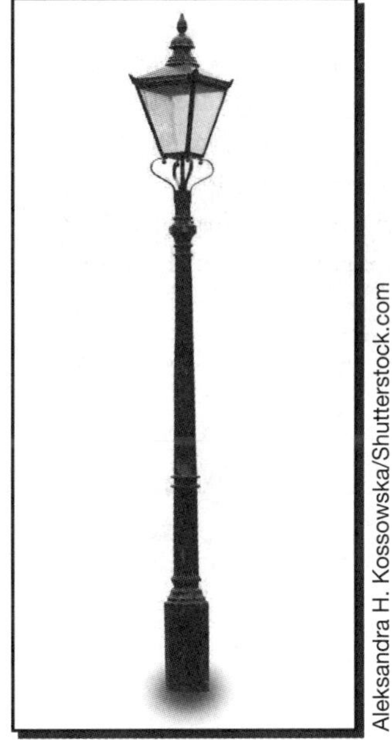

Figure 2-20

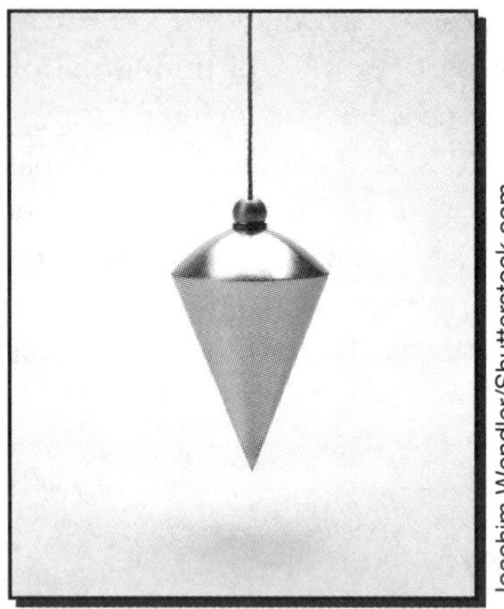

Figure 2-21

The human body operates the same way. All of our limbs are levers, and they adhere to the same rules of physics as any other physical structure.

If you could view a lever from *directly* overhead—looking straight down onto it from above—while it is in its perfectly NEUTRAL position (parallel with gravity/resistance), it would simply look like whatever is on top. Either its base would be "hidden" under its top, or its top would be hidden under its pivot, if the lever were hanging down.

This factor is also true, when you are performing any type of pressing movement. For example, if you could be viewed from directly overhead, while you were performing a *supine dumbbell press*, your forearms and elbow would be "hidden" behind your hand, because they would be directly under your hand, relative to gravity, assuming you are keeping your forearm perfectly vertical.

In Figure 2-22 (a view from above, assuming the exerciser is lying flat on his back), you see that his elbow (the bend of his arm) is hidden under his hand, because his forearm is perfectly vertical (neutral). On the other hand, if this person were to tilt his forearm outward (laterally, away from his midline) the lever would become active in one particular direction—loading the biceps. As a result, you would begin to see the "inside" of his forearm, plus the bend of his arm between the upper arm and the forearm.

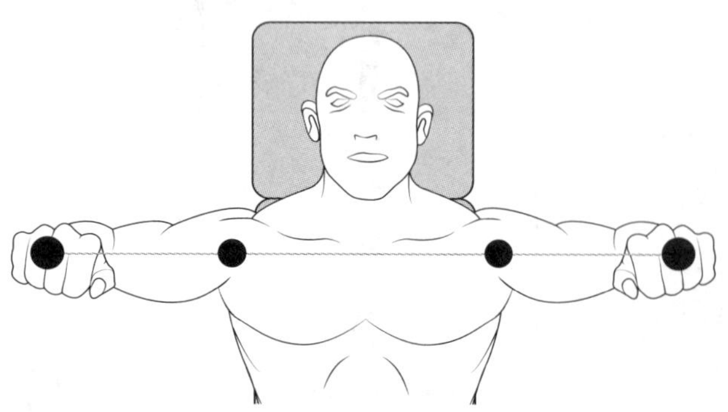
Figure 2-22

If the exerciser were to tilt his forearm inward toward his midline, the lever would become active in a different direction—loading his triceps. In turn, you would begin to see the "outside" of his forearm and elbow.

On the other hand, if the exerciser were to tilt his forearm "internally" (toward his feet), it would become active in yet another direction—loading his infraspinatus and teres minor (the external shoulder rotators). As a consequence, you would begin to see the "extensor" side of his forearm.

If the exerciser were to tilt his forearm "externally" (toward his head), it would become active in yet another direction—loading his subscapularis (the internal shoulder rotator). As such, you would begin to see the "flexor" side of his forearm.

Of course, an exerciser cannot rotate IN and OUT at the same time, nor INTERNALLY and EXTERNALLY at the same time. An individual, however, *can* rotate OUTWARD (laterally) and EXTERNALLY at the same time, or any one of the other combinations. In reality, this sort of thing happens frequently.

As such, when you are performing a supine dumbbell press, it's important to ask yourself (while you are doing the exercise), "Is my elbow directly under my hand?" Furthermore, "Am I allowing my forearm to tilt outwardly or inwardly, externally or internally, or a combination of these two possibilities?" You will find that having your elbow under your hand is best, in terms of maximum power and efficiency, as well as with regard to safety for your shoulder rotators.

It's often difficult to ascertain whether your elbow is under your hand, particularly when you cannot see yourself, as is the case when you are lying on your back on a flat bench. Sometimes, even the view that a mirror gives you is not quite enough to see if a correction is necessary. As such, a mirror does not allow you to see yourself from all sides. All-in-all, it is very difficult to arrange two or three perspectives of your body simultaneously. On the other hand, you need to be aware of how your body should be positioned and try to develop a FEEL for it.

Furthermore, in terms of working with maximum efficiency, you should select exercises that allow the operating lever of your target muscle to cross perpendicularly with the direction of resistance during the range of motion of that exercise. Two examples of this factor would be the forearm during a triceps extension and a lower leg (tibia) during a quadriceps exercise.

As discussed previously, because this does not happen during either *parallel bar dips* or standard *barbell squats*, the efficiency of those exercises is compromised. As such, a "better" version of a triceps exercise would be a *supine dumbbell triceps extension*, while a better version of *barbell squats* (for the quadriceps) would be *leg extensions* or *cable squats*, because these exercises allow the operating lever of the target muscle to be maximally *active* during the movement.

A maximally efficient exercise utilizes a fully active or mostly active operating lever for the target muscle. As noted previously, this factor is defined as a lever that "interacts perpendicularly with the direction of resistance." When this situation occurs, the largest percentage of the weight being used is loaded onto the muscle that operates that lever. As a result, you do not need to use as much weight. In fact, you are unable to use as much weight, compared to less-efficient exercises (i.e., exercises that do not allow the target muscle's operating lever to interact perpendicularly with the direction of resistance).

*In reality, having to use less weight is a sign of efficiency.* It means that you are maximizing the load, while exercising. As such, it is important that you not allow your ego to deter you from doing exercises that obligate you to use "lighter" poundages.

Conversely, an exercise that allows you to use a large amount of weight does so, precisely because it is minimizing the load to your target muscles. It typically does this by either using shorter levers (e.g., using bent arms, instead of straight arms), or reducing the effective length of the primary lever by way of a secondary lever, or by utilizing levers that are only working at a 10, 20, or 30 percent level of efficiency (i.e., mostly "neutral" levers)—or a combination of the these scenarios.

For those individuals who are pursuing muscular development, the wiser/safer/more efficient approach is to utilize maximally efficient levers, which magnify resistance more, because they interact perpendicularly with the direction of resistance. This technique allows you to accomplish more, with less wasted (i.e., unproductive) effort and less risk.

# CHAPTER 3

# MECHANICAL DISADVANTAGE

- ❑ *When a lever (i.e., bone or appendage) is positioned at an angle, such that the muscle is able to pull on it perpendicularly, it is called a "mechanical advantage." This position is the most efficient angle from which a muscle can pull on a bone.*
- ❑ *When a lever is positioned at an angle, such that a muscle is only able to pull on it from an angle that is mostly parallel, it is called a "mechanical disadvantage." Because this is the least efficient angle from which a muscle can pull on a lever, significantly more force is required to produce limb movement, as compared with "mechanical advantage."*
- ❑ *There are various angles BETWEEN perpendicular and parallel from which a muscle can pull on its lever. These angles represent varying degrees of mechanical disadvantage and require increasingly greater amounts of force, given that the angle of pull is more parallel to the bone.*

In Chapter 1, a lever device was introduced to demonstrate the magnification effect of a lever. In this chapter, that same device is used to explain the concept of "mechanical disadvantage."

During the initial experiment, I described how I moved from the first hook on the device (the one farthest from the pivot) to the last hook (the one closest to the pivot). Each time I tested the force required, I pulled straight upward with the scale.

In fact, I was pulling in a direction that was perpendicular to the lever. The lever was horizontal, and I was pulling vertically. Thus, I was pulling from a "*mechanical advantage.*" The reason it is called an "advantage" is because *all* of my effort is being used productively, i.e., to pull the lever in the same direction as it is able to move. In reality, there is no "better" (i.e., more economical) direction from which to pull on a lever.

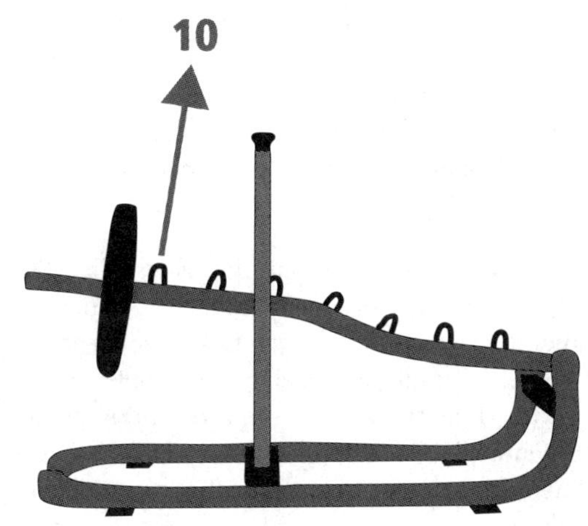

Figure 3-1

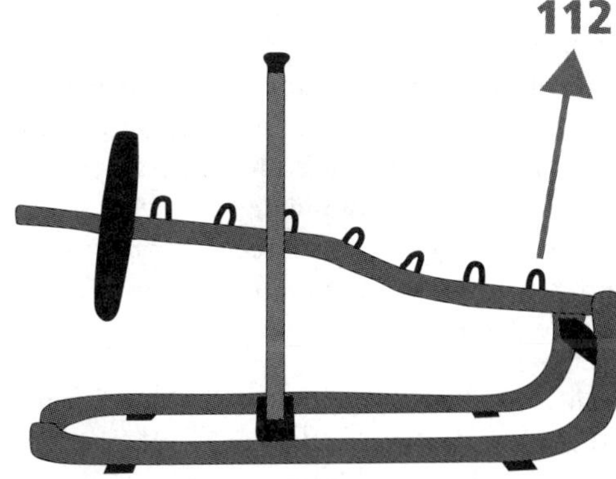

Figure 3-2

The next part of the demonstration involves me pulling from a direction that is NOT perpendicular with the lever. You should note the impact that my effort has on the level of force required. In Figure 3-3, the arrow shows that I am pulling from an angle that is halfway between straight up, and straight in (note the dotted lines), from an angle that is in the middle between the perpendicular angle and the parallel angle, relative to the lever.

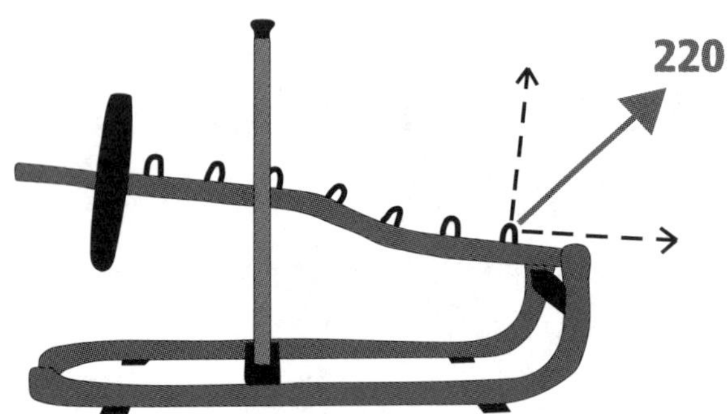


Figure 3-3

The scale demonstrates that this direction of pull requires approximately TWICE as much effort, as does a straight upward pull. Of course, there is still only a 10-pound weight on the end of the lever. The length of this lever magnifies that 10 pounds to 112 pounds, when pulling from a "mechanical advantage." At this point, you can see that that same 10 pounds is further magnified by pulling on the lever from a 45-degree angle, which places it at a "*mechanical DIS-advantage.*"

In fact, any direction of pull that is less than 90 degrees (perpendicular) to the lever will result in an increased force requirement. The force requirement increases proportionately, as the angle of pull approaches the angle most parallel to the lever. The least force requirement is "straight up" (i.e., perpendicular with the lever), while the most force requirement is pulling from an angle that is completely parallel with the lever.

In order to approximate how much of an increased force requirement there is, a simplified calculation, involving percentages, is used. When you pull from a 45-degree angle, you have to produce enough force (effort) so that 50 percent of it equals the amount of the "straight upward" requirement (i.e., a mechanical AD-vantage). The other 50 percent of your effort is unproductively spent pulling the lever inward, toward the pivot. Accordingly, if 50 percent of your effort equals 112 pounds, then the total amount of effort (100 percent) is approximately 224 pounds.

In reality, if you were to pull on the lever from an even "lower" angle, e.g., 20 degrees (relative to the lever), the force requirement would be significantly more. Figure 3-4 shows a 20-degree angle of pull, relative to the lever.

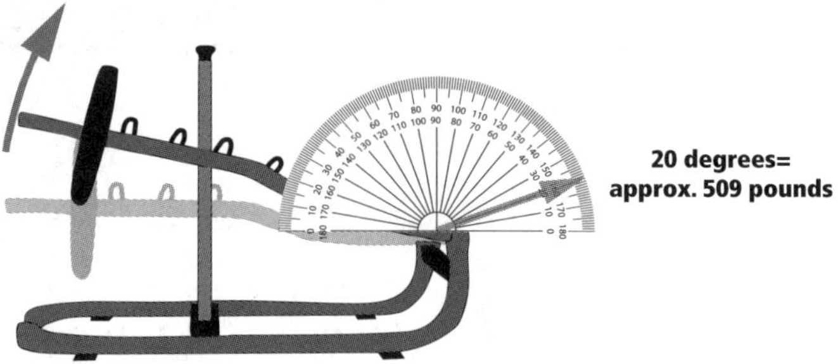


Figure 3-4

As such, 20 degrees divided by 90 degrees = 22 percent, and 100 percent - 22 percent = 78 percent. In other words, approximately 78 percent of the effort being used, when pulling from this angle, is directed INWARD, while 22 percent of the effort is directed upward.

If 112 pounds is 22 percent, then 100 percent is *509 pounds*. Think of that! If you put your arm flat on a table top, and curled a 10-pound dumbbell from that angle, your biceps would have to generate about 500 pounds of force (at the very beginning of the movement), due to the mechanical disadvantage created by having your arm positioned this way (Figure 3-5).

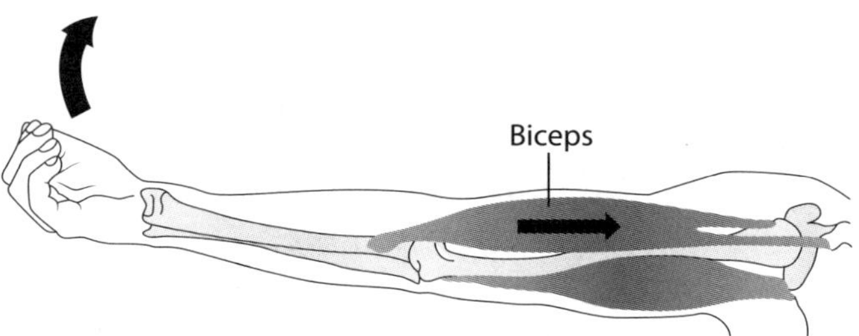


Figure 3-5

While the aforementioned may seem hard to believe, it's true. This factor is a universal physics principle, which applies in all circumstances similar to this. Whether you are building a bridge or trying to develop your body, the concept of a mechanical *DIS-advantage* creating an increased force requirement is an absolute fact.

Although the previous calculation may not be perfectly accurate, it's a reasonably good estimate (without having to use trigonometry). What is most important is to understand that there is a much greater muscle force requirement when a muscle is made to pull on its lever (bone) from a mostly parallel angle, as compared with the muscle pulling on its lever from a mostly perpendicular angle.

The aforementioned scenario is actually one that COMBINES two different resistance magnifications: a mechanical *disadvantage* and a maximally active lever. One relates to the angle of the muscle pulling on its bone, while the other is related to the angle of gravity pulling on the lever. In reality, the muscle force requirement caused by a mechanical *disadvantage* ALONE would be much less, if the operating lever was in a mostly neutral position (i.e., more parallel with gravity, or whatever the direction of resistance happens to be).

## Application During a Standing Barbell Curl

In Figure 3-6, you can see a man performing a *standing barbell curl*. A single line is drawn through his forearm, indicating the bone where biceps attachment would be. A double line is drawn indicating where his biceps would be. You should note that the muscle crosses the elbow joint and attaches onto the radius (one of the two forearm bones). When the muscle contracts, it shortens, thereby bending ("flexing") the elbow joint.

In Figure 3-6 (left), the biceps is pulling on the forearm from an angle that is mostly parallel to it, which shows the point of *mechanical disadvantage*. Then, when the elbow is bent at 90 degrees (Figure 3-6, right), the biceps is able to pull on the forearm from an angle that is mostly perpendicular to the forearm, which shows a point of *mechanical advantage*.

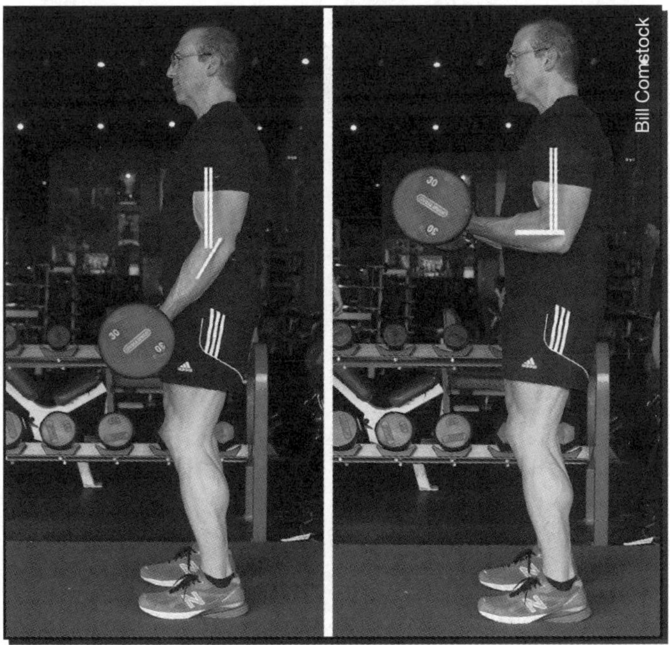


Figure 3-6

During any type of biceps curl (elbow flexion), the biceps always goes through this sequence—i.e., from mechanical disadvantage, to mechanical advantage. Then, once the elbow is bent beyond 90 degrees, varying degrees of *mechanical disadvantage* occur again.

One factor that is convenient, during a *standing barbell* (or dumbbell) *curl*, is that the point of mechanical disadvantage (elbow straight) coincides with the point at which the forearm is mostly neutral. In other words, when the greatest increased force requirement from the mechanical disadvantage exists (at the beginning of the range of motion), some relief occurs in the form of a diminished force requirement from the mostly neutral forearm lever. Then, as the forearm lever increases its degree of "active" (more perpendicular with resistance), the biceps gains a mechanical advantage, thereby providing some relief from the increasingly "active" forearm-lever, in the form of mechanical "economy." To a degree, these two force requirements balance each other out in this exercise.

## When "Mechanical Disadvantage" Meets an "Active Lever"

During a *standing barbell curl*, mechanical disadvantage conveniently meets with a mostly *neutral* lever. It doesn't always happen that way, however.

Have you ever wondered WHY ***preacher*** *barbell curls* are so much more difficult than *standing barbell curls*? It's obvious that you cannot handle as much weight, as when you are doing *standing barbell curls*, especially at the bottom of the range of motion. Yet, it feels too "light" at the end of the range of motion. This is because the biceps' angle of pull on the forearm (mechanical disadvantage) is *not* in sync with the resistance curve that occurs during this movement. It IS, however, in sync, with the *standing barbell curl*.

As you can see in Figure 3-7, the exerciser's forearm is at approximately a 45-degree angle, making it a fairly active lever (halfway between vertical and horizontal). At the same time, his biceps is pulling on his forearm from a mostly *parallel angle*. In fact, his biceps is nearly at its maximum mechanical disadvantage, due to his almost-straight elbows. As was noted earlier in this chapter, this angle of pulling on my demonstration lever (approximately 20 degrees) resulted in an increased force requirement that was approximately *five times* more than what it would be with a 90-degree angle of pull.

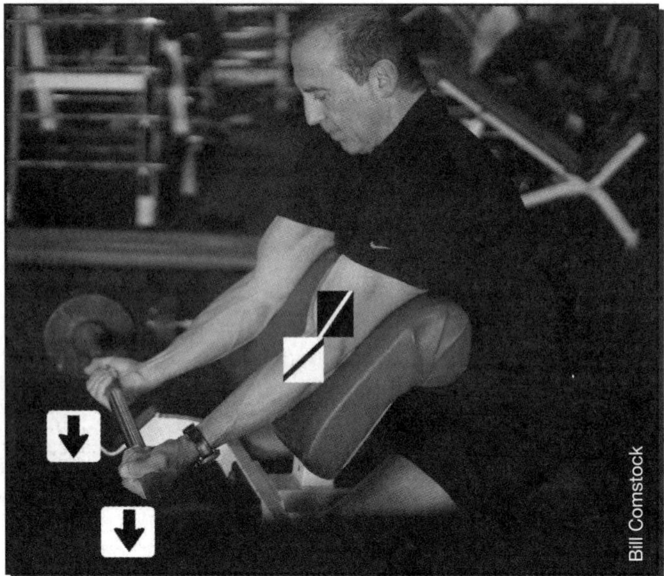


Figure 3-7

When performing *preacher barbell curls*, there are TWO magnifiers of resistance occurring at the same time—both at the beginning of the range of motion. Then, however, when the barbell reaches the top of the range of motion (or close to it), the exercise gets much too easy. This occurs because when the elbow is more fully bent, the biceps gains *mechanical advantage*, which allows it to pull on the forearm from a more perpendicular angle. At the same time, because the forearm is entering a more vertical, neutral position (relative to gravity), the resistance is diminishing. In other words, you're getting "stronger," as the weight is getting "lighter," when you approach the conclusion of this range of motion. The mechanics involved in the *preacher barbell curl* results in too much resistance for the biceps at the beginning of the range of motion and not enough resistance at the end of the range of motion.

The mechanical analysis of a *preacher barbell curl* demonstrates how a change of your upper arm position, relative to the direction of resistance, can drastically alter the benefit and/or risk to the muscles and tendons involved—sometimes for the better, other times for the worse. It also illustrates how these two concepts (an "active" lever and mechanical advantage/disadvantage) sometimes work well together, and other times conflict with each other.

## A Mechanical Disadvantage Only Occurs With "Flexion" Joints and Muscles

Two types of muscle/joint functions exist, excluding rotational joints. The first is a muscle that "bends" a joint, an action also known as a "flexion." In these instances, the joint angle decreases. An example of such a movement would be the *biceps/elbow* joint function. The other is a muscle that "opens" a joint, a function also known as "extension." In these instances, the joint angle increases. An example of such amovement would be the *triceps/elbow* joint function.

Only in circumstances where a muscle flexes (bends) a joint, can there be a mechanical advantage, in the range of motion. Those same muscles also experience mechanical disadvantage (to varying degrees) somewhere else in the range of motion. As such, flexion muscles (muscles that flex a joint) always experience both mechanical advantage and disadvantage. This situation results in a more drastic variation in the potential amount of force required, when flexion muscles are loaded.

On the other hand, extension muscles (muscles that open a joint) never experience mechanical advantage. They always pull on their respective operating levers from a mechanical disadvantage, because the joint angle never bends "toward" the muscle origin. In reality, flexion muscles never have the opportunity to pull on their respective operating levers from a perpendicular angle.

As you can see in Figure 3-8, the biceps is at a mechanical advantage. It is able to pull on the forearm from a perpendicular angle. The triceps, however, can never pull on the forearm lever from a perpendicular angle. The triceps can only pull on the forearm from a mechanical disadvantage, regardless of the degree of elbow bend.

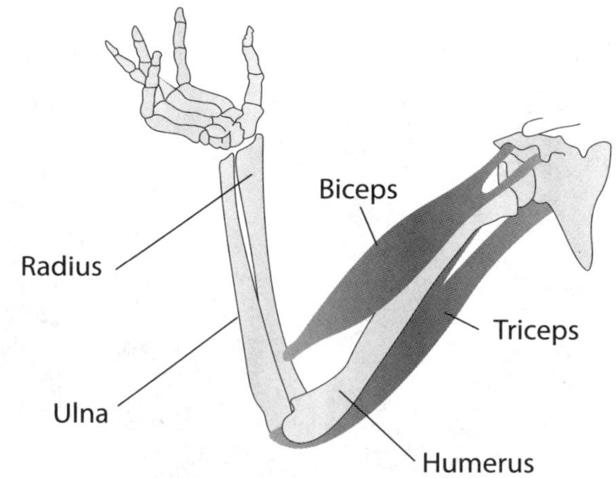


Figure 3-8

Figure 3-9 shows a rare example of a muscle that experiences mechanical advantage most of the time, and only a moderate degree of mechanical disadvantage, some of the time. As you can see, the "calf" muscle, by way of the Achilles tendon, pulls upward on the heel bone from a mostly perpendicular position, most of the time.

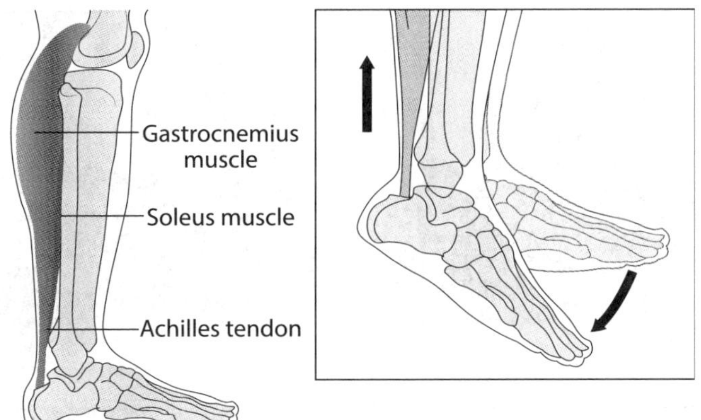


Figure 3-9

In reality, most large anatomical/skeletal movements can be classified as either flexion or extension, such as those involving the elbows, knees, hips, and shoulders. The other type of movement that sometimes occurs is "rotation." Examples of this movement are the humeral rotation, torso rotation, neck rotation, hip rotation (to a limited degree), etc.

In instances involving rotation, the angle of pull by the muscle on the bone could be classified as mostly a "mechanical disadvantage," because the muscle involved can never pull on its "lever" from a perpendicular angle. Even in these instances, however, mechanical disadvantage can be exacerbated, on occasion.

For example, when the humerus (upper arm bone) is externally rotated, while it's alongside the torso, the infraspinatus muscle is able to pull its attachment on the humeral head directly TOWARD its origin, on the inside edge of the scapula. On the other hand, when the humerus is externally rotated, while it is held out, lateral to the torso, mechanical disadvantage becomes dramatically "worse." The infraspinatus is then required to pull in a direction that is different than the desired direction of humeral rotation.

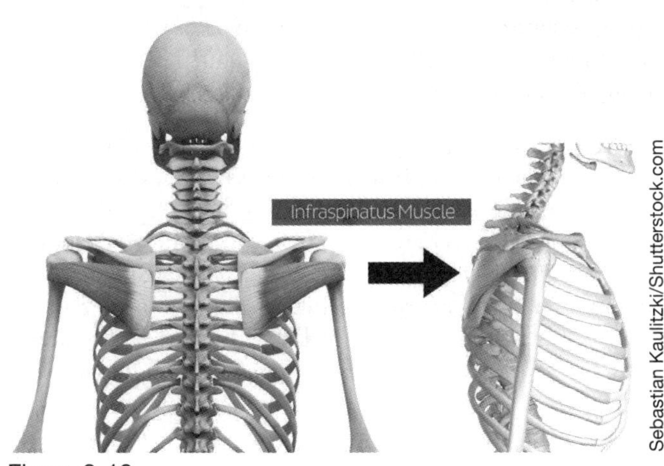


Figure 3-10

Because the infraspinatus can only pull toward its origin, in this type of situation, it must produce about 10 times more force, because only a small percentage of the force can be applied in the direction of the desired humeral rotation. This factor will be explained more fully in Chapter 25.

All-in-all, "mechanical advantage" and "disadvantage" are really descriptions of whether a muscle can, or cannot, pull on its attachment from a perpendicular angle, regardless of how you might classify the type of joint function. As such, the basic matter with which you should concern yourself, is when a mechanical disadvantage is combined (emphasis on the word "combined"), together with a mostly active lever (or other very heavy loading), during a given exercise. This situation drastically increases your risk of injury. Since that is the key issue/concern, it's important to identify the anatomical movements that qualify as "extension" or "flexion."

## List of Muscles That Experience Mechanical "AD-vantage" and "DIS-advantage"

The following flexion muscles are the primary ones that experience a mechanical disadvantage at the early stage of their range of motion, and then a mechanical advantage in the latter phases of their range of motion:

- The biceps brachii (elbow flexion)
- The hamstrings (knee flexion)
- The hip flexors (anterior hip flexion)
- The latissimus dorsi (lateral humeral flexion)
- The pectoralis major (anterior shoulder flexion)

The following extension muscles are the primary ones that always operate with a mechanical disadvantage, i.e., they never experience a mechanical advantage:

- The deltoids/anterior, lateral and posterior shoulder extension/abduction)
- The erector spinae (spinal flexion)
- The gluteus (posterior hip extension)
- The quadriceps (knee extension)
- The triceps (elbow extension)

## Higher Risk of Injury When Training the Biceps, Pecs, Hamstrings, and Lats, Due to Mechanical Disadvantage

An oft-heard expression is "tearing a hamstring," "tearing a biceps," or "tearing a pectoral." Interestingly, these are all muscles with a joint function that "flexes" (bends) a joint.

For some reason, it seems that most muscle tears occur in joint functions where a muscle is able to experience both a mechanical advantage and a disadvantage.

These injuries almost always occur precisely at the moment of greatest disadvantage—when the muscle is fully elongated and the muscle is pulling from a mostly parallel angle on its lever (bone). Of course, it makes sense that a muscle would rupture at this point in the range of motion, because that's when the force requirement dramatically increases.

It is interesting to note that muscles that extend joints don't seem to rupture as often, even though they ALWAYS operate from a mechanical disadvantage. In fact, that is probably the reason why they don't rupture as often. Those muscles are likely accustomed to the greater force requirement. Conversely, muscles that experience both mechanical scenarios operate with a wider range of force requirements, and may have adapted more to operating when the joint is in its mechanical advantage range of motion.

Of course, it's generally true that all muscles are more vulnerable to injury when they are maximally elongated AND maximally loaded simultaneously. The risk of a muscle tear is not very high when a muscle is maximally stretched, WITHOUT a heavy load. On the other hand, as you increase the level of resistance, the risk of injury generally increases in the *extreme parts of the range of motion* (i.e., maximum stretch and maximum contraction). However, a maximally stretched muscle that flexes its joint (e.g., biceps, pecs, hamstrings, etc.), AND is maximally loaded at the point of mostly full elongation, combines the *three* risk factors.

In that regard, it can be helpful to consider three examples of muscle tearing during a biceps exercise, power lifts, and arm wrestling. It's important to note which muscle is injured (whether it's a flexion muscle or an extension muscle) and what the circumstances were at the time of the tear.

❑ Biceps Exercise:

Biceps ruptures are fairly common when the following four circumstances coincide:

- There is a mechanical disadvantage (the elbow is mostly straight).
- A heavy weight is being used.
- There is a mostly "active" lever.
- The palm of the hand is facing upward.

The photos of an exerciser doing a *one-arm preacher curl* (Figures 3-11, 3-12, and 3-13) can help clarify how a rupture occurs.

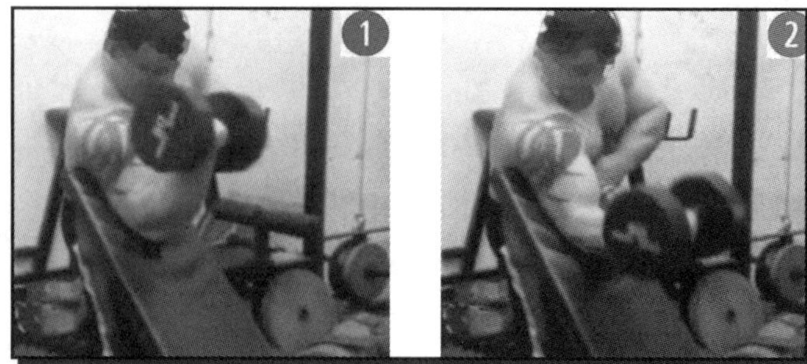

Figure 3-11

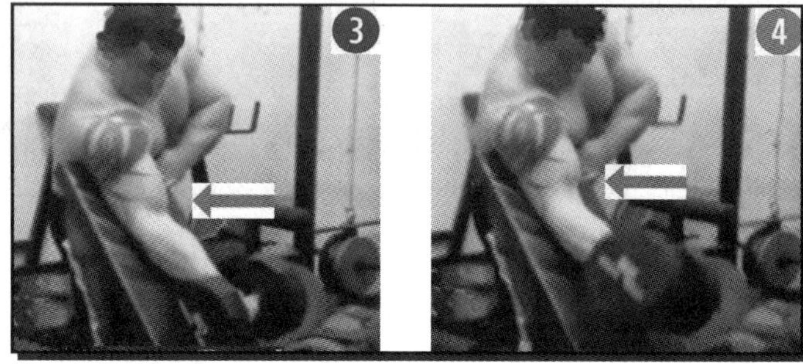

Figure 3-12

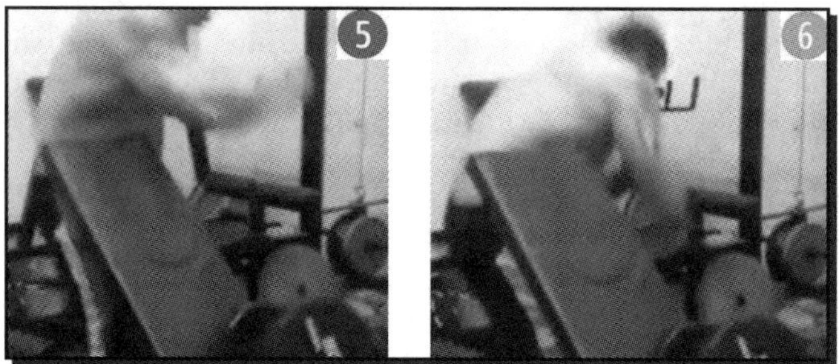

Figure 3-13

In Figure 3-11, the exercise seems to be going along just fine. You should, however, notice what happens between Figures 3-12a and 3-12b. The distal (lower end) of the exerciser's biceps has torn, and suddenly becomes "shorter" in Figure 3-12b, as compared with Figure 3-12a. In fact, this sequence illustrates the most common type of biceps injury—the tendon coming off its attachment on the forearm and sliding up the arm, toward the biceps origin.

At that moment, you can also see a wince on the man's face. This pained look is then followed by him dropping the weight, cringing in pain, and grabbing his right biceps. The biceps ruptured precisely at the point in the range of motion where it entered the area of greatest mechanical disadvantage, when the elbow is nearly straight. At that point, he had the palm of his hand facing upward, and his forearm was at a mostly "active" angle (mostly perpendicular with gravity).

In reality, the biceps is one of the most vulnerable of all the "flexion" muscles. It is worth noting that the elbow "design" appears to require the contraction of the biceps AND the brachioradialis, in combination. This factor may be especially true when the elbow is nearly straight.

In Figure 3-14, you can see that the brachioradialis also crosses the elbow joint, but it does not cross the wrist joint. Therefore, its only function is to assist the biceps in flexing the elbow joint. It is only able to do this as intended, however, when the hand is held in a hammer grip position. When you turn the palm of the hand upward, the brachioradialis is not in the proper position to play as much of a role in elbow flexion. As a result, the biceps is left mostly "un-assisted," and, as such, apparently more vulnerable to rupture, when it's overloaded.

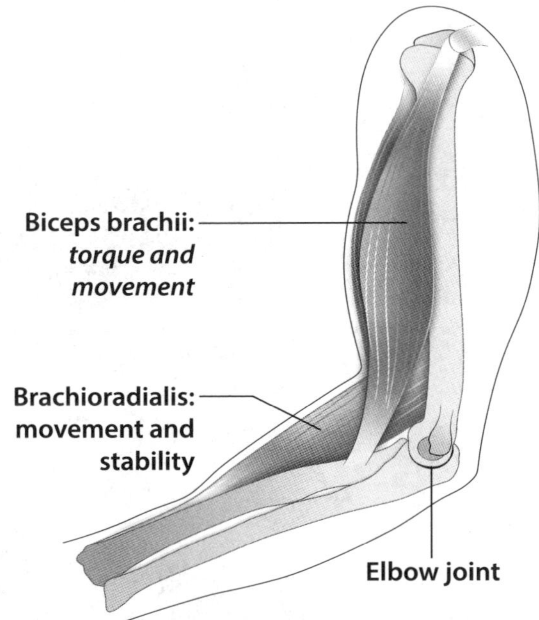


Figure 3-14

❑ Power Lifts:

Figure 3-15 shows a biceps rupture that occurred during a standard "*dead lift*" in a powerlifting competition. You can see the difference in the lifter's biceps between image 2 and image 3. It is obvious that he has torn his left biceps, and the ruptured distal end of the biceps is sliding up his arm.

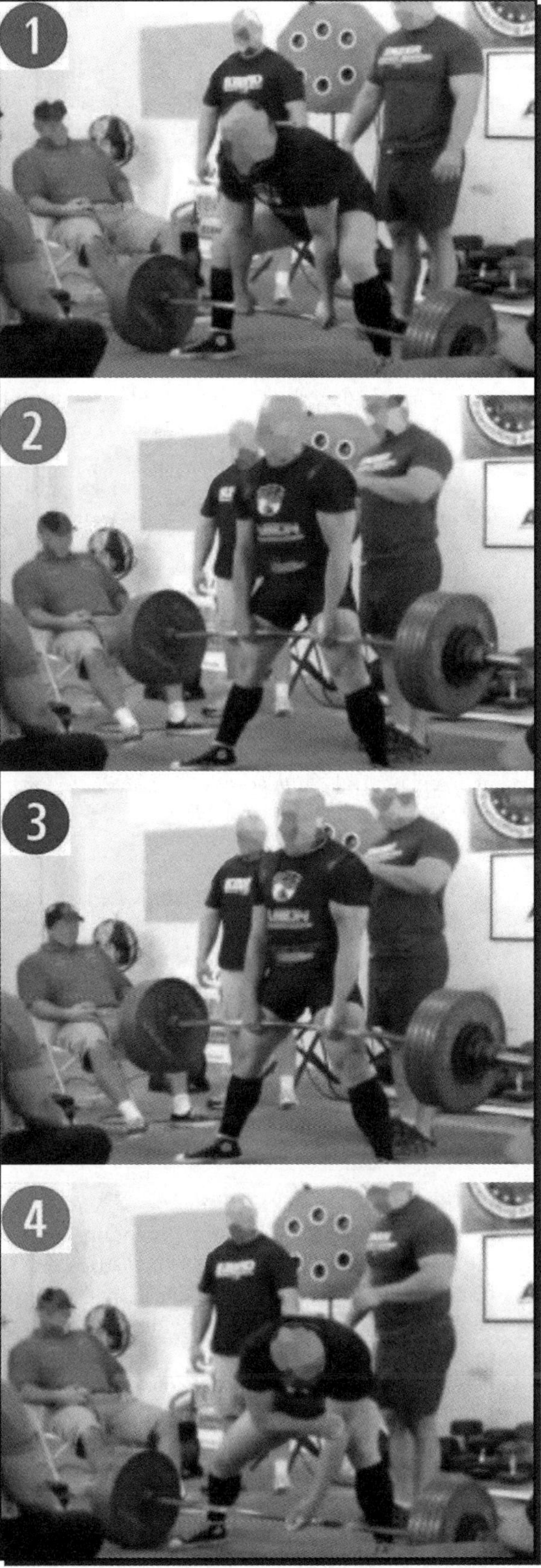


Figure 3-15

You should also note that during this dead lift, the biceps that tears is on the arm that has the palm of the hand turned forward (away from the lifter). The biceps that tears is never on the arm that has the palm of the hand turned backward (toward the lifter). As noted previously, this factor suggests that turning the palm of the hand away (palms "up") virtually eliminates the assistance and the apparent protection of the biceps provided by the brachioradialis. It also demonstrates the vulnerability of the biceps, when the elbow is nearly straight (due to mechanical disadvantage) and is heavily loaded.

When performing a *dead lift*, the forearm is mostly parallel with gravity, suggesting that it is a mostly neutral lever. Of course, lifters intend to keep their arms straight (vertical), but there is often a subconscious tendency to slightly bend the arm, and to pull with the biceps. This action can result in a significant amount of biceps loading.

The degree of the forearm's "perpendicular-ness" only determines the PERCENTAGE of the "available resistance" that is loaded onto the biceps. In other words, if a lifter is *dead lifting* 500 pounds, the potential magnification of his forearm lever length (12X), combined with the *mechanical disadvantage* of a mostly straight elbow, could still result in a 900-pound load to the biceps, EVEN if the tilt of his forearm is only 5 percent from neutral *(500 pounds divided by 2 arms x 12 forearm lever length x 6 mechanical disadvantage x 5 percent active lever = 900 lbs.).*

As such, it is vitally important that when competitive powerlifters perform *dead lifts*, that they keep their elbows fully locked, in order to NOT engage their biceps at all. My recommendation for those individuals who are pursuing physique development and feel compelled to do *dead lifts*, is to use "lifting straps," and keep the palms of both hands facing the lifter.

❑ Arm Wrestling:

Figure 3-16 shows a sequence of photos of a man tearing his biceps during an arm wrestling competition. In the first image, the two competitors are getting their grips set. In the second image, the competitor on the left is pulling the other competitor's arm straight. The competitor on the right is pulling as hard as he can, with a fully extended elbow. Then, pop! In the third photo, you see the torn distal end of the man's biceps sliding up his arm. Then, in the fourth photo, you can see the arm wrestler holding his torn right biceps. Again, the three foreboding typical circumstances are present—the arm is nearly straight, the palm of the hand is turned upward, and the load is significant. A ruptured biceps is almost inevitable.

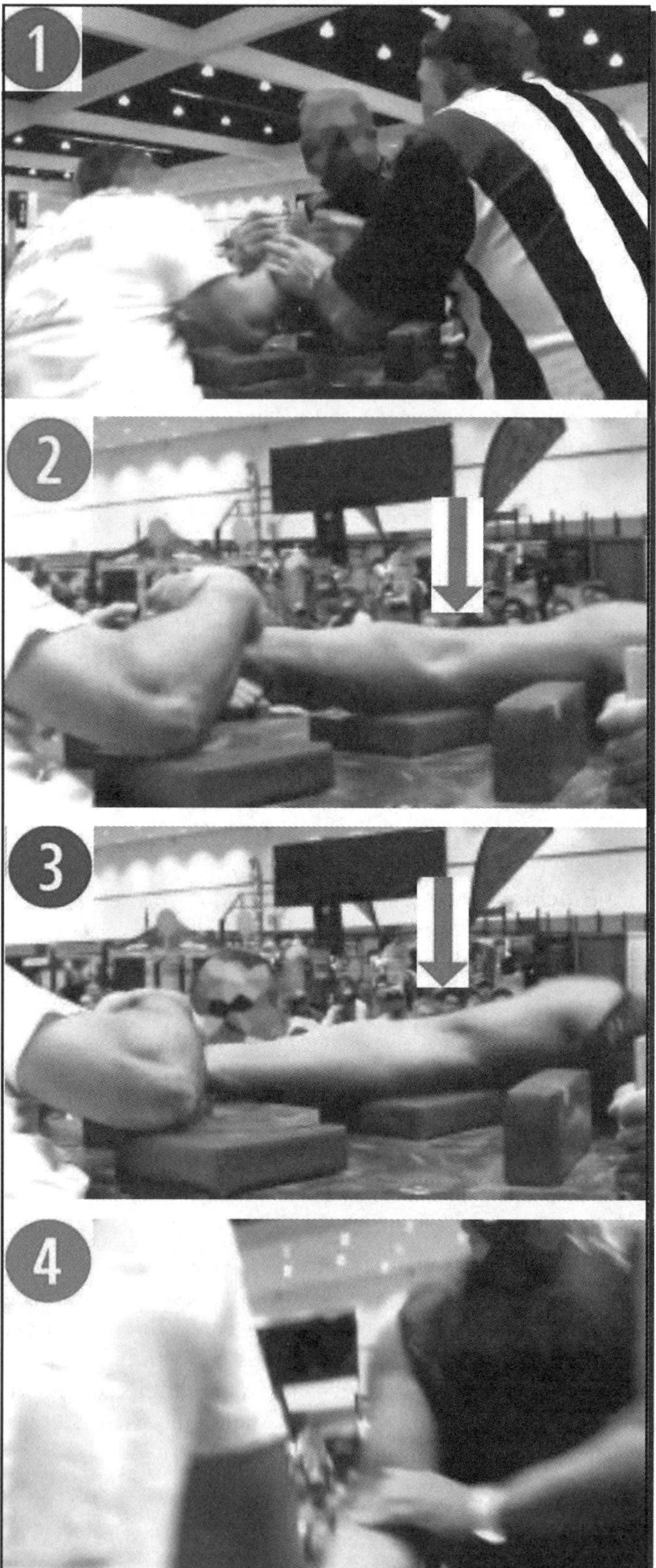

Figure 3-16

## Pectoral Injuries

Another common injury of a flexion muscle, at the point of extreme mechanical disadvantage, is a pectoral tear. This injury occurs most commonly during *bench press* competition, or in preparation for *bench press* competition. On occasion, however, it also happens during physique development training, as well as during "recreational" weight training, when people attempt to do a maximum weight *bench press*.

As you can see in Figure 3-17, the pectoral muscle, which has its origins mostly on the sternum, crosses the shoulder joint and attaches onto the humerus (upper arm bone), about an inch down from the humeral head. When the arm swings out laterally, the angle from which the pectoral must pull on the humerus becomes increasing parallel to it.

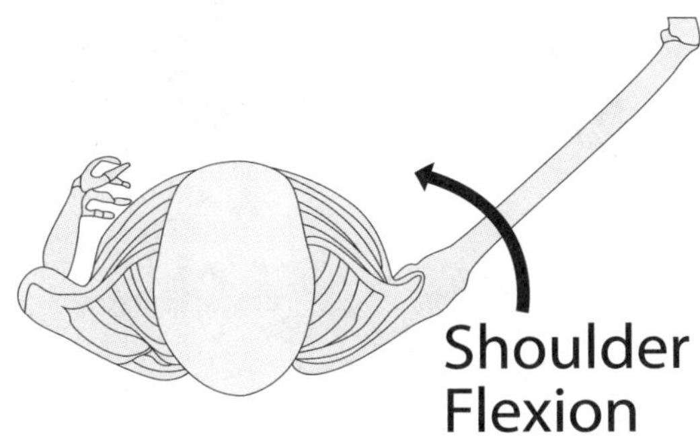


Figure 3-17

When the humerus descends to the point where it is parallel with the ground, it is at its most "active" position—*perpendicular with gravity*. This "heaviest" point coincides with the pectoral muscle pulling from a severe mechanical disadvantage, given that only a small percentage of its effort can be used to move the humerus upward. Most of the pectoral effort involves pulling the humerus inward, toward the sternum.

Doing some simplified math can help clarify what occurs during a 200-pound bench press. It's worth noting how the numbers add up when the humerus gets to the point where it's parallel with the ground—taking into account its *mechanical disadvantage*.

As such, 200 pounds divided by two arms is 100 pounds per arm. The humerus' length magnifies the resistance by a factor of approximately 7. Therefore, the required force (theoretically) is 700 pounds per arm. However, that would be the correct magnification only if the pectorals were pulling on the humerus from a mechanical advantage. Such an action is not possible, however, when the humerus is in the descended position of a *bench press*. In the descended position, the pectorals are pulling on the humerus mostly inwardly, which increases the force requirement by a factor of approximately 6.

100 X 7 (= 700) X 6 = 4,200 pounds

That math is correct. While doing a *bench press* with a 200-pound barbell, the amount of force that each (side) pectoral muscle needs to produce is approximately *4,200 pounds*, when the upper arm is parallel (or slightly below parallel) with the ground. You can do your own calculations and see how *bench pressing* 315 pounds or 405 pounds adds up. When you understand mechanical disadvantage, you realize the enormously increased level of force requirement, and how this situation poses a greatly increased risk of injury to you.

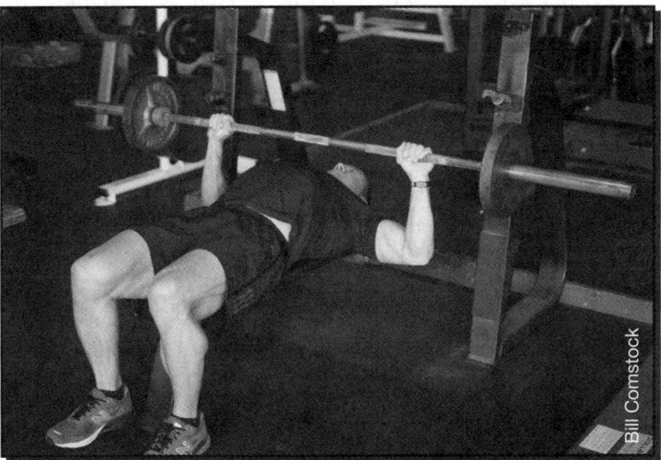


Figure 3-18

In addition to the risk of a tearing a pectoral muscle or tendon during a MAX bench press, there is also some potential risk to the shoulder joint itself, because of the mechanical disadvantage that occurs in the descended position, when performing a bench press. As noted earlier, the *increased force requirement*, which the pectorals experience when the barbell is in the descended position, is approximately six times more than it would be during mechanical advantage. In other words, approximately 1/6 of the pectoral force is moving the humerus upward, while 5/6 of the pectoral force is pulling the humerus inward. As such, using simplified math, it is reasonable to estimate that the humerus is being pulled inward with a force

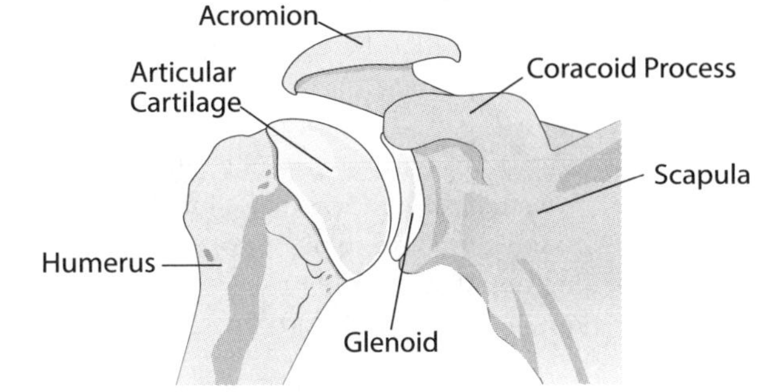


Figure 3-19

of approximately 3,465 pounds (5/6 of 4,200 pounds). Thus, nearly 3,500 pounds of force is pulling the humeral head tightly against the Glenoid socket of the shoulder.

Covering the humeral head is a layer of cartilage. Lining the Glenoid socket is the "labrum" of the shoulder joint. When these two semi-soft surfaces are pressed against each other with great force (for example, the aforementioned 3,500 pounds), the movement of the humeral head against the labrum could eventually create enough friction, over time, to damage one or both of these surfaces.

For individuals whose primary goal is bodybuilding (muscular hypertrophy), this factor should not be as much of a concern, because the primary goal in the pursuit of physique development is NOT to lift maximum poundages. In reality, physique development training is most productive when using a resistance level that allows more than four repetitions, and as many as 20 to 30 repetitions. Lifting maximum poundages for one repetition should not be the primary goal, nor would it be prudent for the person pursuing physique development.

In fact, a torn pectoral is a serious problem. Depending on the circumstances, it is not always possible to surgically repair it. The result of tearing a pectoral muscle or tendon and not being able to surgically repair it would result in some loss of function, as well as pectoral deformity.

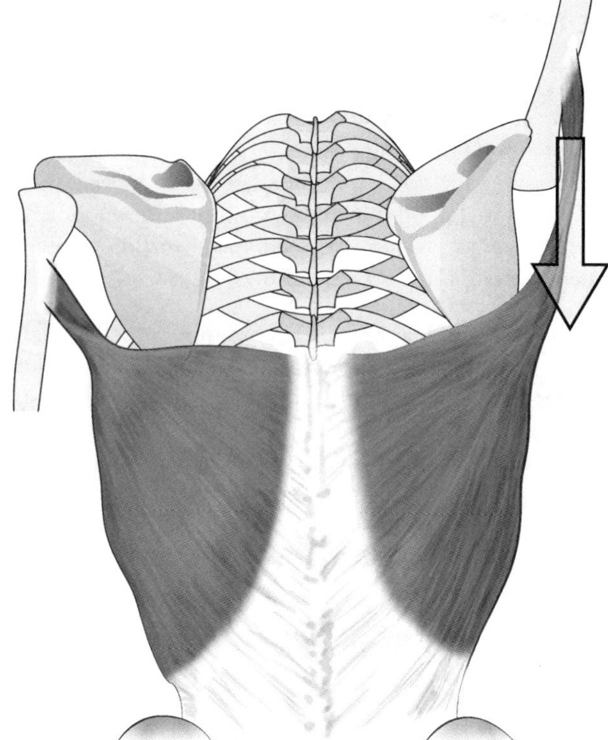

Figure 3-20

## Latissimus Dorsi Injuries

The *latissimus dorsi* is also a flexion muscle, which experiences both mechanical advantage and disadvantage. Most of the time—during day-to-day activity—your lats operate with a mechanical advantage, because you seldom need to reach high and pull down with force.

As you can see in Figure 3-20, this humeral angle creates a mechanical disadvantage, because the latissimus is pulling mostly parallel on its operating lever (the humerus). In contrast, when the humerus is a bit lower (Figure 3-21), the latissimus is able to pull on the humerus from more of an "advantageous" (perpendicular) and safe angle.

Figure 3-22 shows a man hanging from a chinning bar (with a narrow grip), causing his arms to be straight up. When you compare Figure 3-22 with Figure 3-20, you can see that using this type of narrow grip ultimately results in a very dramatic "mechanical disadvantage" for the latissimus. Most people who have used this type of grip can attest to the difficulty of getting out of such a "bottom" position, as well as experiencing some shoulder discomfort during the effort.

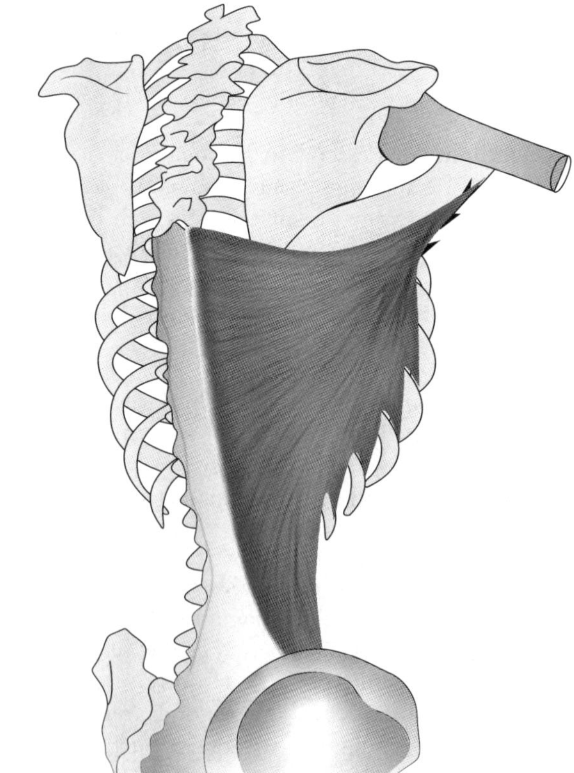

Figure 3-21

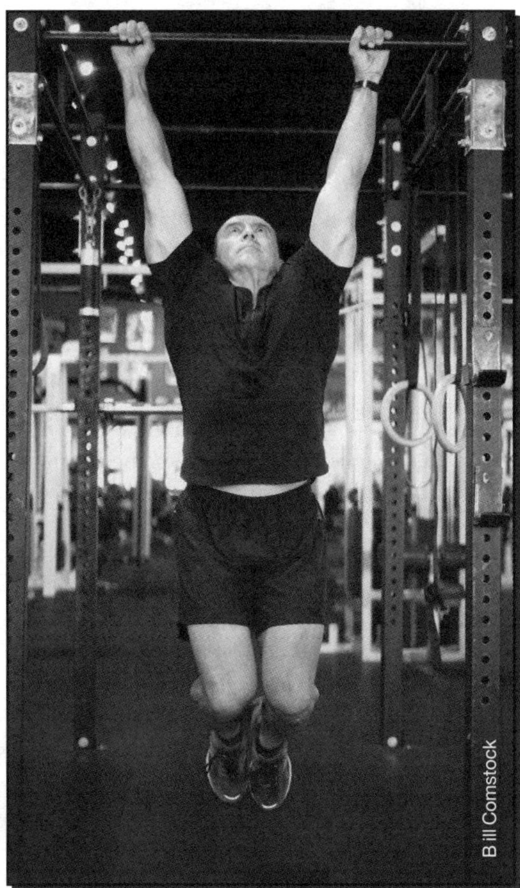

Figure 3-22

This type of narrow-grip chin-up can also cause some degree of "shoulder impingement." "Impingement" is a pinching/squeezing of the supraspinatus tendon between the humerus (upper arm bone) and the acromion process. The "acromion process" is the boney outer-upper edge of the scapula. "Impingement syndrome" (irritation and inflammation of the supraspinatus tendon) occurs when you

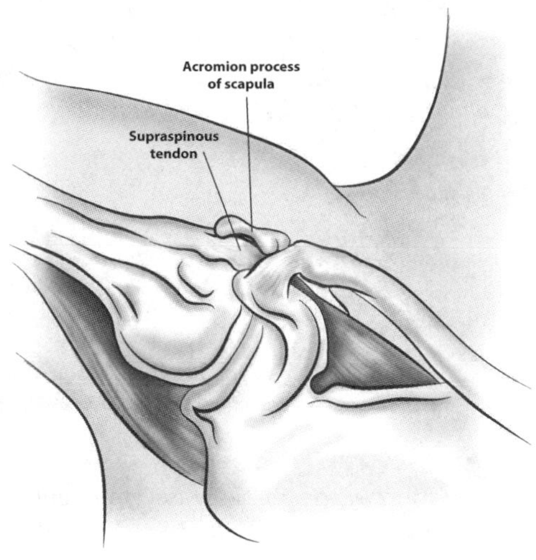

Figure 3-23

repeatedly and frequently move your arms directly overhead. The risk of experiencing this painful condition, however, is not as great when the arms are pulling downward, as it is when they are pushing upward.

All factors considered, the *lat pull-in* (Figures 3-24 and 3-25), is the much better option, as compared with chin-ups or standard lat pulldowns. Not only does a lat pull-in minimize the mechanical disadvantage, it also prevents impingement of the supraspinatus tendon. As you can see in Figure 3-24, the latissimus is pulling on the humerus from a mostly perpendicular angle, rather than from a mostly parallel angle. This angle avoids having the lats entering extreme mechanical disadvantage on the humerus, yet, provides sufficient latissimus muscle elongation, for a full-enough range of motion.

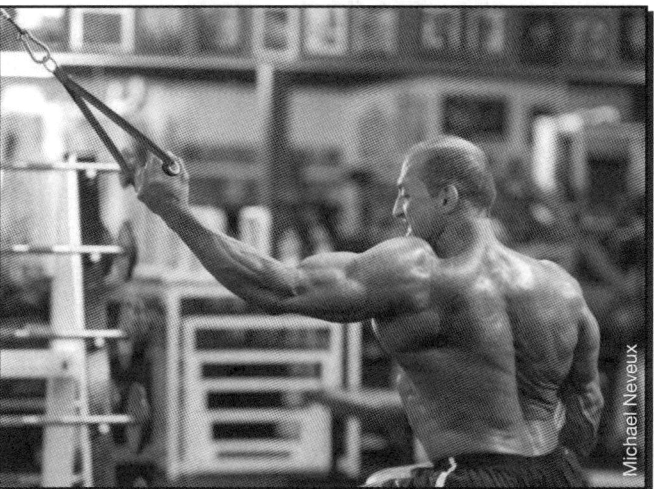

Figure 3-24

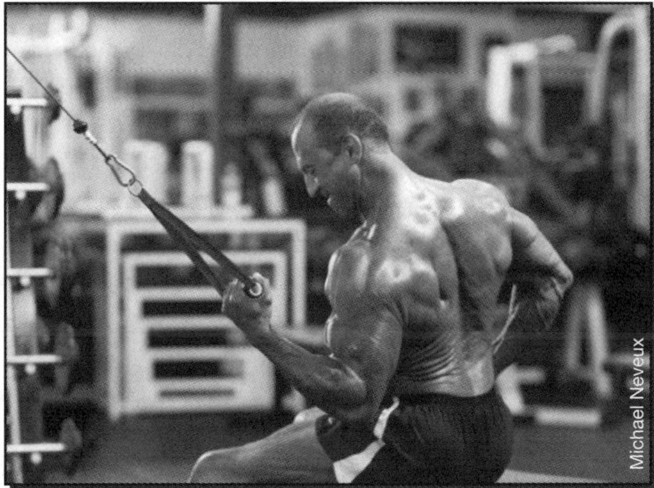

Figure 3-25

## Hamstring Injuries

The hamstrings are also a flexion muscle. In fact, hamstring injuries are very common. They do not occur so much in training for general fitness and physique development, as they do in sports that require sprinting, such as track & field, soccer, football, basketball, etc.

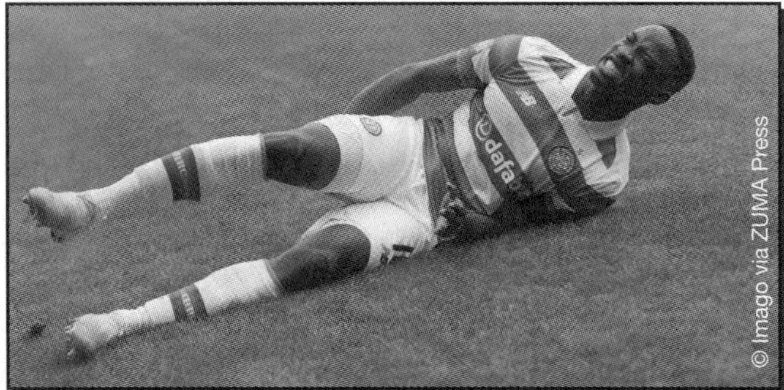

Figure 3-26

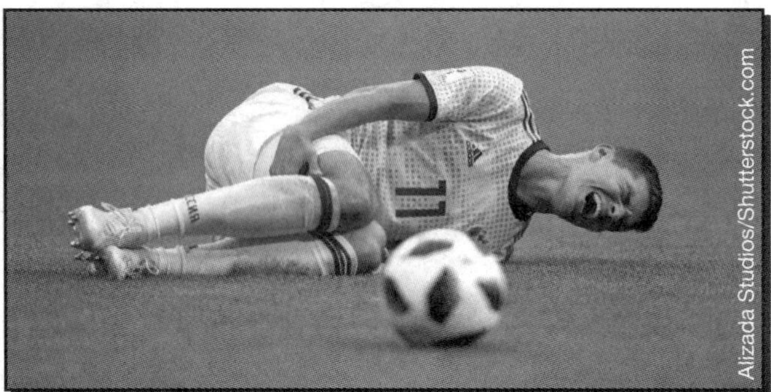

Figure 3-27

Just like with the biceps brachii (of the arm) and the elbow, when the knee is bent at 90 degrees, the hamstring is able to pull perpendicularly on the lower leg, which would entail a mechanical advantage. When the knee is straight, however, the hamstring is only able to pull on the lower leg from an angle that is almost parallel to the lower leg, which is a mechanical disadvantage.

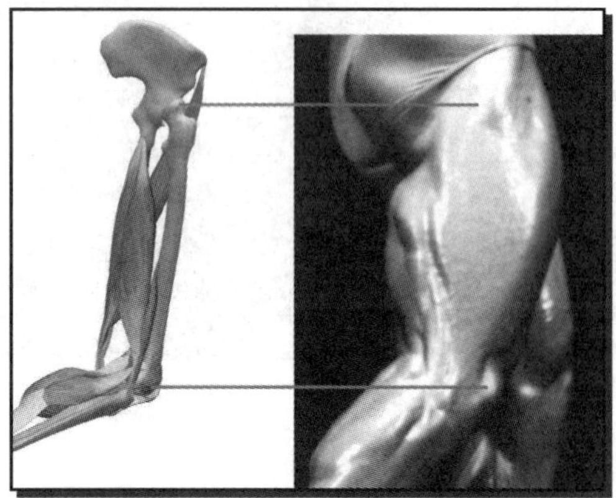
Figure 3-28

During running and jumping activities, it's rare for the lower leg to encounter significant resistance (load), against which it must contract, while the knee is bent at 90 degrees. When sprinting, the knee is usually only bent at approximately 10 or 20 degrees, when the hamstring is required to contract against load. When that resistance exceeds the limits of the muscle or tendon, taking into account the increased force requirement of a mechanical disadvantage, a rupture could occur.

As you can see in Figure 3-29 (upper image), the individual is just coming out of the starting blocks of a sprint. His back leg is propelling his body forward, mostly by way of hip extension. This action requires force that is primarily produced by the gluteus and adductors. The front leg is bent, but is not yet loaded, because it has not yet made contact with the ground. It is preparing to touch the ground. When it does (Figure 3-29, lower image), it will first load the quadriceps. The load will then quickly transfer to the *elongated* hamstrings, with the knee mostly straight. Somewhere, between that point and the point at which the knee is bent to about 20 degrees, is when the highest risk of a hamstr ing injury occurs.

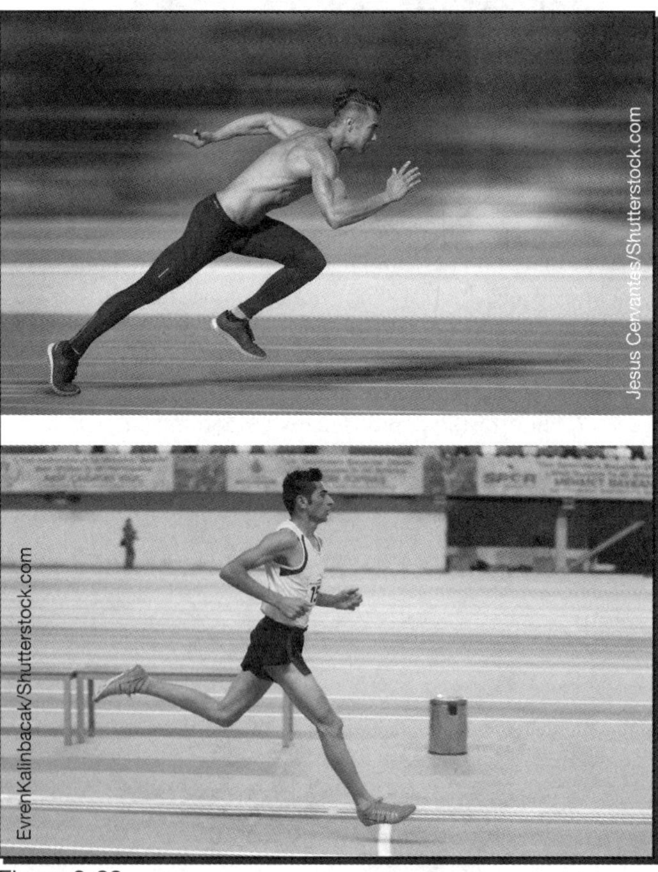

Figure 3-29

In resistance training for physique development, a leg curl machine is typically used to load and work the hamstrings. In reality, while some individuals also perform "stiff-legged deadlifts," that is not a good strategy for hamstring development. This factor will be further discussed in Chapter 22.

The goal of a bodybuilder and a person pursuing "general fitness" is to develop their hamstrings with the least amount of injury risk. It is not to optimize their sports performance. Therefore, it would be wise to prevent the knee from going to the fully straight position, when performing knee flexion exercise (e.g., with *leg curls*) with a heavy weight. Because the "knee-straight" position is when the greatest mechanical disadvantage occurs, it is where caution should be used. It should be noted that allowing the knee to go fully straight, when doing *leg curls* with moderate (emphasis on "moderate") weight, does not present nearly as much risk.

Some *leg curl* machines, currently on the market, have an adjustment that allows "limiting" the range of motion. As such, you can set the machine to stop at the point where the knee is bent at 10 or 15 degrees, thereby preventing the knee from going all the way straight. This feature allows a better (stronger/safer) angle of pull by the hamstrings on the tibia and fibula.

In the photo in Figure 3-30 (taken in 1985), I am seen doing *prone leg curls* on one of the older machines that did not have a "range limiter." To counteract that limitation, I would place a piece of wood (a short "2 x 4" board) between the weights that I was using and those weights I was not (on the weight stack). This step allowed me to stop at a knee-bend of approximately 15 degrees, which kept me from going to fully-straight knees. This degree of knee bend (shown in Figure 3-30) was my starting position, and allowed me to avoid experiencing extreme mechanical disadvantage.

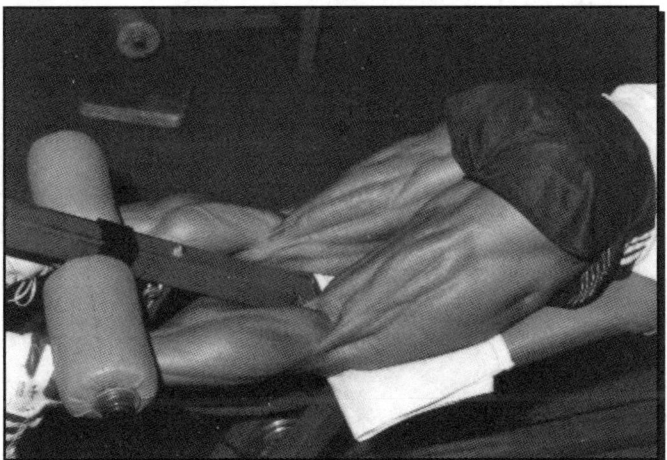

Figure 3-30

One exercise that is often seen in gyms these days, but which has a fairly high injury risk factor, is "*suspension leg curls*"—performed either on a ball or with some type of suspension straps (Figure 3-31). The suspension strap version is more dangerous, because it holds the lower leg at the most distal end—by the heel/foot—which magnifies the load on the hamstrings more than being suspended by the ankles or the calves.

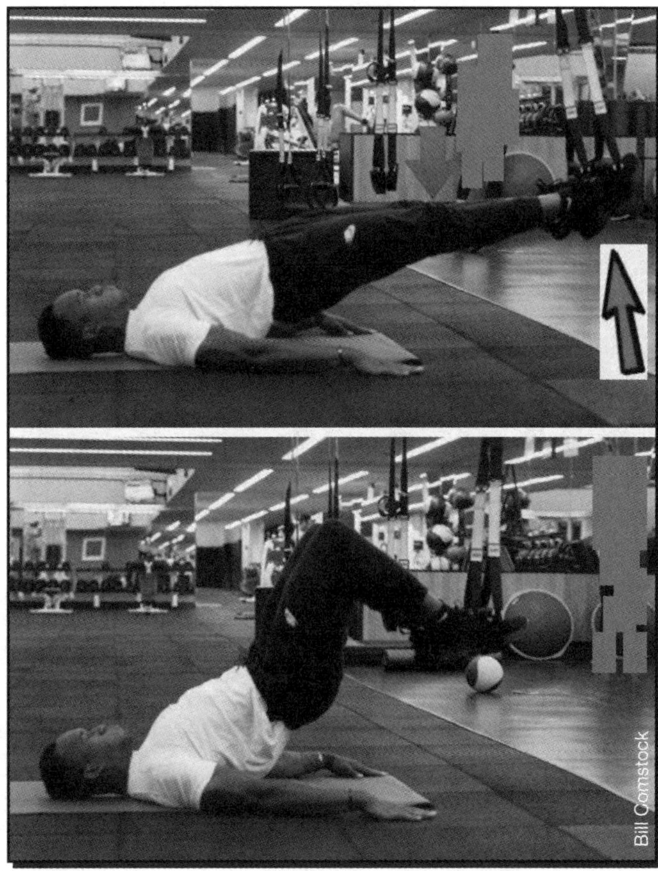


Figure 3-31

Doing some simplified math can help clarify the load placed on the hamstrings in this situation. Assume, for example that the exerciser weighs 150 pounds, and is suspending a third of their bodyweight by way of their feet, which are held in suspension straps, which would result in approximately 25 pounds per leg (50 pounds is 1/3 of 150 pounds of body weight, divided by 2).

The length of the average lower leg is approximately 17 inches (43 cm). That factor would be the first load magnifier (i.e., a 17 to 1 ratio, factoring in the location of the attachment of the hamstrings on the lower leg). As such, 25 pounds per leg X 17 fold magnification = 425 pounds per leg.

The 425 pounds per leg, however, would be the load if the hamstrings were pulling on the lower leg from a mechanical advantage (perpendicularly). On the other hand, when the legs are straight, as they are in Figure 3-31, the hamstring must pull on the tibia from a Mechanical disadvantage. When the hamstrings are pulling on the lower leg from an almost parallel angle, the force required increases by a factor of approximately 6. As a result, the 425 pounds would be magnified to approximately 2,550 pounds per leg. This is the approximate amount of force that each hamstring would have to produce (if you weigh 150 pounds), at the point when the knees are straight, in order to begin the knee flexion during this exercise.

Simply suspending yourself in the "starting position" (when the legs are straight), the amount of downward force that is "trying" to hyperextend your knees is about 425 pounds. Without help from the hamstrings, that amount of load would have to be held by the tendons and ligaments of the knee. As you can see, the stakes are very high in this instance.

What do you think would happen if you attempted to do the exercise shown in Figure 3-31 using just ONE leg? The downward force doubles on the one leg to 850 pounds, which would be the amount of force trying to hyperextend that one knee. At that point, the hamstring of that leg would have to produce over 5,000 pounds in order to begin the knee flexion, as well as to prevent the knee from hyperextending. Needless to say, the heavier a person's body weight is, the more dangerous this exercise is.

This exercise (the two-legged version) might be acceptable for an athletic person who is under the age of 40 and not overweight. In contrast, asking (or recommending) a person who is 60 or 70 years old to do an exercise like this would be very imprudent. In fact, it would be far more dangerous and far more imprudent—to a point of irresponsibility—to recommend this exercise to a person who is 60 or 70 years old, overweight, and unaccustomed to exercising. Arguably, the one-legged version would be seriously taunting fate, at any age.

## Summary

Mechanical disadvantage occurs when a muscle is only able to pull on its operating lever from an angle that is mostly (or entirely) parallel to that lever (limb). This factor occurs in muscles that extend a joint, through their entire range of motion. These muscles include the triceps, quadriceps, glutes, deltoids, etc.

Mechanical disadvantage also occurs in muscles that flex joints, but *only* when the muscle is fully elongated, and the joint is at its most "open" position. During other parts of their range of motion, flexion muscles operate at varying degrees of mechanical advantage, which allow them to pull on their operating levers from a mostly or entirely perpendicular angle. Flexion muscles include the biceps, hamstrings, pecs, lats, and hip flexors.

Muscles that are working at a mechanical disadvantage (pulling on a lever from a mostly parallel angle) require significantly more force than when a muscle is working with a mechanical advantage. The reason for this is that mechanical disadvantage only allows a small percentage of the force the muscle is producing to be applied in the direction of anatomical movement. Most of a muscle's effort would be pulling in the direction of its origin, which would not be the same direction as the desired/required direction of anatomical movement. A muscle can only pull toward its origin, regardless of the direction of anatomical motion the corresponding limb must, or is able to, move.

As such, caution should be used when performing exercises for a flexion muscle, while using a maximally active lever and a heavy weight, when the muscle is fully extend. Examples of this include the following:

- Allowing the elbows to go fully straight during heavy preacher barbell (or dumbbell) curls
- Allowing the knees to go fully straight during heavy leg curls
- Descending too far on heavy supine dumbbell or barbell presses (for the pectorals)
- Allowing the arms to go too high on heavy *lat pulldowns* or *chin-ups*.

# CHAPTER 4

# THE RESISTANCE CURVE

- *A fully "active" lever (i.e., limb) is one that is perpendicular with the direction of resistance, while a fully "neutral" lever (i.e., limb) is one that is parallel with the direction of resistance.*
- *A fully active lever (100 percent perpendicular with resistance) provides maximum load to the muscle that operates it; a fully neutral lever (100 percent parallel with resistance) provides zero load to the muscle that operates it.*
- *The "resistance curve" refers to the variations of resistance that occur between zero and maximum, as the operating lever of a target muscle moves through the arc, which produces angles between parallel and perpendicular with the direction of resistance.*
- *Understanding this concept, and all of its related features, allows individuals to select exercises that are more productive, as well as more safe.*

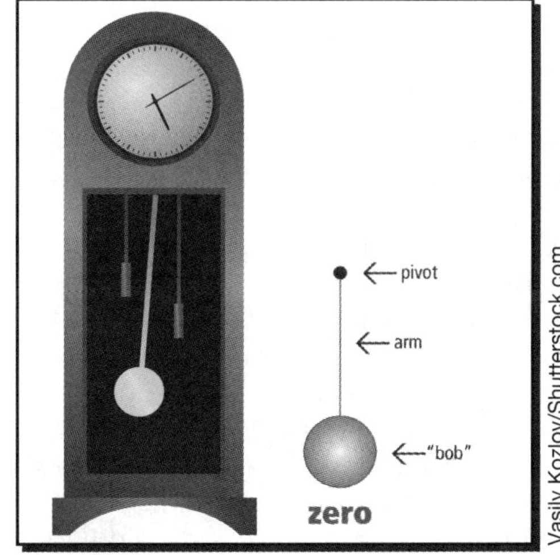

Figure 4-1

## What Is a Resistance Curve?

The "*resistance curve*" is a term that refers to the sequential variations of resistance that occur through a range of motion, as a limb travels through the arc of a given exercise. Specifically, it identifies *where*—in the range of motion of an exercise—the resistance is *more, most, less, and least.*

Hypothetically, imagine that you are standing in front of a large pendulum, like the kind that is typically used in a grandfather clock, shown in Figure 4-1. Like any pendulum, it has a PIVOT, an ARM, and a WEIGHT, which is sometimes called a "bob." Suppose, for example, that this pendulum has not been moved by a clock, nor by any other force. It is just hanging there, motionless. It is not swinging. It is effortlessly maintaining its vertical position, balanced under its pivot.

The reason it is effortlessly maintaining its position is because, as was discussed in Chapter 2, a lever that is parallel with the direction of resistance is neutral. It requires no effort to stay in that position. This position could also be called either the "zero" position or "base" position. The "base" position is the "lowest point in the lower half of a circle." Furthermore, it is also the position that has its "bob" (weight) closest to the source of resistance, which, in this case, is gravity.

For the sake of analysis, say that the weight on the end of this lever ("arm") is 10 pounds. Furthermore, for the sake of consistency, say that the length of the lever arm is 12 inches, similar to the forearm example that was detailed in Chapter 1. As a result, when this lever arm becomes fully "active" (i.e., perpendicular with gravity), it will have the same degree of magnification (12 to 1) that the lever in Chapter 1 had.

If you were to pull this pendulum to the left, with a force that is perpendicular to the lever arm, you would be pulling it with a mechanical advantage (Figure 4-2). If you move this lever to a position that is halfway between the vertical position and the horizontal position to a 45-degree angle (as you know, the horizontal position is the 100 percent "active" position), you are now halfway between vertical and horizontal position. For the sake of discussion, this position is going to be called the "50 percent position," although a trigonometry calculation would reveal a slightly different number. Keep in mind that the underlying purpose of this book is to gain a broad understanding of resistance exercise; it is not to learn trigonometry.

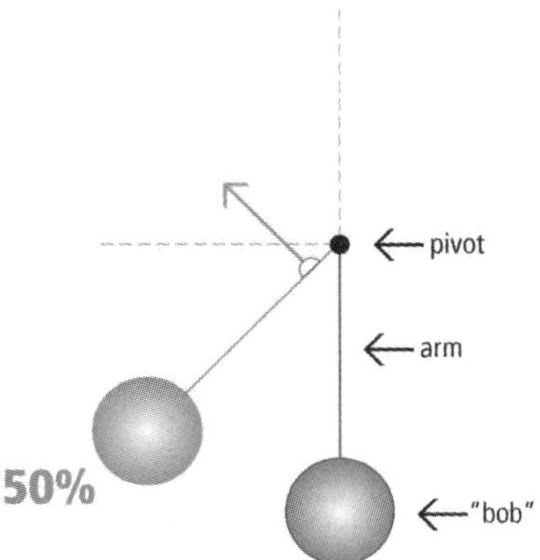

Figure 4-2

"Available resistance" has already been defined as the net amount of load that is produced by the weight being held (attached to the end of the lever), plus the magnification produced by the length of the lever. At this point, the goal is to determine what percentage of that load will be loaded onto the muscle, based on the position of its lever. If the lever (your forearm, for example) is parallel with gravity (i.e., vertical), your biceps would get 0 percent of the "available resistance." On the other hand, if the lever is fully active (perpendicular with gravity), your biceps would get 100 percent of the "available resistance." In turn, if the lever is halfway between vertical (0 percent) and horizontal (100 percent), your biceps would get (approximately) 50 percent of the available resistance. It should be noted that this analysis is very simplified, because mechanical disadvantage also affects the load that is placed on the biceps. The purpose of the diagnosis in this instance is only to examine the angle of a lever, relative to the direction of resistance.

In other words, employing the numbers that were used in Chapter 1, the 10-pound weight resulted in a 112-pound force requirement, when the lever was perpendicular to gravity. Furthermore, a 45-degree (diagonal) lever will result in (approximately) a 66-pound force requirement. Why? Because 66 pounds is half of 112 pounds, and a 45-degree lever is halfway between zero and maximum (112 pounds). Of course, this computation is based on the same set of circumstances that were used in Chapter 1 (e.g., lever-arm length, force-arm distance, etc.). This calculation also assumes there is no "swinging" or momentum involved, just holding the lever arm at that position.

Next, pull the lever farther up, so that it is in the horizontal position (shown in Figure 4-3). This position is the 100 percent position—completely perpendicular with gravity. You are now back to 112 pounds of force required to hold the lever arm at this angle.

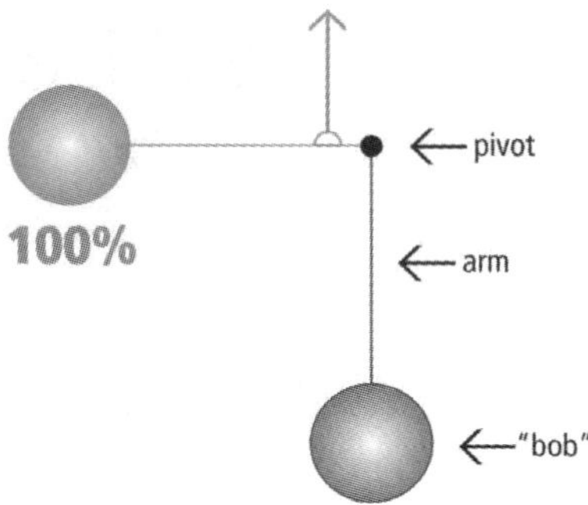

Figure 4-3

The next step in this "experiment" is to move the arm to a 45-degree angle, but on the upper half of the sphere (shown in Figure 4-4). Once again, you are halfway between the horizontal and vertical positions. Accordingly, the force required to hold the lever arm at this angle is (approximately) 66 pounds, which is 50 percent of the "maximum" position.

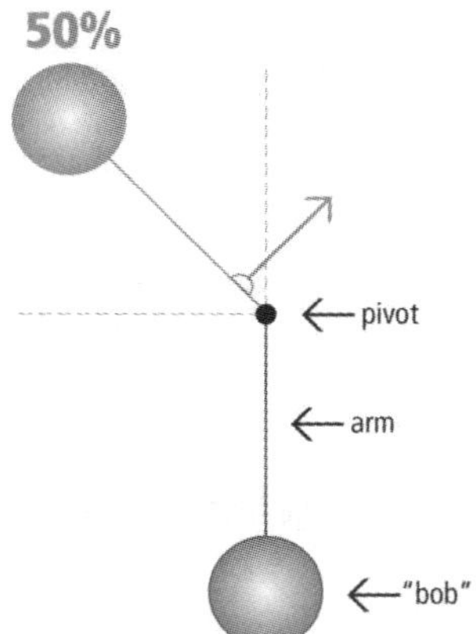

Figure 4-4

It does not matter whether the lever is on the upper half or the lower half of the "circle." A 45-degree angle is the same in either case (assuming no momentum has been created). The reason for this is that the force required is based on the distance from the weight to the pivot, measured vertically. That distance is the same, regardless of which half of the circle (upper or lower) the lever is.

In Figure 4-5, focus your attention on the "bobs" labeled 1 and 2. As you can see by the line drawn through them, their distance from the pivot (identified by the dotted vertical line) is the same. Distance "A" is the same as distance "B."

Technically, this distance is called the "moment arm." Each position would have the same amount of downward force, assuming no momentum (swinging) has been added.

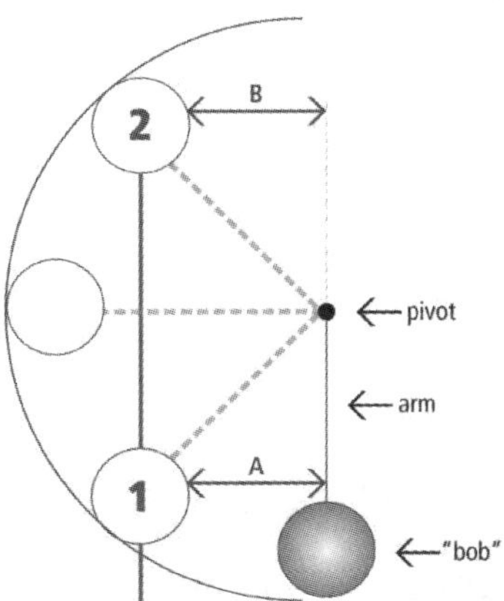


Figure 4-5

In Figure 4-6, the lever arm has been moved to the neutral position that is on the upper half of the circle, a position that is called the "apex." It is characterized as being the highest part of the arc. It is the neutral position that is farthest away from the source of resistance. The lever is in a zero position again, because it is balanced over the pivot.

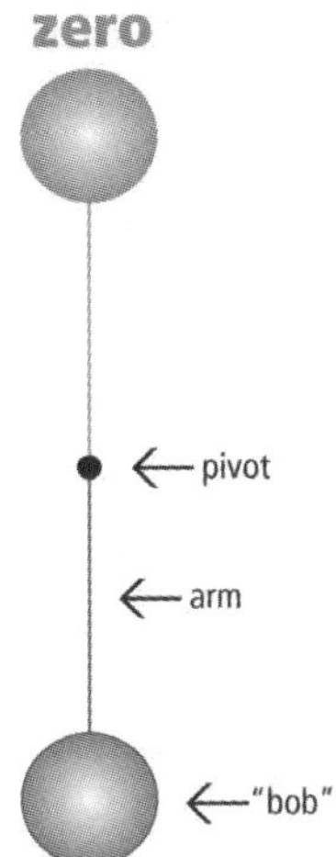


Figure 4-6

This is the resistance curve—the sequential variations of resistance that occur through an arc, as a lever moves through the different angles between parallel with resistance and perpendicular to it. When a lever is 25 percent between parallel and perpendicular, the force required to hold the lever at that position is also (approximately) 25 percent of what that force requirement would be when the lever is at 100 percent, all other factors being equal.

*Note: Once again, it is important to emphasize that one of the basic purposes of this text is not to teach trigonometry, which is what would be used to calculate these sorts of vectors, if the goal was to be as precise as possible. Rather, the purpose of the discussion, in this instance, is to gain a broad understanding of the sequential changes in resistance that occur in resistance exercise, as a lever moves through various angles of resistance.*

It is important to be aware that all exercises have a different resistance curve, depending on the source (direction) of the resistance AND the body's position in relation to the direction of resistance. It should also be noted that *not all resistance curves are equally productive or equally safe.*

There are various TYPES of resistance that play a role in resistance exercise, each of which has a unique set of characteristics associated with it. Without understanding these characteristics, it is impossible to accurately identify the resistance curve of an exercise.

For example, although the two exercises shown in Figures 4-7 and 4-8 utilize the same type of bench, the same seated position on that bench, and the same movement, each of the two exercises is utilizing a different *source* of resistance. As such, each behaves differently. One involves free-weight-gravity (Figure 4-7), which always pull straight downward, thereby creating parallel lines of resistance as the forearm moves through its arc. The other involves a cable (Figure 4-8), which always pulls toward the pulley, resulting in fan-shaped lines of resistance, as the forearm moves through its arc.

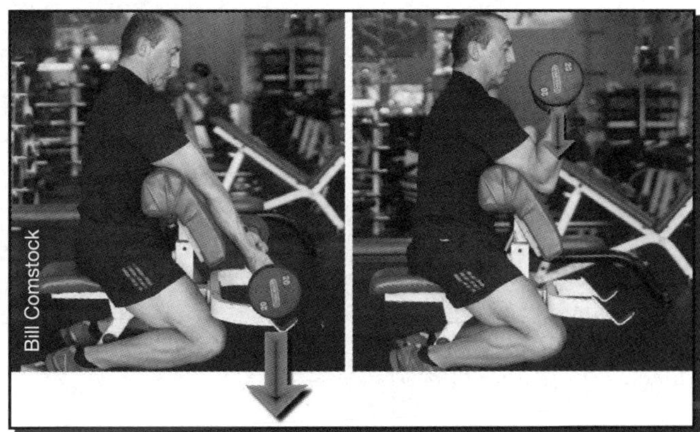


Figure 4-7

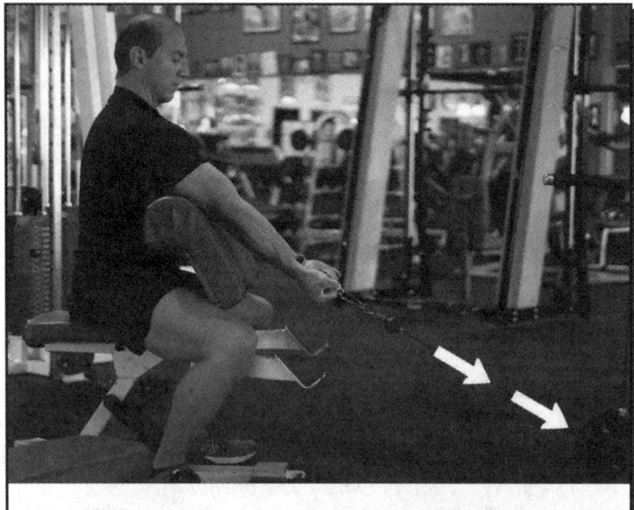

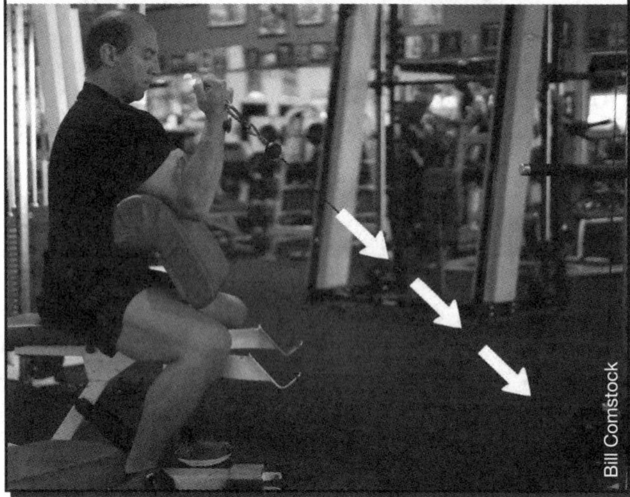


Figure 4-8

One of these two exercises is "very good" (optimally productive and safe), while the other is not as good (less productive and less safe). You'll know which is which, soon enough.

## Types (and Directions) of Resistance

There are at least eight "types" of resistance typically used in resistance exercise. For the most part, each type creates a unique resistance curve, because it provides a different direction or feature of resistance.

❑ "Free Weight" Gravity:

Dumbbells, barbells, and bodyweight exercises (e.g., chin-ups, push-ups, parallel bar dips, TRX, etc.) usually result in a resistance curve that is precisely like that of the aforementioned pendulum. The reason for this is that free weight resistance always results in a "straight down" direction of resistance. Although you cannot SEE gravity, you, of course, know that it always pulls STRAIGHT down. This factor is why a "plum line" is used to determine what is vertical, when constructing a building or other structure.

At any point in the range of motion of an exercise, you can imagine a vertical arrow, pointing straight down, from where ever the weight is. Therefore, a horizontal lever (*i.e., limb*) will always be "perpendicular with resistance," when dealing with "free weight gravity," because gravity is always vertical.

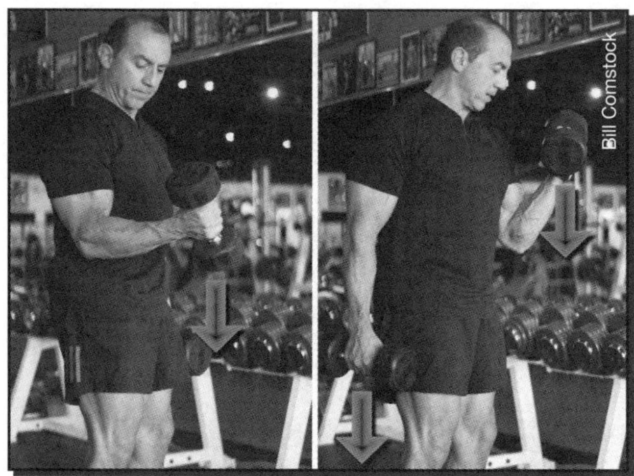


Figure 4-9

❑ Cable Exercises:

Cables produce a direction of resistance that follows the angle of the cable. As such, if the cable is pulling to the left (*horizontally*), rather than straight down (*vertically*), the resistance curve will not be measured the way it would be with a pendulum. A cable REDIRECTS the direction of gravity. For example, it may come from above (*like in a lat pulldown*), because that's where the pulley is. A lever (*i.e., limb*) that is perpendicular with the cable, would be a 100 percent lever.

In Figure 4-10 (*lat pulldowns*), you can see that the weight stack on the machine is being pulled downward by gravity. However, the cable redirects the direction of resistance to the user of the machine, such that it creates an UPWARD direction of resistance for the exerciser, against which he must pull downward. Therefore, the direction in which the cable is pulling would be used to identify the resistance curve.

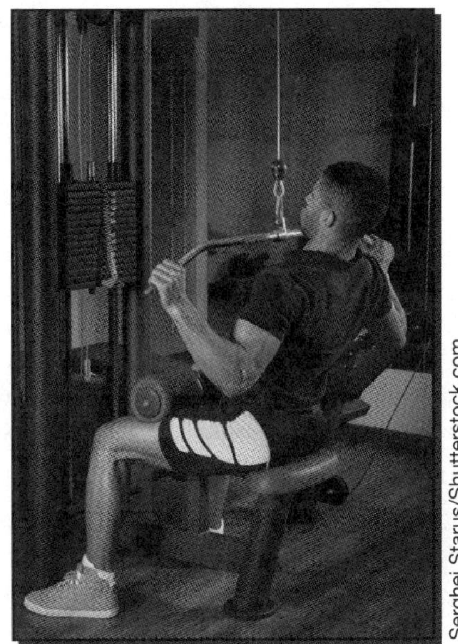

Figure 4-10

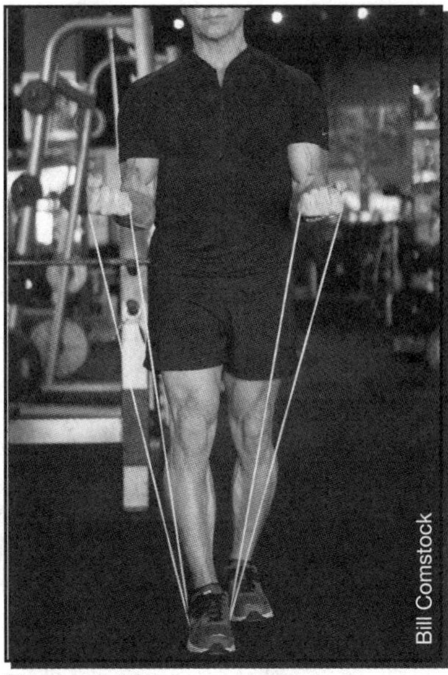

Figure 4-12

❑ Elastic Bands:

Elastic bands are similar to cables, in the sense that the direction of resistance is coming from the location of its origin (i.e., where it's anchored). Unlike cables, however, the resistance that is provided by elastic bands is not consistent. It increases as the band is stretched farther.

There is actually a formula for calculating this resistance: "*Force = (spring constant) x (distance stretched)*. This equation is called "Hooke's Law," named after 17th century physicist, Robert Hooke, who first identified it. Calculating the actual amount of resistance that is provided by an elastic band—at any point in the range of motion of an exercise—would be much more complicated, however. Not only would you have to determine the angle of the limb, relative to the direction of that resistance, you'd also have to calculate the amount of resistance produced by the elastic band as it is progressively stretched.

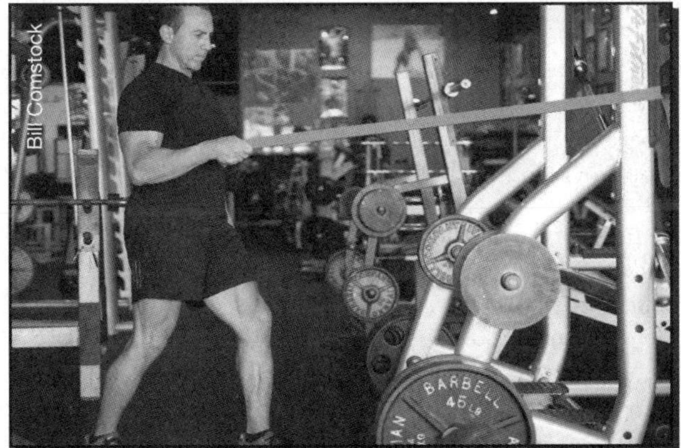

Figure 4-11

Of course, elastic bands are convenient. Because they are light-weight and very portable, they allow a person to do a type of resistance exercise wherever they happen to be. They are NOT ideal, however, from the perspective of muscle development.

Muscles have a "strength curve," which usually allows them to be stronger when they are elongated, and LESS strong when they are contracted (*shortened*). Ideally, the resistance curve of an exercise should accommodate the strength curve of the target muscle. In other words, an exercise should provide MORE resistance when the muscle is elongated, and LESS resistance when the muscle is contracted.

In reality, elastic bands do the opposite. They load the muscle less when the muscle is elongated (i.e., stronger), because the elastic band has not yet been stretched. Then, they load the muscle more as the muscle is shortened (i.e., weaker), because the band is increasing its length and tension.

This feature is an unfortunate aspect of using elastic bands as the resistance source. Such a "backward" resistance curve (*regardless of angle*) is less than optimally productive for muscle building. To a degree, elastic bands are also LESS comfortable and satisfying. All-in-all, using elastic bands tends to leave you wanting more resistance where you're stronger (*in the early phase of the range of motion*), and wanting LESS resistance where you're weaker (*in the latter phase of the range of motion*). Nonetheless, it's important for you to understand the factors involved in evaluating the resistance curve of elastic bands, since they represent one type of resistance exercise.

❑ Machines That Have a Circular Cam:

This type of machine provides an even (*non-varying*) amount of resistance throughout the entire range of motion of a given exercise. An example of this type of machine would be a multi-hip machine (shown in Figure 4-13), which has a cam that is *perfectly circular*, rather than oblong. This design feature causes the cable that is riding on that cam to always be the same distance from the center of the cam. This factor results in an "unchanged" level of resistance, regardless of where the person's limb is in the range of motion.

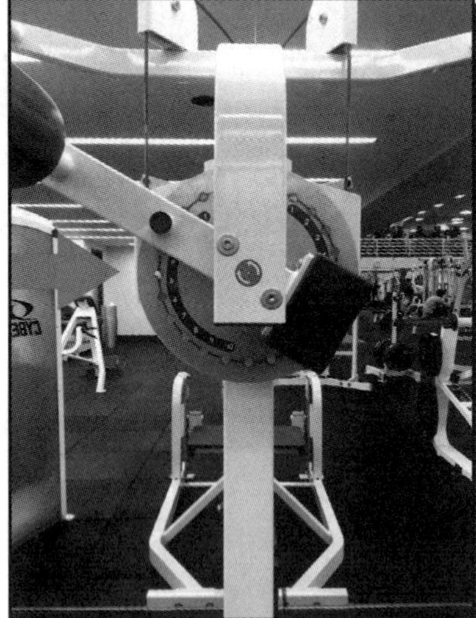

Figure 4-13

❑ Machines That Have an Oblong Cam:

The concept of employing an oblong cam was first introduced by Arthur Jones, the inventor of the original *Nautilus* machine. In fact, the logo for his brand was a (Nautilus) sea shell, because it has an oblong shape. With this type of machine, the resistance increases when the cable rides along the wider part of the cam, and it decreases when the cable rides along the shorter part of the cam.

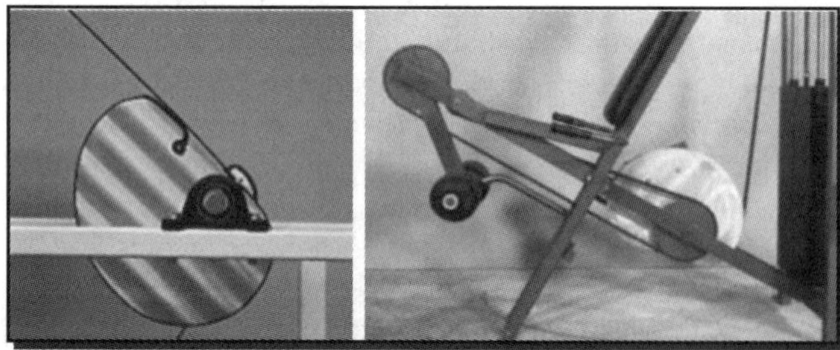

Figure 4-14

Jones' theory was that if a machine's resistance curve matched the strength curve of a target muscle, it would be more effective at developing that muscle. Theoretically, Jones was correct. Sometimes, however, the resistance curve of a particular Nautilus machine did not match the strength curve of the target muscle. Other times, it neglected to account for any mechanical disadvantage that might be occurring in that particular muscle/joint function.

Lastly, not all of the movements provided by Nautilus machines were anatomically "ideal" (i.e., they did not match the ideal motion of a given muscle), although some provided a very good movement. In short, Nautilus machines did not revolutionize the gym equipment industry as much as some people expected that they would. They did not build muscle any better than most other methods of resistance exercise, and they did not always feel "anatomically correct."

"Resistance machines" tend to be especially popular among individuals who are unfamiliar with exercise, because they are easy to use. In general, however, from the perspective of "optimal physique development," they are usually not quite as good as the equivalent exercise performed with either dumbbells or cables. *Leg extensions* and *leg curls* are two notable exceptions, if only because it's impossible to grip anything with your feet, the way you can with your hands.

It should be noted that any kind of "resistance machine" typically requires adjustment for individual height and/or limb-length, as well as correct positioning in the machine. If a person is able to properly adjust the settings, and position their body properly on the machine, the effectiveness of the machine is optimized. On the other hand, incorrect height or limb-length settings, as well as improper body position on the machine, will diminish the effectiveness of a machine.

❑ Machines That Carry the Weight on a Lever Arm:

With this type of machine, plates are loaded onto a lever arm on the machine. Therefore, instead of utilizing your own limb (a forearm, for example) as the reference for where it crosses perpendicularly with gravity, *the lever arm of the machine* would be used to identify where it crosses gravity perpendicularly. Of course, the angle of the machine's lever arm may, or may not, be designed "properly." In other words, it might create either an ideal resistance curve or a compromised resistance curve. You should not assume that all machines are designed properly. Nevertheless, this "lever-loaded" concept is generally good, provided it is designed correctly.

In Figure 4-15, notice that the weight is loaded onto a lever arm behind the user. The angle demonstrated at this precise moment is that the lever arm is rising UP to the maximally active position (perpendicular with gravity), so that the resistance is increasing as the lat muscles are gaining mechanical advantage. This scenario is generally good, although this particular movement is less than ideal, a factor that will be further discussed in Chapter 19.

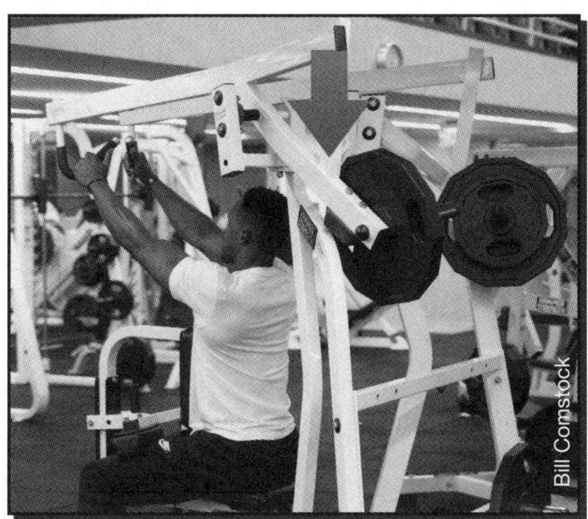

Figure 4-15

In the exercise shown in Figure 4-16, you can see that the weight is loaded onto a lever arm that is at a different angle than that of the user's forearm. All-in-all, this particular design is "good," because of the mechanical disadvantage that occurs in the biceps during this movement. Ideally, you want the resistance to diminish SOME, when your elbow is almost straight, since the "disadvantage" will automatically increase the force requirement. While the particular resistance curve shown in this instance is not quite "perfect," it's fairly good. It would be better, however, if the machine's weight bearing arm was slightly more vertical, when the elbow is fully extended.

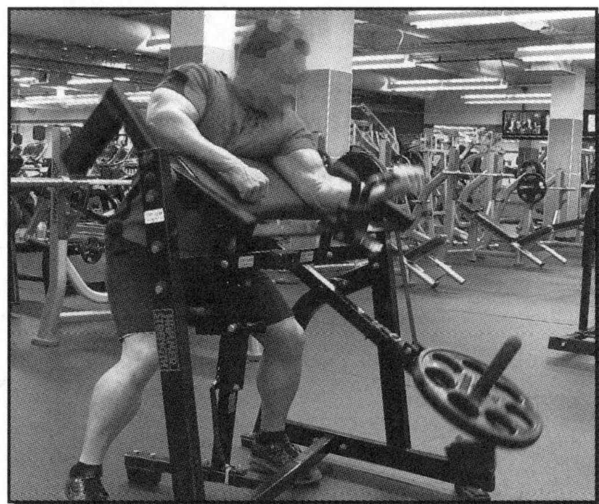
Figure 4-16

❑ Machines That Carry the Weight on a Sled or Carriage:

Rather than moving a weight through an arc, these machines move resistance through a straight line, usually at an angle. Examples of this type of machine would be the *45-degree leg press* (Figure 4-17) and the angled *Smith machine* (Figure 4-18).

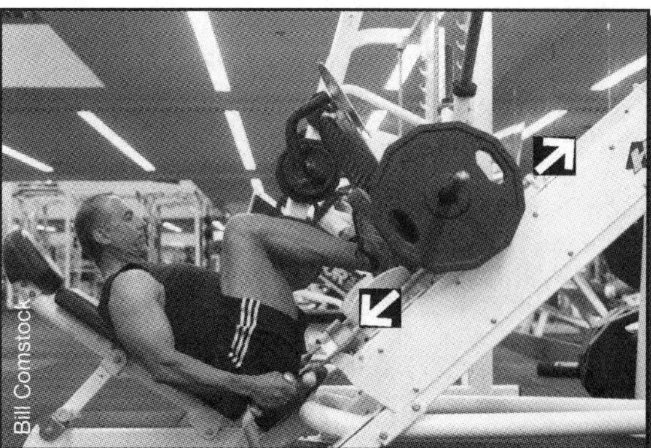

Figure 4-17

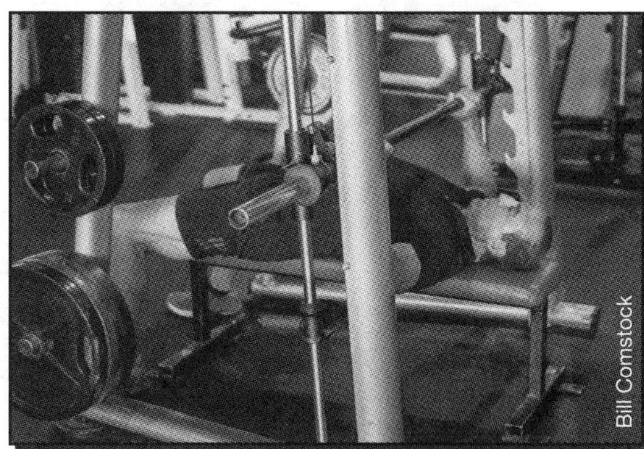

Figure 4-18

With this type of machine, the direction of resistance is the same as the sled's line of travel—parallel with the guide rods of the machine. Any limb that crosses perpendicularly with THAT direction of resistance, would be working as a 100 percent lever. In turn, any limb that is parallel with that direction of resistance would be a neutral (or nearly neutral) lever.

In the *leg press* exercise (Figure 4-17), the tibia (lower legs) are at a 45-degree angle (approximately) with the machine's guide rods, because the feet are placed low on the machine's foot plate. If the foot had been placed higher on the foot plate (as most people typically do), the lower legs would be more parallel with the direction of resistance, making them less "active" (i.e., loading a lesser percentage of the resistance on the quadriceps).

One factor that should be noted with this ANGLED type of machine is that the amount of weight that is actually ON the machine is *not* the amount that is LOADED onto your body. This situation is because the pathway of the sled is not vertical—it's diagonal. Therefore, the amount of weight that is on the machine is reduced by a percentage relative to the degree of the angle.

The more toward horizontal the angle of the guide rods is, the less the percentage of the load that is loaded onto your body. The more toward fully vertical the angle of the guide rods is, the higher the percentage of the load that is loaded onto your body. A carriage that runs along perfectly vertical guide rods (shown in Figures 4-19 and 4-20 will result in 100 percent of the weight bearing downward. This scenario would result in no reduction of the actual load.

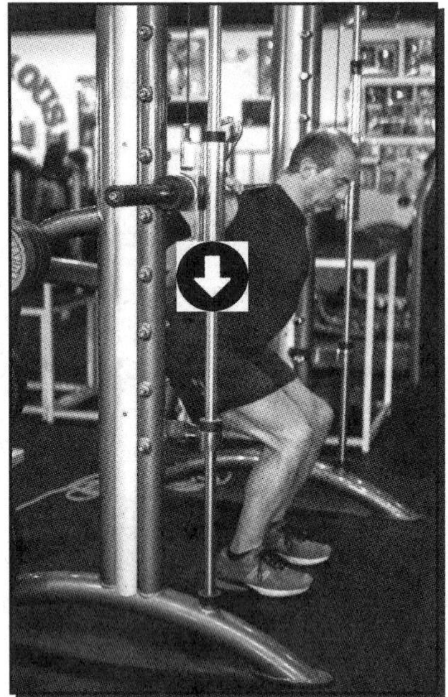
Figure 4-19

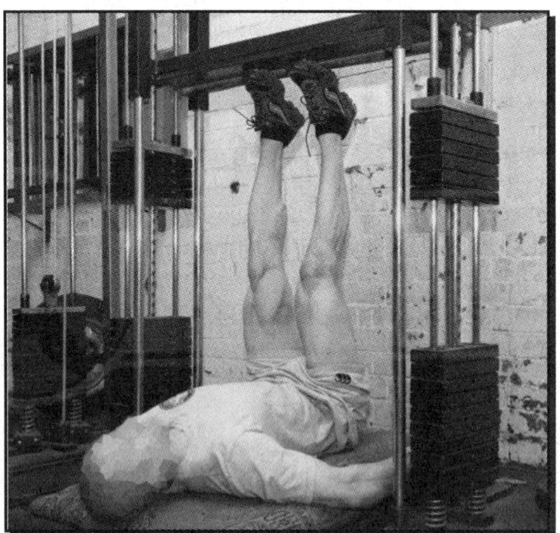
Figure 4-20

It should be noted that there are leg press machines that have a seat that travels horizontally. The resistance that these machines employ, however, comes from a cable and weight stack—not from weights loaded onto a sled, like that of a 45-degree leg press.

The "direction of resistance," when using a machine that has a loaded carriage, is represented by the guide rods of a machine, like the ones shown in Figures 4-19 and 4-20. This factor could be used to identify which limbs (e.g., tibia, femur, humerus, etc.) are "active" and which limbs are mostly "neutral," throughout the range of motion of the exercise.

❑ Pilates Reformer:

Pilates is not usually considered a "physique development" type of exercise. There is still resistance at play in this instance, however, and it follows the same rules.

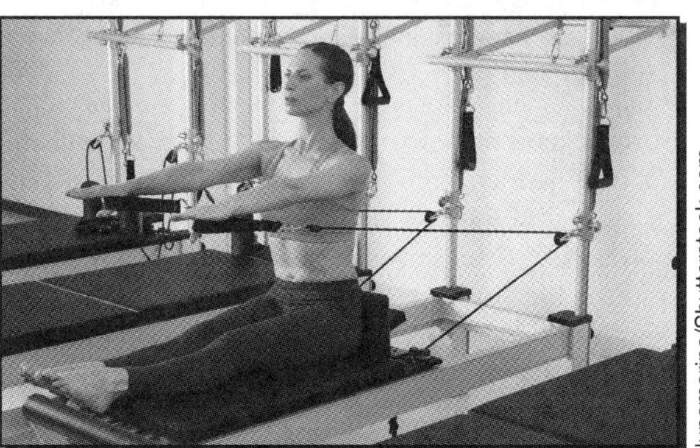
lunamarina/Shutterstock.com
Figure 4-21

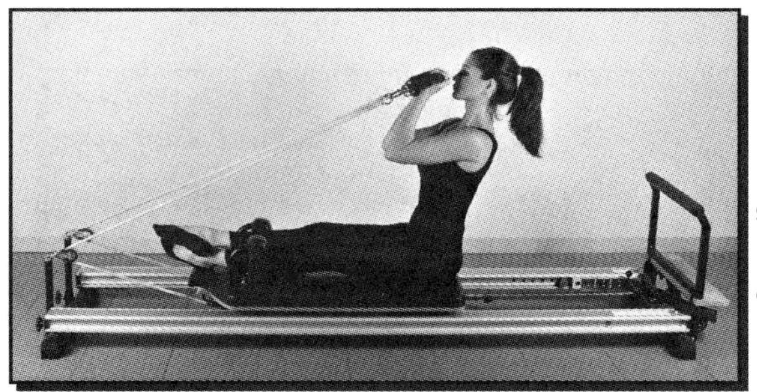
Lucian Coman/Shutterstock.com
Figure 4-22

As is the case when evaluating ANY resistance exercise, the first consideration is the line of pull (i.e., the direction of resistance). Similar to cables and elastic bands, with a Pilates reformer, you can see the line of pull—the rope, coming from the pulley. That is the first clue concerning what the resistance curve will be during all the various exercises typically performed on a reformer.

One of the problems with the resistance provided by a Pilates reformer is that it does not offer any options for directional changes. The exercises that are "designed" to be used on a Pilates reformer are meant to accommodate the design of the machine. In fact, a machine should accommodate the ideal anatomical motions of the human body. The human body has a multitude of anatomical motions, and the reformer cannot accommodate all of those directional requirements.

While it is true that many of the exercises typically performed on a reformer provide some degree of benefit, compared with other exercise alternatives, however, the directions of resistance offered by a reformer are very limited. In reality, the reformer mostly fails to provide the ideal direction of resistance for all of the muscle groups of the human body.

In addition, the resistance curve provided by reformer exercises is also compromised, because the resistance comes mainly from springs underneath the sled. Springs, just like elastic bands, increase their resistance as they stretch, and decrease their resistance as they are allowed to shorten, which, again, is the *opposite* of a muscle's natural strength curve.

The aforementioned does not mean the resistance provided by a reformer has no value. It's just that it does not provide either the ideal direction of resistance nor the ideal resistance curve for optimal muscle development. It has value, but a compromised level of value.

In fact, there are several other types of resistance that also (on occasion) influence the resistance curve. They are not, however, directly related to an apparatus, like a pulley, a machine, or a dumbbell. As such, "momentum," "centrifugal force," and "friction force" add a direction of resistance that could be considered "altered." Although they are invisible to the observer, they are absolutely present, nonetheless. These will be addressed in Chapter 6.

## Manipulating the Resistance Curve

You know that a lever (a limb) that is *perpendicular* with the direction of resistance will load its operating muscle with 100 percent of the available resistance, and that a *parallel* lever will load its operating muscle with ZERO resistance. You also know that a lever that is somewhere between those two points will load the muscle with an amount that is somewhat commensurate with its angle, relative to resistance. As such, a lever that is halfway between being perpendicular with gravity, and parallel with gravity, will load the muscle with approximately half of the available resistance.

Figure 4-23 depicts a circle with a solid line drawn at a 15-degree angle. The dashed line shows a 30-degree angle. The horizontal line shows the position that is perpendicular with gravity. Next, consider a hypothetical situation in which a lever is loaded with 100 pounds. You want to know how much load will be put onto its operating muscle, when that lever is at a 15-degree angle, as well as at a 30-degree angle. Determining the answer will require some simplified math.

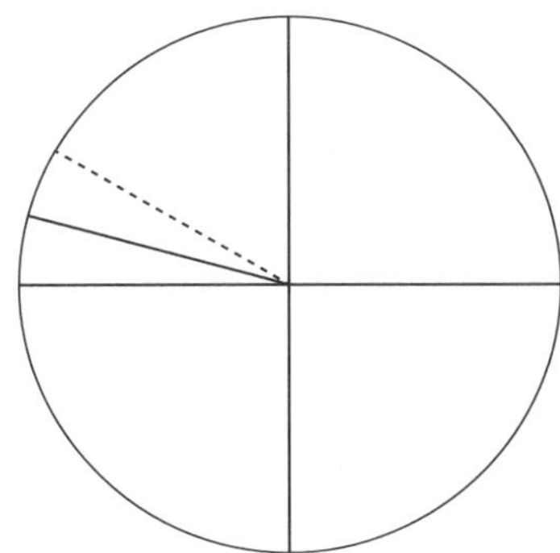

Figure 4-23

A lever varies its resistance between zero (when it's parallel) and 100 percent (when it's perpendicular), over the course of 90 degrees. Accordingly, a 15-degree angle would constitute 16.6 percent of the distance between vertical and horizontal (15 x 100 divided by 90 = 16.6 percent). In turn, a 30-degree angle would constitute 33.3 percent. You should keep in mind that "simplified" math is being employed in this instance—not trigonometry. As such, a lever at a 15-degree angle would load its operating muscle with 83.4 percent of the available resistance (100 minus 16.6 percent), while a lever at a 30-degree angle would load that muscle with 66.7 percent of the available resistance (100 minus 33.3 percent).

Figure 4-24 shows an exerciser doing an abdominal crunch on a bench (which can represent any horizontal surface—e.g., a floor mat, a massage table). In the starting position, his spine (i.e., the operating lever of the abs) is at the horizontal position. Then, in the "crunch" position (bottom image), his spine has curled to approximately a 15-degree angle.

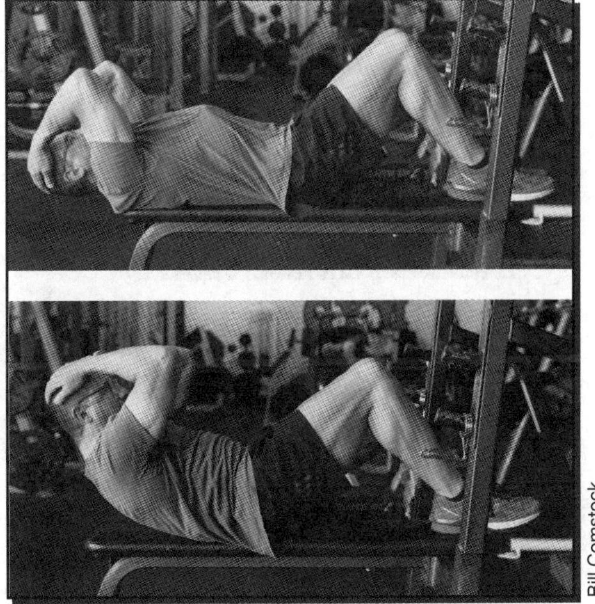

Bill Comstock

Figure 4-24

In order to better understand how the resistance curve is manipulated, compare these two positions to the circle in Figure 4-23. If this exerciser's total weight is 180 pounds, his torso weight may be 100 pounds. Therefore, he's beginning this movement with 100 percent of that 100 pounds, and he's concluding the movement with (approximately) 83 pounds (83.4 percent of that 100 pounds).

Most individuals are aware that an abdominal crunch exercise, performed on the floor (or other horizontal surface), is fairly difficult. In fact, for some people, it's nearly impossible. The degree of difficulty of performing this exercise depends on two factors: a person's torso weight and the individual's abdominal strength. For the average person, doing this exercise—this particular way (i.e., on a flat surface)—is so difficult, that it often prohibits them from doing the exercise correctly.

Ideally, a person should be able to move his torso from the "spine straight" position (while lying on his back) to the "spine fully curled" position (when in the contracted position). On the other hand, when a person weighs too much, or when his abdominal muscle is anything less than "very strong," he simply cannot produce a full range of motion. As a result, the exercise ends up being mostly a head-and-neck movement, rather than a torso/spinal movement.

The simple solution to this dilemma is to lessen the load by *altering the resistance curve.* For example, Figure 4-25 shows the exact same movement, performed at a slight incline angle. In this instance, the exerciser is starting at a 15-degree angle, and ending at a 30-degree angle. Therefore, he's performing this exercise with about 17 percent less resistance than if he were doing it on a floor mat or other flat (horizontal) surface. This reduction in resistance is likely to allow better form, more complete range of motion, and sufficient repetitions. It's also less likely to cause him to "detest" doing this exercise.

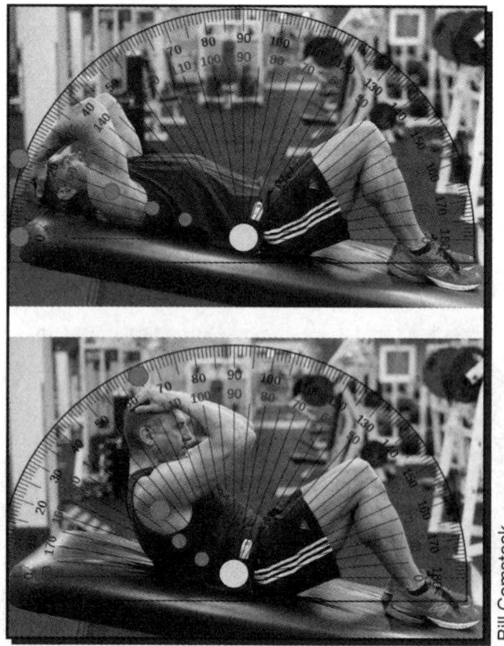


Figure 4-25

The 15-degree angle (and also higher angles) can easily be achieved in a variety of ways, for example, by tilting a massage table, by using an incline bench (and elevating the feet a little bit), or by propping up a simple board against a foot stool or ottoman at home. The higher the angle of incline, the greater the reduction of the load.

There should be no shame in using an incline angle that is set at 45 degrees, if that angle provides a "manageable" amount of resistance for the individual, at that particular stage of the person's fitness. As the person loses body weight, and/or gets stronger, the angle can be lowered. The angle of incline that is selected should allow the person to do (approximately) 20 repetitions with good form, comfortably. While it is important to keep in mind that the resistance level should be challenging, it should not be overwhelming or prohibitive.

> *Note: The original idea of doing abdominal crunches on the floor was based entirely on convenience—not as a "standard test of abdominal strength." There is no logical reason why an assumption should be made that everyone "should" be able to perform abdominal crunches on a flat (horizontal) surface. Of course, if a person is not overweight or has sufficient abdominal strength, performing this exercise from a horizontal position is fine, but that should not be the expected norm. Like any exercise, exercisers must select the resistance level that is* ***comfortable*** *and appropriate for them, at that particular stage of their fitness.*

Some individuals feel that it's "better" to do this exercise on a DECLINE (i.e., head lower than their hips), a position that makes the exercise MORE difficult than doing it on a flat surface. This notion is absurd. In reality, making an abdominal exercise "too difficult" to perform properly will not only compromise development of that muscle—as well as increase the risk of injury—it will also create a sense of defeat. Imagine trying to do a *barbell curl* with a weight that is too heavy to do even one repetition, with FULL range of motion (without the assistance of momentum/swinging/cheating). As a result, you would perform 20 reps, with only 1/4 range of motion, a higher risk of injury, and an unfair perception of weakness. This way of thinking is simply foolish.

In fact, for most people, it is prudent to *reduce* the resistance when performing *abdominal crunches*, in order to make the movement more manageable. In most cases, tilting the angle of an *abdominal crunch* (toward the incline) allows you to reduce the resistance of this exercise just enough to improve the quality of the reps and the productivity of the exercise.

The aforementioned is just one example of how the resistance curve of an exercise can be manipulated, simply by changing the angle of the operating lever relative to the direction of resistance.

## The Ideal Resistance Curve: "Early Phase Loading"

As discussed previously, muscles have an elastic property, such that they typically have more strength potential when they are elongated and less strength potential when they are contracted. This factor is known as a muscle's natural "strength curve."

Accordingly, it is most sensible to select exercises that provide a "resistance curve" that offers the target muscle more resistance during the early phase of the muscle's range of motion—where the muscle is strongest—and less resistance during the latter part of the range of motion—where the muscle is less strong.

> *William Kraemer, Ph.D. (professor of kinesiology, physiology, neurobiology and medicine at the University of Connecticut) and Steven Fleck, Ph.D., (associate professor of health, exercise science, and sport management at the University of Wisconsin—Parkside) explain a muscle's strength curve this way:*
>
> *"At the optimal length [of the muscle fiber], there is potential for maximal cross-bridge interaction and thus maximal force. With excessive shortening, there is an overlap of actin filaments so that the actin filaments interfere with each other's ability to contract the myosin cross-bridges. Less cross-bridge contact with the active sites on the actin results in a smaller potential to develop tension."*

To help clarify the concept of an ideal resistance curve, a simple experiment can be conducted. The objective is to see what happens when two different exercises—both for the triceps—are performed, but with completely opposite "resistance curves."

- Exercise "A": Supine dumbbell triceps extension (Figure 4-26)
- Exercise "B": Dumbbell triceps kickback (Figure 4-27)

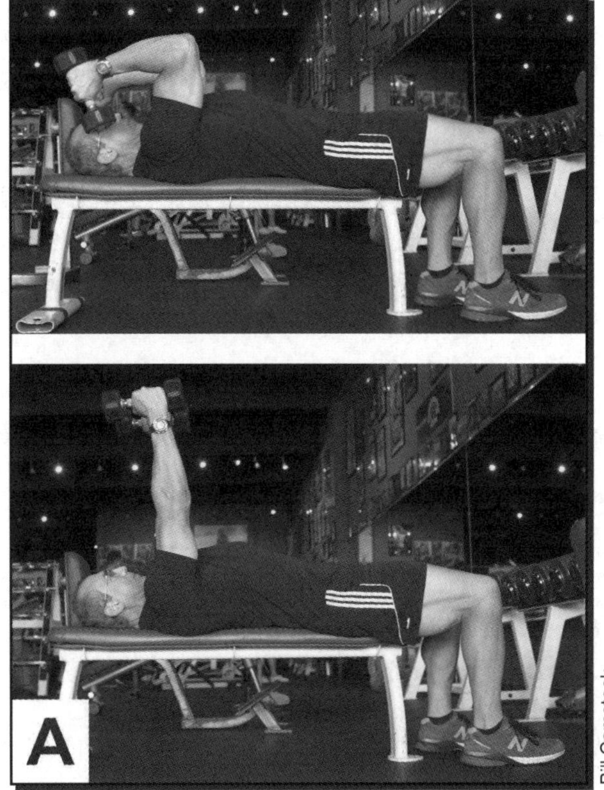


Figure 4-26

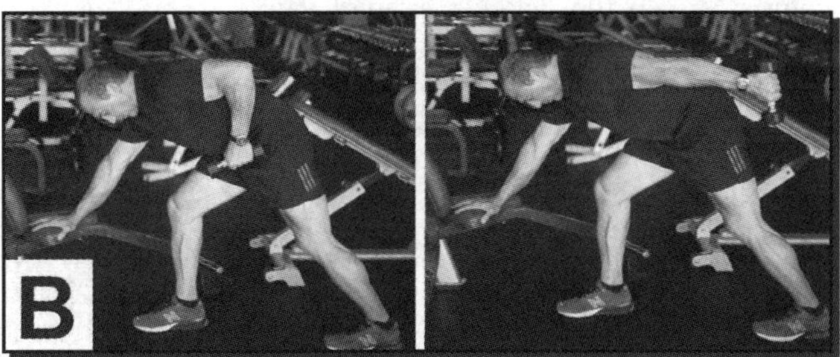


Figure 4-27

Hypothetically, use a 20-pound dumbbell with each of these exercises. You should note that during exercise "A," your forearm reaches the point where it is mostly perpendicular with gravity (i.e., horizontal), when the elbow is bent. During exercise "B," however, it reaches that same point, when your elbow is straight. What you'll discover is that 20 pounds feels relatively easy during a *supine dumbbell triceps extensions* (exercise "A"), while the same resistance feels "awkward" during *dumbbell triceps kickbacks* (exercise "B").

During exercise "A," the resistance curve is such that it loads the triceps more, when the elbow is bent, and the triceps is elongated (strongest), and loads it less, when the arm is extended straight, and the triceps is contracted (weakest). This loading *matches* the strength curve of the muscle. In contrast, during exercise "B," the resistance curve is such that it provides ZERO load to the triceps when the elbow is bent, and the triceps is elongated (strongest), and loads it the most, when the arm is extended straight, and the triceps is contracted (weakest).

In reality, the resistance curve of exercise "B" (*dumbbell triceps kickback*) is the OPPOSITE of the strength curve of the triceps muscle. As a result, the exercise initially feels "too light" in the early part of its range of motion, but then it feels "too heavy" at the conclusion of its range of motion.

As such, because of the natural strength curve of most muscles, it is usually better to select exercises that provide "*early phase loading*," i.e., more resistance in the early part of the muscle's range of motion and less resistance in the latter part of the range of motion.

## Comparing the Resistance Curves of Several "Side Raise" Exercise Versions for the Lateral Deltoids

One of the most common exercises for the lateral deltoids is the "*standing dumbbell side raise*," shown in Figure 4-28. To further throw light on the concept of an ideal resistance curve, examine the resistance curve of this exercise, and see how it compares with the deltoids' strength curve, as well as with other versions of a *side raise*.

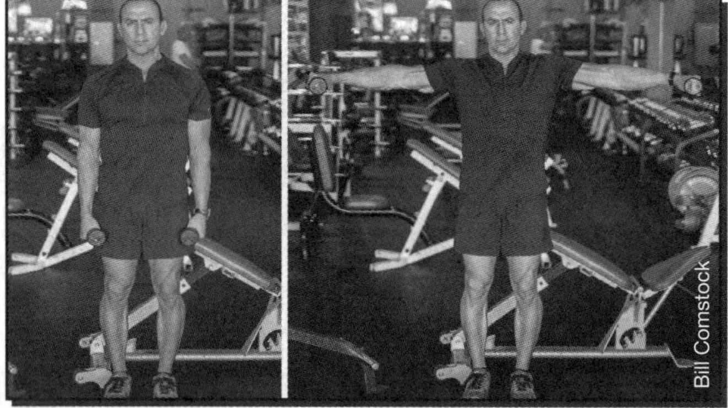


Figure 4-28

The "*standing side dumbbell raise*" begins with the arms down at the exerciser's side, parallel with the direction of resistance (i.e., "free weight" gravity). At this point, the operating lever of the deltoids (the humerus/upper arm) is in the neutral position (image "A" in Figure 4-28). At this stage, the lateral deltoids are entirely unchallenged. This position, however, is where the deltoids are strongest.

Then, as the arms are raised, they encounter increasing degrees of "perpendicular-ness" with gravity, progressively increasing the load on the lateral deltoids. Finally, when the upper arms are parallel with the ground (image "B" in Figure 4-28), they are at their "most active" (most loaded) position. It should also be noted that this position is where the deltoids are weakest.

This factor is very easy to prove. If you use an amount of weight that allows you to hold your arms parallel to the ground, it will feel far too easy during the earlier stages of the movement. On the other hand, if you use a weight that provides a reasonable challenge at the bottom of the movement, it will be impossible for you to hold it at the top.

The resistance curve of a *standing side dumbbell raise* is the *opposite* of the strength curve of the lateral deltoids. This version of a "side raise" fails to provide sufficient resistance at the point where the muscle is strongest (in the early phase of the movement), and then provides too much resistance when the muscle is weakest (in the latter part of the movement).

The "backward resistance curve" that is entailed in the *standing side dumbbell raise* often encourages people to "swing" the weight up, from the bottom to the top, in order to use a weight that feels challenging. They typically begin with a slight forward bend, and then jerk their torso upward (sometimes even going up onto their toes), in order to REACH the top of the movement. But "swinging" the weight (using momentum) is not the solution to a "bad" resistance curve. The solution is either *changing the direction of resistance* OR changing the position of your body relative to gravity.

The "*lying side dumbbell raise*" (Figures 4-29 to 4-31) is an example of how you can reposition your body, so that the upper arms are perpendicular with gravity at the beginning of the movement and parallel with gravity at the end of the movement. During the *lying dumbbell side raise*, the humerus begins the range of motion, when it is parallel with the ground, which means that it is perpendicular with gravity. Therefore, the operating lever of the deltoids (the humerus) is at the 100 percent "active" position in the "early phase" of the movement, precisely where the deltoids are strongest.

As the arm continues on its upward path, the load on the deltoids gradually decreases, as the lever (the humerus) moves toward the neutral (vertical) position. This scenario is acceptable, because the strength potential of the deltoids is also progressively decreasing. The humerus reaches the neutral position, just as the lateral deltoid reaches its weakest phase of the movement. This sequence is a much more productive resistance curve, because it's "early phase loaded."

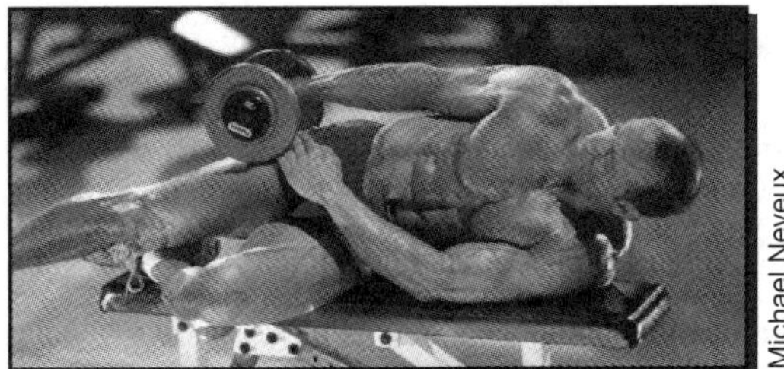
Michael Neveux

Figure 4-29

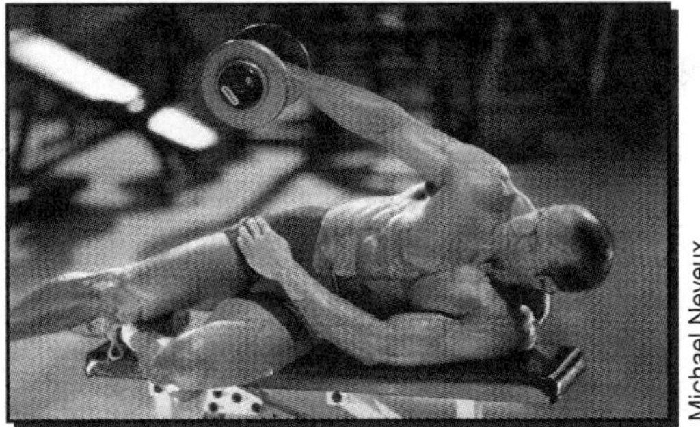
Michael Neveux

Figure 4-30

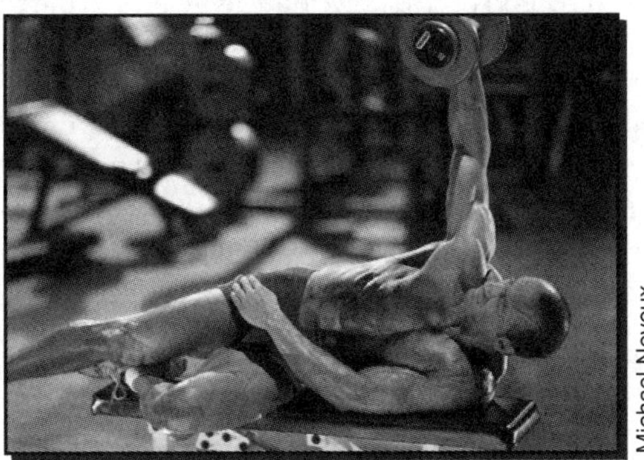
Michael Neveux

Figure 4-31

Another version of a "*side raise*," as it relates to the "resistance curve," is the "*leaning side dumbbell raise*." This exercise has a resistance curve that is even LESS favorable (less productive) than that of the *standing side dumbbell raise*.

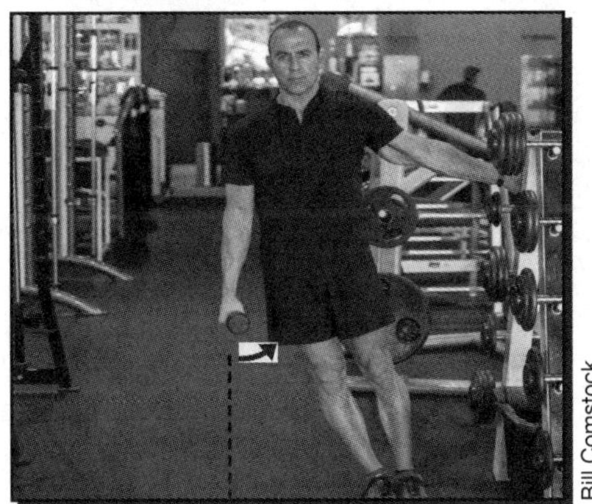
Bill Comstock

Figure 4-32

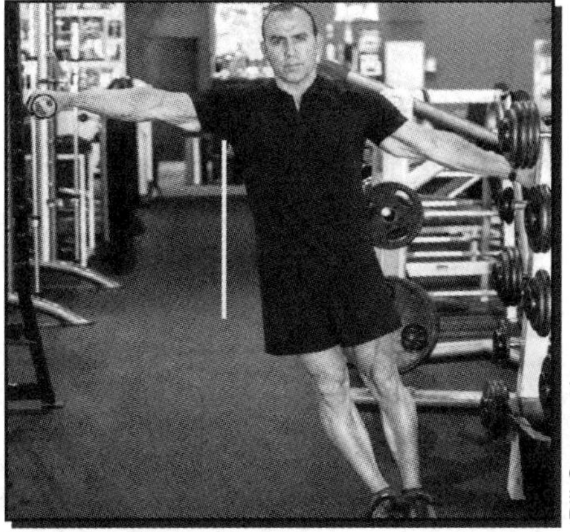
Bill Comstock

Figure 4-33

As you can see, the starting position (arm hanging vertically) skips the first 10 degrees of the range of motion (Figure 4-32). The deltoid's range of motion begins when the arm is actually touching the side of the torso, yet the resistance doesn't start until the arm is vertical—where the line has been placed in Figure 4-32. Accordingly, the earliest part of the range of motion (arguably the most important part) has no resistance at all in this version of a *side raise*. In fact, it doesn't begin providing any significant load until the deltoid is well past the "early phase."

There's also too much load at the top of the exercise, because the deltoid has lost much of its strength potential at that stage. It might not have felt this way to you (*if you've tried this exercise*), because the tendency is to swing the weight up to the top. In other words, it's not so much deltoid force that is getting the weight to the top—it's mostly momentum (*swinging*) that does it.

*Note: If you bring the arm inward, at the bottom, so that it touches the side of your body—trying to not lose any of the range of motion—it's worse. The arm then begins the lateral movement while on the other side of the "base," which means that it will begin with a downward fall—with momentum. As a result, it will swing through the first half of the movement, without much need for deltoid effort. This situation makes a "bad" exercise, even worse.*

A better option, although not quite as good as the *lying side dumbbell raise* (or as good as the *standing side cable raise*, which will be discussed and demonstrated in Chapter 20) is an *incline side dumbbell raise*, shown in Figures 4-34 and 4-35. In other words, angling the torso *away* from the resistance is better than angling the torso *toward* the resistance, as is the case with the leaning side dumbbell raise.

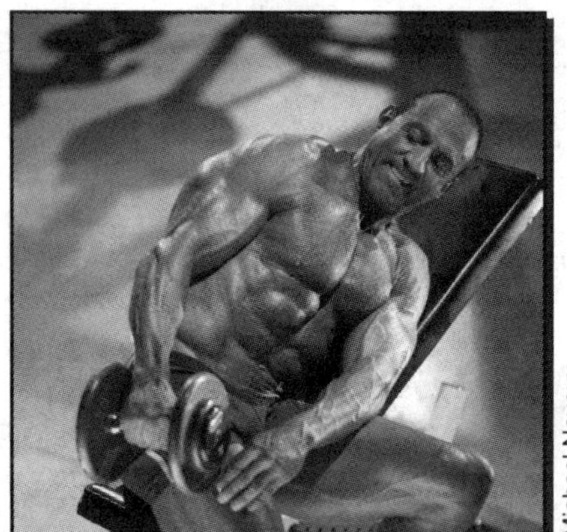

Michael Neveux

Figure 4-34

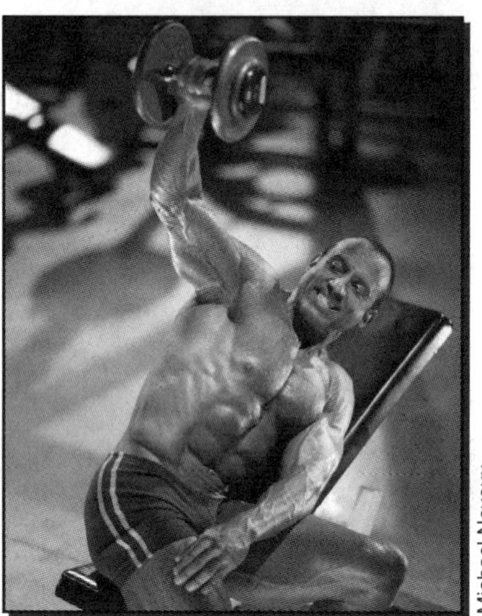

Michael Neveux

Figure 4-35

Using a bench that can be set to about a 15-degree angle (*barely more inclined than a perfectly flat bench*) would provide a nearly ideal resistance curve. A massage table can easily be set at that particular angle. Furthermore, the width of a massage table would also allow for a more stable position. An incline angle like the one shown in Figures 4-34 and 4-35 (45-degree incline) is fairly good, but not ideal.

## Summary

The *direction of resistance*, relative to the position of the body, and relative to the operating lever of the target muscle, is one of the most important factors in evaluating resistance exercise. This chapter deals with how the direction of resistance influences the *resistance curve*, and how you can select exercises that are "early phase loaded," or at least modify them so that they are "early phase loaded." Exercises that are "early phase loaded" are generally more productive than exercises than are "late phase loaded," because they match the strength curve of most skeletal muscles.

Subsequent chapters in this book will explain how the direction of resistance also influences alignment, as well as the *proper position of a target muscle*, relative to the direction of resistance.

The assessment and selection of resistance exercises is predicated on two primary factors—the ideal anatomical movement for a given muscle and the ideal direction of resistance.

The direction of resistance directly relates to the resistance curve of an exercise, and determines if that exercise is mostly productive or mostly unproductive. This factor can only be assessed when you understand that the load on a muscle increases when its operating lever approaches the point of being perpendicular with resistance. It decreases when it approaches the point where it is parallel with resistance; and it loads the muscle with a percentage of the load—between zero and 100 percent—when the lever (your limb) is at various points between parallel and perpendicular with resistance.

CHAPTER 5

# THE APEX AND THE BASE

- *The "apex" is defined as the highest point in an arc, or in the case of resistance training, the point in the arc that is farthest away from the source of resistance. The "base" is defined as the lowest point in an arc, or in the case of resistance training, the point in the arc that is closest to the source of resistance.*
- *When a lever moves through an arc, it sometimes reaches either the apex or the base—both of which are neutral positions, because the lever is then parallel with the direction of resistance.*
- *Moving the lever (or limb) beyond the apex or the base to the other side of the apex or base will result in a transition of the load from one muscle to its antagonist muscle—the muscle that moves that same limb in the opposite direction.*
- *Crossing over to the other side of the apex or base, during an exercise, is usually counterproductive, for the purpose of muscular development.*

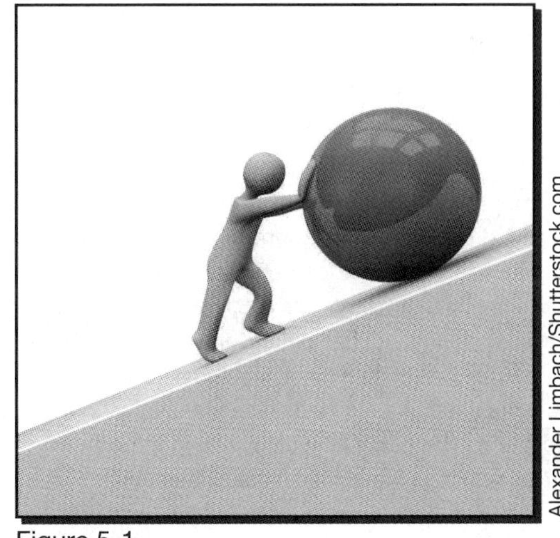

Figure 5-1

## What Defines the Apex and the Base?

Many people remember seeing cartoons in their youth in which two or three characters (for example, the "Three Stooges") are struggling to push a heavy cart up a hill. When they reach the top of the hill, they're able to relax, because the cart is at the "apex" (i.e., top of the hill)—a neutral position. Before actually reaching the top, they would not be able to take a break, because the cart would roll back over them, if they stopped their upward push.

In the typical hypothetical scenario, the "Stooges" pause, while at the "apex," wipe the sweat from their brows, and congratulate each other for their successful effort. At that point, however, one of them accidentally bumps the cart toward the other side of the hill. The cart begins rolling down that other side, with the Stooges chasing after it. This situation offers a profound lesson, which the following example will help illuminate.

Let's say the Stooges were moving "north-bound," as they were pushing the cart up the hill. The upward force they would be using would be required, because they would be pushing away from the downward pull of gravity. After the cart had passed the apex to the other side of the hill, however, the cart no longer needed any "north-bound" force, in order to continue moving in that north-bound direction. It would then roll downhill on its own, pulled downward by gravity. Any attempt to slow down (or reverse) its north-bound (but downhill) movement, would require the application of force in a south-bound direction … toward the apex.

This factor applies in resistance exercise, as well. When the weight is on one side of the apex (or the base), it requires force from one particular muscle. When the weight crosses over to the other side of the apex, however, the force-requirement shifts to the muscle that is on the *other side* of that limb.

You should note that at this point in this book, as you progress through various principles of physics, you'll notice that each successive chapter dovetails with previous (or future) chapters. While they are separate principles, they all interconnect. For example, in the previous chapter, we discussed the "resistance curve" and how it relates to the apex and the base. Now, as the "*transfer of load*" is discussed, which occurs when a lever crosses over from one side of the apex or base to the other side of the apex or a base, the principles of "opposite position loading" (Chapter 8) and "reciprocal innervation" (Chapter 11) are automatically involved.

"Opposite position loading" refers to the fact that the resistance placed on a lever always loads the muscle that is on the same plane as the direction of resistance, and is positioned directly opposite the pull of the loaded lever. "Reciprocal innervation" refers to the fact that one muscle OR the opposite ("antagonist") muscle can work at any given time. As such, two opposing muscles (like biceps and triceps) cannot contract simultaneously.

## Transference of Load After Crossing the Apex or Base

In order to help clarify this principle, it can be beneficial to more closely examine the "transition of load" that occurs when a lever crosses over to the opposite side of the apex or the base. In Figure 5-2, you see a circle. In reality, what you are really looking at is *four separate arcs*, plus a pivot in the center, where the vertical and horizontal lines meet. Two of the arcs are the left and right halves of the sphere. The other two arcs are the upper and lower halves of the sphere. The horizontal line represents the point at which a lever is perpendicular with resistance, where it would be "maximally active." The vertical arrows indicate the direction of resistance (gravity). You should notice that the horizontal line ("A") is perpendicular with those arrows, while the vertical line ("B") is parallel with those arrows.

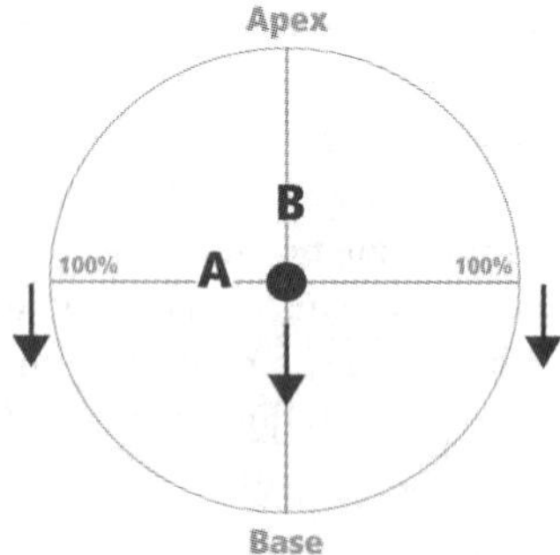


Figure 5-2

When you lift weights, there is always a pivot—a place around which the anatomical movement rotates. Once the pivot and the direction of the resistance have been identified, you can then establish where the base and the apex are. At that point, you can decipher the sequential variations of resistance that occur when your "limb" (e.g., a forearm) travels on the left or right side of the circle, as well as on either the upper half or the lower half of the circle. You can also determine onto which muscle the load will transfer, when that limb crosses over, beyond the apex or base.

In Figures 5-3 and 5-4, you see the first part of a demonstration that shows what occurs when a limb is on the upper half of this sphere. In Figure 5-3, the forearm is at the apex position, so it's neutral. Therefore, neither the biceps nor the triceps are loaded. The weight in the exerciser's hand is balanced directly over the pivot (the elbow).

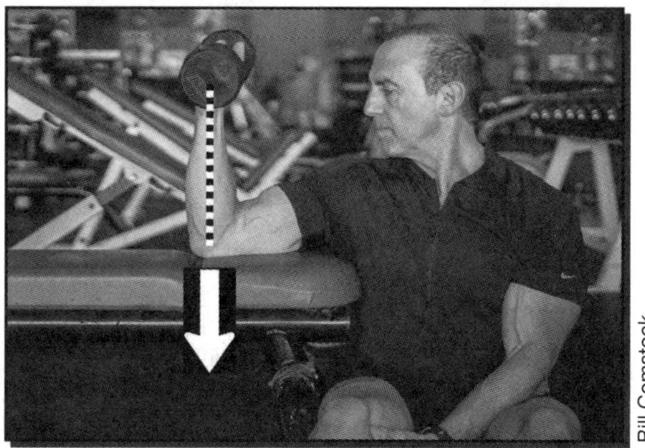


Figure 5-3

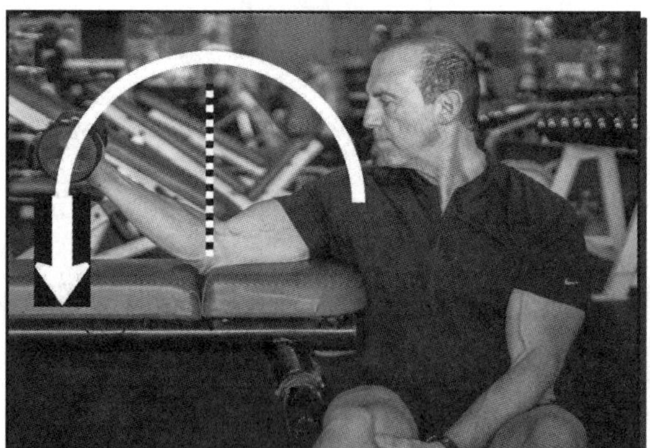


Figure 5-4

In Figure 5-4, however, the forearm is tilted to the left side of the upper sphere. In doing so, the forearm has become an active lever, loading the muscle that is on the "opposite side of the lean," which is the biceps. When the forearm initially departs from the apex position, it begins with very little resistance. As the forearm enters into progressively more perpendicular angles with gravity, the load on the biceps increases. Eventually, the forearm reaches its "maximally active" position, when it is 100 percent perpendicular with gravity (horizontal).

*Note: Of course, the demonstration illustrated in Figures 5-3 and 5-4 is not meant to be an actual biceps exercise. It is only meant to illustrate how the resistance curve functions on the upper half of the sphere. It also illustrates why a movement like this would NOT be a particularly good exercise for the biceps, as you shall soon see.*

Ideally, the biceps should be able to go through its entire range of motion—from full extension to full contraction—with SOME degree of resistance. This particular arc, however, only provides resistance through the first 60 percent of the biceps' ROM. The biceps load becomes neutral at the apex, thereby leaving the other 40 percent (the final part of the range of motion) without any opposing resistance.

In Figure 5-5, the forearm has tilted to the right side of the upper sphere. In doing so, it has crossed over to the other side of the apex, thereby causing a transfer of the load from the biceps to the triceps. In other words, biceps force is no longer required on this (right) side of the apex, because the weight in the hand will now "fall" in that direction, if not halted, held, or reversed by the triceps. On the right side of the apex (when viewed from this angle), the biceps is not at all challenged. In fact, it's forced to relax. This is because—as you'll see in Chapter 11—when the triceps is activated, the opposing muscle is deactivated by the central nervous system.

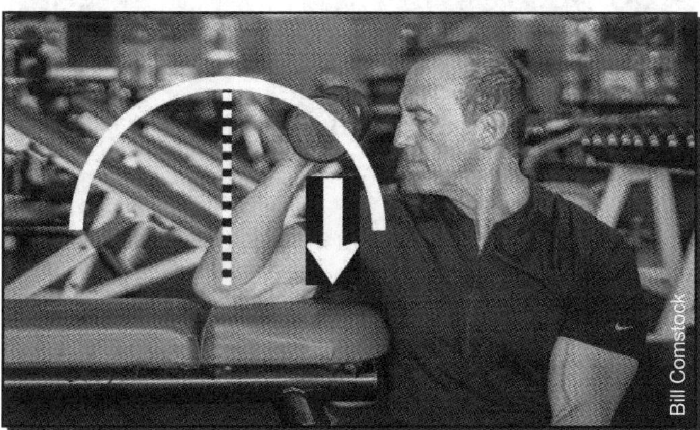

Figure 5-5

One of the reasons this would NOT be considered a good biceps exercise is because the apex occurs in the middle of the range of motion. As was previously pointed out, the biceps would only be active for about half of its range of motion. Likewise, when the load transfers to the triceps, after it crosses the apex, the triceps would only be active for half of its range of motion. Some people may think this is a "good" movement, because it allows both the triceps and the biceps to work, but neither muscle is worked well, because neither muscle is provided resistance through its full range of motion.

Next, it can be helpful to look at how the resistance curve operates on the lower half of the sphere. In Figure 5-6, you can see the forearm hanging straight down from the elbow. This positioning is similar to the standard "pendulum." The forearm lever is now in the "base" position—neutral, "hanging" (without effort from the biceps or triceps) from its pivot (the elbow).

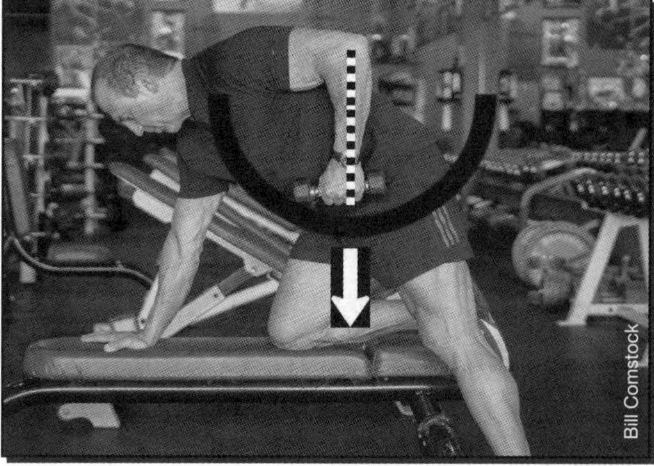

Figure 5-6

In Figure 5-7, you can see that the forearm has been tilted to the *right* side of the lower sphere, thereby loading the triceps. At this point, with the forearm about halfway between the base and the position that is perpendicular with gravity (horizontal), the triceps is loaded with about 50 percent of the available resistance.

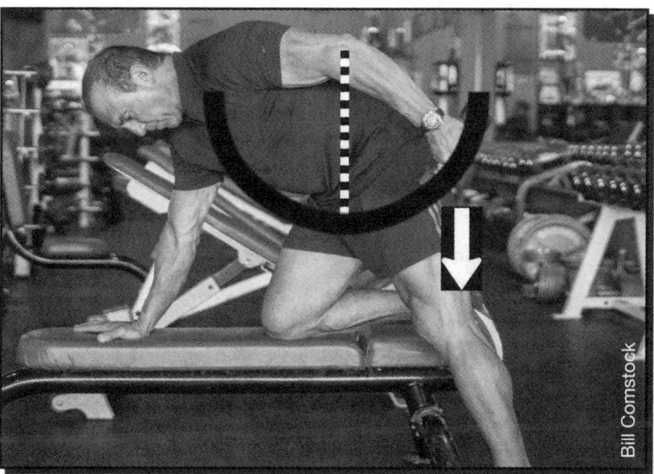

Figure 5-7

In contrast, in Figure 5-8, the forearm has been tilted to the *left* side of the lower sphere, thereby loading the biceps (which is on the opposite side of the triceps), because the forearm has crossed over to the other side of the base. At this point, the exerciser is "pulling" the weight (toward his shoulder), rather than "pushing" the weight (away from the shoulder). Again, neither the biceps nor the triceps are experiencing resistance through their entire range of motion, so neither the biceps nor the triceps are getting an optimally productive resistance curve. As such, this is NOT a good triceps exercise.

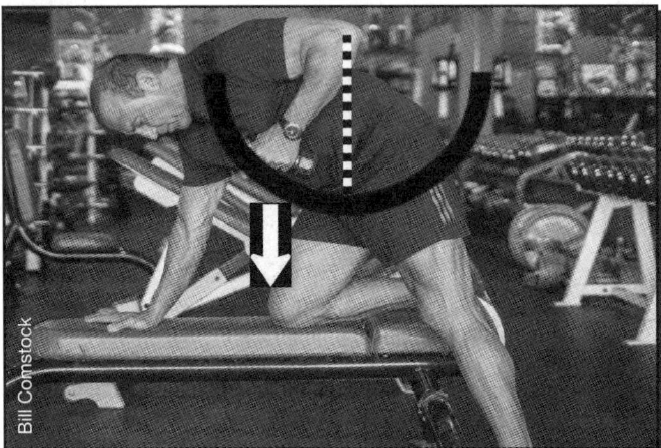

Figure 5-8

Of course, as is often the case when a person performs a *triceps kickback*, if the forearm is allowed to simply DROP from the triceps-extended position (with the rate of descent not being controlled by the triceps), it causes the forearm to swing past the base by sheer momentum, thereby reducing the need for muscular force. Then, once the forearm has reached the position closest to the shoulder, the weight is again allowed to DROP and swing the other way. This scenario again relieves the triceps of having to generate as much (if any) force. Needless to say, this situation is unproductive and foolish. In essence, the forearm simulates a playground "swing"—moving more by momentum, than by deliberate muscular force. This makes a "bad" exercise even less productive.

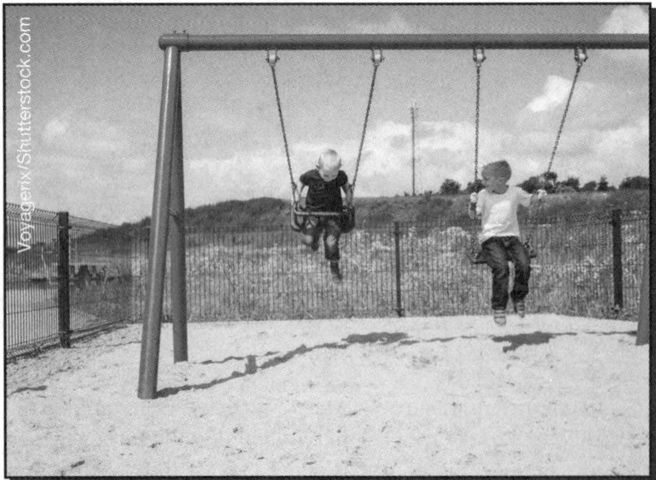

Figure 5-9

You should notice that the tendency to "swing" (allowing the use of momentum) *only* occurs on the bottom half of the sphere, when the lever crosses the base. It does not happen on the upper half of the sphere, when the lever crosses the apex.

You should also be aware that on the lower half of the sphere, the resistance increases, as a weight is moved upward from the base to the horizontal line. On the upper half of the sphere (Figure 5-10), however, the resistance decreases, when a weight is moved upward from the horizontal line toward the apex.

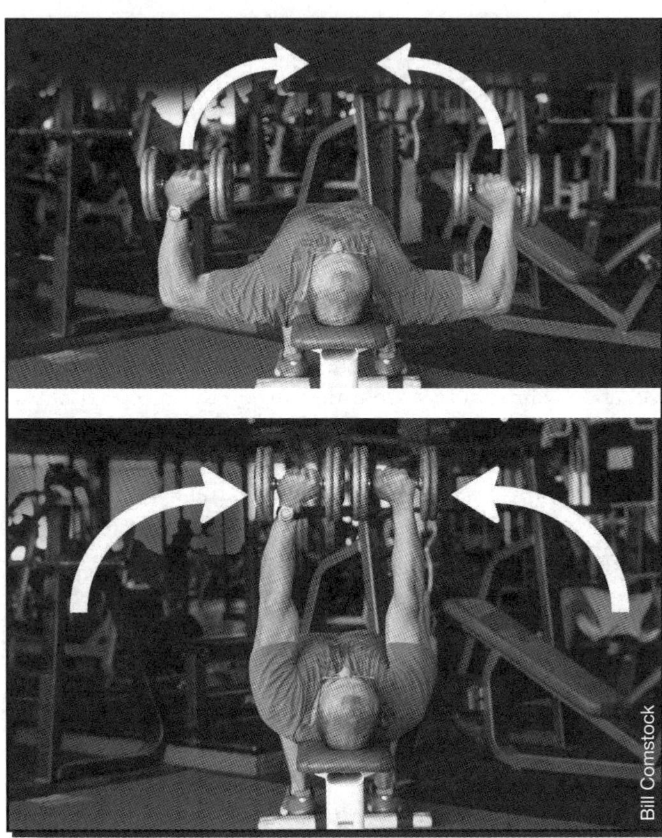

Figure 5-10

In the exercise shown in Figure 5-11, (an individual doing a *bent-over rear dumbbell raise* for the posterior deltoids), you can more easily see how the upper-arm levers are moving through the lower half of the sphere. The movement starts at the base and then moves toward the horizontal position. The resistance increases, as the arms (levers) move upward through this range of motion.

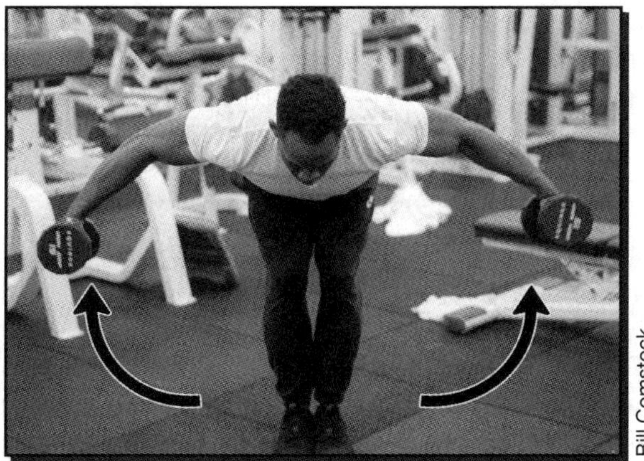

Figure 5-11

## The Four Resistance Quadrants

At this point, it can be helpful to look again at the "sphere" (Figure 5-12). You can see the pivot in the center, as well as both the left and right arcs and the upper and lower arcs. You should notice that each "quadrant" is a point of *transition*—of one type or another.

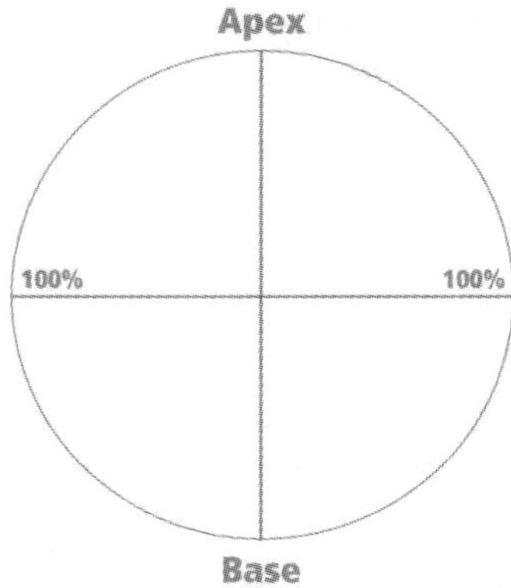

Figure 5-12

When a lever (i.e., limb) moves from the base, up toward the horizontal line on the left (image A in Figure 5-13), the muscle moving that limb experiences an increasing resistance. Once that lever passes that "quadrant" (the horizontal line), however, the muscle experiences a decreasing level of resistance, as the lever moves toward the apex (image B in Figure 5-13). That's one transition.

Then, when that lever (limb) continues PAST the apex (moving clockwise), another transition occurs (image C in Figure 5-13). The muscle that caused that limb to rise up to the apex (on the left side of the sphere) would then NO longer be active, once the lever passes the apex. Instead, the antagonist muscle, the muscle that controls that lever in the opposite direction, becomes active and controls the movement in the clockwise direction. That's the second transition.

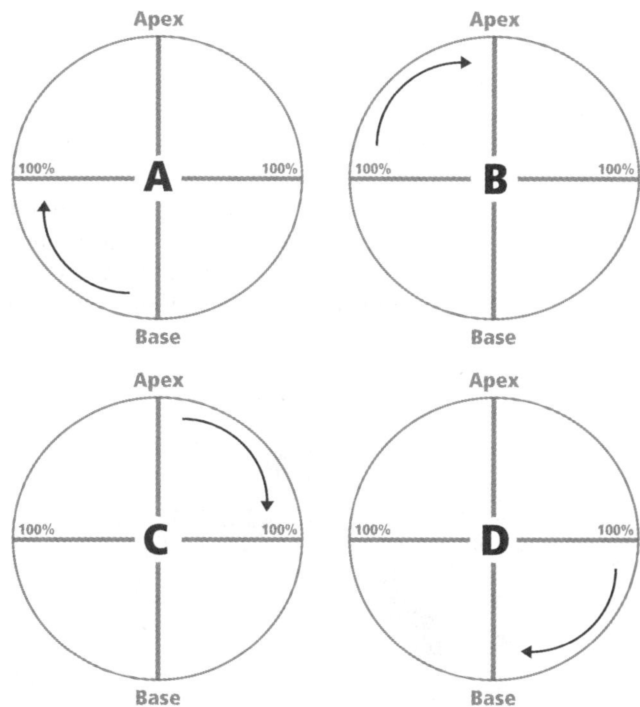

Figure 5-13

The second muscle, which is now controlling the descent, experiences an increasing level of resistance, until it reaches the horizontal line. Once it crosses that horizontal line (image D in Figure 5-13), however, the resistance begins decreasing. That's the third transition. The fourth transition would be when the lever passes the base again and starts the cycle anew—utilizing the opposite muscle again.

## Application

When you work a muscle during an exercise, it is best to use a resistance curve that provides resistance for that muscle throughout most (if not all) of its range of motion. Ideally, it would be best for the exercise to have a resistance curve that is "early phase loaded," i.e., providing more load to the target muscle in the beginning (during the first-third of the range of motion) and then progressively diminishing during the latter two-thirds of the range of motion. This would match the strength curve of the muscle—challenging it when it can best handle it, and easing off when it can least handle it.

As a consequence, performing an exercise that causes the target muscle's operating lever to encounter the base (or the apex) midway through its range of the motion, will drastically compromise the benefits of that exercise. In other words, the muscle will only have an opposing resistance for a fraction of its full range of motion, and then the load will transition to the muscle that is on the opposite side of that limb. Then, the opposing muscle will also only be loaded for a fraction of its range of motion.

At this point, consider the triceps kickback (Figure 5-14). Pictured is a person performing this exercise in a way she believes is completely correct. This illustrates, to a degree, the level of misinformation that has occurred over the last century. Just because this exercise is commonly performed, and performed in this manner, does not mean it is biomechanically "good." Many people perform this exercise as one of multiple exercises for their triceps, believing that each exercise contributes something "different" to that muscle. This assumption, which is absolutely false, will be further discussed in Chapter 17.

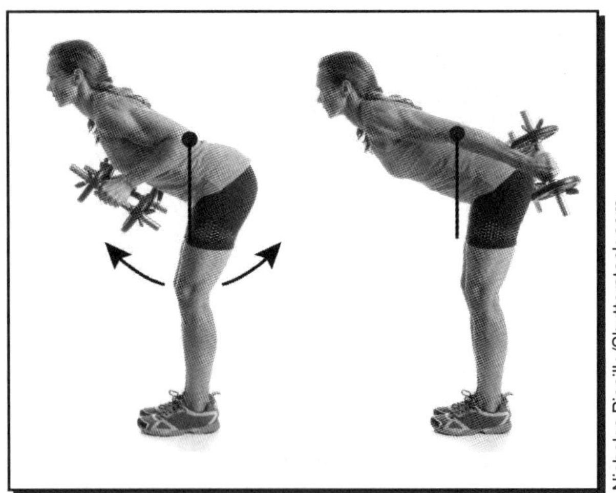

Figure 5-14

In the left image in Figure 5-14, a vertical line has been placed, starting at her elbow (the pivot). As you can see, her forearm has already crossed over to the left side of the base—the side on which the biceps would be activated, if "swinging" wasn't what brought it beyond the base. This slight activation of the biceps would completely shut off triceps activation, as a result of "reciprocal innervation" (which will be discussed in Chapter 11). Needless to say, that factor would be very counterproductive, since the exercise is meant to be a triceps exercise.

During this exercise, when the elbow is bent at 90 degrees, the forearm is in vertical (neutral) position, which means that the triceps is not getting ANY load at that point. However, that is the point in the range of motion where the triceps is "strongest" (i.e., has the most strength potential). Furthermore, the triceps is not getting ANY activation (or load) during the first-third of its range of motion. Arguably, that is the most important part of a muscle's range of motion.

As the elbow is extended, the forearm becomes more and more "active," thereby increasing the load on the triceps. This situation is also counterproductive, because the triceps loses strength during the latter part of the range of motion. That is the phase (in the ROM) when the triceps has the least strength. As such, the resistance curve of this exercise is the opposite of the triceps' strength curve—it's the opposite of what's ideal. This is another reason why this is NOT a good triceps exercise.

As discussed previously, certain exercises, including the triceps kickback exercise tend to encourage "swinging" the weight (because the forearm is traveling through the lower half of the arc, and because it's crossing past the base), which deprives the triceps of having to work deliberately, a factor that further compromises the potential benefit from doing these particular exercises. This circumstance illustrates the problem with selecting an exercise that has a base in the middle of the range of motion of the target muscle, which is yet another reason why this is NOT a good triceps exercise.

*Note: There is still another problem with the triceps kickback that is unrelated to the apex/base issue. In this exercise, the posterior deltoid is holding the upper arm in place, in a horizontal position. When the elbow is bent, the posterior deltoid is loaded with an amount of weight that is produced by the weight held in the hand, plus the magnification of the upper-arm length. When the arm is straightened, however, the amount of load on the posterior deltoid doubles, because of the length of the arm has doubled (given that the forearm acts as the secondary lever of the posterior deltoids). In other words, the posterior deltoid gets more load during a triceps kickback, than the triceps does. Yet, it's not a good exercise for the posterior deltoid, because it's entirely isometric. All-in-all, this exercise has a very high "cost" of effort, with very little reward.*

## Another Example

Figure 5-15 shows an example of what happens, when the forearm crosses over to the other side of the apex. While doing an *overhead triceps extension*, the triceps are loaded, as long as the forearm stays on the left side of the apex (when viewed from this angle). When the forearm reaches the apex, the triceps is no longer loaded, because the forearm has reached the neutral position. Yet, the triceps has not completed its range of motion at that point, and the elbow has not yet fully straightened. On the other hand, allowing the forearm to cross over to the other side of the apex (in an effort to complete the range of motion), transitions the load to a different muscle. At that point, it would be the anterior and lateral deltoids that would prevent the arms from falling farther forward.

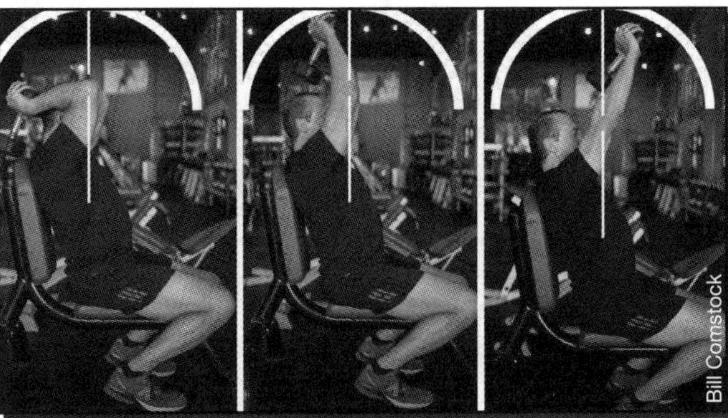


Figure 5-15

The problem during this exercise begins with the fact that the upper arms are not vertical. When the elbows are fully extended, the forearms and the upper arms always form a continuous line. As a result, if the upper arms are slanting forward (as they are in Figure 5-15), the forearms will also slant forward, when the elbows are fully extended.

Trying to position the upper arms vertically, while sitting at this angle, would be very uncomfortable for the shoulder joint. One solution would be to allow the torso to be more reclined (using an incline bench). This technique would allow the shoulders to be in a more comfortable position, and yet still enable the upper arms to be vertical. This factor would then allow the forearms to stay on the left side of the apex (as opposed to not going beyond the apex), when the elbows are fully straight.

*Note: The "overhead triceps extension" exercise is not more beneficial than triceps exercises that allow the arms to be down, alongside the torso. Accordingly, the key issue of how to perform this exercise, without having the forearms cross beyond the apex, yet still have the humerus in a comfortable position, is academic. This factor will be further explained in Chapter 21. This example, however, allows you to see what happens any time a lever (i.e., a limb) crosses beyond the apex.*

## How the Apex and/or Base Interact With a Secondary Lever

In Figure 5-16, you see an individual performing a *one-arm dumbbell row* exercise. In this exercise, his forearm acts as the secondary lever to his humerus. This situation is due to the fact that the weight must be held by hand, which is attached to the forearm. The humerus is the primary lever for the lats.

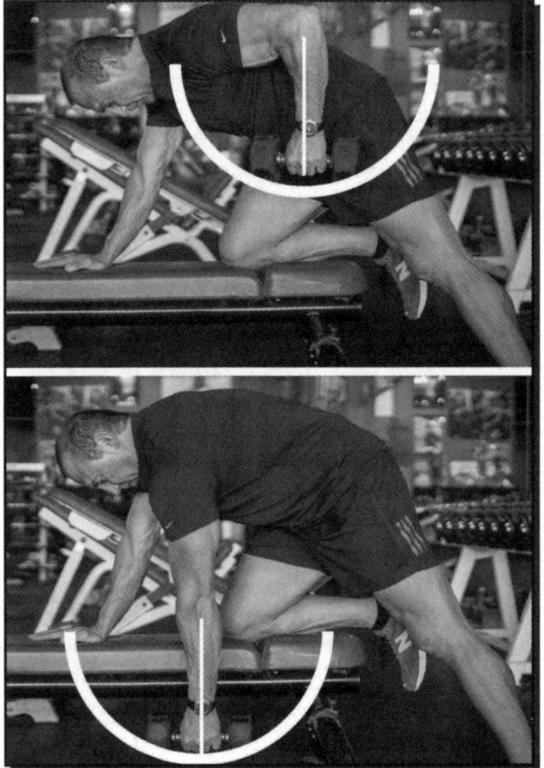


Figure 5-16

The forearm must participate, even though the target muscles do not connect directly to the forearm. The weight cannot be directly connected to (held by) the humerus. Therefore, the forearm—as the secondary lever in this exercise—acts as a "connector" between the weight and the humerus.

A vertical line, starting at the elbow, has been placed in the image to highlight where the forearm should be (ideally), relative to the base position. The base is neutral. Ideally, the forearm should be maintained in the neutral position during this exercise. The forearm should be kept perfectly vertical throughout the entire movement.

In reality, however, since you usually cannot see your forearm when you're doing *one-arm dumbbell rows*, you may not be aware of whether or not the forearm is perfectly vertical throughout the range of motion. As such, people often tend to tilt their forearm *forward* (toward their shoulder) when doing this exercise, because it makes the exercise seem easier. In fact, this action effectively shortens the upper-arm lever, thereby reducing its magnification of the weight being used. It also activates the biceps a bit, although that is not nearly as relevant as the fact that the goal of the exercise (to work the lats) is compromised by allowing the secondary lever to shorten the primary lever.

There is a little "trick" that can be applied in this instance, however. Once you know that allowing the forearm to cross over to the either side of the base transfers the load to the muscle of the opposite side, you can correct any forearm tilt while you're performing the exercise. If you FEEL fatigue in the biceps (while doing this exercise), you can deliberately cause your forearm to tilt "back" (toward your butt) instead, which will shut off the activation of the biceps. This adjustment will also slightly extend the upper-arm lever, rather than shortening it. This adjustment would increase the magnification of the humerus a bit, which would load the target muscle more. Of course, this step requires the ability to SENSE fatigue, in one muscle or the other. In reality, some people are better able to do this than others.

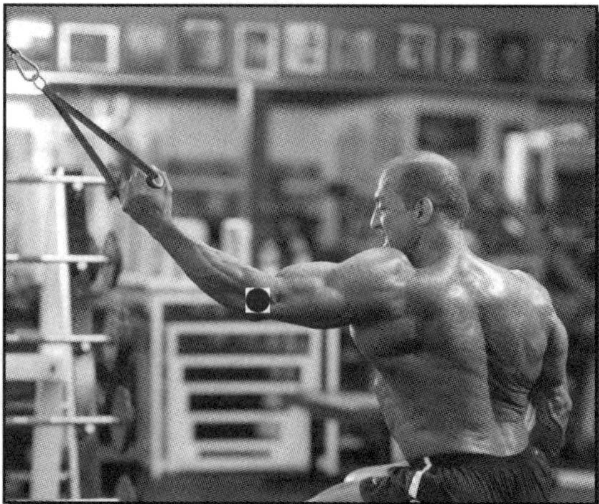
Michael Neveux

Figure 5-17

The same "adjustment" can be made during the exercise (Figures 5-17 and 5-18)—the *one-arm lat pull-in*. If you feel fatigue in either the biceps or the triceps, while doing any exercise that is intended for the lats, it is an indication that you are failing to keep that lever (the forearm) perfectly "neutral"—parallel with the direction of resistance. When doing *one-arm lat pull-ins*, the direction of resistance is the cable, not vertical "free weight" gravity.

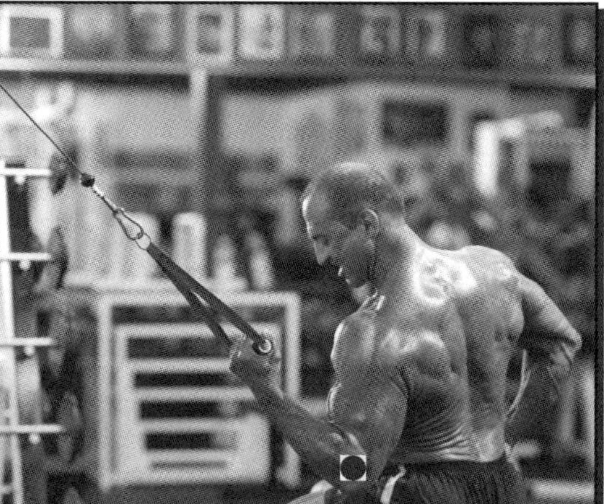
Michael Neveux

Figure 5-18

When you're using a cable resistance, the base is that which is parallel with the cable and closest to the pulley (image B in Figure 5-19). The apex would be directly opposite the base, parallel with the cable, but farthest from the pulley (image A in Figure 5-19). The elbow is the pivot. Furthermore, what was previously called the "horizontal lines" are now whatever angle is perpendicular with the cable (the line in Figure 5-19). All of the same rules of "transition of load" still apply.

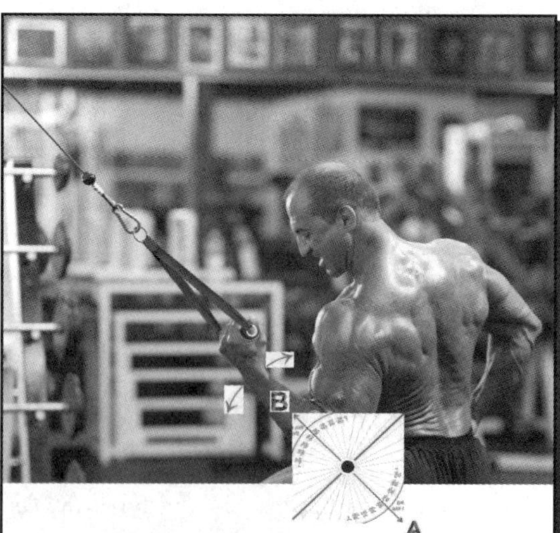

Michael Neveux

Figure 5-19

If you feel fatigue in your biceps, when you perform this exercise, you need only tilt your forearm (slightly) to the other side of the base, and it will de-activate the biceps. Instead, it will activate the triceps a bit. Ideally, neither the biceps nor the triceps should be very involved in a latissimus exercise, because the forearm should ideally be kept in a neutral position. However, if you find that excessive biceps fatigue or triceps fatigue is compromising the movement, you need only tilt your forearm toward the other side to make the exercise more comfortable.

## Summary

In the previous chapter, the fact that the base and the apex are part of the resistance curve was discussed. In this chapter, you learned that when a loaded lever crosses over to the other side of the base or apex, it results in a "*transition of load.*" This transition *always* shifts the load directly to the muscle that is on the opposite side of that lever. For example, in the images that are part of Figure 5-20, you can see a man in three positions. In the center image, his torso-lever is at the apex, balanced directly over the pivot. In this case, his torso is acting as the operating "lever" of his obliques. In the vertical position, his torso lever is neutral. As a result, neither of his oblique muscles (neither right side nor left side) are loaded.

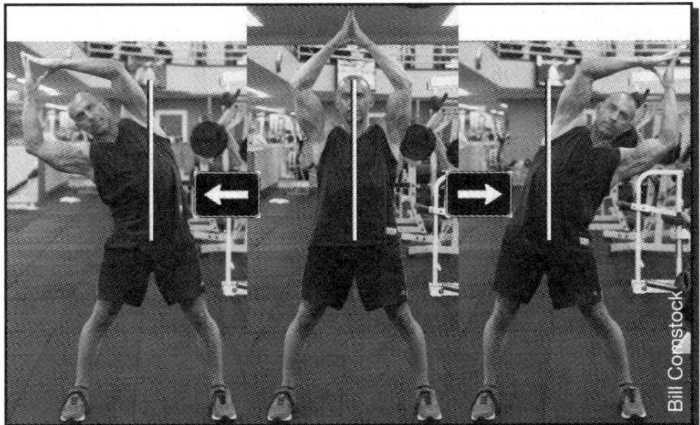

Figure 5-20

When he tilts his torso to his right side (left image), the weight of his torso loads the oblique muscles (external and internal obliques) that are on the LEFT side of his waistline. The principle that "whichever muscle is positioned directly opposite resistance, will be most loaded" will be further discussed in Chapter 8. In this example, because his left obliques are positioned on the opposite side of his right-leaning torso, they are loaded by the weight of his torso. Then, when he tilts his torso to his left side (right image), crossing past the apex, the weight of his torso *transfers* to the oblique muscles that are on the RIGHT side of his waistline.

The two sides (right obliques and left obliques) cannot both be loaded at the same time, because each is the "agonist/antagonist" of the other. We'll learn more about this concept in Chapter 11.

This transition of load is typical of what happens whenever a loaded lever (i.e., limb) crosses the apex or the base, during an exercise. Whenever this happens, among the questions you should ask yourself are the following:

- *Am I aware that I am crossing the apex (or base) right now, and that the load has shifted to the antagonist muscle?*
- *Am I aware that this transition of load usually compromises the benefit of this exercise to my target muscle?*
- *Is there a better way of achieving my objective of optimally loading the target muscle?*

The exercise shown in Figure 5-20 (*bodyweight side-bends*) is not an especially good exercise, unless your objective is simply to stretch the obliques and provide them with a moderate level of resistance for only half their range of motion. If your objective, however, is to really "work" (to develop) your oblique muscles, this version of *side bends* is not optimally productive, because of this "apex crossing" feature.

The exercise shown in Figure 5-21 (*side bends with lateral cable resistance*) illustrates the ideal solution for eliminating the apex that exists in the aforementioned version. By adding a cable resistance that originates from the side (from an angle that is perpendicular to the torso), you create a much better resistance curve. In this version, the vertical torso position is no longer "neutral," because the downward force of gravity is NOT the primary resistance source. In this instance, the exerciser is loading his right oblique muscles, using a left pulling resistance, and is providing resistance to his target muscle through its entire range of motion. Of course, each side must be worked separately. After you perform a set of repetitions for the obliques on one side, you must turn around, grasp the cable handle with the other hand, and work the obliques on the other side.

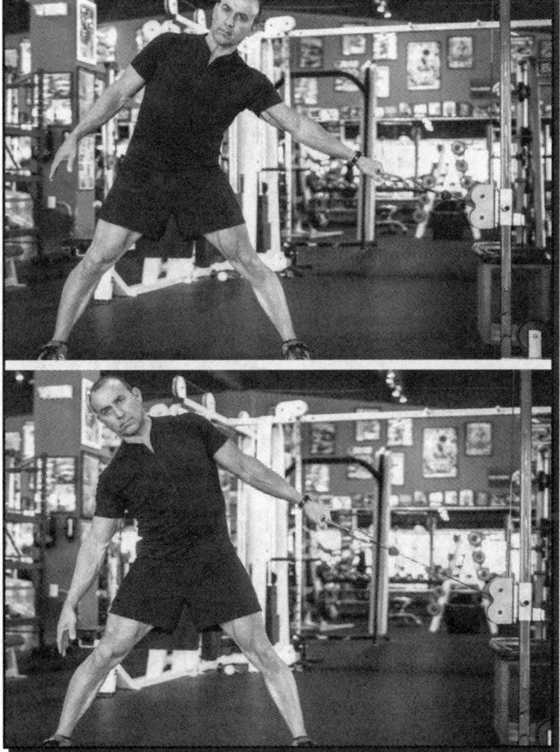

Figure 5-21

A similar situation occurs when an individual performs *torso rotation with a cable,* shown in Figure 5-22. In this scenario, the exerciser is rotating his torso toward the right, against a *left-pulling resistance,* which is the correct way of doing this exercise. The complete range of motion in this exercise encompasses a distance from a fully rotated torso angling right to a fully rotated torso angling left. As such, a left-pulling cable resistance provides load through that entire range. Then, the exerciser must turn around, which will provide resistance from the opposite side of the exerciser, against which the concentric torso rotation is performed in the opposite direction.

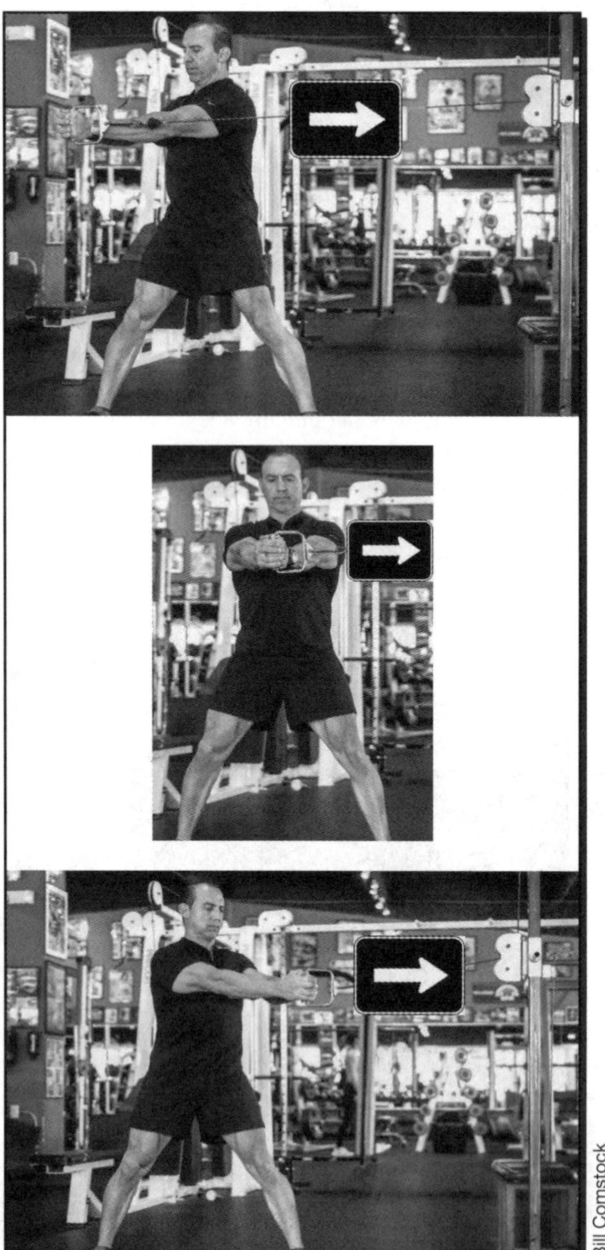


Figure 5-22

The middle image in Figure 5-22 is the midway point of the movement, which is the point where the greatest resistance will occur, in this scenario. That is also the point where the lever (his extended arms, acting as the secondary lever of the torso) meets resistance (the cable) perpendicularly.

On the other hand, if the cable resistance were pulling straight forward (rather from the left side or the right side), that center photo would be the neutral/base position. If that were the case, rotating to the left or to the right, from that center position, would only provide resistance for HALF the range of motion for each side's oblique muscle. It would also fail at providing resistance for either side, at the most critical point in the range of motion.

As yet another example, if you were seated on a bench, with your torso perfectly upright (vertical), your torso would be positioned at the apex (middle image in Figure 5-23). In this position, it is neutral, balanced over the pivot (which is

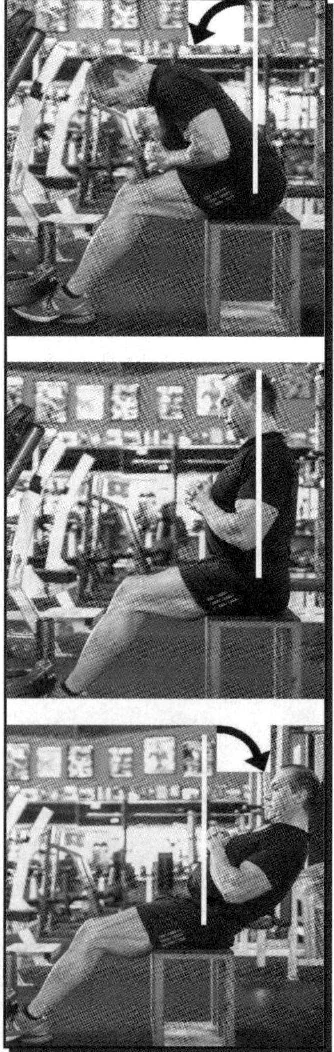


Figure 5-23

your pelvis). If you then tilt your torso to the posterior side of the apex (bottom image in Figure 5-23), you would load the abdominal muscles, because they are positioned on the opposite side of the torso's tilt. In turn, if you tilt your torso to the anterior (front) side of the apex (top image in Figure 5-23), the load transitions to the opposite side of the torso—the erector spinae ("lower back" muscles). The erector spinae would then be the muscles that are positioned on the opposite side of the torso's tilt.

The apex and the base are neutral positions, but they are also the point at which the load transfers from the muscle that is on one side of the "limb" to the opposing muscle(s) on the opposite side of the limb. As such, knowing when your operating lever (limb) is at the apex or base provides you with several advantages. Not only does it allow you to make a better exercise selection, you'll also be using better form during certain exercises. It also provides you with the ability to manipulate exercises by adjusting your body position or the direction of resistance, in order to achieve maximum benefit from your efforts.

# CHAPTER 6

# PRIMARY AND SECONDARY RESISTANCE SOURCES AND OTHER FORCES

- *When you do "resistance exercise," you typically use a variety of types of resistance, including free weights, cables, machines, body weight, etc. There are also other sources of resistance that are not obvious, like "friction force" and "momentum." Furthermore, more often than you realize, you combine a variety of resistance sources in a single exercise.*
- *An obvious example of the aforementioned is barbell squats. In this exercise, the "primary resistance" you're using is your own body weight, to which you add a "secondary resistance" source (e.g., a barbell), which combines with your body weight.*
- *Sometimes, the "primary resistance" and "secondary resistance" are both bearing in the same direction, as is the case with barbell squats. Other times, however, the two resistances are bearing in different directions, which influences the mechanics of the exercise.*
- *Understanding how these various sources of resistance—as well as other forces—combine and produce a mechanical result that is different from that which may seem obvious, is an important aspect of understanding biomechanics.*

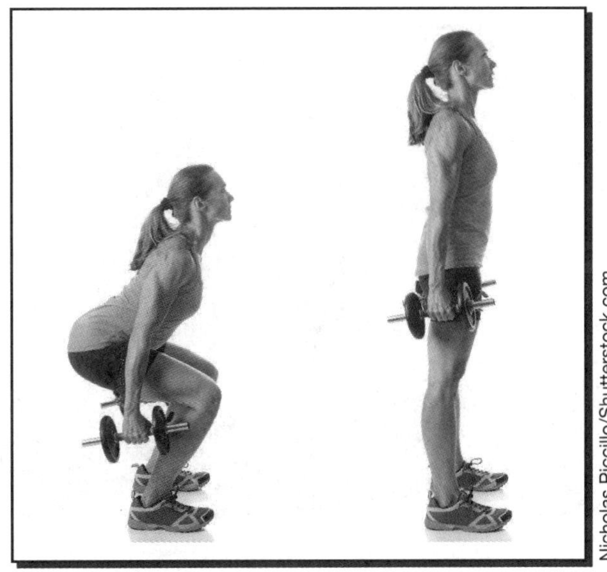
Nicholas Piccillo/Shutterstock.com

Figure 6-1

## What Defines a Secondary Resistance?

When you perform "body weight" exercises, e.g., *free hand squats, chin-ups, push-ups, parallel bar dips, ab crunches,* etc., it's clear that the source of resistance is your own body weight. On occasion, you may add a "secondary resistance" source, by putting a barbell on your shoulders or a chain with a weight around your waist, or by holding a pair of dumbbells. In cases like these, you have two sources of resistance, both of which may seem to be acting as one. They don't always "act as one," however. In fact, even the placement of the secondary resistance can influence the mechanics of the exercise.

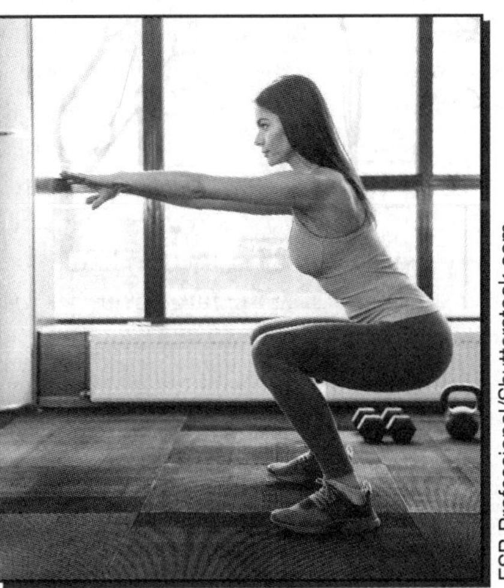
ESB Professional/Shutterstock.com

Figure 6-2

For example, in Figure 6-1, the exerciser is holding a "secondary resistance" source in her hands. Since the hands are attached to the arms, and the arms are attached to the highest part of the torso, the weight of the dumbbells also makes the *torso* more "active" (as a weighted lever), as compared with no added weight being held in the hands. In other words, where the secondary resistance is held plays a role in which muscles are loaded, as well as to what degree they're loaded.

As you learned in Chapter 1 ("Primary and Secondary Levers"), holding the arms (with dumbbells) farther out in front of you would essentially "lengthen" the torso (as a lever), while holding the arms (with dumbbells) farther back would essentially "shorten" the torso (as a lever). This technique would have the effect of loading the "erector spinae" MORE, in the first scenario, or LESS, in the second scenario. As such, using the second scenario during *dumbbell squats* would be wise, because it would relieve the lower back, while still providing the additional downward load that an exerciser seeks for the quads and glutes.

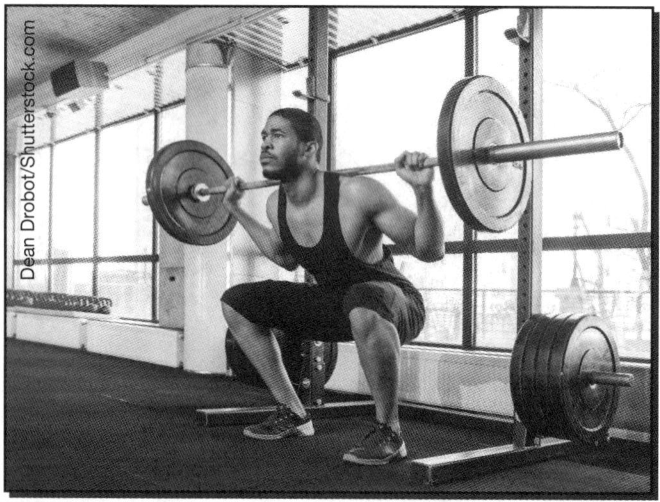


Figure 6-3

Conversely, holding a barbell on the shoulders (Figure 6-3) makes it impossible to shift the secondary resistance forward or backward. The weight of the barbell is placed high on the torso-lever, thereby magnifying the load on the lower back much more. Furthermore, adding a barbell to the squat also adds a downward compressive force directly on the spine, which must also be factored into the assessment of the exercise. As such, adding a secondary resistance, as well as where that resistance is placed, can significantly affect the mechanics of an exercise, separate from simply loading the target muscles more.

## When a Secondary Resistance Pulls a Different Direction Than the Primary Resistance

On occasion, you use resistance from a cable as your primary source, and a (separate) secondary resistance is pulling in a direction that is *opposite* that of the cable. For example, when you do a *lat pulldown*, the direction of the *primary* resistance is upward—toward the pulley. On the other hand, there is a *secondary* resistance (though much lighter), pulling in a different direction. While the cable is pulling your arms upward, the weight of the *lat pulldown* bar, plus the weight of your arms, is being pulled downward by gravity. In essence, the weight of the bar, as well as that of your arms, is "assisting" your downward effort. In fact, it is *subtracting* from the upward pull provided by the cable.

A hypothetical example can help clarify the issue. Say that you're using 100 pounds on the *lat pulldown* machine. The *pulldown* bar weighs 20 pounds, while the weight of your arms could be another 20 pounds (average 10 pounds per arm; the average human arm is 5.3 percent of a person's total body weight). In other words, that's 40 pounds that is being subtracted from the weight you're using on the machine. In essence, the weight with which the lats (and other assisting muscles) are loaded may only be 60 pounds (not factoring in the magnification of arm length, etc.). Of course, when you do this exercise, you simply select the weight that you feel is challenging, automatically compensating for the subtraction of weight that is caused by the weight of the bar and your arms.

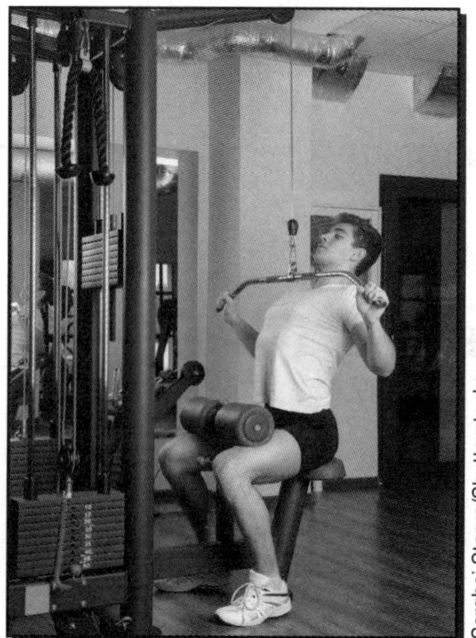


Figure 6-4

Other examples also exist in which the primary and secondary resistance sources are pulling in directly opposite directions. For example, when you do *triceps pushdowns* with a cable (top image in Figure 6-5), you are pushing downward against an upward resistance. However, the weight of the pushdown bar, plus that of your forearms, is being pulled downward. This total SUBTRACTS from the load used on the pulley. Conversely, when you do *standing cable curls* (bottom image in Figure 6-5), the weight of the bar, plus that of your forearms ADDS to the downward resistance of the cable.

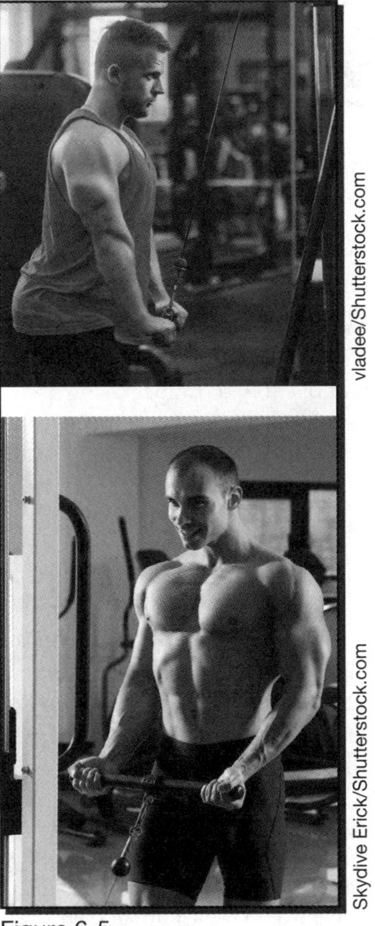
vladee/Shutterstock.com
Skydive Erick/Shutterstock.com

Figure 6-5

Of course, this factor is true for any exercise in which you are either pulling upward or pushing downward against a pulley or machine. For example, *leg extensions* and *seated leg curls* create a similar situation. With *leg extensions* (top image in Figure 6-6), the weight of the machine's lever arm, plus the weight of your lower leg, are ADDED to the resistance you've selected on the machine, because you are moving all of it upward. On the other hand, when you do *seated leg curls* (bottom image in Figure 6-6), the machine's lever arm, plus the weight of your lower legs, are SUBTRACTED from the weight you've selected on the machine. Although the machine's resistance is being pulled upward, the weight of the machine's lever arm, as well as that of your lower legs, is being pulled downward.

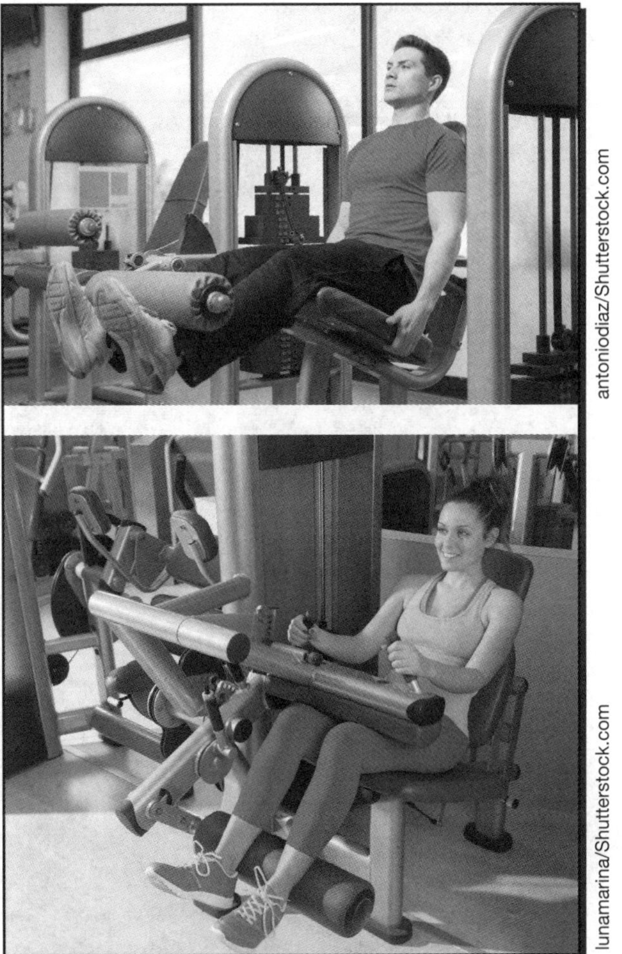
antoniodiaz/Shutterstock.com
lunamarina/Shutterstock.com

Figure 6-6

In situations like the aforementioned ones, the secondary resistance source either "adds to" or "subtracts from" the primary resistance source, but the mechanics of the exercise are not altered much, if at all, by the secondary resistance source. On the other hand, there are times when the direction of the *primary* resistance and of the *secondary* resistance are not simply "up" or "down." When the directions of resistance are not utterly opposite, but multi-directional, it significantly alters the mechanics of an exercise. This factor could be good, if planned and intentional, or it could be bad, if accidental (unintentional and uninformed).

## Composite Direction of Resistance

The exercise shown in Figure 6-7, *cable squats*, has two different resistance sources. Normally, when you perform squats, your body weight is considered as the "primary" source of resistance. As such, any added weight would be considered the "secondary" source. In the exercise in Figure 6-7, while you can still call the cable resistance as the "secondary" source, the direction of the cable resistance is what makes this exercise so unique and beneficial. As such, it can easily be argued that the cable is the "primary" resistance.

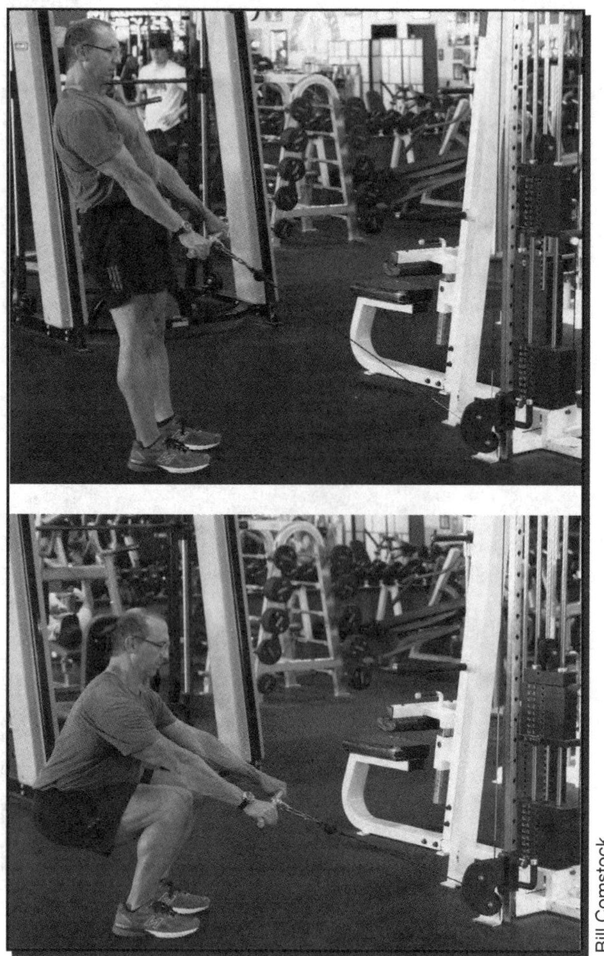

Figure 6-7

Of course, because both directions of resistance are present simultaneously, an exerciser needs to play an active role in coordinating the two, in terms of balance. The lighter the cable resistance is, the more upright a person is able to stand. The heavier the cable resistance is, the more an individual needs to lean backward in order to prevent being pulled forward/off balance. It is interesting to note that the more the exerciser leans backward (as necessitated by the amount of cable resistance), the more beneficial the angle is for quadriceps loading.

The direction of the cable pull varies between 40 degrees and 20 degrees, depending on how far back you stand, and whether you are in the standing position or the descended position. For the sake of this analysis and explanation, let's just use the average of 30 degrees.

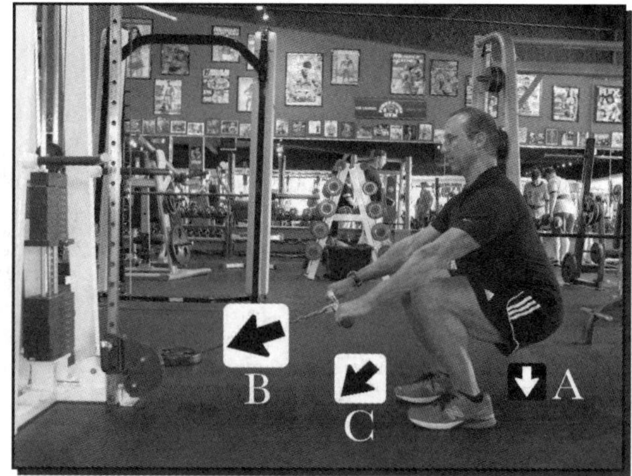

Figure 6-8

The exerciser's body weight, which is about 200 pounds ("A" in Figure 6-8), and the additional 100 pounds of weight coming from the cables ("B" in Figure 6-8) are pulling in two different directions. The two, however, meld into one "composite" direction of resistance, somewhere around 60 degrees ("C" in Figure 6-8). The exact angle of the composite resistance would depend on the ratio between your bodyweight and the amount of cable resistance being used. The less weight that is used on the cables, the closer the composite direction shifts toward 90 degrees (vertical). The more weight that is provided by the cables, the closer the composite direction shifts toward 30 degrees (the angle of the cable).

The basic purpose of *cable squats* is to provide a more perpendicular direction of resistance, relative to the tibia (the operating lever of the quadriceps), than typically occurs during a standard *barbell squat*. As such, any amount of forward pulling cable resistance (used as a secondary resistance) would be better than the purely straight-down direction of resistance encountered during regular *barbell squats*.

In reality, a *straight-down-only* direction of resistance does not cross the tibia perpendicularly enough to qualify as an "excellent" direction of resistance for a quadriceps exercise, unless you are very novice. Adding a secondary resistance that pulls "slightly downward, but more forward" is an excellent strategy for enhancing the load on the quadriceps.

It's important to recognize that these two directions of resistance ("A" and "B" in Figure 6-8) BLEND together, creating a new direction of resistance that is neither 90 degrees ("straight down" gravity) nor 30 degrees (the average angle of the cables). Of course, this composite direction of resistance is invisible—like gravity. On the other hand, you need to be aware of this factor in order to accurately assess the exercise, based on how perpendicular the direction of resistance is, relative to the tibia.

There is another type of force at play, as well, during cable squats. It's called "friction force," which refers to the fact that there is a forward "sliding" effect that is trying to occur at the level of the feet. You can actually feel your feet sliding forward inside your shoes. The grip of the shoe tread on the rubber floor mat prevents you from sliding forward, which is referred to as "friction force." This factor will be further explained toward the end of this chapter.

There is another example that can help clarify how you can strategically separate the primary and secondary resistance sources, so that you are better able to load the target muscle, while simultaneously reducing or eliminating the load that could strain a non-target muscle. For example, when you do *bent over rear deltoid raises* with dumbbells (Figure 6-9), your goal is to target the posterior deltoids. In this case, the *primary resistance* of the exercise is the dumbbells, which is intended to load the posterior deltoids. The lower back, however, is also being loaded by the weight of those dumbbells, PLUS the weight of the torso itself (*the secondary resistance*). In fact, the lower back is loaded more than are the posterior deltoids, because it's getting both loads. Since the secondary resistance (the weight of the torso) is not contributing any load at all to the posterior deltoids, it would be wise to eliminate it.

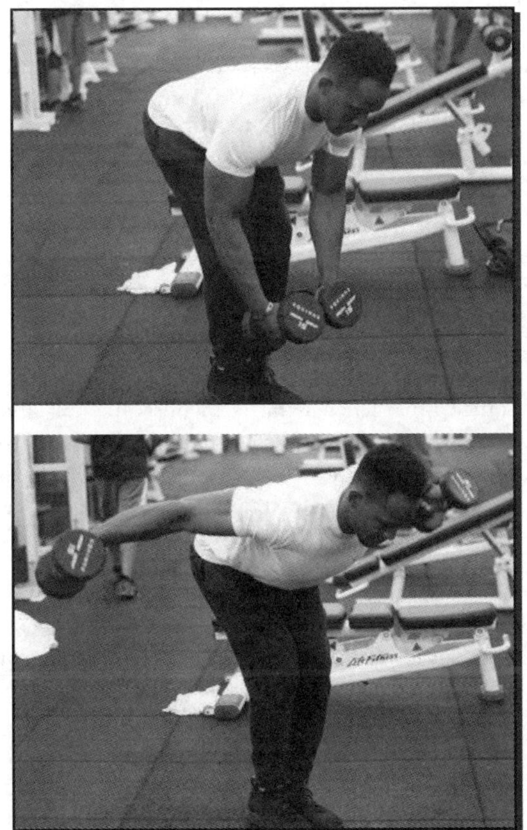
Bill Comstock

Figure 6-9

One possible solution to this issue is shown in Figure 6-10. While it's the same exercise, with regard to the posterior deltoids, using a bench as support relieves the lower back of some of the torso weight. The torso weight cannot be entirely eliminated this way, so the lower back is still loaded, to some degree. This version of the exercise, however, is still significantly more safe than the version detailed in Figure 6-9, even though it is not very comfortable for the head and neck. Furthermore, this version of the exercise requires finding a bench that is the appropriate height, i.e., about the height of the hips.

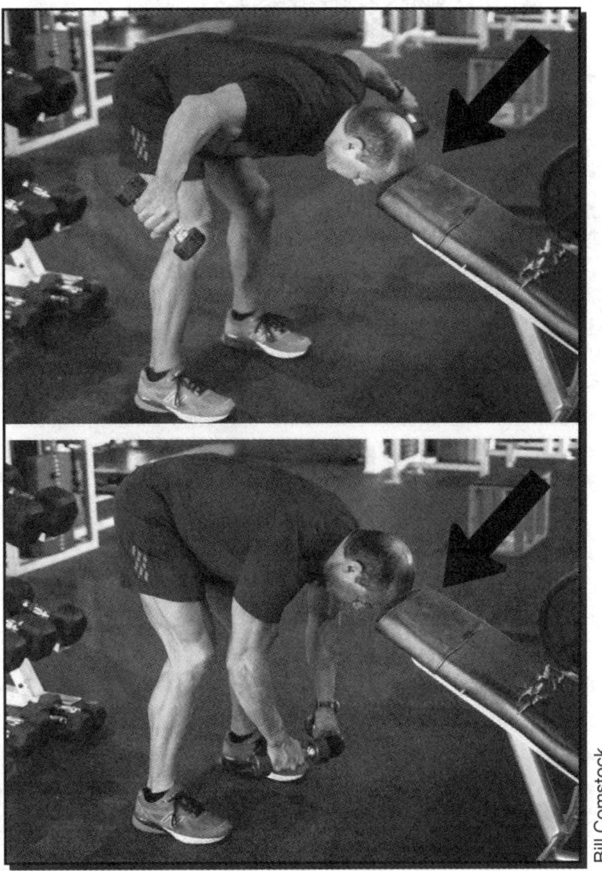
Bill Comstock

Figure 6-10

Although this exercise is more safe on the lower back (as compared to the version shown in Figure 6-9), it is still not a "great" posterior deltoid exercise. This shortcoming is because both of the aforementioned versions are "*late-phase loaded.*" Both of these exercises are "lightest" at the beginning of the range of motion (because the arms begin vertically at the neutral position). That, however, is where the posterior deltoids are strongest. Subsequently, the resistance is "heaviest" at the end of the range of motion (because the arms are then horizontal—perpendicular with gravity), which is where the posterior deltoids are weakest.

Figure 6-11 shows a third version of a rear deltoid exercise, performed with cables. The *primary resistance* source is the cables, and, as you can see, they are coming from two different directions. At first glance, it might appear as though two primary resistance sources exist—one for each posterior deltoid (left and right). In reality, however, each posterior deltoid only has one primary resistance source.

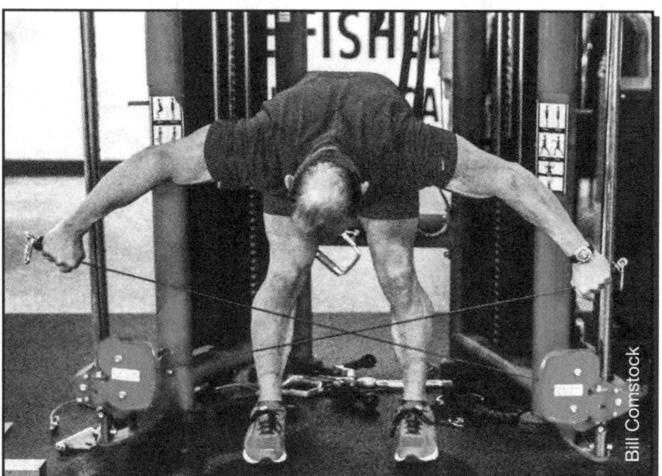

Figure 6-11

The direction of resistance provided by the cables in Figure 6-11 is significantly better than that which is provided by the dumbbells (free weight gravity) in the previous two examples. This improvement is because it provides more early-phase loading of the posterior deltoids. On the other hand, you still have some degree of load on your lower back. It's less than that of the first example (Figure 6-9), because the two cables are not pulling straight down. As such, they are pulling from an angle that is more from the sides, than straight down. This situation produces a composite downward resistance that is approximately half of that which the dumbbells would produce. Still, this factor, combined with the weight of the unsupported torso, makes this exercise less-than-ideal, due to excessive lower back strain.

Figure 6-12 shows another version of this exercise. While it has the same movement and a similar resistance curve for the posterior deltoids as the version shown in Figure 6-11, this one is performed while lying supine on a flat bench. In this version, the *primary resistance* is that which is coming from the cables. The torso weight has been eliminated. It is no longer a factor in this version. As such, the erector spinae is no longer loaded. You are now in a comfortable position from which you can focus on targeting the posterior deltoids.

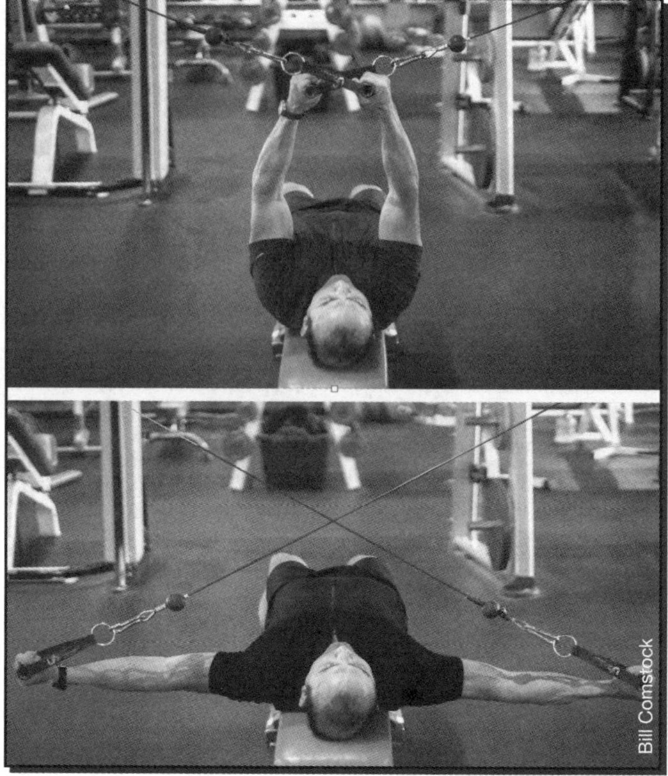

Figure 6-12

There is a new *secondary resistance* source in this instance, however—the weight of the arms (and the handles, although it isn't much). In fact, this resistance source existed in the three previous versions of the exercise. In those cases, however, it was adding to the posterior deltoid resistance. In the version shown in Figure 6-12, the weight of the arms (and handles) is subtracting from the posterior deltoid resistance, because the primary resistance (the cables) is pulling upward, while the weight of the arms and handles is being pulled downward.

Of course, this deficit is fairly inconsequential, and can easily be compensated by a small increase in the weight selected on the weight stack. As such, this exercise provides a productive resistance curve for the posterior deltoids, without the problems associated with your torso weight overloading your lower back.

In reality, the aforementioned exercise is not necessarily "the best" posterior deltoid exercise, although it is relatively good. A better option will be discussed in Chapter 20 ("Deltoids"). The primary purpose of comparing the three versions of the aforementioned exercises is to show how primary and secondary resistance sources affect the mechanics of an exercise. It also illustrates how you can manipulate the two (or three) resistance sources, so that you can make the best exercise selections.

## Improperly Adding a Second Resistance Source

In Figure 6-13, you can see an individual performing this exercise correctly (even though this is not the "ideal" exercise for the obliques). He is holding a dumbbell in his right hand only. He is not also holding a second dumbbell in his left hand.

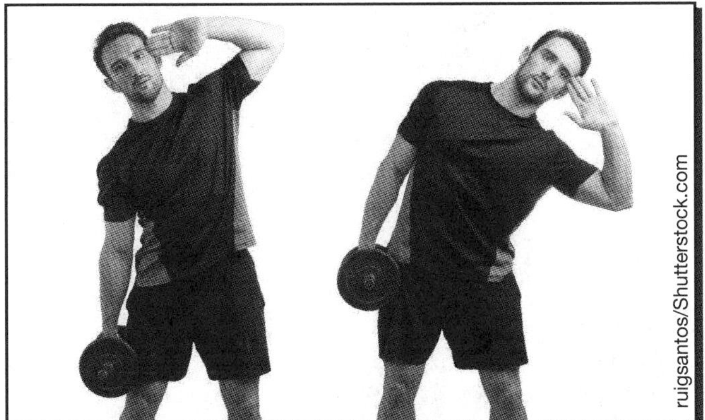


Figure 6-13

Holding the dumbbell in his right hand causes his torso to be weighted TOWARD the right side, which causes the LEFT "obliques" (the muscles on the left side of the waist) to work in opposition of the pull toward the RIGHT. That is how an exercise for the obliques is meant to work.

This exercise must be performed in two stages, because each "oblique" pulls in the torso in the OPPOSITE direction. The left oblique muscles are challenged ("worked") by a weight that is held in the right hand, and pulls the torso to the right. In contrast, the right oblique muscles are challenged by the weight that is held in the left hand, and pulls the torso to the left.

Despite the obvious logic of this, you occasionally see people in the gym performing this exercise while holding TWO dumbbells at the same time—one in each hand (Figure 6-14). The addition of the second dumbbell significantly compromises the exercise. The two dumbbells simply cancel each other out.

This situation creates an effect similar to that of a "seesaw" (Figure 6-15). The two sides neutralize each other, so that ZERO force is required by the oblique muscles of either side. The dumbbell on the left helps pull up the dumbbell that's on the right, while the dumbbell that's on the right helps pull up the dumbbell that's on the left.

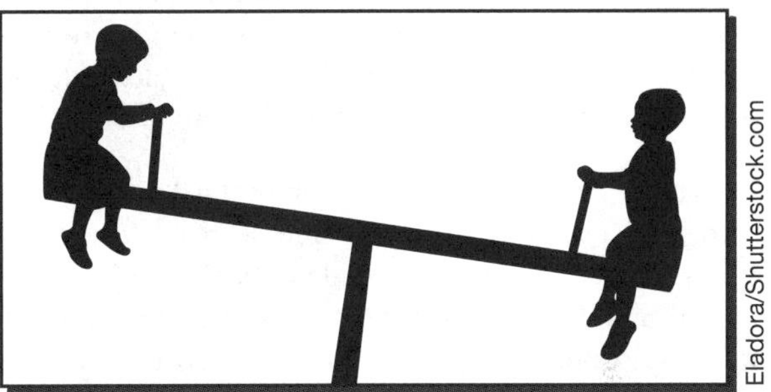


Figure 6-15

While neither side's obliques are benefiting much from this, the straight downward pull of the two dumbbells isometrically loads the upper trapezius muscle fibers, unnecessarily and unproductively. It also produces additional downward compression on the spine. In other words, this "two-dumbbell" version of a *side bend* produces virtually no benefit to the target muscles (the obliques), while needlessly straining the trapezius and spine.

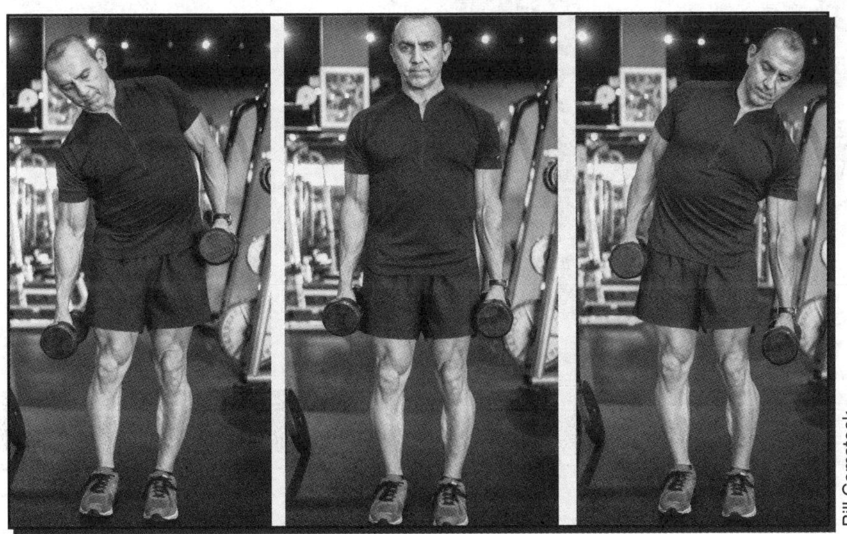


Figure 6-14

## Centrifugal Force and Momentum

In addition to the two resistance sources previously discussed (body weight, as well as the additional resistance of "free weight," cable or machine), there are several other forces that sometimes play a role in resistance exercise. These other forces are not visible, nor are they obvious. On the other hand, they greatly influence many of the exercises that are performed with weights.

"*Centrifugal force*" is a force that is generated as a consequence of rapid circular movement. You'll recall Isaac Newton's First Law of Motion: "*An object at rest stays at rest, and an object in motion stays in motion with the same speed and direction, unless acted upon by an unbalanced force.*" This form of "resistance" comes from a particular movement "wanting" to continue along the path it has been launched, as it is rotating around an axis.

A clear example of this factor is the "hammer throw" (Figure 6-16), an event that is often seen in "track & field" contests. In this event, the athlete begins with a circular swing of a weighted ball that is attached to a cable that is connected to a handle, which he holds. A representation of this centrifugal force is what you see in Figure 6-17—the weighted ball moving away from the thrower as he is performing the event, and then when the ball is finally launched. As such, the weighted ball "wants" to continue outward, in a straight line, from each and every point in its circular trajectory.

That outward force is counterbalanced by the athlete leaning his body weight away from the weighted ball's trajectory. His body weight and backward lean, referred to as "*centripetal force*" in this scenario, are opposing the ball's trajectory, until the handle is released.

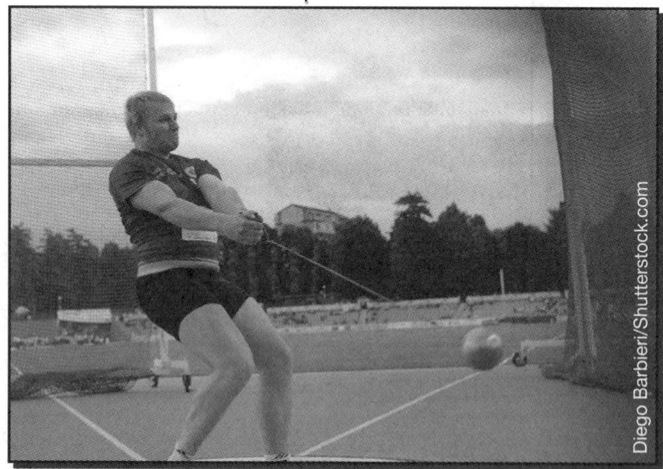


Figure 6-16

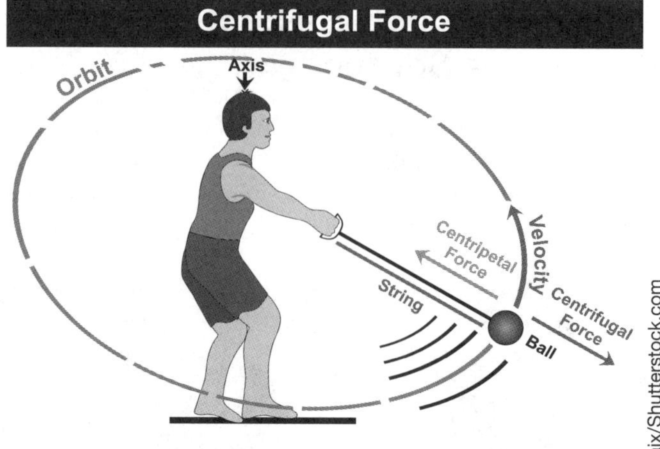


Figure 6-17

In reality, centrifugal force is not commonly found in conventional weight training, because you rarely "swing" anything circularly, around an axis. On the other hand, centrifugal force is seen in some kettlebell exercises, like the one in Figure 6-18.

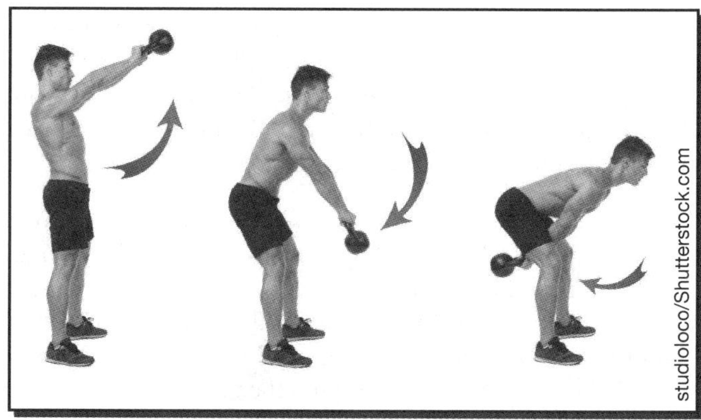


Figure 6-18

In order to assess an exercise like the one in Figure 6-18, you would need to consider the weight of the kettlebell, the speed of the swing, the trajectory of the ball, and the position of the limbs through that trajectory, in order to understand which muscles are loaded, how much they are loaded, and when (through the swing) they are loaded. As you can see, the direction of resistance is not linear. It is not vertical. It is curved, like that of a hammer throw.

Although this particular exercise would not be considered a good "bodybuilding"/muscular development exercise, it is a relatively good general conditioning exercise. It stimulates the quads, glutes, adductors, and erector spinae. It does not stimulate the shoulders (deltoids) as much as it might appear, because the swing upward is mostly generated by the propulsion created by the lower body (see "momentum" in Chapter 14).

This exercise also stimulates the cardiovascular system. When performing this exercise, perfect form is required, or else there is a high risk of lower back injury.

In reality, most of the exercises performed in the pursuit of muscular development are linear and very deliberate. They do not involve "swinging"—nor should they.

"*Ground reaction force*" and "*friction force*" are two types of force that are commonly found in resistance training exercises. In fact, they often interplay with each other. As such, Newton's Third Law of Motion states that "*for every action, there is an equal and opposite reaction.*" This law describes very accurately how these two types of force operate in resistance exercise.

In Figure 6-19, you can see a man pulling on a rope. In the top image, the rope is attached to a wall. In the bottom image, the rope is attached to an elephant. In both instances, the scale measures the same amount of force (500 N). In the example involving the elephant, it's obvious that the elephant is pulling with a force that is equal to the force generated by the man. What is *not* so obvious, is that the wall is also "pulling" with a force that is equal to the force being generated by the man.

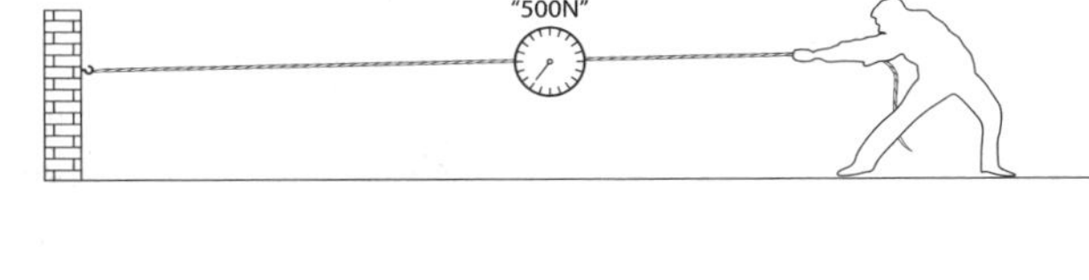


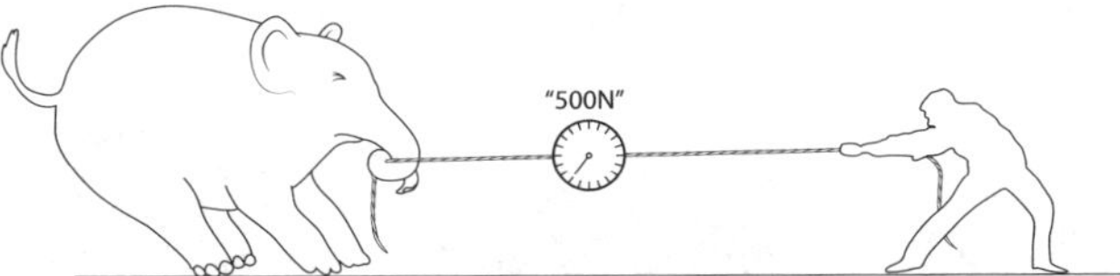


Figure 6-19

(Note: N = "newtons" / one newton = 0.22 pounds / one pound = 4.44 newtons)

You might argue that the wall is not "actively" pulling. In fact, the wall is actually "resisting" an amount of force that is equal to that which is provided by the elephant. A wall that is "resisting" a force is the same as a force that is provided by a living creature or by a barbell. The amount of force the man encounters is identical. As such, "ground reaction force" is essentially the force created by the ground, or by any other solid object or brace, as it resists a person's "push" or "pull."

In Figure 6-20, you see a man performing a barbell squat with 225 pounds on his back. That amount of weight, combined with his own body weight (assume that it's 190 pounds), totals 415 pounds. In essence, he is pushing downward, against the ground, with that amount of force.

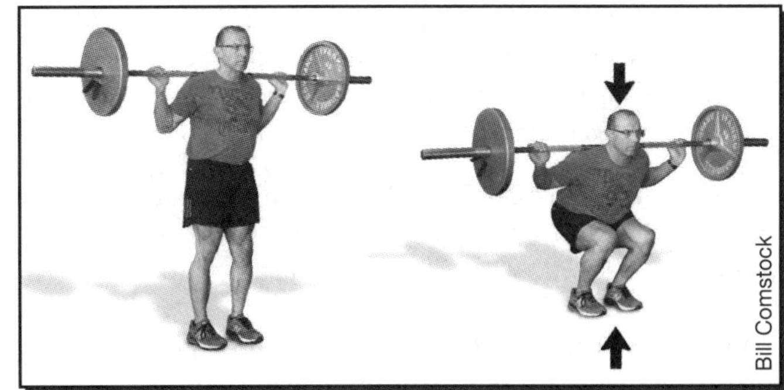


Figure 6-20

The ground below his feet is supporting that amount of weight. Basically, the ground is *exerting* 415 pounds of upward force, to match the amount of force with which the man is pushing downward. The ground is not sinking under him, as would happen if the ground was "pushing" upward with LESS than 415 pounds of force. Nor is the ground rising under him, as would happen, if the ground was "pushing" upward with MORE than 415 pounds of force.

It is worth noting in the aforementioned example that in addition to the ground matching the *amount* of force the man is producing, it is also matching his *direction* of force. Since he is "pushing" straight downward, the ground is "pushing" straight upward.

The following illustrates an instance in which "friction force" often interplays with "ground reaction force." In Figure 6-21, you can see a sprinter coming out of the "starting blocks." The reason sprinters use starting blocks is to prevent any backward slide of their feet, when their legs produce the explosive backward force that results in their forward propulsion. Thus, the secured starting blocks become part of the "ground," against which the runner applies a certain amount of force, in the particular (downward/backward) direction you see in Figure 6-21. In response, the "ground" (which now includes the starting blocks) delivers an "*equal* and *opposite*" amount of force, by resisting any backward slide.

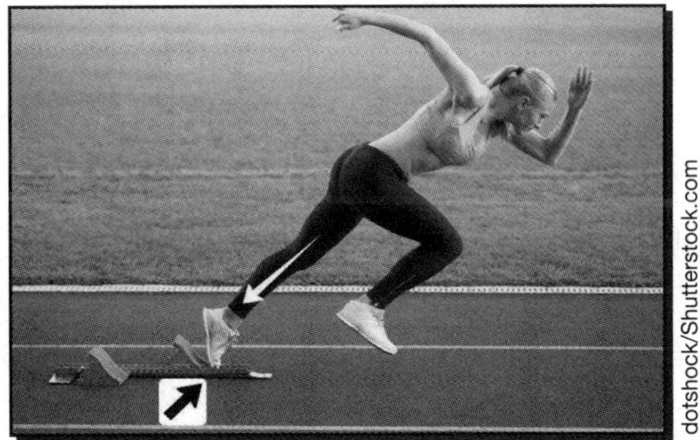


Figure 6-21

In other words, "ground reaction force" could be defined as follows: *An immovable "brace" against which another force is applied (even when it's not part of the actual "ground"), which results in an equal (amount) and opposite (direction) of force.*

In reality, the slightly backward force produced by the sprinter's forward propulsion is called *"friction force."* As you can see, however, it combines with the upward force of the ground and jointly produces an *"opposing force."* From a mathematical standpoint, the amount of friction force (being horizontal) and the amount of ground reaction force (being vertical) equals a *direction of force* that is exactly opposite the *direction of thrust* produced by the athlete.

In an assessment of resistance exercise, this factor matters immensely, because the direction of a person's effort (pushing or pulling) must be factored into the calculation, especially when there's some kind of "brace" involved, or when the direction of thrust is not directly opposite gravity.

Consider, for example, the exercise *"squats against the wall with a Swiss ball"* (Figure 6-22). An assumption might be made that the direction of resistance, during this exercise, is straight down—like "free weight gravity"—but it is not.

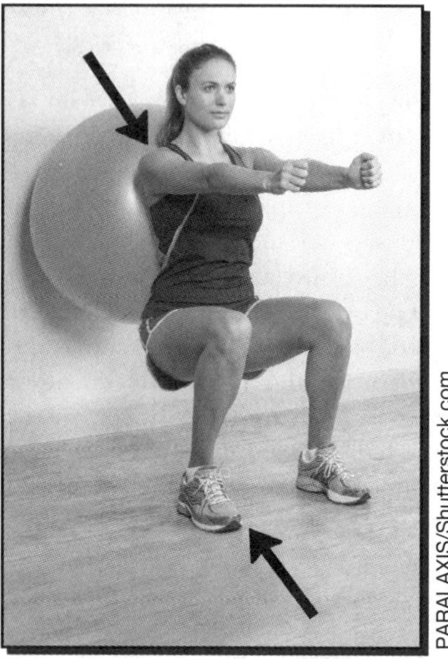


Figure 6-22

Unlike the example of the man performing a standard barbell squat, the direction of the exerciser's thrust in Figure 6-22 is NOT straight upward. This individual's thrust is angled upward and slightly backward, approximately 20 degrees from vertical. Therefore, her application of force against the ground is not straight downward. Instead, her application of force is downward and slightly forward.

Therefore, the *direction of the opposing force* (ground reaction force plus friction force) is upward and slightly backward, directly opposite the man's direction of force. This different direction of opposing force is significantly different than that which is produced during a *standard barbell squat.*

The *direction of resistance* always determines which levers (limbs) are active, and to what degree they are active. As such, the exercise shown in Figure 6-22 (*wall squats with a Swiss ball*) cannot be evaluated using a vertical direction of resistance. The direction of resistance is *actually* produced by the ground reaction force, combined with the friction force, and—in the case of the aforementioned example—results in the angle of force indicated by the arrow pointing upward. THAT is the direction of resistance of this exercise. As such, it is what should be used to evaluate how "active" the tibia and femur are during the various stages of this exercise's range of motion.

Consider another example of how an individual's "direction of effort" (resulting from situational friction force combined with gravity) influences the mechanics of a resistance exercise. For example, during a standard *bench press*, you typically exert a degree of lateral pushing combined with upward pushing. This factor is why barbells are knurled, and why you often use chalk to prevent your hands from sliding laterally along the barbell. If the bar was slick (no knurling), and you oiled the bar, you would quickly realize that you are pushing laterally, to some degree. Your grip on the knurled bar (and maybe some chalk) creates a "brace," which prevents your hands from sliding laterally along the bar. This factor acts like the starting blocks, used by the aforementioned sprinter.

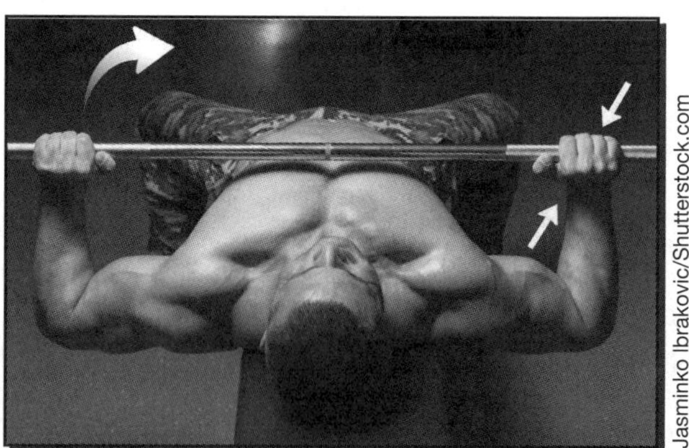


Figure 6-23

The diagonal arrow on the right side of the image in Figure 6-23, indicates the only direction in which the person is able to push, in this particular situation. The curved arrow on the left side of the same image shows the direction in which the arm COULD move, if this person were using dumbbells. On the other hand, when you're using a barbell, you are not able to "pull" the weight *inward* (toward the sternum/the origin of the pectorals). The grip on the barbell prevents it. It only allows an upward/*outward* (semi-horizontal) direction of force. Since the exerciser's direction of "push" is upward and slightly outward (toward the side), the resulting "direction of resistance" that is produced is downward and slightly inward—as indicated by the diagonal-downward arrow.

This downward and slightly inward "direction of resistance" factors into the evaluation of whether his forearm and upper arm are "active," and to what degree they are "active." This is the reason there is triceps participation during a bench press, despite the forearm tilting outward from the apex. This same elbow and forearm position, during a supine dumbbell press, would result in biceps activation—not triceps activation.

The same factor occurs when performing *wide-grip push-ups*, shown in Figure 6-24. Because the force this exerciser is producing originates FROM his shoulder, and because his hands are fixed ("braced") on the ground, his direction of force must be applied in a diagonal (lateral and downward) direction. He cannot push vertically (straight down) from this angle. The opposing resistance that is produced by this set of circumstances (gravity, plus his slightly lateral direction of effort, plus the brace of his hands against the ground) is directly opposite the arrow that is on the image at an upward angle. THAT is the resultant direction of resistance in the wide-grip push-up, which is the factor that you must reference in order to evaluate which muscles are loaded and to what degree they are loaded.

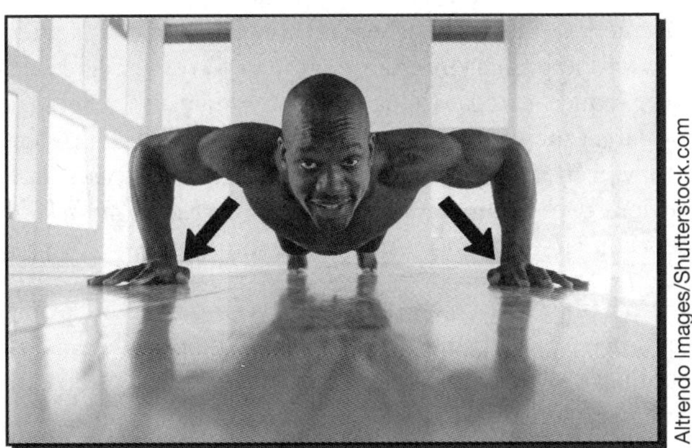


Figure 6-24

Whenever you evaluate an exercise, you not only have to ask yourself "in which direction is the resistance?" but "in which direction is the application of effort?" and "is there a brace opposing it?" In many instances, "friction force" and "ground reaction force" combine, thereby producing an altered direction of resistance. That factor then becomes the guide in determining an exercise's resistance curve. That is the direction of resistance, against which you'll compare the angle of the limbs to determine which muscles are loaded and to what degree they're loaded.

## Momentum Meets Ground Reaction Force and Friction Force

Figures 6-25 and 6-26 provide two versions of a *lunge*—one in which the person steps forward, and one in which she steps backward. In the first example, the *forward lunge* produces a certain amount of forward momentum, which combines with the downward pull of gravity and creates a slightly forward-and-down trajectory. This forward-and-down trajectory is met (once the foot plants on the ground) with a ground reaction force that is precisely in the opposite direction of that slightly forward-and-down trajectory. It's approximately a 70-degree upward-and-backward force. Compare that direction of force (represented by the arrow in Figure 6-25) with the angle of her tibia and her femur.

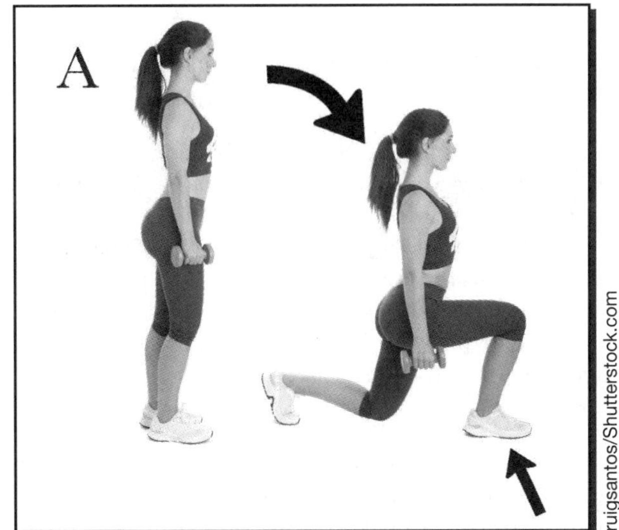



Figure 6-25

Next, look at the second example of a lunge (Figure 6-26). This image shows that a *backward lunge* produces a bit of backward momentum, which combines with the downward pull of gravity and creates a slightly backward-and-down trajectory. This slightly backward-and-down trajectory is met (once the foot plants on the ground) with a ground reaction force that is precisely in the opposite direction of that slightly backward-and-down trajectory. It's approximately 70 degrees upward-and-forward. Compare that trajectory (represented by the arrow in Figure 6-26) with the angle of her tibia and her femur.

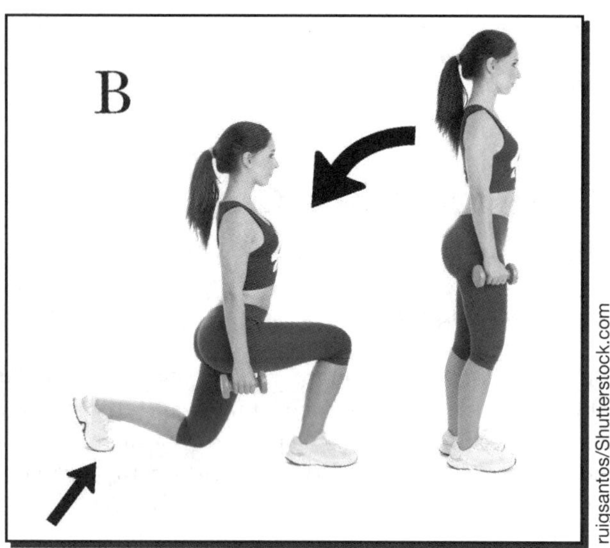

Figure 6-26

When evaluating each of these two types of *lunges*, you should use this altered direction of resistance (the arrows in both Figures 6-25 and 6-26) to determine which version loads the quadriceps more and which loads the gluteus more. More specifically, you should compare the angle of the tibia of both legs, as well as the angle of the femur of both legs, as they relate to the aforementioned arrows.

As such, you can easily see that the forward lunge would load the quadriceps of the front leg more than the backward lunge, because the tibia of the front leg is more perpendicularly front-loaded with its arrow, than the tibia of the backward lunge is with its arrow. The backward lunge, however, would load the gluteus of the front leg more than the forward lunge, because the femur of the front leg is more perpendicularly loaded with its arrow, than the femur of the forward lunge is with its arrow.

Of course, you should also factor in the direction of force that you must produce in order to return back to the original standing position. The forward lunge requires a sort of front leg "knee extension," in order to propel your body up and back. In contrast, the backward lunge requires more of a front leg "hip extension," in order to propel your body up and forward.

The aforementioned demonstrates how the addition of momentum can create a change in the opposing force, (i.e., the altered direction of resistance, based on the combination of ground reaction force and friction force). This altered direction of force relates directly to which levers are more or less "active," and, therefore, which muscles are more or less loaded. It also demonstrates how a person's direction of thrust must be factored into the biomechanical assessment of an exercise.

## Summary

Whenever you perform any kind of movement, against any kind of opposing force (resistance), you should always be aware of whether there is a secondary resistance, as well as maybe even a tertiary resistance, in play. You should also be cognizant of whether those additional sources of resistance are simply adding to the primary source, subtracting from the primary source, or altering the mechanics of the exercise.

Furthermore, you should be mindful of whether the additional source(s) of resistance is working in your favor (adding additional stimulation to the target muscle), or detracting from the benefit of the target muscle, or simply creating unnecessary strain or risk of injury. Two or three directions of resistance may blend together and become one single (composite) direction of resistance, one that is different from the direction of resistance that may appear to be in play.

When an additional resistance source (e.g., dumbbells, cables, machines or limb weight, or the interplay with momentum, ground force reaction and friction force) provides "resistance" in a direction that is not simply straight down (as occurs with "free weight gravity"), the modified direction of resistance needs to be taken into consideration, in order to determine which levers (limbs) are more or less active.

In most instances, the secondary resistance—or its placement on the body (where or how it is held)—will alter the effect of the primary resistance, at least to some degree. It will either reduce it, negate it, or add to it. It may also activate other non-target muscles in ways that would likely not be productive. It may even increase the risk of injury. In some cases, like the previous two examples—*cable squats* and *cable rear deltoids*—the secondary resistance can be used strategically.

Whether you refer to body weight as the "primary" resistance source, and the added resistance (e.g., barbell, dumbbells, cables, elastic bands, etc.) as the "secondary" resistance source, is irrelevant. What matters most is that you understand that there is more than one resistance source involved in most exercises. The weight of your body, your limbs, handles, bars, machine carriages, momentum, "ground reaction force," and "friction force" should always be considered in order to accurately assess an exercise.

# CHAPTER 7

# ALIGNMENT

- *In the context of resistance exercise, striving to keep the direction of movement, the direction of resistance, and the angle of the operating lever of the target muscle, as well as the origin and the insertion of the target muscle—all on one plane—significantly improves efficiency.*
- *When this situation occurs, all or most of the "load" (resistance) being used during that exercise is directed toward the target muscle. When that occurs, joint distortion (strain) is minimized or eliminated, and the unintentional loading of smaller, non-target muscles is reduced, which significantly decreases injury risk.*
- *When the aforementioned markers are not in alignment, a percentage of the load is diverted away from the target muscle and loaded onto smaller/weaker muscles. Furthermore, joint distortion often occurs, which further increases the risk of injury.*

When you see someone doing a *standing barbell curl* (for their biceps), you take for granted that as that person pulls upward, gravity is pulling directly in the opposite direction (i.e., downward), along the same plane.

The plane through which the forearm (as the operating lever of the biceps) travels is aligned with the direction of resistance, as well as with the origin and the insertion of the biceps. In addition, the angle of the forearm is in alignment with these markers. This alignment is *not* an incidental aspect of the resistance exercise. In fact, it is essential for maximum efficiency.

In Figure 7-1, notice that the forearm travels through the plane that aligns with the biceps origin and the biceps insertion. The trajectory of the forearm (traveling up or down) is on the same plane as the downward resistance, which is as it should be. The same factor can be said for all "good" exercises, even though the importance of this principle is often overlooked.

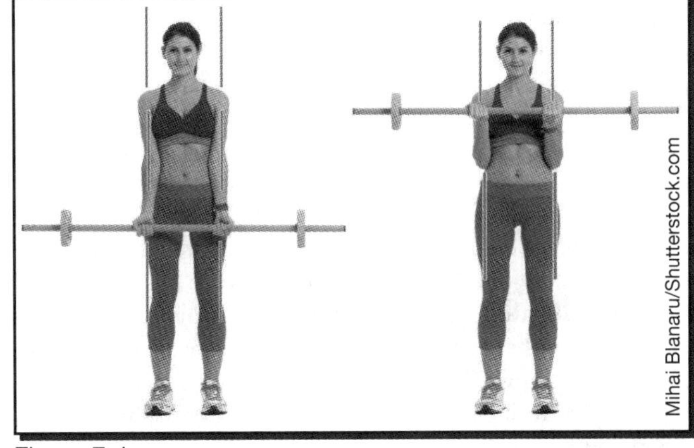


Figure 7-1

For example, when you do triceps pushdowns (Figure 7-2), you again comply with this principle, even though you may not be entirely aware of it. The cable provides an *upward* resistance, and you "oppose" it by pushing directly opposite (i.e., *downward*) through the same plane. That plane also aligns with the origin and insertion of the triceps.

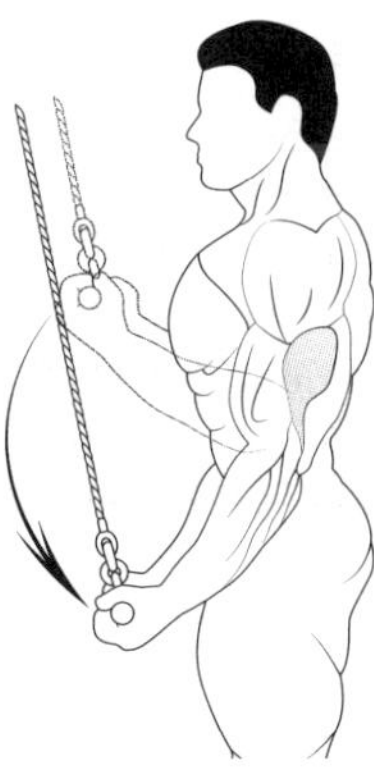

Figure 7-2

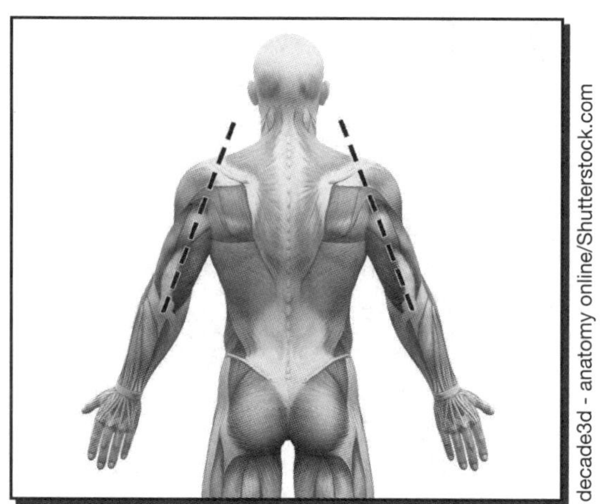

Figure 7-3

## The Consequence of Misalignment

Of course, there are degrees of compliance and non-compliance, based on how well you're doing the exercise (i.e., exercise "form"). Perfect alignment gives you maximum efficiency. The more out of alignment these factors are, the more the efficiency of the exercise is compromised.

Chapters 18 through 25 closely examine the origins and the insertions of all the physique muscles, as well as the direction of those muscle fibers. These chapters also look at the apparent design of the joint over which those muscles cross. These factors help inform you of what is the "primary function" of those muscles—what constitutes the "ideal anatomical movement" of those muscles. This factor suggests the ideal "pathway" the operating levers of those muscles should take during a "good" exercise, one that is intended to develop those muscles.

Therefore, this chapter does not devote too much time discussing muscle origins and insertions. Rather, the focus of this chapter is on the alignment of the three other factors—the *direction of movement*, the *direction of resistance*, and the *angle of the operating lever* of a target muscle.

## Alignment of Movement and of Resistance

The concept of "resistance exercise" is based entirely on the principle of challenging a muscle with an opposing resistance, thereby causing it to adapt (to strengthen). If it were it not for an opposing resistance, a muscle would not be challenged.

An "opposing resistance" refers to a load that is pulling in the opposite direction of a movement. This factor may seem like a very obvious requirement, yet you often see people using a resistance that is NOT pulling directly opposite their movement, during an exercise.

In Figures 7-4 and 7-5, you can see "*torso rotation with a weighted ball.*" The muscles that produce this *horizontal* movement in this exercise are mostly the internal and external obliques. They are assisted a bit by "iliocostalis," which is part of the erector spinae group (which runs alongside the spine) and the transverse abdominis.

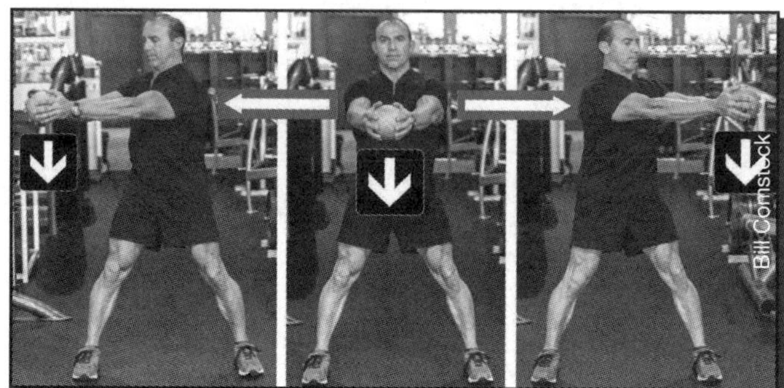

Figure 7-4

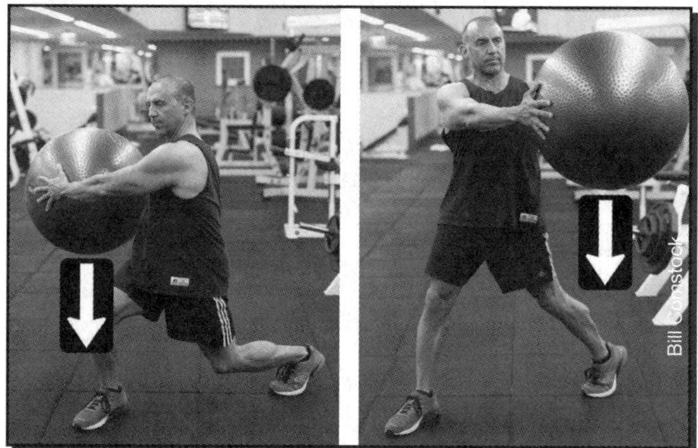

Figure 7-5

As mentioned, this rotation of the torso is *horizontal*—left to right. The resistance provided by the weighted ball, however, is vertical. The ball is being pulled downward by gravity. Therefore, the horizontal movement and the muscles that produce that motion are entirely unchallenged by this downward pulling resistance. There is no "opposition" to the horizontal movement. Ideally, the muscles that produce torso rotation should be made to work AGAINST a resistance that pulls opposite the direction of movement.

During this (ill-conceived) version of a torso rotation exercise, the muscles that are preventing the ball from falling toward the ground are the ones that are being challenged by the weight of the ball—namely the deltoids, biceps, trapezius, lower back, etc. It is important to note that these muscles are *not* the focus of the exercise. Nor is this exercise the ideal way to work these muscles.

In fact, this exercise, as shown, produces virtually no benefit to the *torso rotation* muscles, and very little benefit to the other muscles. This exercise is as foolish as it would be if a person were to lie down on their side and perform a dumbbell curl (Figure 7-6). The direction of movement and the direction of resistance are not on the same plane.

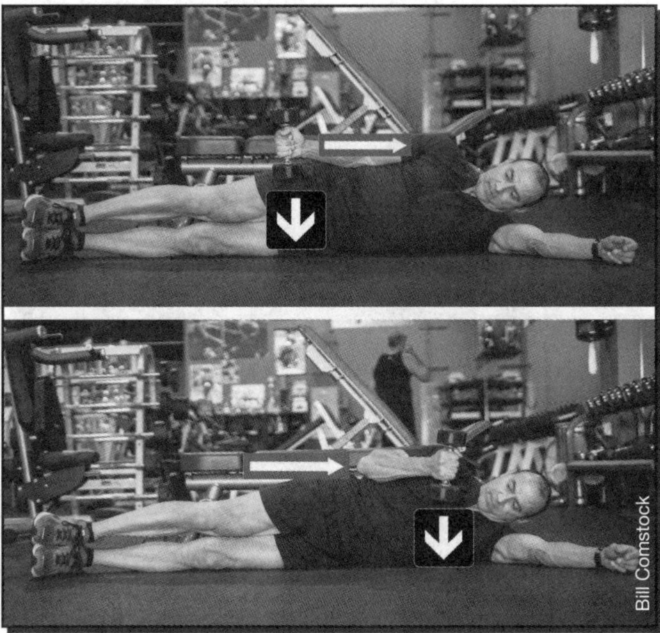


Figure 7-6

The solution is simple. The exerciser should switch from using a weighted ball to a cable that pulls from *either* one side or the other (Figure 7-7). You then rotate the torso in the opposite direction of the cable's pull. You should be aware that this rotation must be performed in TWO separate movements, because it's TWO separate muscles. The left side muscles rotate the torso to the left, and the right side muscles rotate the torso to the right. Each direction of movement requires its own opposing resistance. Then, there is alignment.

Another exercise that people often do, which also lacks alignment, is the one shown in Figure 7-8. This exercise is meant to benefit the rotator cuff muscles of the shoulder, but this horizontal movement cannot possibly be challenged by a vertical resistance. The resistance SHOULD come from the opposite direction of the movement.

The weight the exerciser is holding in his hand in Figure 7-8 is being pulled downward. It is being prevented from falling by the biceps, but this exercise is not meant to be for the biceps. Meanwhile, the rotator cuff muscles are encountering ZERO opposition to their movement, even though they are the intended target of the exercise.

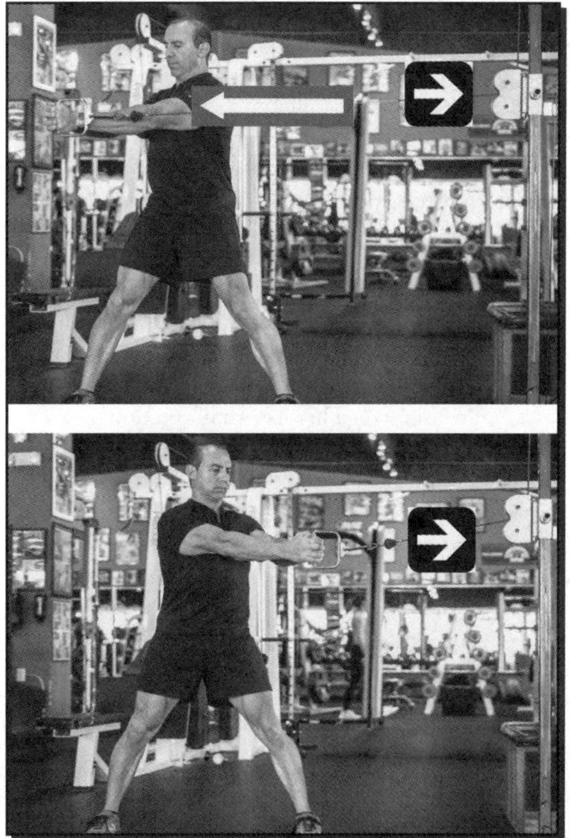


Figure 7-7

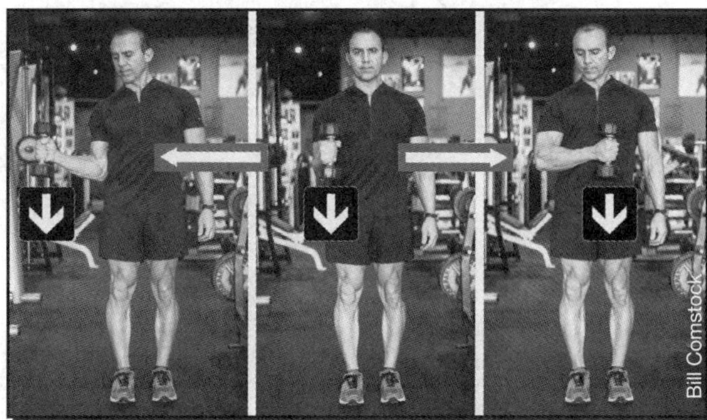


Figure 7-8

In reality, he is performing two separate movements, although he may be entirely unaware of it. He is doing an *inward rotation* of the humerus (upper arm bone), as well as an *outward rotation* of the humerus. These two motions are produced by two different sets of muscles. As such, the way this "pseudo-exercise" is being performed, neither of these two movements is challenged. In fact, what he is doing produces almost no benefit whatsoever to the target muscles (i.e., the internal and external shoulder rotators).

In order to work the "*internal* shoulder rotators," you must work against an outward-pulling resistance. In turn, in order to work the "*external* shoulder rotators," you must work against an inward-pulling resistance. These are two separate directions of movement, each of which requires its own separate, opposing resistance. The two directions of movement (internal and external shoulder rotation) cannot be challenged simultaneously.

Figure 7-9 shows an "*external humeral rotation*" being performed with this person's right arm. The resistance (in this example) comes from an elastic band, which is pulling from the exerciser's left side. He then rotates his arm to his right, against that resistance. This external rotation movement is thus challenged by the resistance that is pulling "internally." He would then turn around and perform the same movement with his left arm, with the resistance pulling from the right. As you can see, the movement and the resistance occur along the same plane. They are in alignment.

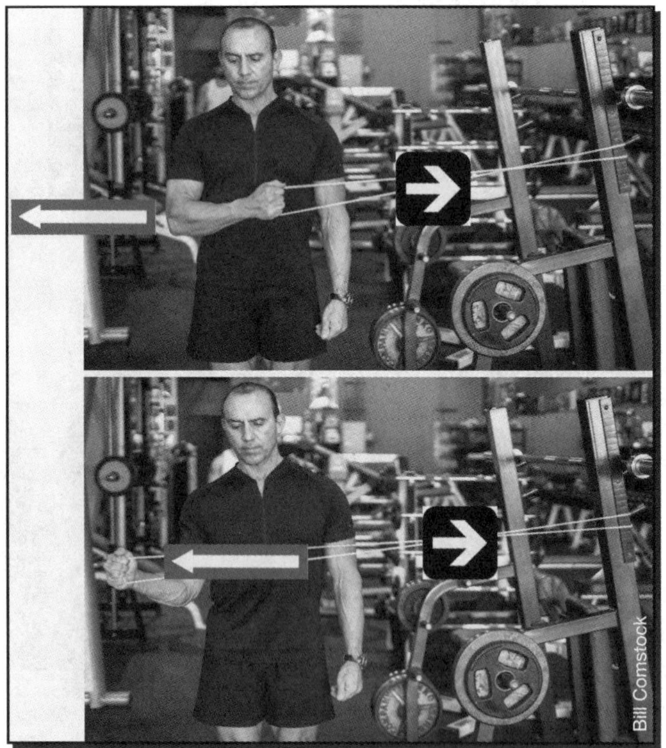


Figure 7-9

After having done both "external rotation" movements (right arm and left arm), a person might then choose to perform the two "internal rotation" movements for his right and left arm, also with an opposing resistance (Figure 7-10). In this instance, you can see the resistance (arrow) coming from his right side, while he rotates his arm "internally" (toward his left) against the opposing resistance. He would then switch sides and do the same movement with the other arm.

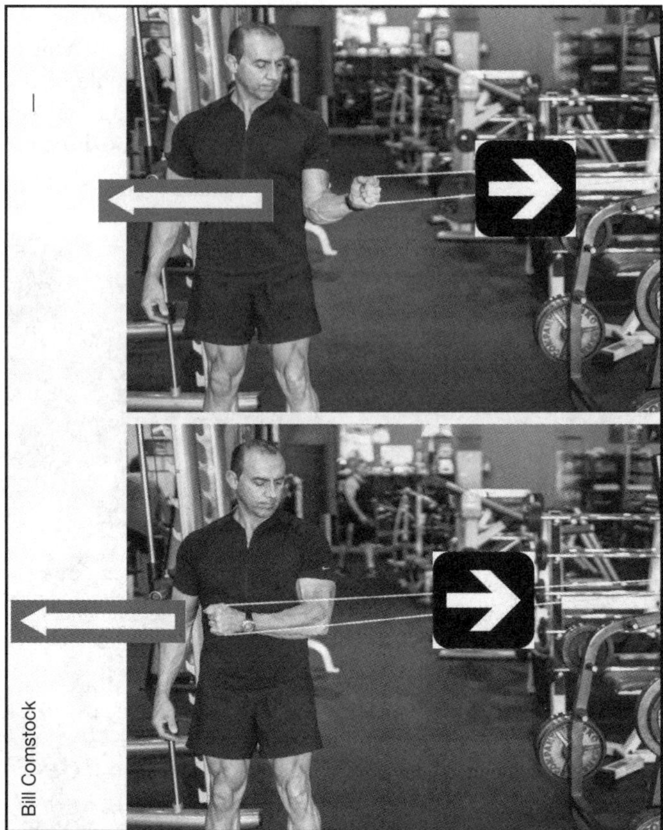


Figure 7-10

Again, as you can see, ALIGNMENT exists between the direction of movement and the direction of resistance. They are both on the same plane.

This exercise can also be performed using conventional pulleys (cables). What is essential is that the resistance originates from a direction that is directly *opposite* the concentric movement. As a rule, muscles should be made to work against an *opposite* direction of resistance.

In the aforementioned examples, it was established that a horizontal movement performed with a vertical resistance does not benefit the muscle producing the horizontal movement. However, misalignment is not always as obvious as that.

In Figure 7-11, you can see a man performing a supine dumbbell press improperly. The reason it's "improper" is because his *direction of movement* is NOT on the same plane as the *direction of resistance*. He is moving his arms at an angle that is approximately 20 degrees from the vertical line, but the *direction of resistance* is perfectly vertical. You can also see that the trajectory of his humerus (which is the operating lever of his target muscle, the pectorals) is also not aligned with the direction of resistance.

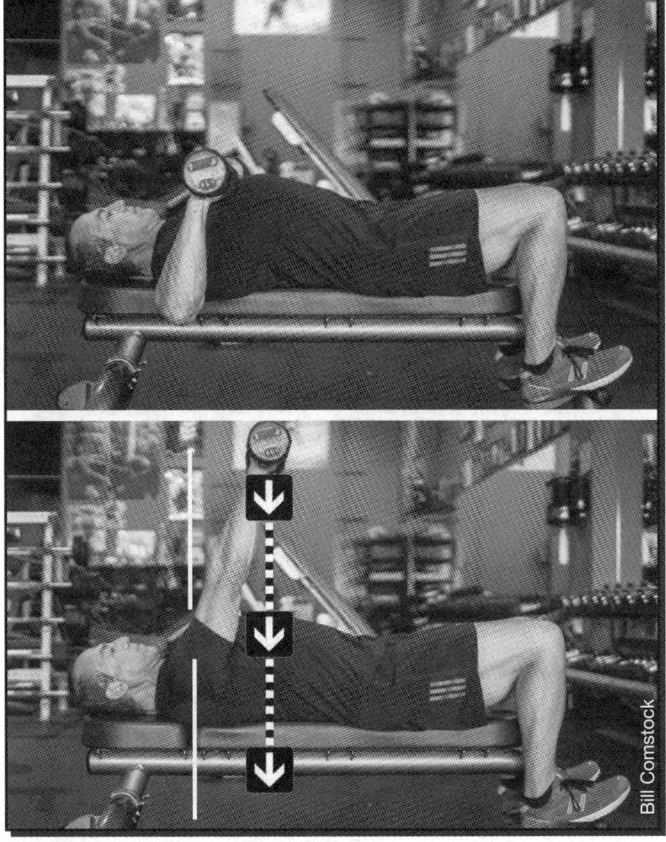

Figure 7-11

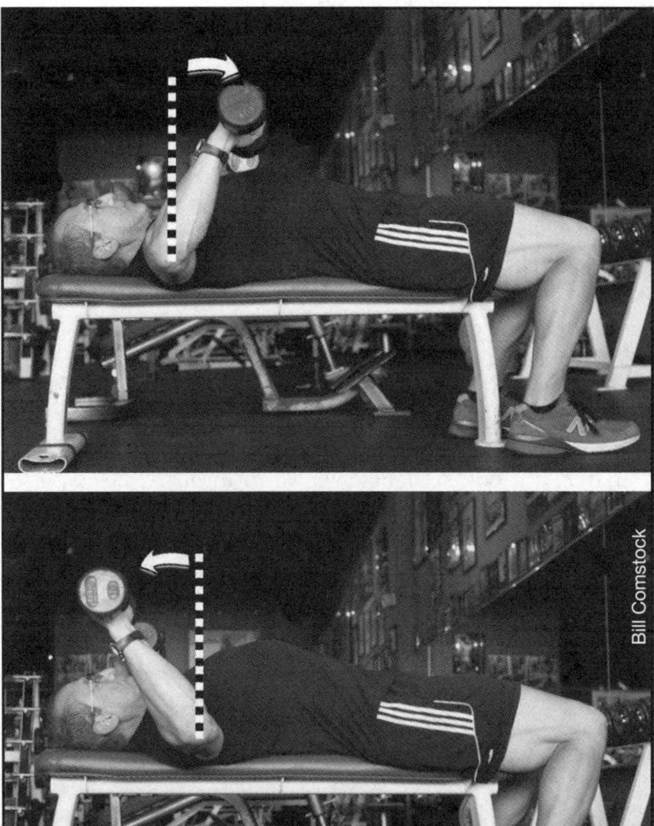

Figure 7-12

This misalignment is less obvious than in the previous two examples. Nevertheless, there is still a lack of alignment occurring. Because this misalignment is not as drastic as the "vertical and horizontal" examples previously mentioned, the degree of compromise is not as great. However, it's still significant. Rather than getting ZERO benefit from this example (Figure 7-11), there is about a 20 percent reduction of load to the target muscle. Furthermore, the amount of load that is reduced from the target muscles (in this case, the pectorals) is shifted over to other weaker, non-target muscles, as well as to the joints.

In addition, by moving the operating levers (upper arms and forearms) in a direction that is not on the same plane as the direction of resistance, a person causes the secondary lever (which would otherwise be neutral) to become active in a potentially injurious way. In Figures 7-12 and 7-13, you can see what happens when you inadvertently tilt the forearm toward your feet and head, while intending to perform a *supine dumbbell press*.

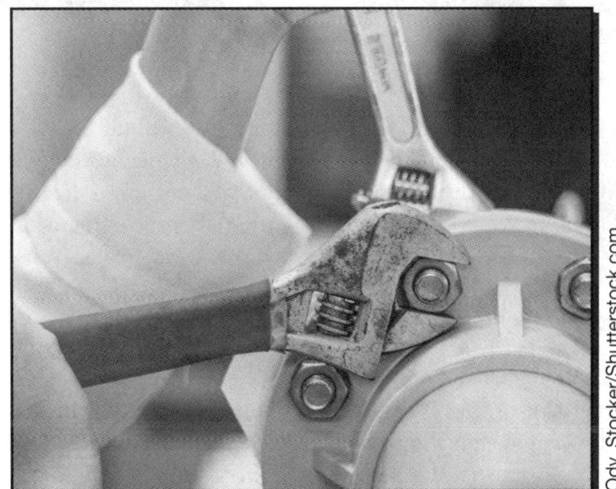

Figure 7-13

By failing to keep the forearm aligned with gravity (during a *supine dumbbell press*), the forearm acts as a wrench when the elbow is bent. It causes rotation (internal or external, depending on which of the two misalignments is occurring) of the humerus in the shoulder socket. This factor forces the smaller, weaker rotator muscles to prevent further misalignment, which could easily strain them in the process.

As discussed previously, perfect alignment in resistance exercise also requires that the *origin* and *insertion of the target muscle* be aligned with the direction of movement, as well as the direction of resistance and the operating levers (primary and secondary) of the target muscle.

In Figure 7-14, you can see what this would look like if you were to look straight downward, through the plane of resistance (gravity) and the direction of the movement, when alignment is correct. As you can clearly see, there is also alignment with the pectoral muscle's origin on the sternum (A), and its insertion on the humerus (B).

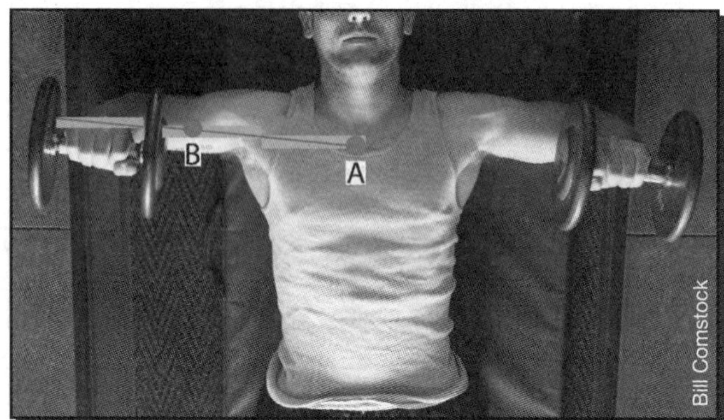

Figure 7-14

This alignment is not a coincidence. It is the only way to load a target muscle, without diluting the resistance, without diverting a portion of the load to unintended muscles and without joint distortion (twisting). Any deviation from this alignment would result in a proportional diminishment of the load to the target muscle, and a commensurate transference of the load to other, non-target muscles, as well as (possibly) some degree of joint strain.

In Figure 7-15, you can see a side view of the perfect alignment that is also shown in Figure 7-14. From this angle, you can see that the upper arms (the primary levers), as well as the forearms (the secondary levers), are also aligned with the shoulder joint, and with the origin and insertion of the pectorals, as well as with the directions of resistance (gravity) and movement.

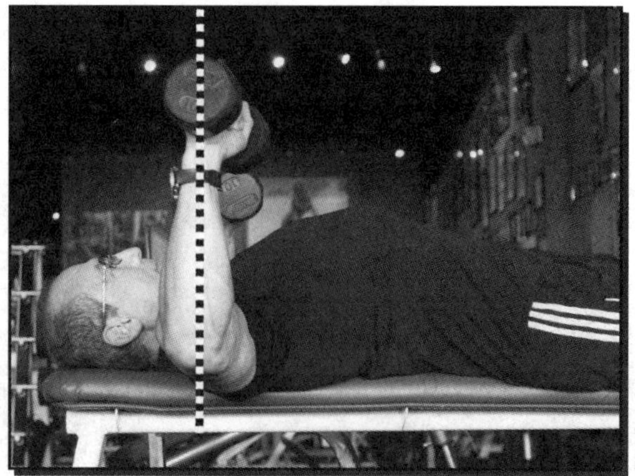

Figure 7-15

At this point, it can be helpful to look at another exercise—*supine dumbbell triceps extensions*. Again, the focus should be on examining the exerciser's alignment, as well as the absence of alignment. While you're at it, you should also note which angles of viewing are best for checking the alignment of an exercise.

Figure 7-16 provides a side view of this exercise. This view allows you to see the resistance curve, the point in the range of motion at which the forearm "crosses" perpendicularly with gravity. From this angle of view, you can see where the operating lever is most "active," and least "active." What you cannot see, however, from this angle of view, is whether or not there is perfect alignment.

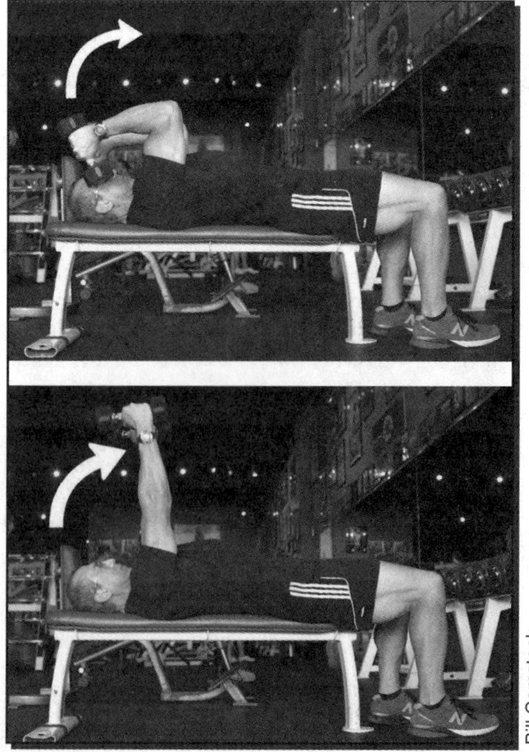

Figure 7-16

## The Viewing Plane of Alignment

When viewing an exercise for the purpose of checking *alignment*, you should view it from a perspective that enables you to see the "planes" of movement and of resistance, as represented by straight lines. The side view in Figure 7-16 allows you to see the arc of the resistance curve, but not the "plane" of either resistance or the movement.

If you go back up and review Figure 7-1 of the woman doing the *barbell curl*, you'll notice it's not a side view. That perspective, when viewing this particular exercise, is why you are able to draw a straight line through both the plane of movement and the plane of resistance.

The same factor was true when analyzing the *triceps pushdown*. A side view would allow you to see the *arc* of the resistance curve, but not the *planes* of resistance and of movement. A front view, however, would allow you to see the plane of resistance and of movement, as represented by straight lines. An overhead view would also allow you to view both of these.

In Figure 7-17, you can see the plane through which gravity pulls, as well as the plane through which the movement travels (i.e., the trajectory of the forearms)—both viewed as straight lines. The first indication of whether the exercise is properly aligned is to see whether those two planes (lines) overlap with each other and appear as one line, as is the case in Figure 7-17.

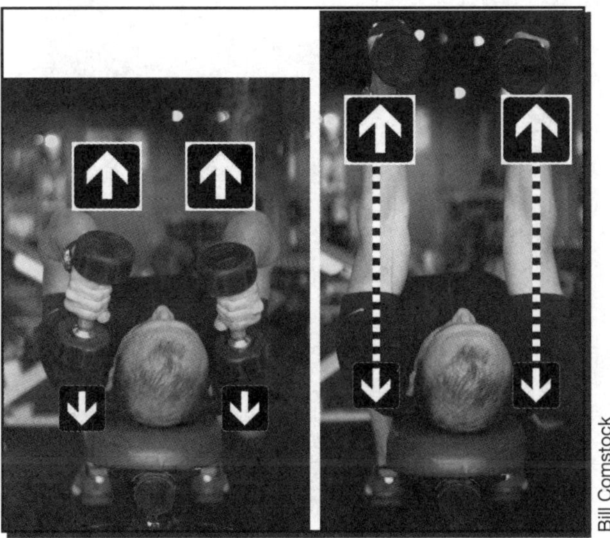


Figure 7-17

The arrow pointing up (indicating concentric movement) and the arrow pointing down (indicating the direction of resistance) are on the same plane. Notice that the origin of the triceps (located on the posterior side of the shoulder) and the insertion of the triceps (located on the olecranon process of the forearm, just below the elbow) are also on that same plane. This exercise is in perfect alignment.

Figure 7-18 shows an overhead view of the same exercise. Again, you see a line that represents the plane through which the anatomical pathway of movement occurs, as well as the direction of resistance. That same line (one for each arm) overlaps with the origin and insertion of the triceps, as well as with the operating lever of the triceps (the forearm). Once more, this view shows perfect alignment.

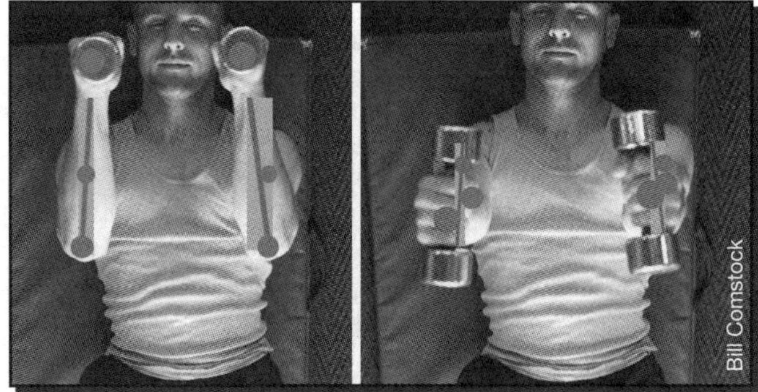


Figure 7-18

Next, Figure 7-19 provides a view of what *misalignment* looks like, from an advantageous perspective, when examining the *supine dumbbell triceps extension*. You can clearly see the *vertical* "down" arrow, representing the direction of gravity, is not on the same plane as the diagonal trajectory of the forearm.

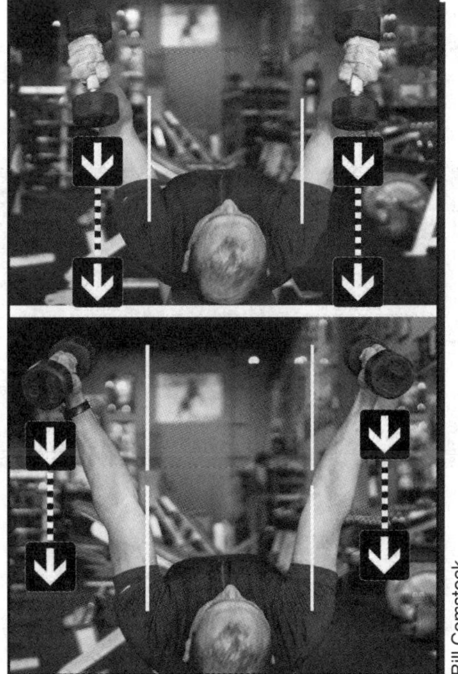


Figure 7-19

Since the elbow is a "hinge" joint and can only extend in one direction, the direction of movement automatically follows the angle of the upper arm. Accordingly, although the origin and insertion of the triceps is aligned with the direction of movement (diagonal), the origin and insertion are not aligned with the direction of resistance (vertical gravity). The operating lever of the triceps (the forearm) is also not aligned with the direction of gravity.

Since the humerus and forearms are not vertical (as is the direction of gravity), they are now loading—and straining—the rotator cuff muscles. In addition, due to the lateral tilt of the upper arms, the pectorals are now slightly loaded. Where is the load on those two (non-target) muscle groups coming from? *It's being subtracted from the triceps load.*

The lack of alignment causes a diminishment of the load on the triceps, and diverts that load to the pecs and the internal shoulder rotators. This loading of the pectorals and of internal shoulder rotators is not contributing to the benefit of the triceps. Furthermore, it's also not necessarily productive for the pecs and the internal rotators. It's not enough load, nor sufficient range of motion, to adequately stimulate the pecs. It's also not the best way to exercise the internal rotators, given that it could easily strain the internal shoulder rotators.

In Figure 7-20, you can see this misalignment from a different perspective. The weights are being pulled straight down, through the plane of gravity. The origin and insertion of the triceps, however, are not aligned with the direction of resistance, as in the previous example. Furthermore, in this version, the concentric movement is not—and cannot be—vertical, because the forearm must follow the outward tilt of the humerus. As a result, the pathway of the forearm's motion is slightly diagonal, while the direction of resistance is vertical—not in alignment.

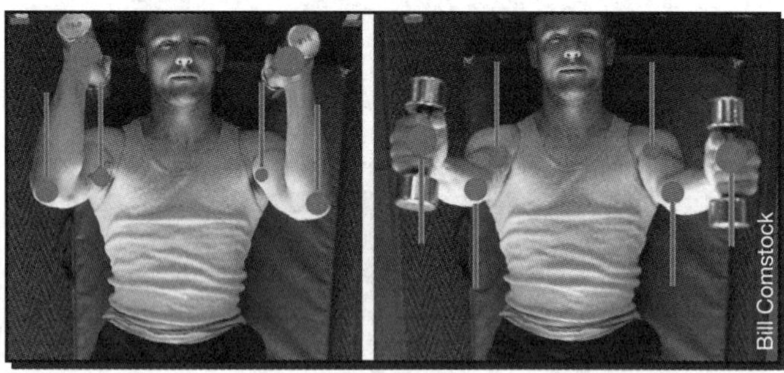

Figure 7-20

This lack of alignment results in a lack of efficiency, i.e., higher cost/lower benefit. For example, a person using this type of improper alignment, during a *supine dumbbell triceps extension*, will spend "X" amount of energy, but will waste about 20 percent of that energy on non-target muscles (unproductively) and joint strain. Perfect alignment would load the triceps more efficiently, with little or no risk of injury or strain.

The issue of whether or not the direction movement and of the direction of resistance are on the same plane is almost always present, *even if an exercise does not qualify as an "ideal anatomical movement" for a particular muscle.* Having the direction of the movement and the direction of resistance on the same plane is vital for preventing the twisting of joints, and the inadvertent loading of smaller muscles that may not be able to handle the load that's being diverted to them.

For example, in Figures 7-21a-c, you see three different directions of movement. Figure 7-21a shows a straight forward direction of movement, as well as the fact the pulley (the direction of resistance) is on the same plane as the direction of movement. You can also see that the humerus and forearm are on that same plane. As such, this is good alignment.

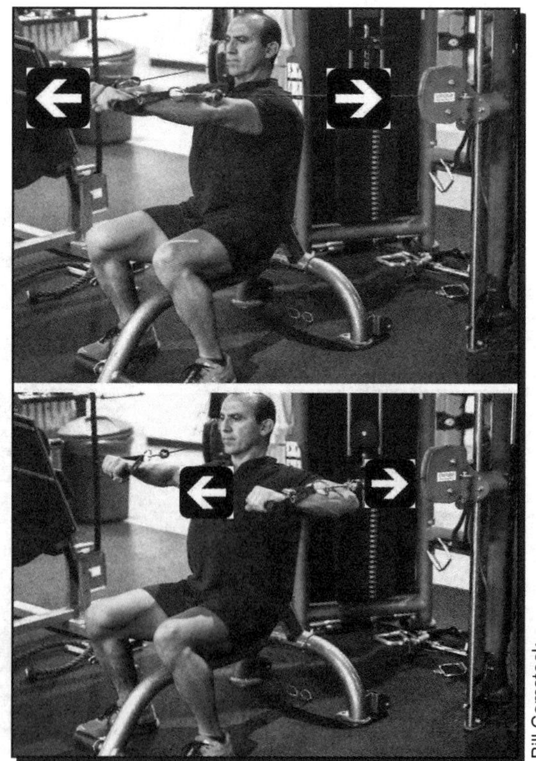

Figure 7-21a

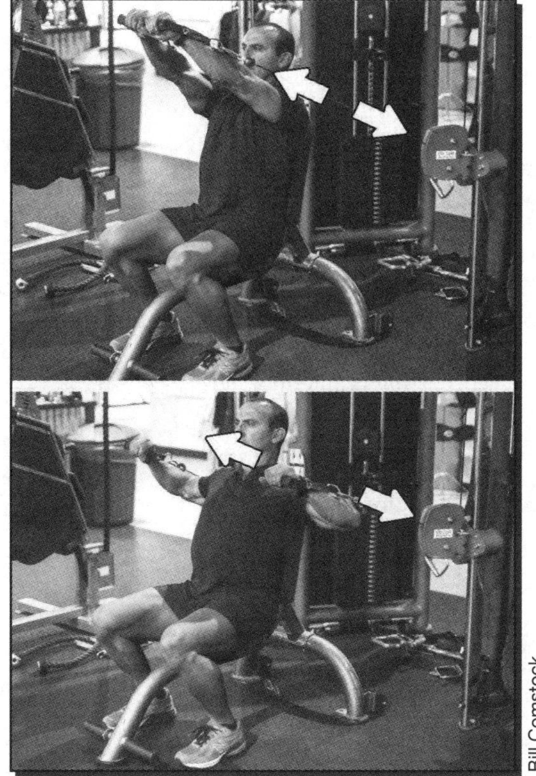


Figure 7-21b

In Figure 7-21b, the direction of movement has changed to a slightly upward (incline) angle. Notice, however, that the pulley has been lowered, so that the direction of resistance is still on the same plane as the direction of movement. The cable (indicating the direction of resistance) is also on the same plane as the humerus and the forearm. As a result, there is no humeral torque (twisting of the shoulder joint). This is also good alignment.

In Figure 7-21c, the direction of movement has been changed to a slight "decline" angle. Notice, however, that the pulley has been raised, so that the direction of resistance is still of the same plane as, and parallel with, the direction of movement.

This illustration allows you to see that, regardless of the direction of movement, it's always important to ensure that the direction of resistance is "directly opposite" (and in alignment with) the direction of movement.

As you'll soon learn, an *incline angle chest press* is not a good movement. Nevertheless, at least the direction of resistance was adjusted to accommodate the change in the direction of the concentric movement.

> *Note: The incline angle press is often used for working the pectorals, but it is not a very good exercise, as will be more fully explained in Chapters 17 and 18. The aforementioned illustrations, however, are primarily intended to show how anatomical movement should always be directly opposite the direction of resistance.*

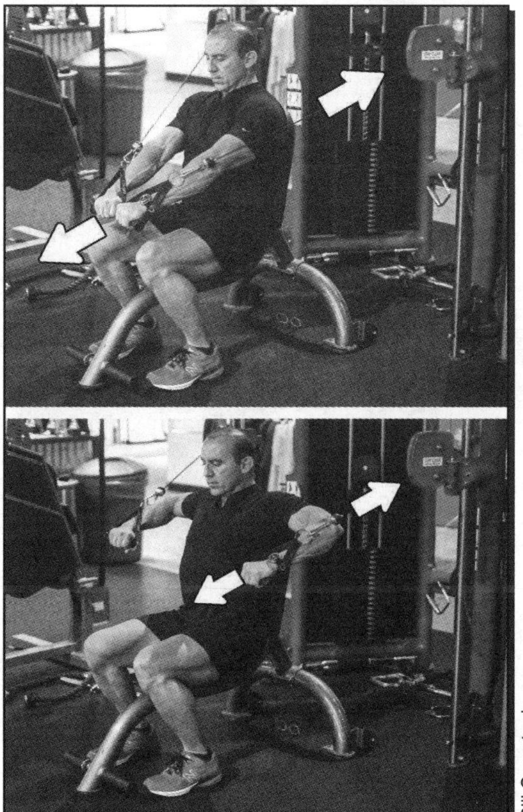


Figure 7-21c

## Summary

In order to fully grasp the essence of proper biomechanics in resistance exercise, one of the first things to understand is the importance of having the movement of an exercise to be challenged by an "opposing" resistance. The primary objective of resistance exercise is to challenge a muscle. As such, the only way that can happen is when resistance pulls in a direction that is opposite the direction of movement (i.e., during dynamic exercise).

The more "directly opposite" the resistance (perfect alignment), the greater the percentage of that resistance will be loaded onto the target muscle. The less "directly opposite" the direction of resistance is, the more that load will be diluted from the target muscle and transferred over to non-target muscles. It is also more likely that joint strain will occur.

The more close to perfect alignment an exercise has, the more efficient it is. This factor translates to more load on the target muscle and less wasted energy/unproductive effort. As you'll see in Chapters 18 through 25, where various exercises for individual muscle groups will be analyzed, one of the primary factors used to determine the efficiency of an exercise is alignment. Whether you are working the latissimus dorsi, the posterior deltoids, the middle trapezius, the pectorals, or the anterior deltoids, a *good* exercise will always have proper alignment.

Alignment must be viewed as a plane—a straight line, drawn through the direction of resistance, the direction of movement, the origin and insertion of the target muscle, and the levers involved in that action.

Some exercises are only slightly misaligned, and thus dilute the benefit (to the target muscle) by only 10 percent or 20 percent. Of course, that 10 percent or 20 percent of the load is redirected somewhere else, often to smaller muscles and joints. This redirection may not be enough to cause injury, but it's certainly not as good as performing an exercise with perfect alignment. On the other hand, some exercises are so lacking in alignment that they dilute the benefit (to the target muscle) by as much as 90 percent or 100 percent (e.g., *torso rotation with a weighted ball*).

An argument could be made that all movements are productive, to some degree, even in the absence of alignment. A better argument, however, could be made that it's good to know precisely which muscles are being loaded, and that those muscles are being intentionally loaded, and that no dilution of that load is occurring unintentionally.

It's also good to know when an elevated risk of injury exists. Understanding how alignment works in resistance exercise is essential for determining that.

# CHAPTER 8

# OPPOSITE POSITION LOADING

- *In order for a target muscle to be maximally loaded by a resistance that you've selected for an exercise, that target muscle's origin(s) must be positioned directly opposite the direction of the resistance. If a target muscle's origin is NOT positioned directly opposite resistance, it will NOT be fully loaded by that resistance.*
- *Whichever muscle is positioned directly opposite the direction of resistance WILL be the most loaded, whether it is intended or not. If a non-target muscle is mistakenly positioned directly opposite the resistance, it will be MORE loaded than the target muscle.*

Consider the "Leaning Tower of Pisa." Suppose it is your job to prevent that edifice from falling, using a very strong rope and sufficient physical strength. On which side of the Tower would you position yourself with that rope? The answer is, "*directly on the opposite side of the Tower's lean.*" In fact, it would be mostly unproductive for you to stand anywhere else.

As such, the most productive place for you to position yourself, with your rope, in order to prevent the Tower from falling, is EXACTLY opposite the direction of the Tower's tilt. If the Tower were leaning (falling) directly north, you must position yourself directly south, in order to be most effective, because that is where the *greatest percentage of the load* would be, of a North-falling Tower. A very small percentage of the north-falling load would be on the east side or the west side of the Tower.

Consider this factor from a different perspective. For example, hypothetically say that you have a rope, and you throw it over a tree branch. Then, you grab hold of both ends of the rope, and pull them straight down, in a 6:00 direction (relative to a clock). Where (on the tree branch) would the greatest rope pressure be, due to your 6:00 direction of pull? It would be at the 12:00 mark—directly opposite your direction of pull.

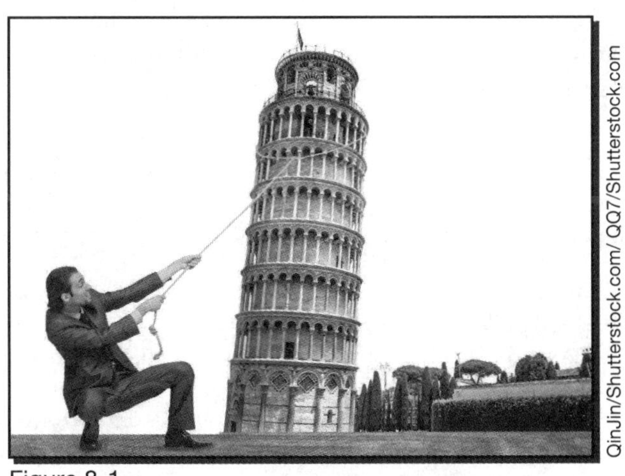
QinJin/Shutterstock.com/ QQ7/Shutterstock.com

Figure 8-1

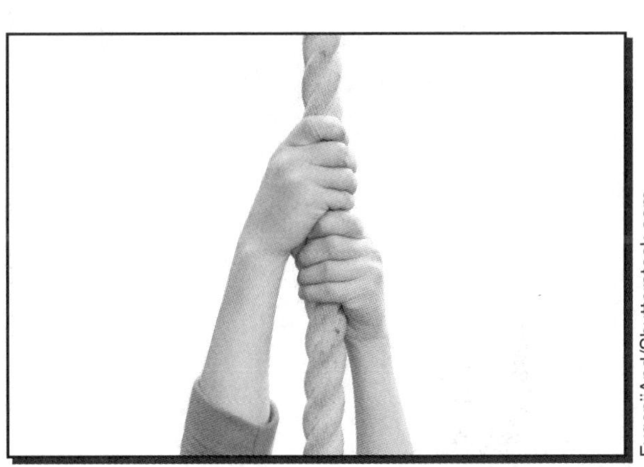
EvgeniiAnd/Shutterstock.com

Figure 8-2

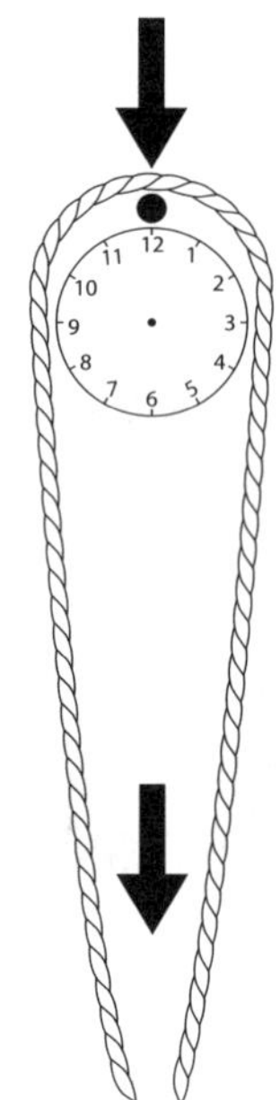


Figure 8-3

Although there would be a small amount of rope pressure on the branch, at the 3:00 position and 9:00 position, it would be a fraction of the amount—maybe as little as 25 percent—of the pressure that would be at the 12:00 position. Obviously, ZERO rope pressure would be on the 6:00 position of the tree branch, because the rope isn't even touching the 6:00 position of the branch.

Next, let's say that you actually WANT to apply the greatest pressure on the branch at the 1:30 position. You will NOT be able to do that, by pulling in a 6:00 direction. You would need to change the direction of your pull, relative to the branch. In order to deliver the greatest amount of your force (load) onto the 1:30 area of the branch, you need to pull from a 7:30 direction (Figure 8-4).

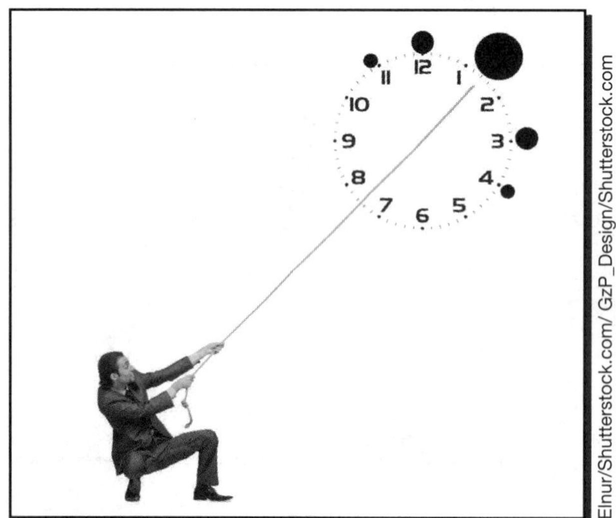


Elnur/Shutterstock.com/ GzP_Design/Shutterstock.com

Figure 8-4

## The Load Is Always Greatest Opposite the Direction of Resistance

This physics principle is universally true, and resistance exercise is no exception. On the other hand, many traditional exercises FAIL to provide the *ideal direction* of resistance for the muscle you intend to work. Or, you FAIL to position the target muscle at the best angle, relative to the direction of resistance. As a result, only a small percentage of the available resistance is delivered to the target muscle, while a larger percentage of the load is delivered to a muscle that you do not intend to load.

To be clear, it is the ORIGIN of the target muscle that should be positioned directly opposite resistance. This is based on the fact that "all muscles pull toward their origins." If the origin of your target muscle is not positioned opposite resistance, that muscle will be compromised in its ability to fully participate in the pulling of that load.

For example, hypothetically, you are performing an exercise that provides a 12:00 direction of resistance, but the origin of your target muscle is not at the 6:00 position. Instead, it is in the 4:00 position. The result will be that your target muscle will only get about half as much load as the muscle that is at the 6:00 position. Whichever muscle is in that 6:00 position will be the most loaded, even though it may NOT be the muscle you most want to work.

## Proper Positioning of a Muscle Relative to Resistance

Since the early days of bodybuilding (the late 1800s), individuals wanting to work the muscles of their upper and middle back have typically performed various types of *"rowing"* exercises, including the *bent-over barbell row, one-arm dumbbell row, t-bar row,* and *low pulley row*—to name a few. Today, over 100 years later, little has changed, in terms of which exercises are *thought* to be "the best," for the development of the upper and middle back. *None* of the standard rowing exercises, however, are maximally efficient, because they all fail to comply with the principle of "opposite position loading."

Next, look at the mechanics of a typical rowing exercise, with three factors in mind—1) the *direction of resistance*, 2) the position of the target muscle's *origin*, and 3) the direction of the exercise's *movement*.

In reality, most rowing exercises typically provide a FRONT-pulling resistance, like the *low pulley row*, shown in Figure 8-5 from an overhead view. In this instance, the image shows a "12:00 direction of resistance." Based on the aforementioned principle, the greatest load from this direction of resistance will fall on whichever muscle origin is in the 6:00 position—directly opposite the line of resistance. Hopefully, that will be the muscle you most intend to work.

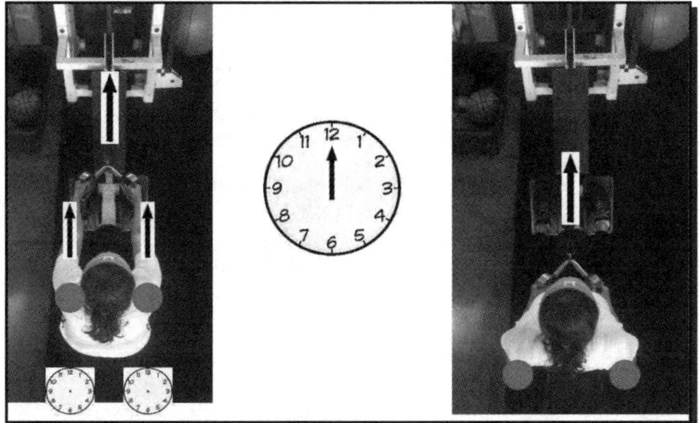
Figure 8-5

In the images that encompass Figure 8-5, a dot has been placed at that 6:00 position. As you can see, its focus is the rear deltoids (and, to a lesser degree, the teres major).

The origin of the latissimus muscle fibers, as well as the middle trapezius muscle fibers, is on the spine. The spine is positioned at 4:00 of the left arm, and 8:00 of the right arm. As such, the latissimus and the trapezius will only be loaded with about half as much load as the rear deltoids are getting.

Figure 8-6 allows you to see this situation more clearly. As such, when the arms are stretched forward, they will each be holding a resistance that is coming from the 12:00 angle, when the exerciser is performing a *low pulley row*. The two midsize arrows indicate the frontward pull of resistance—"the 12:00 direction." To reiterate, the latissimus and the trapezius both originate on the spine. The two smaller arrows pinpoint the only direction those muscles can possibly pull, because they are pulling on the arms and scapula (respectively) *toward* the spine. The largest arrows designate the direction in which the arms must move (i.e., opposite resistance), when rowing. Clearly, the arms are NOT pulling toward the spine. Rather, they are pulling in a 6:00 direction. In fact, the muscle that mostly pulls the arms in that particular direction is the posterior deltoids.

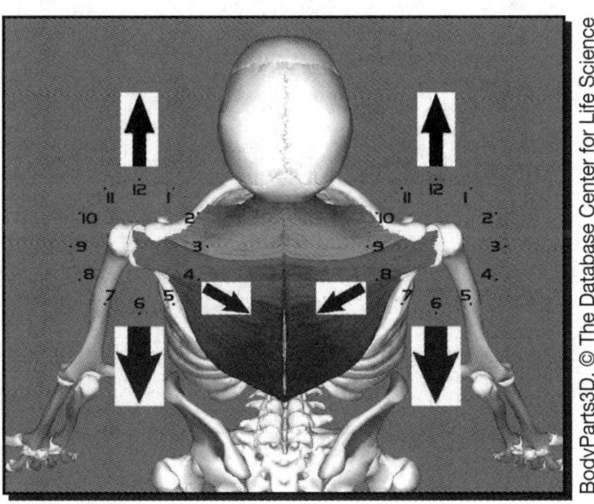
Figure 8-6



The trapezius and the latissimus cannot contribute much toward a 6:00 direction of pull. The left latissimus and trapezius pull in a 4:00 direction, while the right latissimus and trapezius pull in an 8:00 direction (when a person is facing a 12:00 direction).

The previous chapter discussed ALIGNMENT. It was established that there needs to be alignment between the direction of resistance, the direction of movement, and the origin and the insertion of the target muscle. THAT is clearly *not* happening when you perform a standard rowing movement, with a forward-pulling resistance.

To help clarify the point, think of the "Leaning Tower of Pisa." You would not stand on the east side nor on the west side of the Tower in order to be in the BEST position from which to pull the rope in the southward direction—opposite the northward fall of the Tower. In other words, the latissimus and the trapezius (which are your target muscles during this exercise) are NOT in best position to be the dominant force during an exercise that provides a forward-pulling resistance.

As a result, other muscles are forced to be the dominant load bearers, because they are better positioned. In Figure 8-7, you can see the posterior deltoids and teres major—the only two muscles that are positioned directly opposite the forward-pulling resistance. Accordingly, these two muscles will end up getting the majority of the load, during any standard rowing exercise.

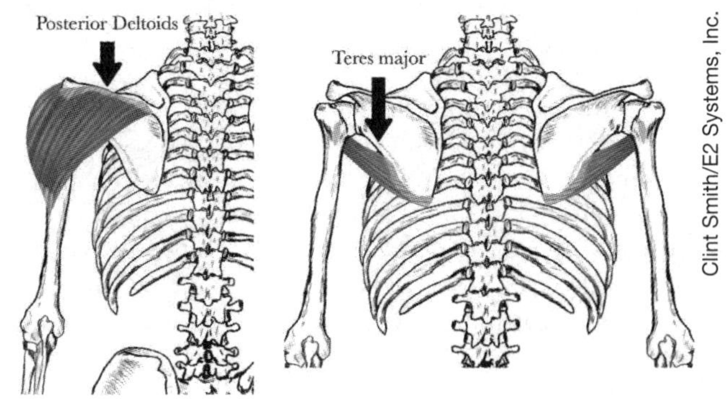

Figure 8-7



Separate from the issue of "loading" is the issue of movement. You should ask yourself, which muscle is creating this movement? Consider the marionette doll, shown in Figure 8-8.

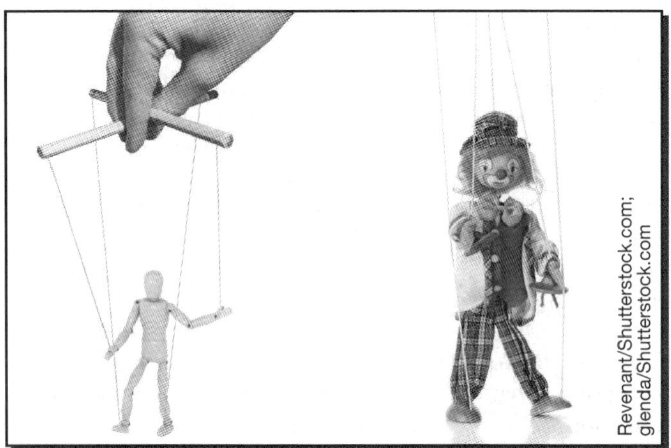


Figure 8-8

If you were a puppet master, controlling the movement of a puppet's arms, and you wanted to make the puppet perform a "rowing motion," from which direction would you pull the string that is attached to its arm? You would have to pull from a position that is along the same path as the movement you are creating. You would have to pull in a 6:00 direction (posteriorly), because that is the direction opposite the frontward pull of the cable.

You would NOT pull on the left arm from a 4:00 angle, nor would you pull the right arm from an 8:00 angle. Yet, that is the only angle from which the lats and the middle trapezius can pull. Furthermore, that is what you are unrealistically expecting to happen, when you perform a low pulley row (or any other frontward-loaded rowing exercise).

That topic will be explored much more fully in Chapters 18 through 25. At this point, however, it's worth noting that the two most significant muscles of the "middle and upper back" are the lats and the trapezius. They occupy the largest areas of the back.

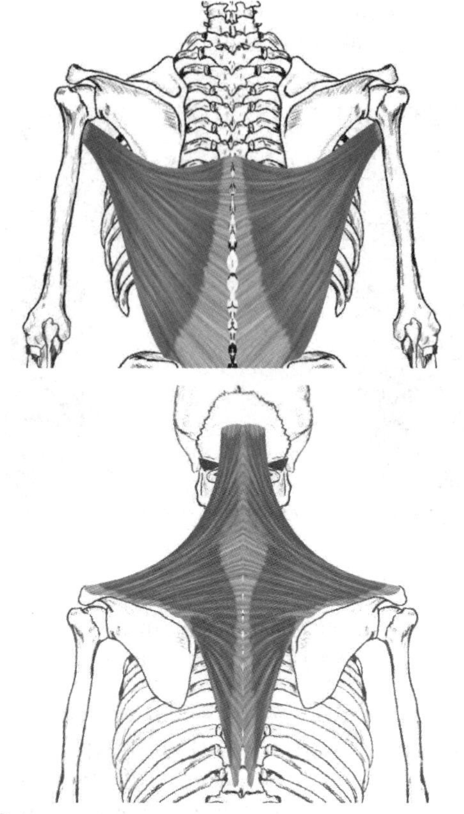


Figure 8-9

As you can see, the lats (Figure 8-9, top image) and the trapezius (Figure 8-9, bottom image), both originate on the spine. Therefore, both of these muscles pull toward the spine—toward their origins. They are obviously *not* well-positioned to participate much in a movement that entails the arms pulling straight backward. Nor would they be the muscles that are the most loaded, because a straight forward resistance does not pull directly opposite their origins.

Since the direction of movement during standard rowing exercise is not toward the origin of the trapezius, nor toward the origin of the latissimus, neither of these muscles will be the primary beneficiaries of a standard rowing exercise. Of course, you can "try" to squeeze your shoulders together at the conclusion of each repetition, but that would constitute a different *direction of movement*, from that of your arms. It's very difficult to create more than one direction of movement during an exercise that has a single direction of resistance (as all exercises do), especially when the weight is heavy. Even if you could squeeze your shoulders together at the conclusion of the arm movement, a straight forward direction of resistance would still not fully load either the lats or the middle traps.

It should also be noted that the trapezius fibers DO NOT connect to the arms at all (Figure 8-10). As a consequence,

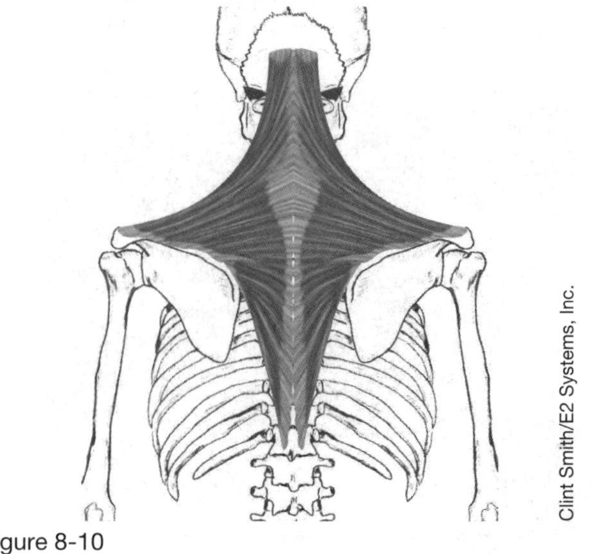


Figure 8-10

the trapezius is UNABLE to participate directly in the "arm part" of a rowing movement. This muscle originates on the spine and attaches to the outer part of the scapula (shoulder blade). Its primary function is to pull the scapula inward, toward the spine. As such, the trapezius cannot pull on the arms. The trapezius can only stabilize the scapula (during a standard low pulley rowing exercise)—a minor role, compared to the dynamic work of the posterior deltoids and teres major when moving the arms.

The next time you see someone doing a seated cable row (Figure 8-11) in the gym, watch how their primary motion is the arms pulling backward. It's nearly impossible to pull in any direction other than straight backward, when doing a rowing motion with a straightforward pulling resistance. "Straight back," however, is not where the lats originate, and it's also not where the middle trapezius originate. Thus, it's difficult to consider a *seated cable row* (or any rowing exercise) as an exercise that primarily works the "upper and middle back."

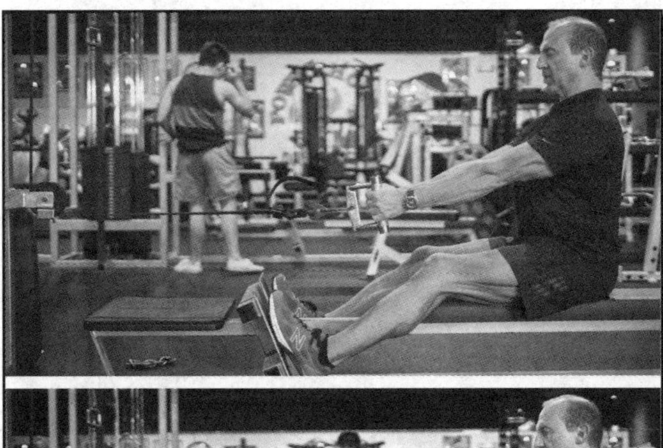

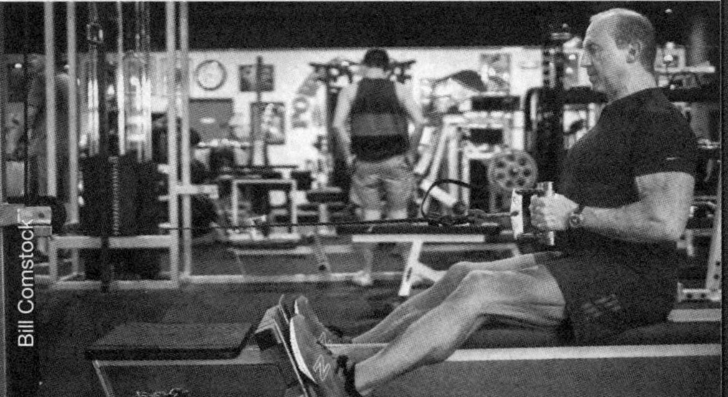


Figure 8-11

In order to fully load the lats and the middle traps, the resistance must originate from a more lateral (side) angle. Since the lats and the middle traps are positioned (approximately) at 4:00 (left arm) and 8:00 (right arm) positions, relative to a 12:00 facing torso, the ideal direction of resistance should come from approximately the 10:00 (left arm) and 2:00 (right arm) angles.

There is another muscle that is positioned directly opposite a forward-pulling resistance when doing a *seated cable row*—the "lower back" (erector spinae), shown in Figure 8-12. This muscle is optimally loaded, given that *whatever muscle(s) is/are positioned directly opposite resistance will be the most loaded, whether you intend it to be or not.* The forward pull of the cable transfers through the arms, which pulls the torso lever forward. Were it not for the erector spinae muscles (running up the entire length of the spine), the torso would fall forward like a rag doll during this movement.

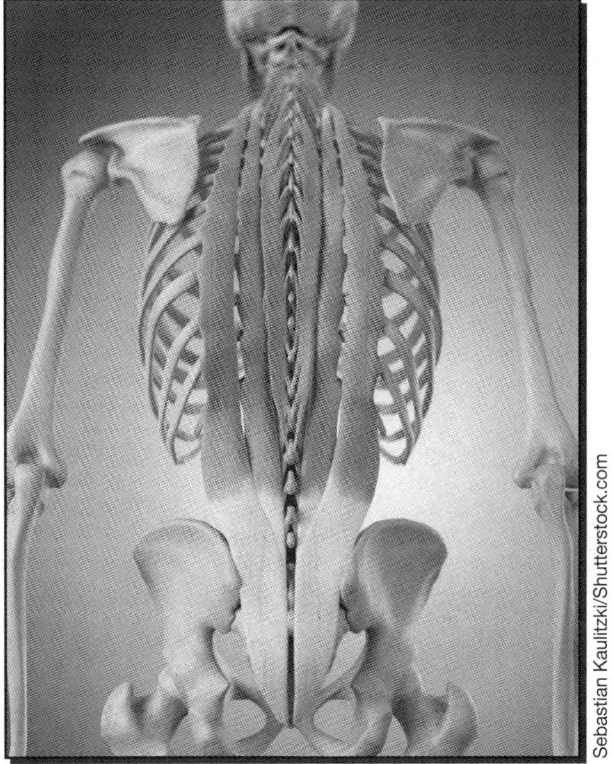


Figure 8-12

Certainly, it is NOT the intention of someone performing a *seated cable row* to maximally load their lower back, but that is exactly what's happening with a forward-pulling resistance. The lower back is receiving *100 percent* of the forward-pulling load, unless you are using some kind of chest-supported rowing machine.

In addition to the erector spinae (muscle) possibly being "overloaded," there is also the possibility that you might round your spine forward, when performing an unsupported *rowing* exercise (e.g., *seated cable row,* unsupported *T-bar row,* or *bent-over barbell row*). An overly rounded spine, combined with a heavy forward resistance, could result in a "herniation" of a spinal disc. The herniation could then press on a nerve, causing severe back pain.

In Figure 8-13, the "A" arrow indicates the forward pull of a standard, unsupported *rowing* exercise. The "B" arrow indicates the area that is vulnerable to injury during a heavy, forward-pulling *rowing* exercise that not "chest-supported." Figure 8-14 shows a herniated disc in the lumbar region of the spine. It also shows the "pinched nerve," which is a disc bulge pressing against the nerve.

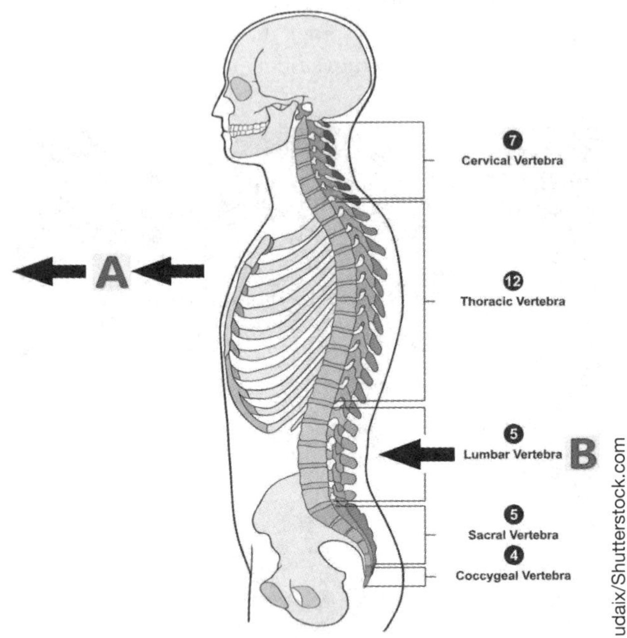


Figure 8-13

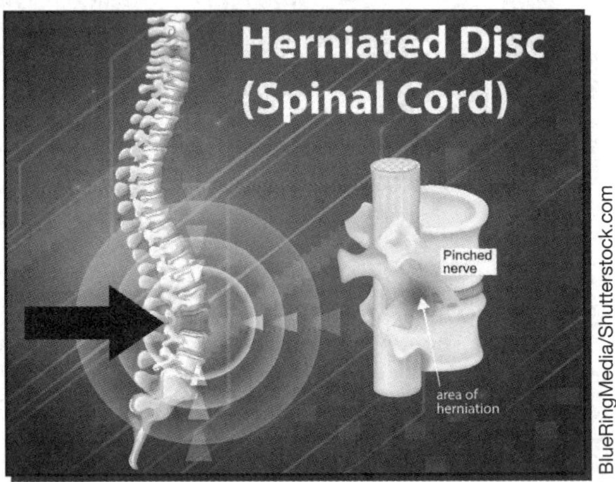


Figure 8-14

Despite the traditional belief that *rowing* exercises are good for the lats and upper back muscles, most standard *rowing* exercises load the posterior deltoids and the lower back much more than they load the latissimus and the middle trapezius. In reality, the latissimus and middle trapezius only get about 40 to 50 percent of the load that's being used. That's extremely inefficient. As such, the "cost" (effort and potential injury risk) is far too high, and the "reward" (development of the lats and mid-traps) is far too low for any standard rowing exercise to be considered a "good" exercise for the latissimus or the middle trapezius.

The *bent-over barbell row* (Figure 8-15) is perhaps the *worst*, least efficient of all the *rowing* exercises, because—in addition to the direction of resistance being incorrect, and the direction of anatomical movement being technically incorrect (for the lats and middle trapezius)—there is also the issue of an unproductive secondary resistance. As such, the lower back has to sustain the weight of the torso, in addition to the weight of the barbell, which loads the lower back even more than the *low pulley row* does.

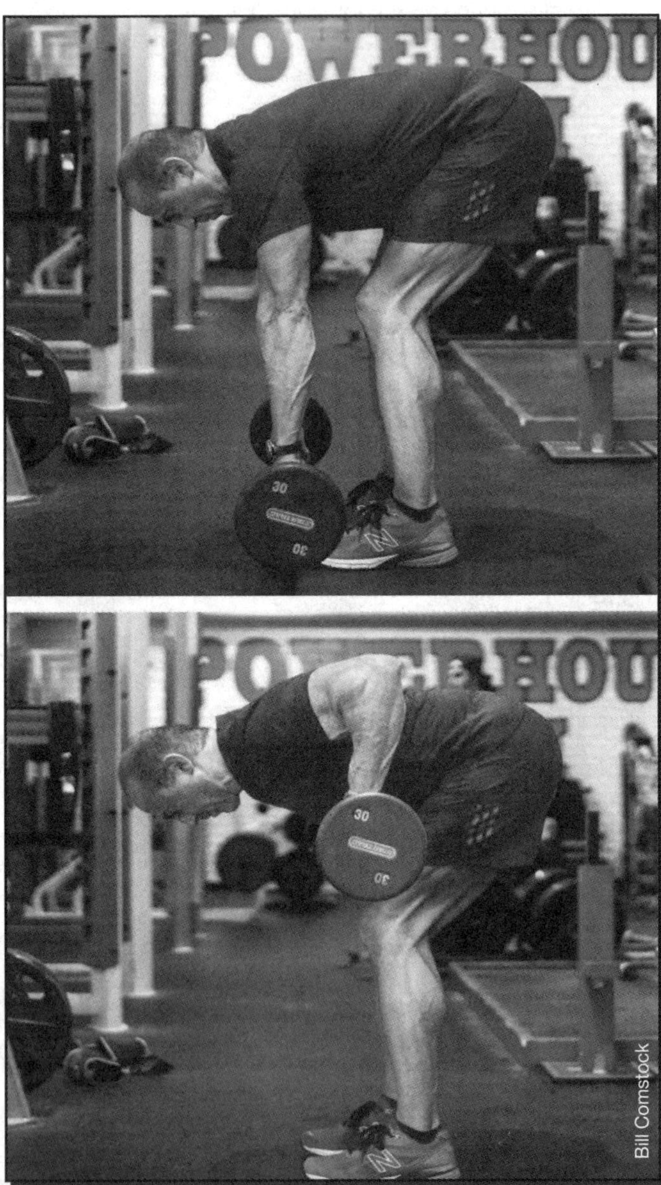


Figure 8-15

To optimally work the lats and/or the middle trapezius, the concentric movement should be inward (starting from an *outward* angle), while the direction of resistance should be directly OPPOSITE the muscle origins, coming from a somewhat lateral angle (on each side). An ideal alternative for working the lats and the middle trapezius is shown in Figure 8-16.

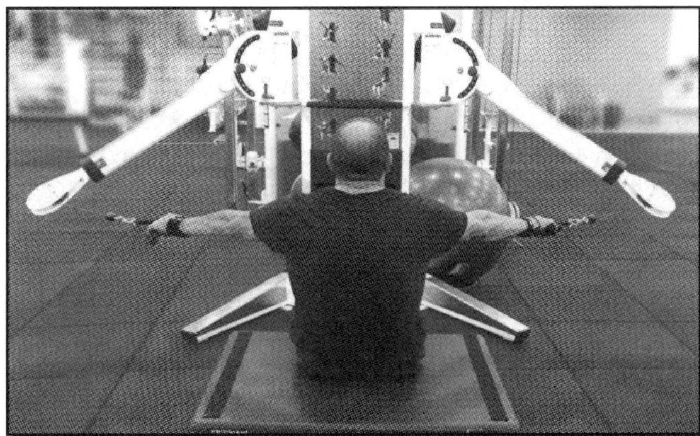
Figure 8-16

In Figure 8-16, the direction of resistance, which is coming from a 45-degree angle (from each side), is now originating from a position that is opposite the origins of both the trapezius and the latissimus. Furthermore, because the posterior deltoids are now positioned less opposite the direction of resistance, they are loaded much less. In turn, the directions of humeral and scapular movement are more inward, toward the spine, as well as in line with the muscle origins, as it should be.

The combined pull (left cable and right cable) produce a composite forward pull that is approximately 30 percent LESS than a straight forward resistance, thereby relieving strain on the lower back. In other words, this exercise provides more of what you want—which is to load and work the lats and trapezius—and LESS of what you don't want—to load the posterior deltoids and lower back.

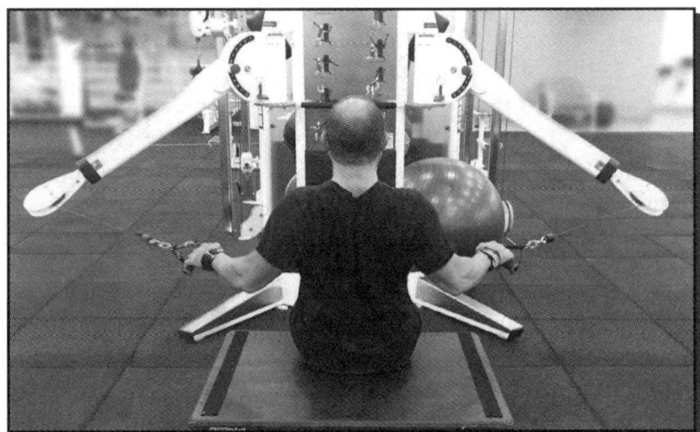
Figure 8-17

I refer to this movement as "*scapular retraction.*" Even though it also involves a small degree of arm movement, it is mostly a scapular (shoulder blade) movement. I hesitate to call it "rowing," because this exercise does not (and should not) produce an emphasis on the arm movement that is typified by the rowing action used on a boat.

The primary emphasis in this instance should be on shoulder (scapular) movement, releasing the scapula forward (Figure 8-18), and then retracting them, pulling the shoulder blades back and inward, toward the spine (Figure 8-19). The reason there should only be a secondary emphasis on the "arm" part of the movement is because the focus, in this instance, should be on the middle trapezius—not on the lats.

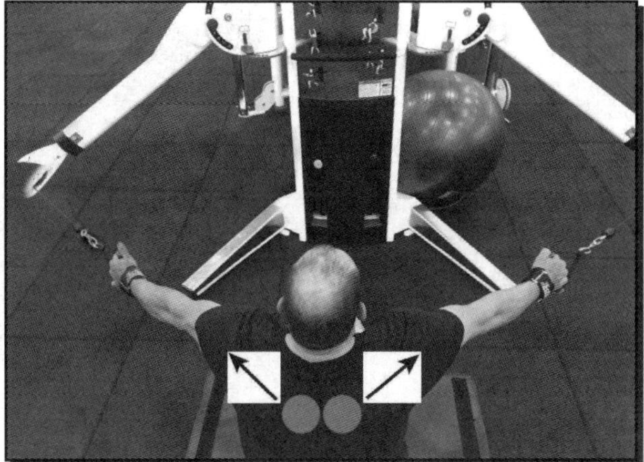
Figure 8-18

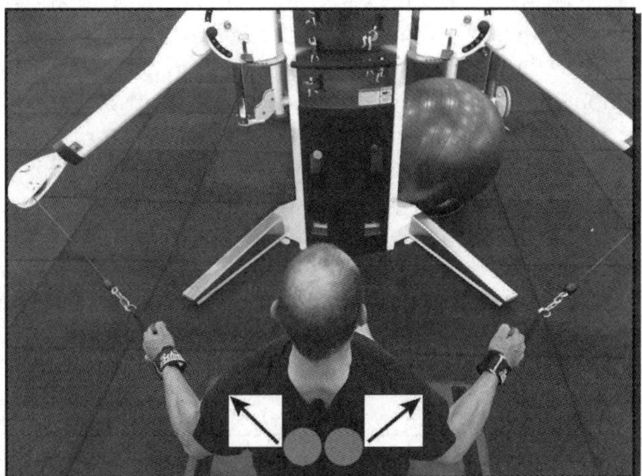
Figure 8-19

The lats mostly pull the arms downward, from a slightly more elevated angle than this. In fact, there is another, far better exercise for the lats. While "*scapular retraction*" involves some degree of latissimus activity (mainly the highest fibers), it is not enough to be a "stand-alone" exercise for the lats. This exercise, however, is the absolute best middle/lower trapezius movement, due to its emphasis on scapular retraction and its ideal "opposite position loading."

The following is another example of how "opposite position loading" is not provided for a chosen target muscle. In fact, the principle applies across the board, in every single resistance exercise you do, whether you realize it or not.

The exercise illustrated in Figure 8-20—a *"barbell front raise"*—has always been considered an "anterior deltoid" exercise. In reality, however, it is NOT a very good exercise for this muscle. One of the primary reasons for this shortcoming is that it is not "opposite position loaded."

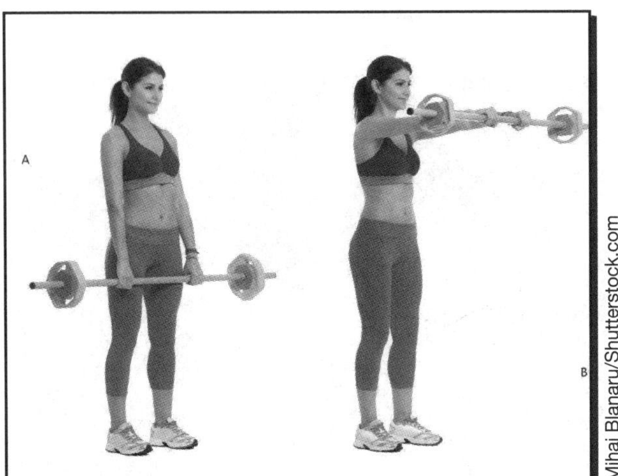


Mihai Blanaru/Shutterstock.com

Figure 8-20

Figure 8-21 offers a similar version of this exercise, performed with dumbbells instead of a barbell. The anterior deltoids have been outlined, so you can observe their position, relative to the direction of resistance. Are the anterior deltoids positioned directly opposite resistance? The answer is, *no*—not quite. The resistance is pulling straight down, in the 6:00 direction. As you can see, however, the anterior deltoids are not positioned at 12:00, as they should be. The exerciser's right anterior deltoid is positioned at 2:00, while his left anterior deltoid is positioned at 10:00. As a result, his anterior deltoids will only receive about 40 percent of the load, which is a very low percentage of load, considering the anterior deltoids are the primary target of the exercise.

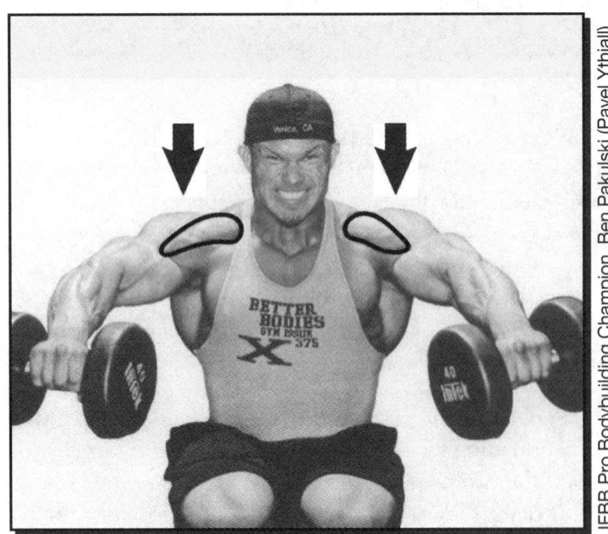


IFBB Pro Bodybuilding Champion, Ben Pakulski (Pavel Ythjall)

Figure 8-21

In Figure 8-22, the lateral deltoids are outlined. Are the lateral deltoids positioned directly opposite resistance? The answer is, *yes*—much more so than the anterior deltoids. Therefore, they'll receive most of the load. As a result, the lateral deltoids will benefit more from this exercise, even though it's intended to be an anterior deltoid exercise.

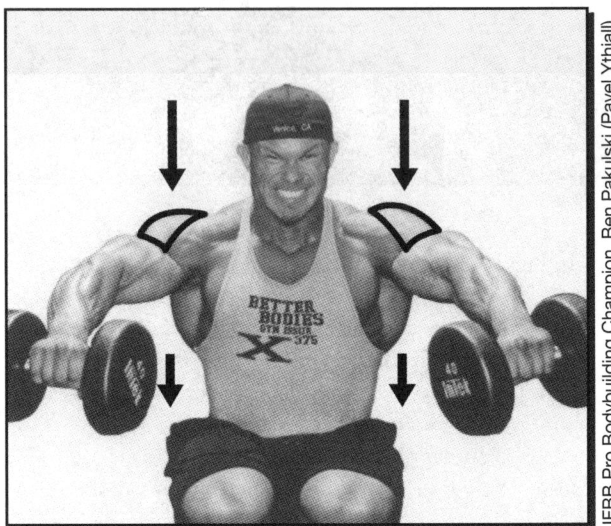


IFBB Pro Bodybuilding Champion, Ben Pakulski (Pavel Ythjall)

Figure 8-22

To reemphasize a point previously made, the direction of the *movement* is not what causes a target muscle to be LOADED. The direction of the *resistance* determines which muscle is most loaded. Whichever muscle is directly opposite the direction of resistance will be the most loaded, regardless of the direction of movement.

In order to LOAD a target muscle, you must deliberately position that muscle so that it is opposite the direction of resistance. In order to do that, you must either change the position of the body (or position of the limb) relative to the direction of resistance or the direction of resistance relative to the body (or the limb).

The degree of humeral (upper arm) rotation plays a role in this instance, although it is not the only factor. By causing the palms of the hands to face downward (as they are in Figure 8-22), the humerus is rotated such that the elbows are pointing laterally (to the sides). This "inward" rotation of the arms causes the lateral deltoids to face upward—opposite resistance.

Conversely, turning the palms of the hands either toward the midline of the body (hammer style) or upward causes the elbows to point downward (instead of to the sides), and rotates the humerus externally. This action causes the lateral deltoids to rotate out toward the sides (away from the opposing resistance), and rotates the anterior deltoids to the 11:00 position, which is closer to ideal. This location places them in a position to get the highest percentage of load from the downward resistance.

As a comparison, look at this version shown in Figure 8-23. The person is still in the upright position, and gravity is still the direction of resistance. The only change is the external rotation of the arm, such that the palms are facing inward, and the anterior deltoid has rotated into a better position to OPPOSE the downward direction of resistance. While this is a better position for the anterior deltoids, it's still not the ideal way to work them.

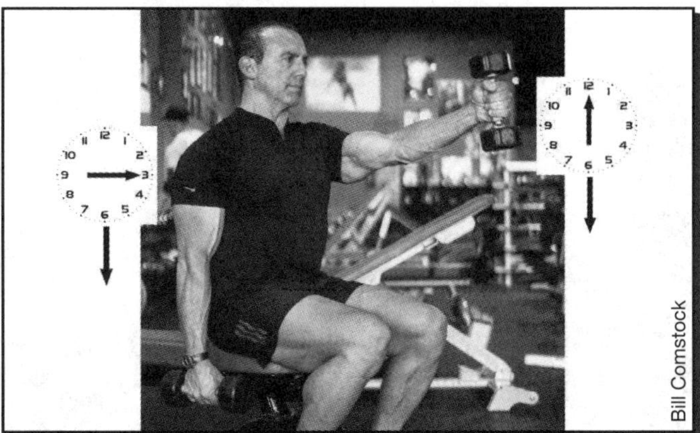

Figure 8-23

Notice that the anterior deltoid is not in the 12:00 position *until* the arm is raised up. At the beginning of the movement, the anterior deltoid is in the 3:00 position (which is NOT opposite resistance). In other words, the target muscle is not fully opposing resistance UNTIL the end of the range of motion. Therefore, the "resistance curve" is not ideal. As such, the anterior deltoids are not being "early phase loaded." Rather, they are being loaded at the end of the range of motion, where a muscle is typically weaker. Furthermore, they are unchallenged in the early phase, where the muscle is strongest.

As you learned in Chapter 5, it's better to load the *early* part of the range of motion, because a muscle is stronger when it's elongated. The muscle is usually weakest at the end of its range of motion.

So, although we corrected the position of the target muscle by rotating the humerus externally (in Figure 8-23), the "resistance curve" still needs to be improved. As a result, in order to make the exercise "ideal," you need to change the direction of resistance, relative to the torso, so that the movement is "early phase loaded."

The exercise demonstrated in Figures 8-24 to 8-26—"*supine dumbbell front press*"—is much closer to the ideal mechanics for the anterior deltoid. The palms of the exerciser's hands are facing upward (toward his head) and his elbows are pointing downward (toward his feet). This technique rotates the humerus, such that the anterior deltoids are in line with the opposing resistance. Furthermore, because the resistance is now coming from behind the exerciser ("posteriorly"), rather than from the direction of his feet (like when someone is standing or sitting upright), the resistance curve is much better. This exercise provides most of the load during the early phase of the range of motion and less load during the latter part of the range of motion.

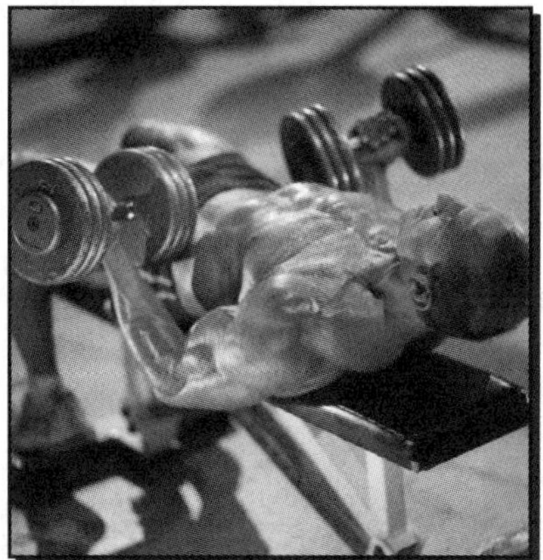

Figure 8-24

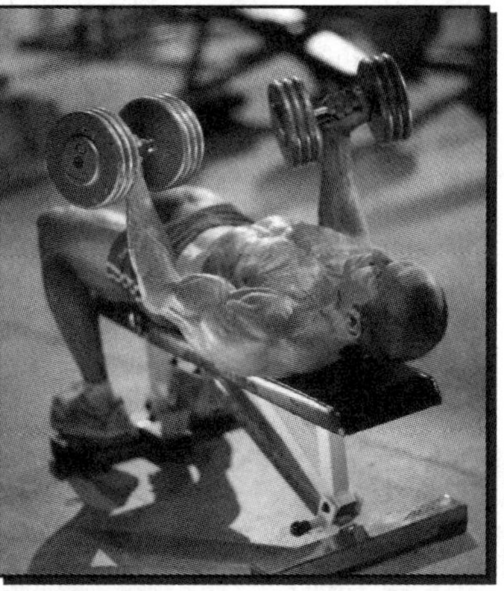

Figure 8-25

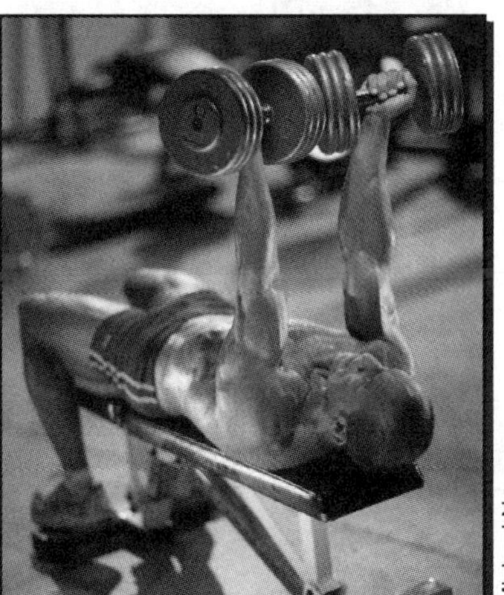

Figure 8-26

Of course, the anterior deltoids don't "know" whether the elbows are straight or bent. The anterior deltoids only pull on the humerus, and don't "care" whether the person is using a longer lever (straight arm/more magnification) with a lighter weight, or a shorter lever (bent arm/less magnification) with a heavier weight. In other words, this exercise could be done either way. Using a bent arm (i.e., a pressing motion), however, bypasses the potential strain on the biceps and biceps tendon (when using a straight arm), so the *pressing* motion is the better option in this instance.

## Summary

Understanding the principle of "opposite position loading" allows you to identify which muscles are loaded during an exercise, and which ones are not. It also enables you to determine how much (approximately) a muscle is loaded, on a percentage basis.

If a muscle is directly opposite resistance, it is positioned to receive the largest percentage of the available load. If it is positioned to the side of the opposing resistance, it may only be loaded with half, or a quarter, of the available resistance. As such, by positioning a target muscle directly opposite resistance, as well as positioning non-target muscles so that they are not opposite resistance, you are able to maximize your efforts and minimize wasted energy.

In the beginning of this chapter, the question could have been asked, "If the Tower is leaning directly north, where would the greatest load be?" The unequivocal answer would be, "directly south"—opposite the direction of the Tower's lean. In other words, if your goal is to get the most amount of load on a specific target muscle while exercising, you should position that muscle directly opposite the direction of resistance.

In Figures 8-27 and 8-28, the exerciser is performing a "lying side dumbbell raise." In this instance, think of the exerciser's right arm as a "mini tower." When this "tower" moves from the vertical position and begins to "lean" (hypothetically "north," as shown by the compass placed on the exerciser's arm), it will load whichever muscle is positioned opposite that lean. In this instance, that's where the lateral deltoid is positioned— on the "south" side. The load would not be on the front deltoid nor on the rear deltoid, which could be regarded as the west position and the east position, respectively.

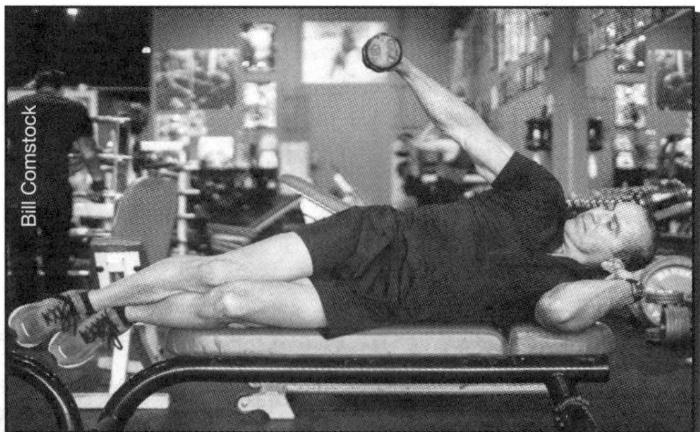

Figure 8-27

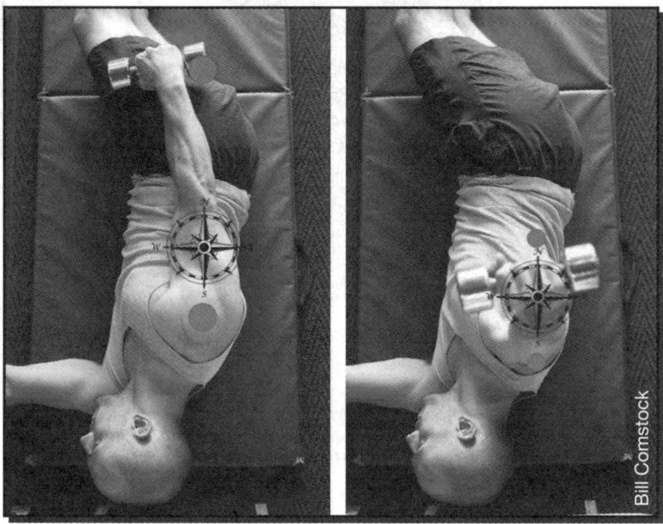

Figure 8-28

This factor is precisely what makes this exercise a "lateral deltoid exercise." The "falling" (lowering) of the exerciser's arm is opposed (resisted) by the muscle that is positioned opposite the tilt of his arm—exactly as if it were a "leaning tower."

Subsequently, the concentric "lifting" of the exerciser's arm occurs as a result of his lateral deltoid pulling this "mini tower" in a direction that is opposite its direction of "falling." Again, this is just like the example of the "Leaning Tower of Pisa."

In Figures 8-29 and 8-30, the exerciser's arm (this "mini tower") has been tilted in a *western* direction. As a result, the load shifts to the *east* side of this "tower." Because the posterior deltoid is positioned there, it becomes the load bearer. In causing this "tower" to lean to the "west" (instead of "north"), the exerciser has selectively loaded a different muscle (different from the previous example), by simply changing the direction of the lean of this "tower."

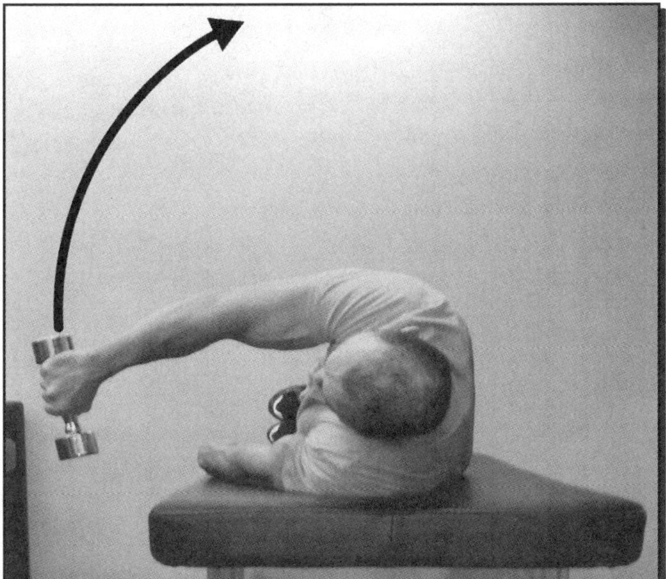

Figure 8-29

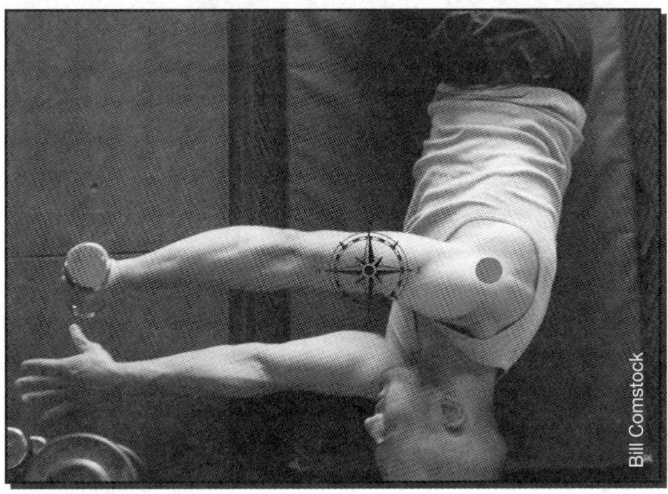


Figure 8-30

What do you suppose would happen if this "tower" (the exerciser's arm) had been leaned in a direction that is BETWEEN the north and the west direction, i.e., in a northwestern direction, as shown in Figure 8-31? The load would then be shared between the two muscles—partially on the lateral deltoid and partially on the posterior deltoid. Each muscle would bear a percentage of the load. In other words, they would be cooperating with each other, in a combined effort. Neither of them, however, would be working as much (or as well) as each muscle could, if the "tower" (the arm) was leaning entirely north or entirely west.

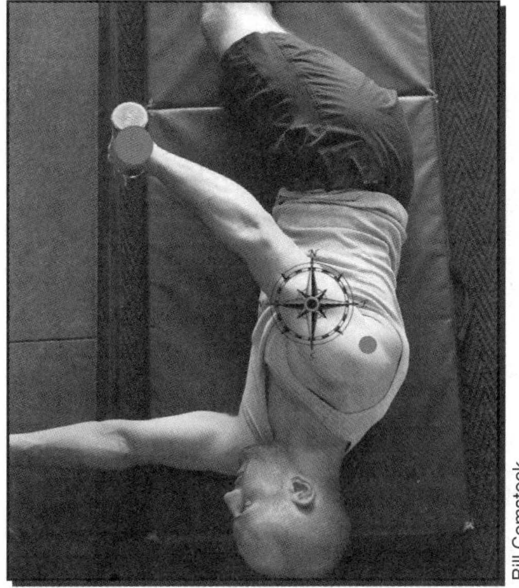


Figure 8-31

As you can see, this rule of opposite position loading coincides perfectly with the principle of alignment, which was discussed in the previous chapter. Perfect alignment requires that the direction of resistance be on the same plane as the direction of movement, on the opposite side of the concentric motion, as well as on the same plane as the origin and insertion of the target muscle.

CHAPTER 9

# "DYNAMIC" VS. "STATIC" MUSCLE CONTRACTION AND RANGE OF MOTION

- *"Dynamic" muscle contraction occurs when a muscle lengthens and shortens against resistance. This type of muscle contraction causes the joint over which that muscle crosses to bend (flex or extend), thereby producing anatomical movement.*
- *"Static" muscle contraction (aka "isometric" muscle contraction) occurs when a muscle holds tension, without lengthening or shortening. Instead of causing the joint to flex or extend, the muscle holds that anatomical position, without movement.*
- *Generally speaking, dynamic muscle contraction is considered more productive for the purpose of muscle growth/physique development, as compared with static muscle contraction. It is also believed to be more "functional," from a strength-building standpoint.*
- *Dynamic muscle contraction requires "range of motion" (movement)— though not necessarily "full" range of motion. However, for muscle-building purposes, a longer range of motion is more productive than a very short range of motion, generally speaking.*

When you speak of "bodybuilding" and/or weight training programs, the issue of "sets and reps" is usually included in the conversation. The concept of "repetitions per set" is a system of measurement. Theoretically, it could be considered a "dose" of muscle stimulation, part of which the weight being used is also a factor. Various studies have demonstrated adaptation differences between the use of "high reps" versus "low reps," but both utilize the principle of motion and both have benefits.

For the purpose of muscular development, repetitions of motion, during resistance exercise is considered an established and important part of resistance exercise. Repetitions of movement against an opposing resistance automatically implies "*dynamic*" exercise.

## The Difference Between Dynamic and Static Muscle Contraction

Muscle contraction *without* (notice emphasis on "without") movement is referred to as "*static*" or "*isometric*" exercise. The reason isometric exercise is not used much, if at all, in either bodybuilding or general fitness, is because it has been proven to be not as productive as dynamic exercise. Not only does it not "build" (grow) a muscle as well, its strength stimulation is also limited primarily to the particular point in the range of motion where the limb (joint) is held static. As such, it produces less "full range" strength benefits, as compared with dynamic exercise. In reality, isometric exercise is most often used in physical therapy programs, as a way of introducing "resistance" exercise to specific muscles, while avoiding the movement of a joint, which may be injured or is being rehabilitated.

Figure 9-1 shows an example of *static* pectoral muscle contraction. In this instance, the pectoral muscle is contracted, without the shoulder joint movement that is typical during standard (dynamic) pectoral exercises. The hands are simply pressed against each other, thereby causing the pectorals to experience static muscle tension.

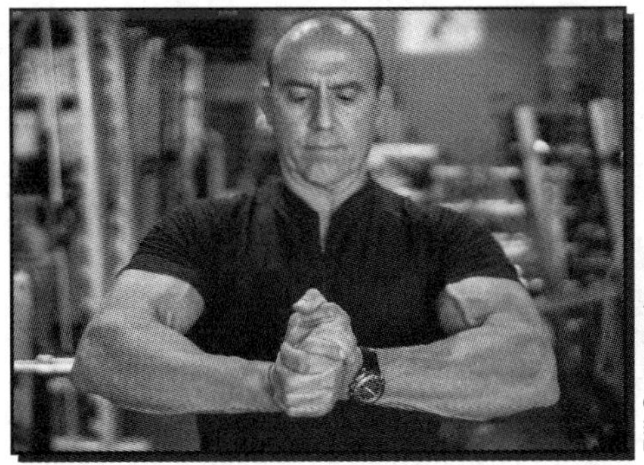
Bill Comstock

Figure 9-1

There is no "range of motion" nor any "reps," with isometric exercise. Instead, muscle tension is typically held for a predetermined count (e.g., 20 seconds, 30 seconds, etc.). When a person is pushing against their own opposing force, or against an immovable object (e.g., a wall), there is no way of establishing how much force is being used, because there is no actual weight being held. In such cases, there is no particular force threshold that needs to be met. An individual simply uses their own judgment with regard to the degree of force applied.

In Figure 9-2 (left image), you can see a man performing an isometric anterior deltoid exercise. He is pressing the hand of his left arm forward against an immovable post, thereby creating static muscle contraction of his anterior deltoid. In Figure 9-2 (right image), the man is performing an isometric posterior deltoid exercise. He is pressing the elbow of his right arm posteriorly against the immovable post, thereby creating static muscle contraction of his posterior deltoid. These exercises are typically employed in shoulder rehabilitation, because they avoid moving the shoulder joint. (*Note: There are other muscles that also participate in both of the aforementioned exercises, although to a lesser degree.*)

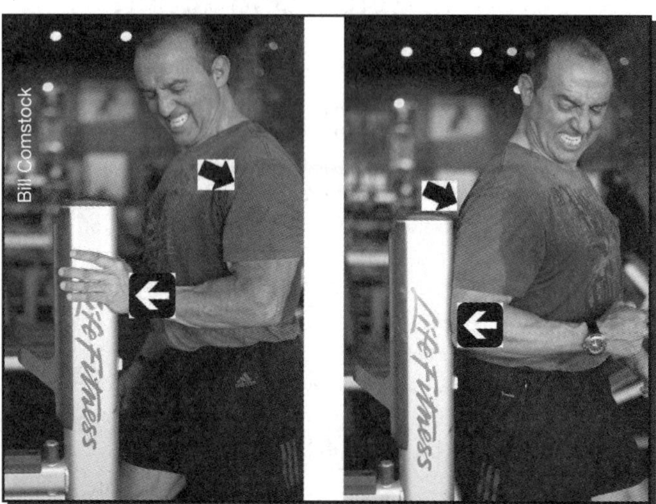

Figure 9-2

Isometric exercise can also be performed with free weights. For example, you could hold a pair of 10-pound dumbbells out to the sides (Figure 9-3), with your arms straight, for a specific time count (e.g., 30 seconds). Or you could hold a barbell, with your elbows bent at 90 degrees, at the mid-point of a barbell curl, for a pre-determined time count (Figure 9-4). Using weights establishes a threshold of force to be met, which enables you to better gauge how much force is being used, as well as whether your level of strength is improving.

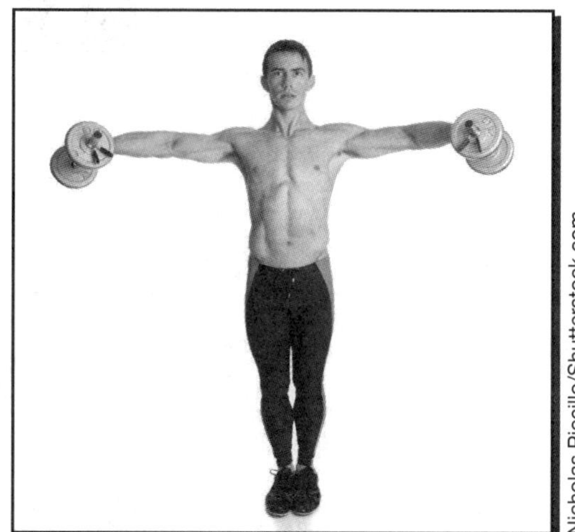

Figure 9-3

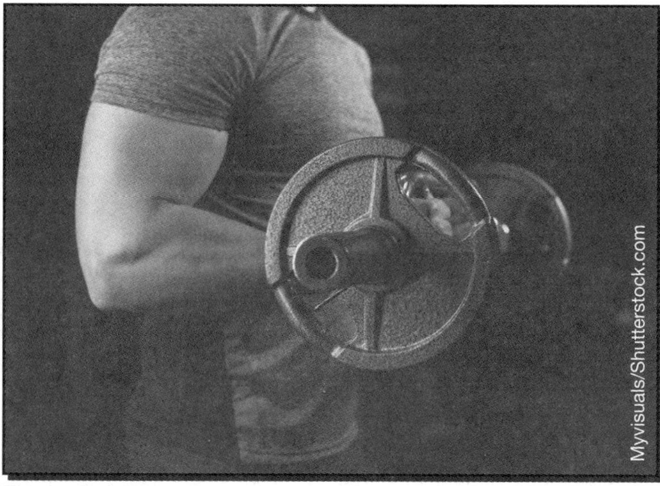

Figure 9-4

When rehabilitating an injury, *dynamic* muscle contraction (i.e., exercise with joint movement) may not be feasible, because the injury may limit joint mobility. As such, the concept of challenging a muscle, without causing a joint to move, has merit in those circumstances.

From a functional standpoint, however, performing exercise WITH joint movement produces a more useful benefit, because it increases strength through a muscle's entire range of motion. Furthermore, since dynamic exercise involves elongation of muscles (stretching) against resistance, the flexibility of the muscles involved tends to improve, as does joint mobility.

In terms of *muscle growth*, numerous studies have shown that using isometric exercise is less productive for the purpose of muscle building, as compared with the use of dynamic resistance exercise. Furthermore, there has never been a competitive bodybuilder of any renown who has developed their physique, by way of isometric exercise. In reality, if outstanding muscular development could be achieved by using isometric exercise, it would be considered standard procedure by now. Yet, not a single person has ever achieved a significant level of muscular development, using isometric exercise as their primary form of training.

Resistance exercise often involves a combination of *dynamic* contraction for the target muscle, while the stabilizing muscles work *isometrically* to maintain posture. For example, in Figure 9-5, you can see a man performing a *standing barbell curl*. His biceps are performing dynamic muscle contraction—lengthening and shortening, elongating and contracting—as they bend (flex) his elbows. Other muscles, however, are isometrically stabilizing his upright position.

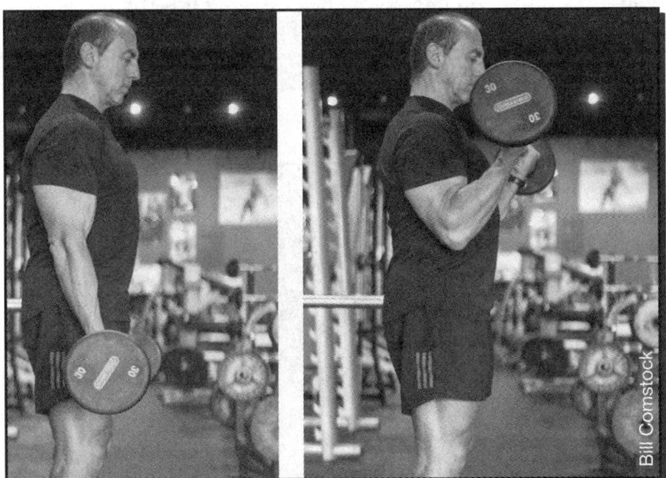


Figure 9-5

His "lower back" (erector spinae) is holding static tension, to prevent him from being pulled forward by the front-loaded torso. His trapezius is loaded by the "opposite position loading"/downward resistance of the free weights. His gluteus and hamstrings are also maintaining isometric tension, while helping him to maintain rigid posture against the forward pulling barbell. His forearm flexor muscles are working isometrically, in keeping his hands in line with his forearms, while the barbell "tries" to bend his wrists back. His fingers are also working isometrically as they maintain a static-tension grip on the barbell. Even the muscles of his calves and feet are in some degree of static muscle activation.

The stabilizing muscles only participate isometrically, and thus do not get stimulation that is very productive for growth, nor for strength gains through their full range of motion. The target muscle (i.e., the biceps, in this case) should be performing dynamic muscle contraction—using *full range* of motion—in order to optimize muscular gains.

As you'll learn in Chapters 13 and 14, the isometric muscle contraction experienced by stabilizing muscles, during a given exercise, can be referred to as "peripheral recruitment." To a degree, almost all resistance exercises require some degree of peripheral muscle recruitment.

## Using Dynamic Tension for Target Muscles and Isometric Tension for Stabilizing Muscles

Ideally speaking, all exercises should be like the *standing barbell curl* (Figure 9-5). With exercises like that, the intended target muscle (the biceps, in this instance) is the muscle that works dynamically, while all the stabilizing muscles merely work isometrically.

On occasion, however, people mistakenly cause the *target* muscle to work isometrically, while a *non-target* muscle works dynamically. When this situation occurs, the target muscle gets less benefit than do the non-target muscles.

The *standing barbell curl* is considered a "biceps exercise," and not a "lower back exercise," for good reason. The stabilizing effort (isometric contraction) that is provided by the "lower back" is not productive enough to qualify the *standing barbell curl* as a "lower back exercise."

On the other hand, a *lying leg raise* (Figures 9-6 and 9-7) is generally considered an abdominal exercise, even though the abs are *mostly stabilizing* the spine during the exercise. In fact, the abs do NOT lift the legs, because the abs are not even connected to the legs. The "hip flexors" are lifting the legs and are, therefore, doing dynamic work. They are NOT, however, the target muscle. This is an example of causing a non-target muscle (the hip flexors) to work dynamically, while the target muscle (the rectus abdominis) works mostly isometrically, which is foolish.

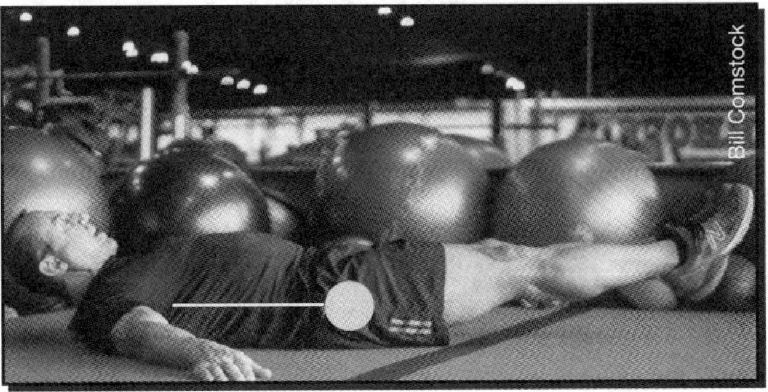


Figure 9-6

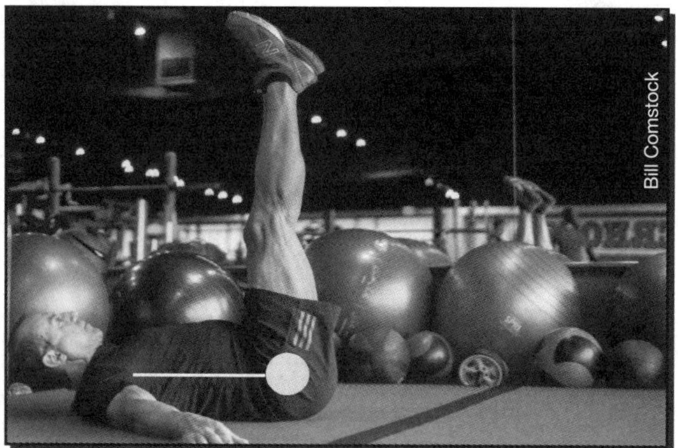

Figure 9-7

With regard to the aforementioned, in Figures 9-8 and 9-9, you can see the rectus abdominis (the "abs"). This muscle originates on the pubic bone of the pelvis. It then reaches up and attaches onto the front part of the lower ribs. It does not attach to the legs at all. Do you see any part of the abs connecting to the leg bones in these illustrations? Of course not. Since the abs do not connect to the legs (the femur bones), the abs simply cannot play an active role in "raising the legs."

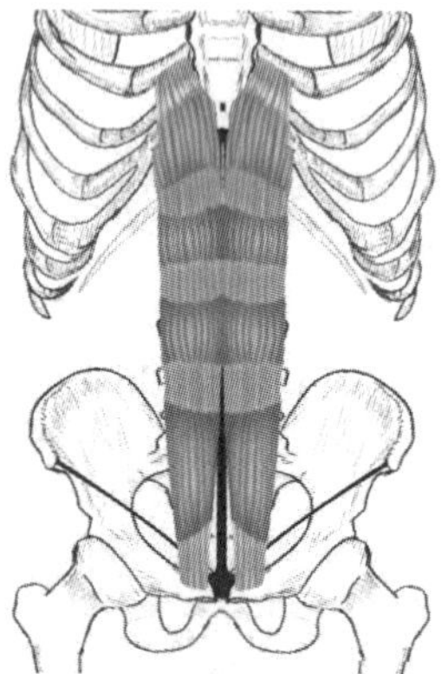

Figure 9-8

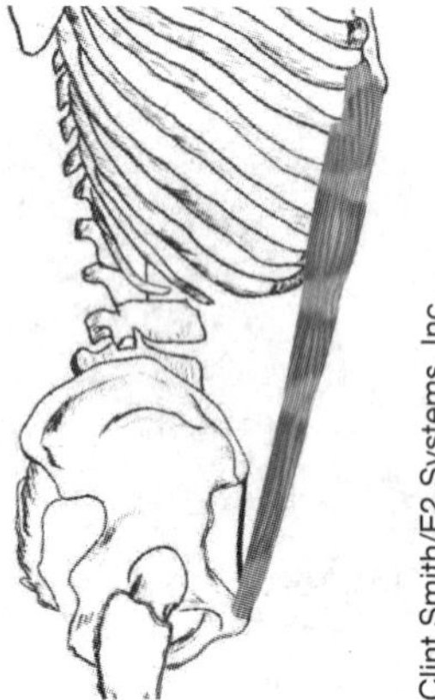

Figure 9-9

Arguably, if the fitness industry wants to call *leg raises* an "ab exercise," then *barbell curls* should be called a "lower back exercise." Otherwise, leg raises should be called a "hip flexor exercise." The name of the exercise should be based on the muscle that is doing the MOST work—the muscle that is working dynamically. It's patently ridiculous to name an exercise based on a muscle that only works isometrically to stabilize the posture, while another (less-prioritized) muscle does the majority of the work.

In reality, any type of *leg raise*—whether it's performed while lying flat on the floor, or while hanging from a chinning bar, or while suspended on a "Roman chair" (Figure 9-10)—is an extremely inefficient abdominal exercise, because the abs are not working dynamically. Some individuals would argue that a leg raise is considered an "ab exercise," because the pubic bone should be pulled forward—toward the rib cage—as the legs are raised. Theoretically, this action would cause a small degree of spinal flexion, which is the action that the rectus abdominis produces. The hip flexors would, still, however, be producing more motion, and would therefore be more engaged than the abs.

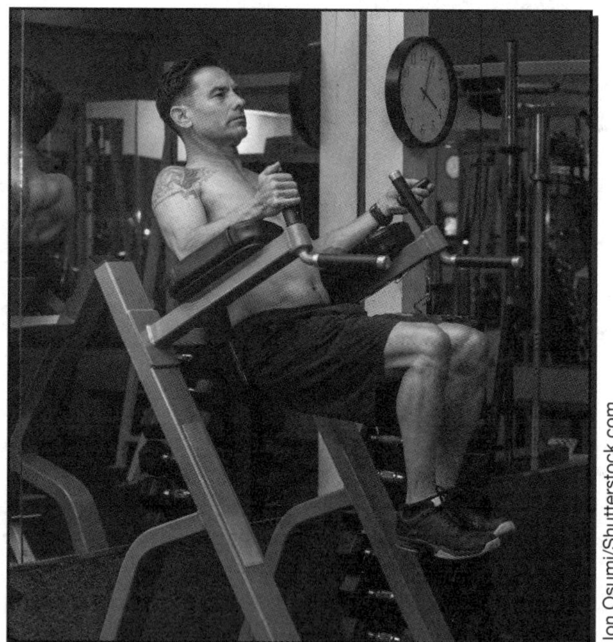

Figure 9-10

As you'll see more clearly in Chapters 23 (Hip Flexors) and 24 (Abs), however, it's extremely difficult for the abs to function properly during a leg raise. This is because the hip flexors are trying to *arch* the spine, while the abs are trying to *flex* (curl) the spine. The result is that the abs are not able to fully contract, because the hip flexors are preventing spinal flexion.

The criteria that determines which muscle is working dynamically versus isometrically is JOINT MOVEMENT. In that regard, you have to first identify where the joint movement is occurring, and then determine which muscle(s) cross(es) that particular joint. As such, in order to deliberately cause a target muscle to contract dynamically, you need to know which joint to bend, and then cause that joint to bend during the exercise.

In the abdominal exercise shown in Figures 9-11 and 9-12, the action is a deliberate bending (flexing) of the mid-spine, because that is the action that is produced by dynamic contraction of the rectus abdominis. The spine is made up of multiple joints, and they must bend, for the abs to contract. By flexing (forward-bending) the mid-spine, the insertion of the abs (on the front of the ribs) is brought toward the origin of the abs (on the pubic bone of the pelvis), thereby producing muscle contraction (shortening).

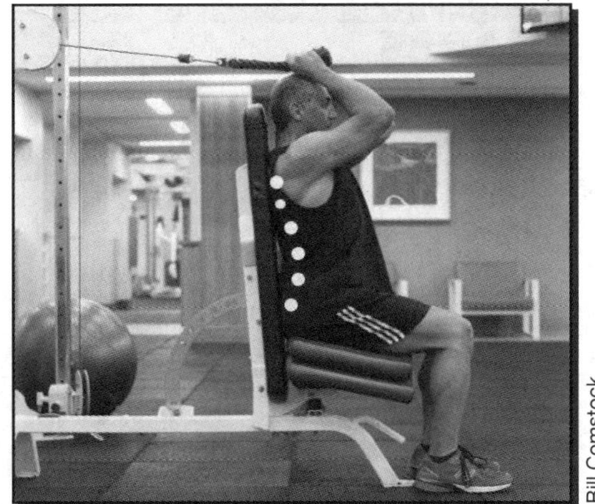

Figure 9-11

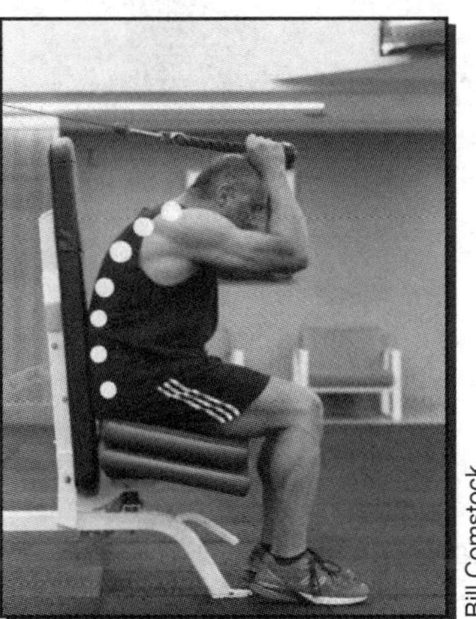

Figure 9-12

Compare the degree of *spinal flexion* (bending) that occurs in the aforementioned exercise, with the amount of spinal flexion that occurs in the first example of a *leg raise*.

It is also worth noting that the entire rectus abdominis is working in this case—from top to bottom. This concept will be explored more fully in Chapter 10 (The "All or Nothing" Principle of Muscle Contraction), as well as in Chapter 24 (Abs).

The exercise shown in Figures 9-13 and 9-14—a "*lower back extension*"—is another example of a person bending the "wrong" joint for the proposed target muscle. This exercise is typically intended for the erector spinae (the muscle that runs from the lower back up to the top of the spine). The erector spinae, however, extends the spine; it does not extend the hips. Yet, it is the hip joint that is primarily being moved in this exercise.

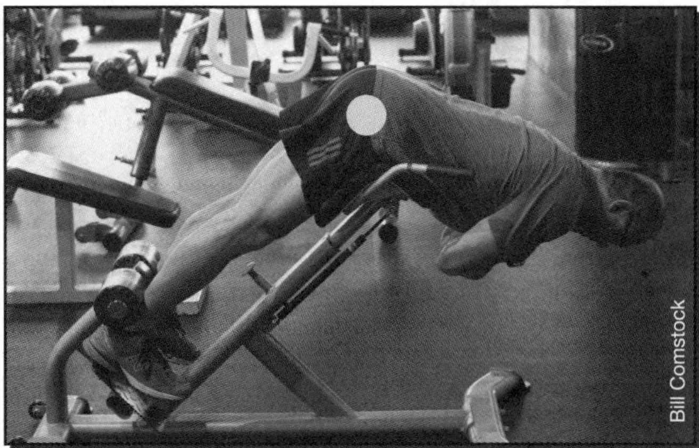

Figure 9-13

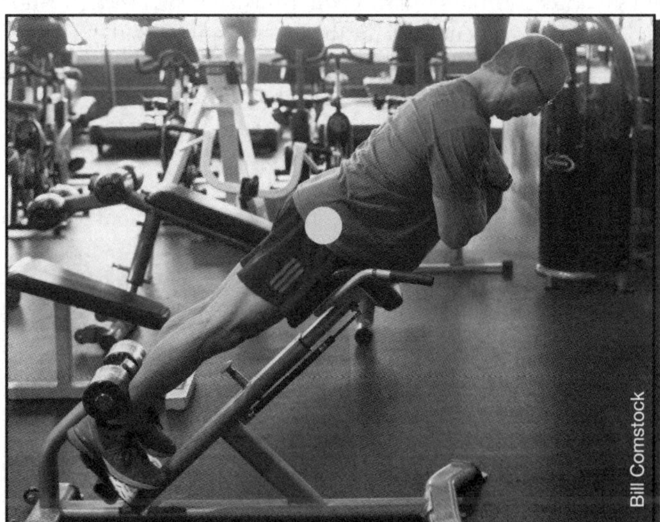

Figure 9-14

During this exercise, the torso (spine) is typically held in the same position throughout the exercise. Thus, the erector spinae work mostly *isometrically* to maintain (hold steady) that torso position. Meanwhile, the glutes (with some help from the adductors and hamstrings) are extending the hip joint—*dynamically*. Therefore, the intended target muscle of the exercise (the erector spinae) is getting less stimulation than the non-target muscles (the glutes, adductors, and hamstrings). This is another example of how individuals sometimes mistakenly use *dynamic* (i.e., superior) muscle contraction for a muscle that is NOT their target muscle, while using *isometric* (i.e., inferior) muscle contraction for the muscle they most want to prioritize.

> *Note: In this context, "inferior" refers to stimulation that is LESS likely to produce muscle hypertrophy, as well as less likely to produce strength through a broad range of motion. In turn, "superior" refers to stimulation that is MORE likely to produce muscle hypertrophy.*

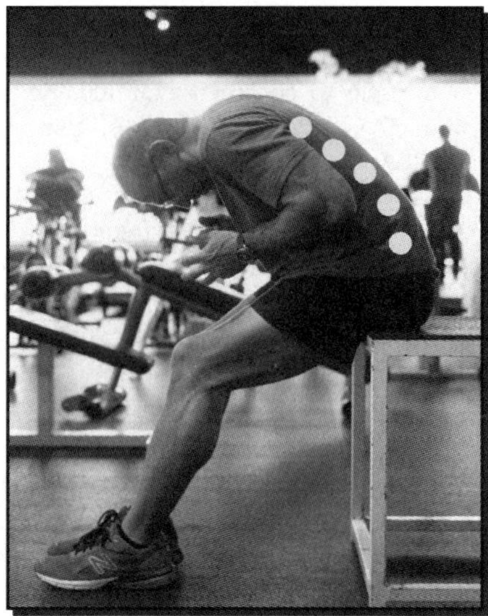

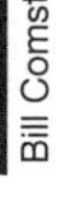


Figure 9-15

Some people might think, "since the aforementioned exercise provides better stimulation for the gluteus, why not just use it and regard it as a gluteus exercise?" All-in-all, that proposition isn't a bad idea, provided people are *knowingly* using it that way. On the other hand, the glutes are generally much stronger than the resistance this exercise normally provides, or allows.

In fact, this exercise (in Figure 9-14) is very similar to a *deadlift*—with a slightly different resistance curve and straighter legs. If the objective is to maximally load the glutes, the challenge is to do so without overloading the spine and the erector spinae, which will be discussed at greater length in Chapter 23. Either way, neither the *low back extensions* nor *deadlifts*, are as beneficial for the erector spinae as they are for the gluteus, given that in both exercises, it's the hip joint that is doing most of the bending, rather than the spine.

If your goal is to target the spinal erectors (aka the erector spinae), you'd be wise to use a dynamic exercise, instead of an isometric exercise. In order to work the spinal erectors dynamically, you need to bend the SPINE—not the hip joint. This action can be done very easily, without much involvement of the hip joint. In fact, it would be a good strategy to not involve the hip joint much, when attempting to develop the erector spinae, because spinal extension is best performed with undivided attention. Most people tend to be out of touch with the way their spine moves, so they typically lack the coordination to do it well. With a little practice, however, spinal coordination and spinal mobility can be greatly improved.

The exercise shown in Figures 9-15 and 9-16 is a "*seated torso extension*." When performing this exercise, the range of motion begins when the spine is forward-rounded ("flexed") position, which elongates the erector spinae. Then, the spine is arched ("extended"), which contracts the erector spinae. This sequence will be further explained in greater detail in Chapter 24.

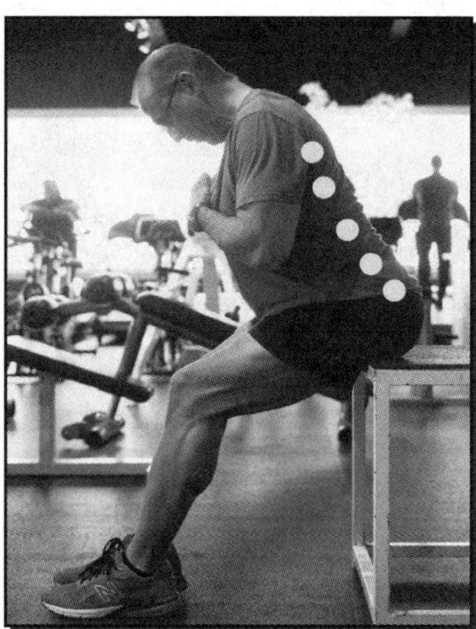

Bill Comstock

Figure 9-16

When performing the *seated torso extension*, the movement is primarily in the spine (the dots indicate spinal movement), and much less at the hip, as compared with the standard "*low back extension*." This would cause the target muscle (the erector spinae) to work dynamically. It's also important to notice that the exerciser is staying entirely on the left side of the apex. He is not crossing over to the right side. Thus, he is complying with the rule of "opposite position loading," as well as the rule of not crossing over to the other side of the base or the apex.

Care should be taken, when doing this exercise, to not "overround/overflex" the spine, nor to "overarch/overextend" the spine. The spine IS made to move, but, just like any joint, it has limits as to how much it can move safely. You should never force excessive joint motion, and that includes spinal movement. Certainly, however, some degree of spinal movement is better than no movement at all, in order to achieve the goals of improved muscular development, as well as improved mobility.

Accordingly, when considering "*dynamic* versus *isometric*" as part of your exercise analysis, you should ask the following questions:

- "Which muscle are you intending to target with this exercise?"
- "Which joint is moved by the muscle you are intending to target?"
- "Is the joint that is operated by the muscle you are intending to target the one that bends most (or exclusively) during this exercise?"

If the joint that is crossed by your target muscle is NOT the joint that moves most during a given exercise, then you are failing to use dynamic muscle contraction for your target muscle. You are also probably activating a non-target muscle *more* than your target muscle. The target muscle should be producing the actual movement. It should not merely be holding its joint steady, while another non-target muscle does most of the actual work at a different joint.

Another (final) example of this type of "error," can be seen in the gym when someone attempts to perform a *cable triceps pushdown*, with the intention of working their triceps muscle. Because they are unaware of how to do the exercise properly, they sometimes mostly bend at the shoulder joint, while keeping their elbows mostly straight (Figure 9-17). Of course, the correct form when performing *triceps pushdowns* requires that the elbows bend, and the shoulder joint be held still (Figure 9-18).

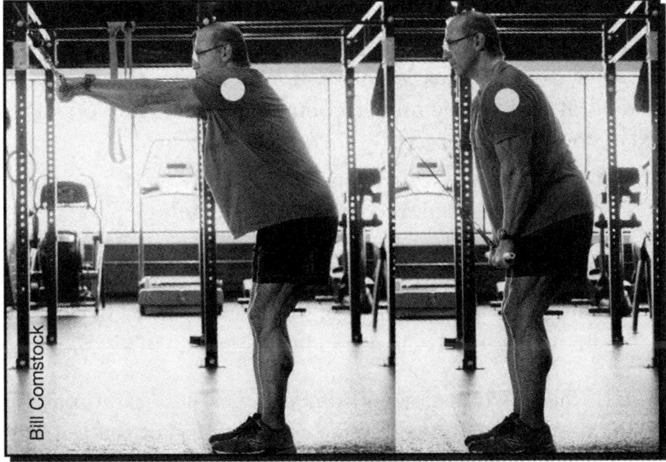

Figure 9-17

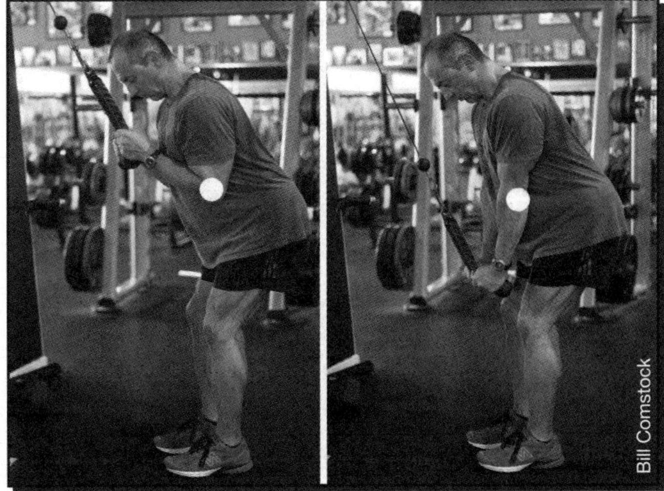

Figure 9-18

*Note: Of course, I am referring to individuals who are intending to work their triceps. This situation is not to be confused with people who are performing a "straight arm pulldown" for their lats.*

Performing a *triceps pushdown* with this kind of improper form (Figure 9-17), does engage the triceps muscle, but only *isometrically*. The triceps works to keep the elbow in a rigid position, by way of static tension. Meanwhile, the muscles that cross the shoulder joint—principally the latissimus, the posterior deltoids, and the teres major—are the ones that are producing the downward movement, by bending ("adducting") the shoulder joint.

The reason the example shown in Figure 9-17 would be considered "incorrect," as a triceps exercise, is because tensing the triceps isometrically is NOT as productive as contracting the triceps dynamically. Similarly, the rationale for performing *dynamic squats*, with movement (Figure 9-19), is because they develop the quadriceps and the gluteus better than *static squats*, without movement (Figure 9-20).

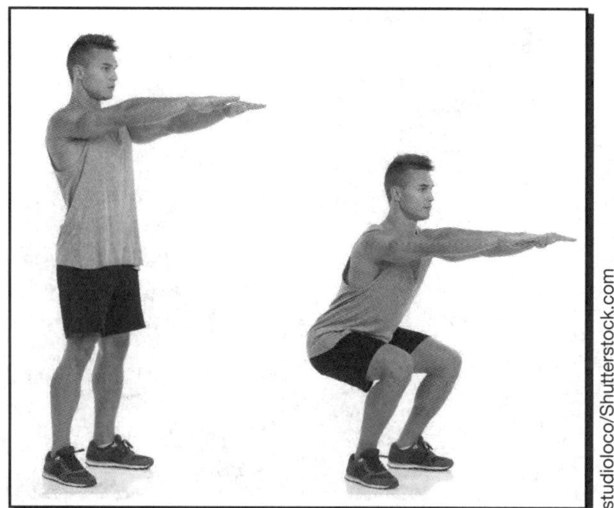
studioloco/Shutterstock.com

Figure 9-19

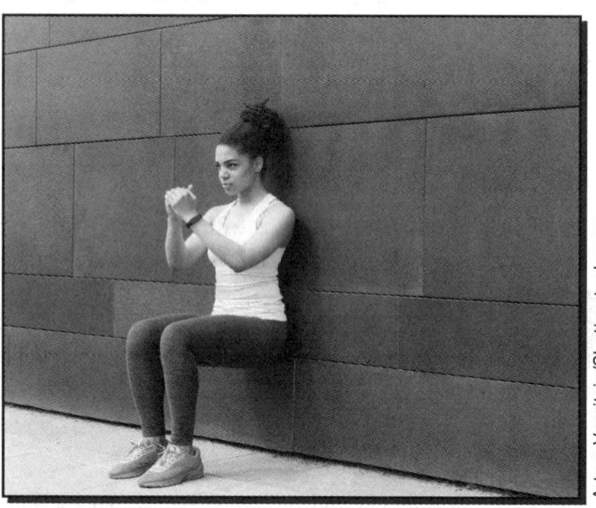
Artem Varnitsin/Shutterstock.com

Figure 9-20

In reality, the dynamic versus static comparison holds true in virtually all situations, as the following examples illustrate:

- *Flat bench dumbbell presses*, performed with movement, are more productive for the development of the pectorals than a *static* (no movement) *push-up*.
- *Torso rotations*, performed with movement—against an opposing resistance, are more productive than a static torso hold, with resistance.
- *Side bends*, moving against an opposing resistance, is more productive than a *static side plank*.
- *Ab crunches*, performed with movement (Figure 9-21—top images) using bodyweight or resistance provided by a cable, is more productive for development of the abs than are static *planks* (without movement, Figure 9-21—bottom image).

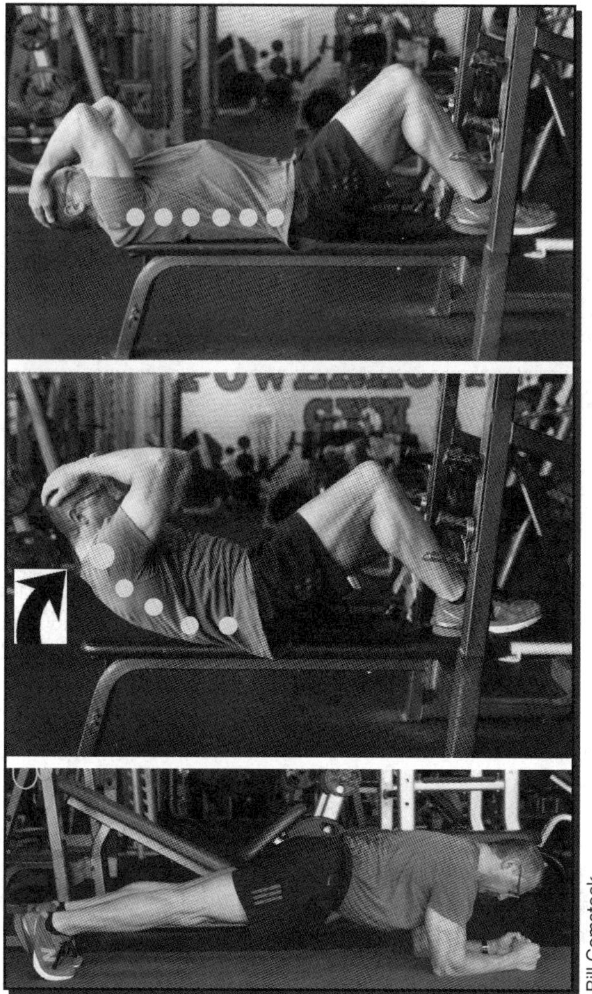
Bill Comstock

Figure 9-21

All factors considered, dynamic muscle contraction is more productive than static muscle contraction, for the goal of visible muscle development, and for increasing strength through a full range of motion. While static muscle tension is better than no muscle contraction at all, it's not nearly as beneficial as dynamic muscle contraction. There are only two exceptions to this precept:

- A joint injury or other physical anomaly is preventing or inhibiting normal freedom of movement.
- A person's goal is to maximize the strength of a muscle in one specific position. For example, a boxer may want to improve the "rigidity" of his torso, in order to provide him with better resilience to receiving punches in the ring.

In these two instances, isometric muscle tension may be preferable over dynamic muscle contraction. For the purpose of general fitness and muscular development, however, dynamic exercise is preferable over isometric exercise.

## How Much Range of Motion Is Enough?

Up to this point, the discussion has entailed comparing "movement" (dynamic) with "no movement" (isometric exercise). The next key issue that needs to be addressed is, "*how much* movement is ideal—or sufficient?" It's relatively easy to compare full range of motion with zero range of motion. It's not so easy, however, to establish an absolute guideline about *how much* range of motion is ideal.

Everyone has seen people in the gym carelessly doing exercises with very abbreviated (short) ranges of motion. It's logical to assume that an insufficient range of motion will compromise the benefit of the exercise. After all, a range of motion of 10 percent is almost "isometric." On the other hand, is 100 percent range of motion absolutely necessary—or even "best"? Is 100 percent range of motion always safe? Is 80 percent ROM as effective as 100 percent ROM? At what point (percentage-wise) does a reduced range of motion become insufficient?

A muscle's "full" range of motion could theoretically be defined as being from the point at which it is most elongated to the point at which it is most shortened. On the other hand, it's clear (to those individuals who have been participating in the sport of bodybuilding for decades) that using 100 percent "full" range of motion is not *necessary* for optimal muscular development. In fact, it often has potential risk. Is there such a thing as an "ideal" range of motion, expressed as a percentage of a muscle's complete range of motion? The answer depends on a number of variables, including the following:

- The resistance curve of a particular exercise
- Whether a "muscle/joint" experiences mechanical disadvantage during the early part of its range of motion
- The amount of weight being used in a given exercise (represented as a percentage of maximum effort for that muscle)
- The skeletal limitations of the joint being operated
- Whether or not a muscle has been warmed up

Chapter 3 discussed the mechanical disadvantage that occurs when the biceps is pulling on the forearm from a parallel angle, when the elbow is straight. As such, it would be risky to perform a 100 percent full range of motion (full extension) on a *preacher barbell curl* (Figure 9-22), while using a weight that represents anything more than about 70 percent of the biceps' maximum effort. This limitation exists because of the mechanical disadvantage that prevails, combined with a resistance curve that provides too much resistance at the beginning of the movement. This combination could easily jeopardize the safety of the biceps tendon, if a significant amount of weight were used.

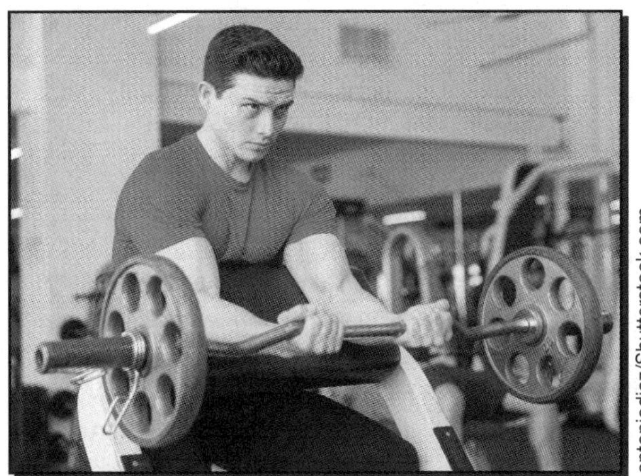
antoniodiaz/Shutterstock.com

Figure 9-22

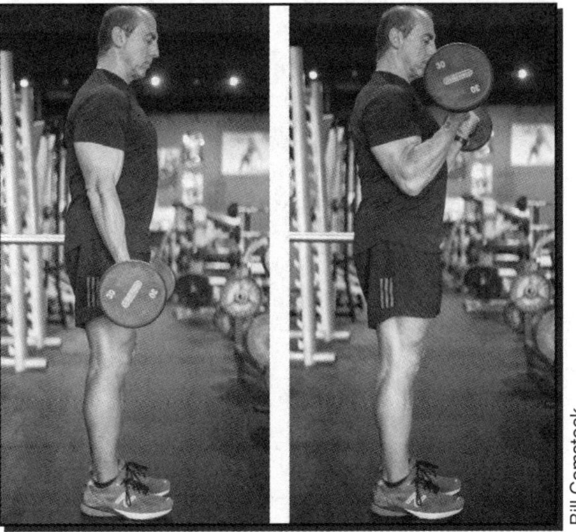
Bill Comstock

Figure 9-23

It would not be risky, however, to perform a 100 percent full range of motion when doing a *standing barbell curl* (Figure 9-23) with that same weight, because when the forearm is parallel to gravity (at the beginning of the range of motion), there is no load on the biceps. As such, the mechanical disadvantage that occurs during *standing barbell curls* would not pose any injury risk. Accordingly, a person could thus use a weight that requires maximum effort, with full range of motion, without much risk at all, when doing a *standing barbell curl.*

Furthermore, it would not be risky to perform a full extension on a *preacher barbell curl* if the weight being used was "light" (less than 30 percent of maximum effort, approximately). As such, you can see how the factors combine to determine when "full range of motion" is safe, and when it's not. Similarly, determining "enough" or "too much" ROM is also subject to other factors, including momentum, repetition speed, and whether there is an apex or base at the beginning or at the end of the range of motion.

All of these factors combine and determine what the "appropriate" range of motion might be for a particular exercise under those specific circumstances. Because each exercise has a different set of mechanical circumstances, each exercise would require its own parameters, with regard to the range of motion that would be considered ideal.

Nevertheless, basic "range of motion" guidelines can and should be established at this point, since this chapter deals with "dynamic muscle contraction," a topic that automatically implies range of motion. In that regard, the following factors apply:

- It is known that skeletal muscles have more strength potential when they are elongated, versus when they're shortened/contracted. Therefore, it's reasonable to assume that the early part of the range of motion is more productive than the latter part of the range of motion. Accordingly, as a rule, it is logical to conclude that if you are going to abbreviate an aspect of the range of motion of an exercise, it's better to abbreviate the latter part of the range of motion, rather than the early part.
- It is known that there can be some degree of increased injury risk at the maximum stretch position of a muscle, especially if the weight being used is "very heavy" (i.e., a level of resistance allowing fewer than six repetitions to be performed, generally). This factor would be further exacerbated if there is a mechanical disadvantage occurring at that point. Accordingly, as a rule, caution should be employed during the most elongated 10 to 20 percent of the range of motion, on exercises that load heavily in the early phase—especially if the weight being used is "heavy," and if there is mechanical disadvantage occurring.
- The final 10 percent of a muscle's range of motion seems to be the least "productive," from the perspective of hypertrophy (growth). In other words, a muscle generally has the least strength potential in the final phase. In fact, it's often difficult to even reach the latter part of the range of motion, when using a weight that sufficiently challenges the early phase of the repetition. Furthermore, there seems to be a bit more risk, especially in the joints that extend, like the elbows (triceps extension) and knees (quadriceps/leg extensions), in the final degrees of full extension. As such, you need to be careful upon full extension, or abbreviate that final part by about 10 percent.
- This leaves the middle 80 percent of the range of motion, which seems to be "always safe," as well as "always productive."
- During the first few repetitions of a set—when the muscle is least fatigued—it is good to move through as much range as possible, assuming it's within your comfort range (no pain or discomfort). On the other hand, as the muscle becomes more and more fatigued, and less capable of doing its full range of motion, it's "acceptable" to lessen the range of motion to whatever is necessary, even if it's only 50 percent of the normal movement. This factor should be determined, however, only by necessity—not by "laziness" or carelessness. It should be dictated by a greatly diminished physical ability—not by lack of willingness. As such, you should reduce the range of motion, when you must, if your only other alternative is to stop completely. You should never start a set, however,from the very beginning, using only 50 percent range of motion.
- You should never use so much range of motion that it distorts a joint to a painful degree, takes a limb significantly beyond its "normal" ranges, or contorts the body into extremely "unnatural" positions. An extreme stretch, as part of the "weighted" range of motion of an exercise, has never been associated with greatly enhanced muscle growth. In the extreme stretch position, there is a reduced potential benefit, as well as a drastically increased risk of injury.

All "physique" muscles (and joints) will be analyzed in Chapters 18 through 25, to ascertain each muscle's "ideal" range of motion.

## A Bit of History: The Marketing of Isometric Exercise

In the early 1920s, a man calling himself "Charles Atlas" (real name: Angelo Siciliano) began promoting an exercise program called "*dynamic tension*," a regimen that was based entirely on isometric exercise. The irony, in this instance, is that he called his course "dynamic." In reality, it was the opposite of dynamic exercise.

In the program that Atlas marketed, a person would perform a series of exercises—all without weights and *without movement*. The exercises were all static holds, wherein a person would simply hold a tensed position—pressing or pulling against either immovable objects (e.g., a wall or floor) or their own opposing force.

His advertisements (Figure 9-24) became iconic: A cartoon showing a scrawny man on the beach, bullied by a larger, more muscular man, embarrassing him in front of his girlfriend. The scrawny man then buys the "*Dynamic Tension*" course, and after a short while (i.e., "*in only 15 minutes a day*"), he miraculously transforms himself into a muscular "he-man." He subsequently returns to the beach and punches the bully in the face, thereby winning the admiration of his girlfriend.

In his advertisements, Charles Atlas publicly claimed that he had developed his physique using this very same static tension exercise course. In the process, he became the poster boy for isometric exercise, of that era. His claims, however, were not entirely truthful. He actually developed his physique by performing traditional (dynamic) weight-lifting exercises, which involved movement.

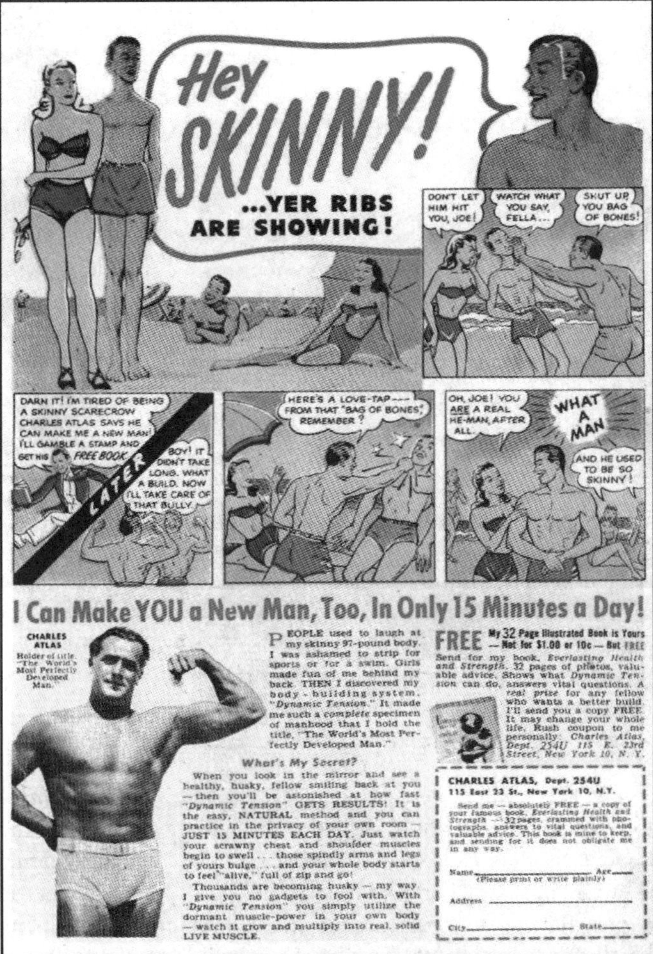

Figure 9-24

In a 1918 edition of a magazine called "*Liederman*," it was reported that "Atlas" performed a one-arm overhead press with a 236-pound weight. A separate 1920 edition of that same magazine stated that he did a one-arm press with a 266-pound weight. Clearly, he trained and developed his physique using weights and *movement*.

Of course, he realized the marketing appeal of selling a course that "*anyone could do, without any equipment, in the comfort and privacy of their own home.*" The exercises were relatively easy to understand and easy to do, as compared with the more intimidating and complicated, traditional weight-lifting exercises. According to reports in the early 1940s, he had sold over 400,000 courses—at $30 each. If those figures

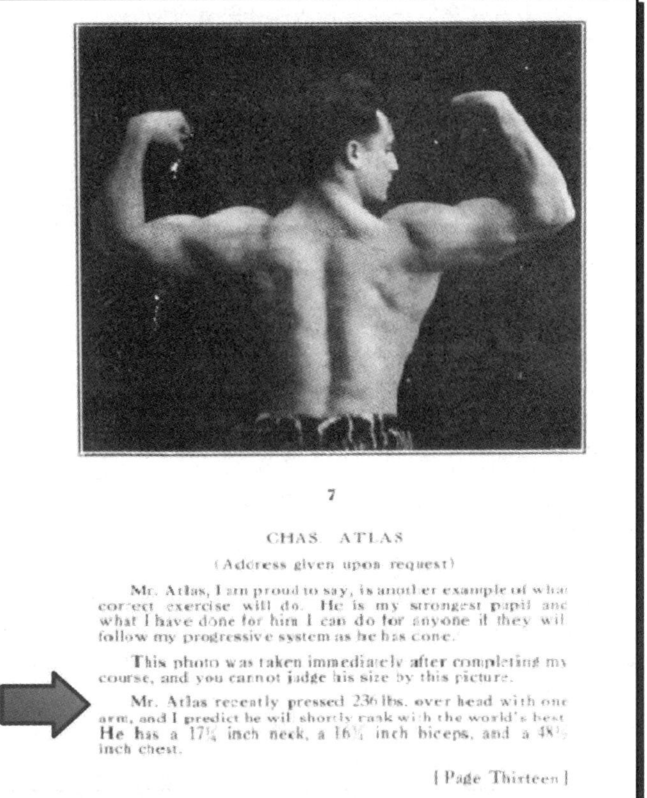

7

CHAS. ATLAS

(Address given upon request)

Mr. Atlas, I am proud to say, is another example of what correct exercise will do. He is my strongest pupil and what I have done for him I can do for anyone if they will follow my progressive system as he has done.

This photo was taken immediately after completing my course, and you cannot judge his size by this picture.

Mr. Atlas recently pressed 236 lbs. over head with one arm, and I predict he will shortly rank with the world's best. He has a 17¼ inch neck, a 16½ inch biceps, and a 48½ inch chest.

[Page Thirteen]

Figure 9-25

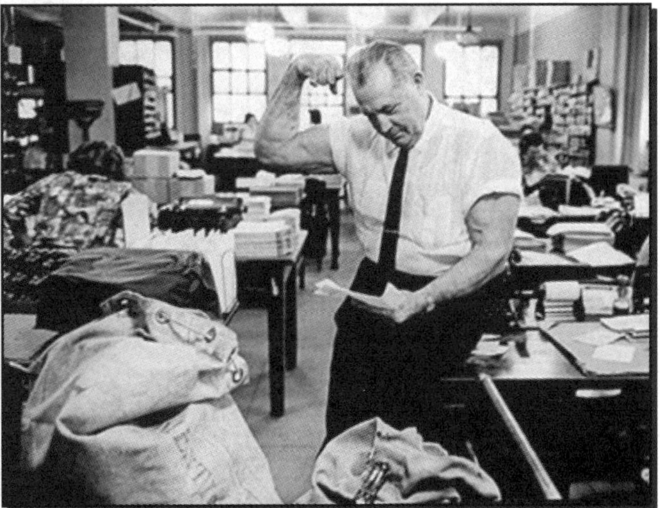
Figure 9-26

are correct, "Charles Atlas" and his business partner made over $12 million, which would have been a staggering amount of money in those days.

Obviously, in those "low-technology" days, very few people knew that Charles Atlas had actually not developed his physique using only the program he was selling. Today, this scenario might be considered "false advertising." There was no way of researching such things back then. Even today, there are many products that are marketed as "miraculous," despite the fact that they could not possibly produce the results that the manufacturers claim.

To his credit, Charles Atlas was a dedicated fitness practitioner and exercised diligently his entire life. Even at the age of 75, he was known to do a daily morning exercise routine that included 50 knee bends, 100 sit-ups, and 300 push-ups (all of which are dynamic exercises, it is worth noting). He was also a devoted husband and father. Less to his credit, however, is the fact that he was a profit-motivated person, who realized that many people were willing to pay a price to "learn" how to be strong and muscular, even if what they were "learning" was more fantasy than reality. As such, he appeared to take full advantage of the situation.

If you were told today that the aforementioned exercises would develop a very muscular physique, you might not believe it. In fact, you might suspect that you were being fed propaganda. On the other hand, are you really any wiser now? Are you less likely to believe a "*too good to be true*" notion about getting fit, without skepticism? It appears not. In fact, the same deceptive marketing of fitness programs and methods occurs today, arguably on an even larger scale.

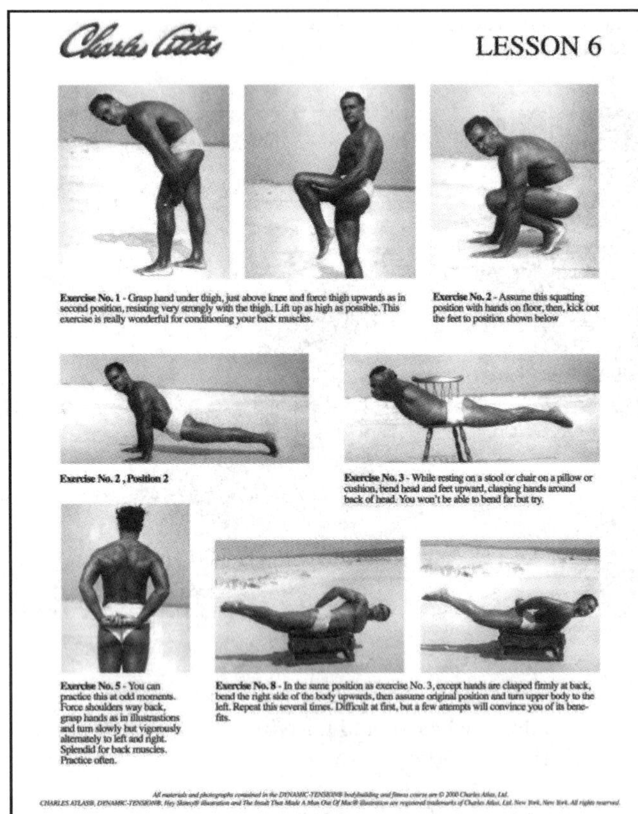


Figure 9-27

In fact, the fitness industry is more commercially driven now than ever before. There will never be a shortage of people willing to sell a program that cannot possibly deliver the results promised. Nor will there ever be a shortage of people who are gullible enough to buy an exercise method that promises miraculous, yet totally unrealistic, results.

Whether you're a student or a teacher of exercise, you should know which exercises have more benefit and which ones have less benefit, as well as which ones have more risk and less risk. As such, you should not believe, nor create the false impression, that all exercises—and all exercise methods—are equally productive, and therefore are all interchangeable.

## Summary

For purposes of physique development, visible muscle growth, and strength gains through a muscle's entire range of motion, *dynamic resistance* exercise is better than *isometric resistance* exercise. Furthermore, using a longer, mostly complete range of motion, when performing resistance exercise, is more effective for increasing muscle size and strength, as compared with using a shorter range of motion.

A study* published in the *Journal of Strength & Conditioning Research* concluded that increases of muscular size, as well as muscular strength, were greatest in a test group that used the longest range of motion (note: the exercise tested was the squat). This factor was true even though the group using the shorter range of motion utilized 10 percent to 25 percent more weight (resistance), than the group employing the longer range of motion.

When evaluating an isometric exercise, like the *plank*, for example, you should consider the energy cost versus the benefit of that exercise, as compared with using dynamic exercise options. For example, the plank causes isometric contraction of the rectus abdominis, the quadriceps, and the hip flexors. As a result, you might conclude that since there are three muscle groups working at the same time that the exercise is "good" because it saves time. On the other hand, the benefit of isometric contraction is very compromised, while the energy cost of loading three muscles simultaneously is very high. This situation results in the exercise having a very poor cost/benefit ratio.

Would you consider holding a straight-knee position on a leg extension machine to be a "good exercise" for the quadriceps? Of course not, at least not compared with performing full range of motion repetitions on that same machine. Therefore, the isometric participation of the quadriceps during a *plank* is not as productive as dynamic exercise for the quads (e.g., leg extensions, squats, etc.).

*(*January 2014 - Volume 28 - Issue 1 - p 245-255*)

The primary goal of performing *planks* is for the benefit of the exerciser's rectus abdominis. The isometric tension (of the abs) that occurs when doing planks, however, is less productive for abdominal development, than is dynamic abdominal exercise, e.g., *seated cable crunches* or *incline ab crunches.* Since isometric exercise is not productive enough to achieve visible muscular development of the pectorals, the quadriceps, the deltoids, etc., why would you think that isometric exercise for the abs is "as good as" (or "better than") dynamic exercise for the abs?

Many exercises require isometric stabilization from certain muscles, while the target muscle works dynamically—a situation that is perfectly acceptable. It is important, however, to do this "correctly," ensuring that the target muscle(s) is working dynamically (with joint movement), while the stabilizing muscles are working isometrically (without joint movement).

CHAPTER 10

# THE "ALL OR NOTHING" PRINCIPLE OF MUSCLE CONTRACTION AND THE MYTH OF "SHAPING" A MUSCLE

- *When a muscle fiber contracts, it does so from origin to insertion.*
- *It is impossible for only part of a muscle fiber to contract, or for one end of a muscle fiber to contract more forcefully than the other end of the muscle fiber, by the selection of exercises.*
- *Either the entire length of the muscle fiber contracts or it does not contract at all.*

Like so many human endeavors, bodybuilding is filled with folklore—beliefs that are based more on wishful thinking, than on fact or logic. People often believe that certain exercises will change the shape of a muscle—beyond simply making it larger—in ways that would make it more aesthetically pleasing. In reality, that viewpoint is physiologically impossible.

It is also common for people to assume that every person with an amazing physique developed their body with "advanced" insight. As a result, another assumption is often made that every exercise a "very fit" person performs has been selected by that person because it's 100 percent effective. People also assume that the ultra-fit person had full control over the shape their body has taken. These are all incorrect assumptions.

People typically do a number of different exercises for each muscle. So, it is common to assume that all those exercises contributed equally to the end result. That would be yet another incorrect assumption. This analysis is not to suggest that the person with an amazing physique has not worked hard, or that they didn't have some degree of insight into what they were doing.

In reality, exercises are NOT all equally productive. This is an absolute fact. As such, the ultimate shape of a person's muscles—after they've been developed (hypertrophied)—is mostly predetermined by genetics. The shape of your muscles, after they've hypertrophied as a result of performing resistance exercise, is not entirely of your choosing.

When your muscles grow, they become a larger version of what they were when they were smaller, generally speaking. One analogy that is particularly applicable, is that a circle is still a circle, even when it's bigger. It doesn't become a rectangle. Similarly, this factor is also true with regard to muscular development.

## What Is the "All or Nothing" Principle?

In a way, muscles are similar to ropes or elastic bands. For example, if you tie a rope around a tree and pull on it (Figure 10-1), the rope will be evenly taught through its entire length. It cannot be more slack, or more taut, anywhere between you and the tree. The tension is evenly distributed along the entire length of the rope. Muscles operate the same way.

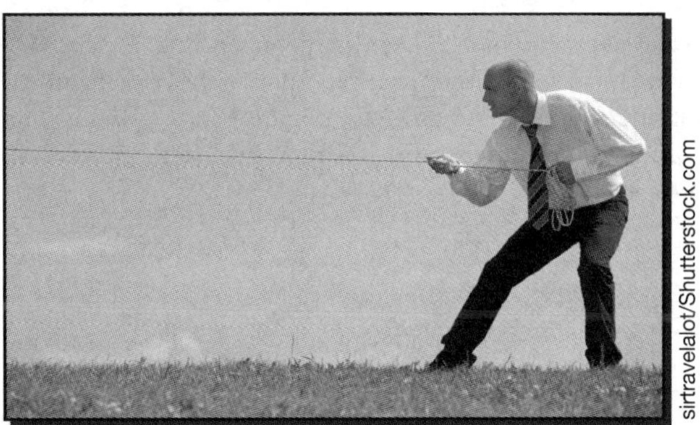
sirtravelalot/Shutterstock.com

Figure 10-1

Perhaps, you may be thinking that that scenario might be true, when one end of the rope is anchored to a stationary object, like a tree. You might think that it would be different, if both ends were mobile. By exploring what happens during a "tug-of-war," when both ends of the rope are free to move, we can lend clarity to this line of thinking.

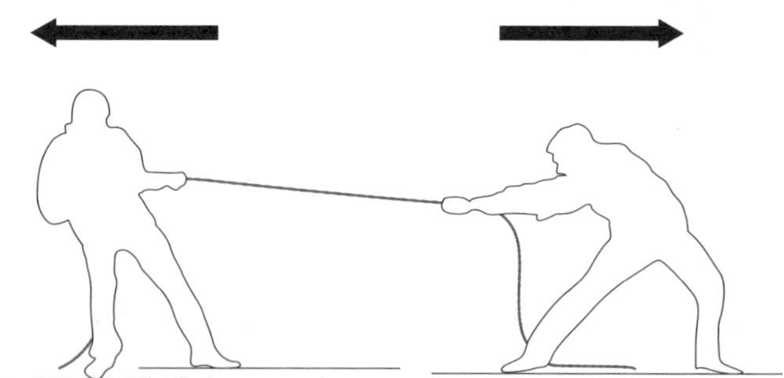

Figure 10-2

If the individual on the right (Figure 10-2) were "winning" (i.e., the entire rope moving more toward him), would the rope be more taut closest to him? No, it would not be. It does not matter who's "winning." It does not matter whether the rope is moving more toward the left or to the right. Either way, the rope will have the same tension through its entire length, from one end to the other.

In reality, it's "all or nothing." Either the entire length of the rope has equal tension, or no tension exists anywhere on the rope. It is impossible to pull on the rope in any way, such that more tension is on one end, and less tension is on the other end. If the amount of force increases, it increases evenly everywhere on the rope. If it decreases, it does so evenly throughout the entire length of the rope.

The same factor is true with muscles. Any muscle that is required to contract against resistance will have the muscle tension evenly distributed through the entire length of the muscle fibers, from the origin (where it's anchored) to the insertion (where it connects). The reason a muscle is able to produce skeletal movement is because of the evenly distributed contraction that causes the muscle's origin and insertion to move closer together.

❑ "Inner" and "Outer" Pectorals?

For years, a myth has been perpetuated that a *dumbbell press* (Figure 10-4) works the "inner" portion of the pecs (Figure 10-3, left side), and that *a dumbbell flye* (Figure 10-5) works the "outer" portion of the pecs (Figure 10-3, right side). This presumption is completely *false*.

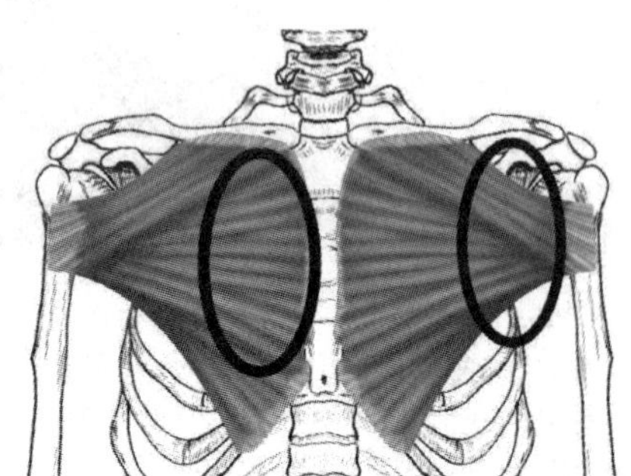

Clint Smith/E2 Systems, Inc.

Figure 10-3

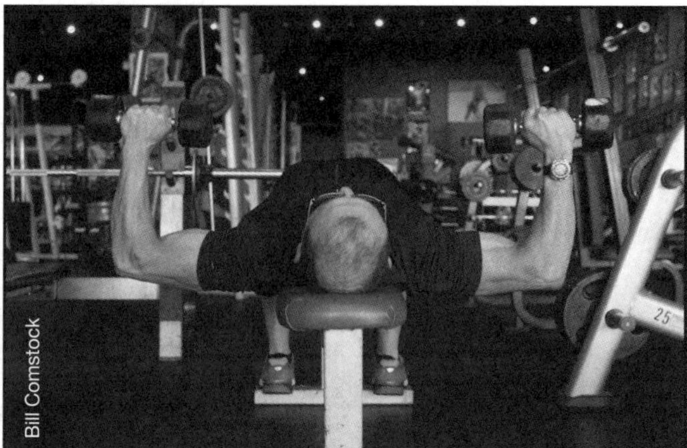


Figure 10-4

As you can see (Figure 10-6), the (sternal) pectoral fibers run from the sternum (center of the chest) to the humerus (the upper arm bone), like continuous "ropes." Regardless of whether the elbow is bent more or bent less, the pectoral muscle pulls the humerus toward the sternum in the exact same way. In fact, the pectoral muscle doesn't even "know" the position of the elbow. The pectoral fibers simply "know" the amount of load—regardless of whether it's a product of a longer lever (e.g., fly/straight arm) or a shorter lever (e.g., press/bent arm).

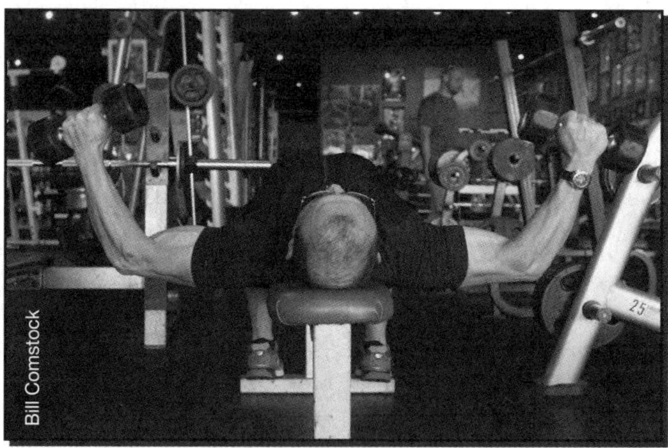


Figure 10-5

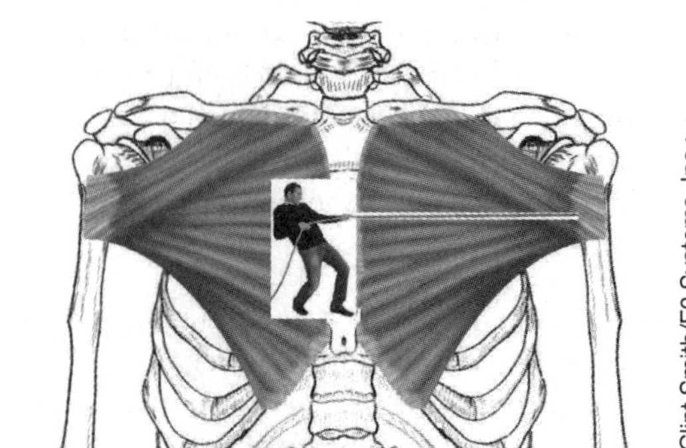

Clint Smith/E2 Systems, Inc.; eelnosiva/Shutterstock.com (inset)

Figure 10-6

The only difference between the two versions (Figures 10-4 and 10-5) is the "effective length" of the operating lever (i.e., the upper arm, plus its "secondary lever," the forearm). A longer effective lever (elbows less bent) magnifies resistance more, which requires that less weight be used. A shorter lever (elbows more bent) magnifies resistance less, which allows more weight to be used. Either way, however, the pectoral fibers that are working, are contracting evenly—from origin to insertion. There's simply no way for a person to selectively load, or contract, the "inner" part of the Pectorals more than the "outer" part of the pectorals (or vice versa), while performing any kind of pectoral exercise.

### ❑ "Upper Abs" and "Lower Abs?"

The "all or nothing" principle of muscle contraction also applies to the abs, although not to the same degree as it does in all the other skeletal muscles. This point will be explained in more detail in Chapter 24, during a specific discussion of the rectus abdominis.

Many people talk about the "lower abs." In fact, if you were to do an Internet search on "lower abs," you would find thousands of articles discussing "how to work the lower abs." In reality, however, there is no "lower ab," as a separate muscle. Furthermore, even if a person could emphasize that lower region of their abdominals, it would not produce the result most people expect.

Figure 10-7 shows a side view of the rectus abdominis. It is a single sheet of muscle that originates at the pubic bone of the pelvis and attaches onto the frontal part of the lower ribs. When the muscle contracts, it pulls either the front of the ribs toward the pelvis, or the pelvis toward the ribs. The muscle doesn't "know" which end is moving toward which end. This situation is analogous to the previously noted tug-of-war. It does not matter who is "winning" the tug-of-war. Either way, the "rope" has even tension throughout.

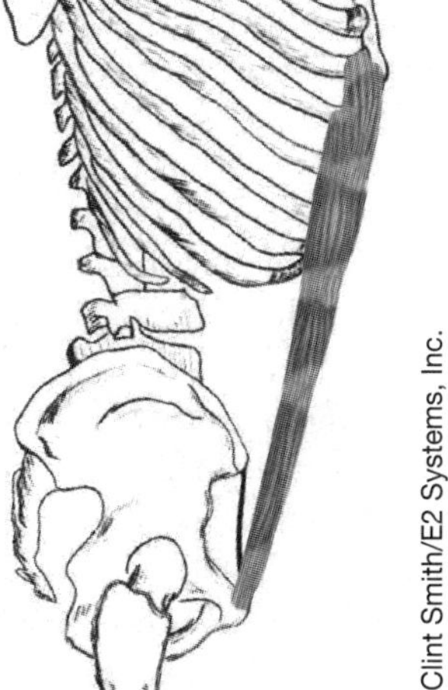

Clint Smith/E2 Systems, Inc.

Figure 10-7

The purpose of muscle contraction is to pull the origin and the insertion toward each other, thereby producing skeletal movement. The function of the rectus abdominis is to produce "spinal flexion." This skeletal movement would not occur unless the entire rectus abdominis—from origin to insertion—contracted.

You cannot *only* contract the "upper abs," *nor only* the "lower abs." You also cannot contract the "lower abs" a bit more than the "upper abs." There is no such thing as an exercise that allows you to do that.

Furthermore, it is impossible to add another "row" of abs, and it is equally impossible to selectively "dissipate" the fat that has accumulated in that lower region, by way of any exercise. As such, the effort to emphasize "work" on the lower region of the midsection is misguided anyway.

> *Note: The upper area of the abs always contracts with a bit more force than the lower area of the abs. This factor will be further explained in Chapter 24. Regardless, this circumstance is not something over which you have any control.*

### ❑ Making Biceps More "Full?"

In the 1960s, a man named Larry Scott (Figures 10-8 and 10-9) dominated the bodybuilding scene. He won Mr. California in 1960, Mr. America in 1962, and Mr. Universe in 1964. He then won Mr. Olympia in 1965 and again in 1966. Although he had an excellent overall physique, he was especially known for his arms—his biceps, in particular. They were big, of course, but they were also unusually "full." By this, it means that his biceps went all the way into the crook of his arm, whereas the biceps of most people stop about a half an inch before the crook of the arm.

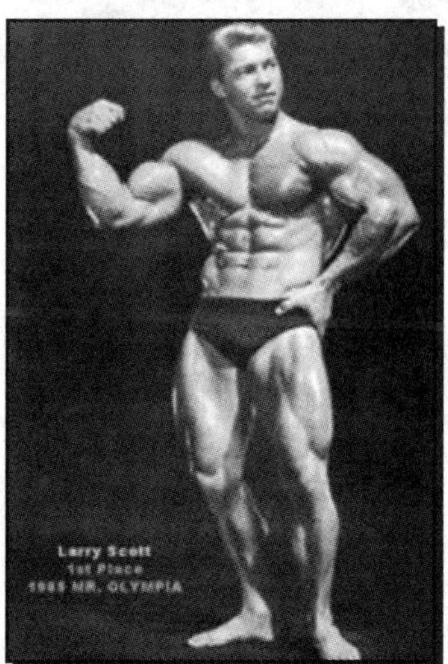


Figure 10-8

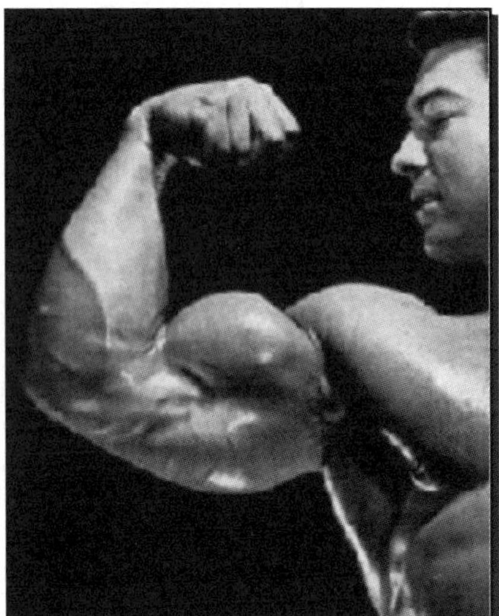
Figure 10-9

People assumed that Larry Scott must be doing a special exercise, to cause his biceps to be so full. Interestingly, he did have a "favorite" exercise, which is known as the "preacher curl" (Figure 10-10). As a result, many individuals assumed that this particular exercise was responsible for the fullness of his Larry Scott's biceps. In fact, the exercise subsequently became known as "Scott curls"—a term that is still used today by some of the "old schoolers."

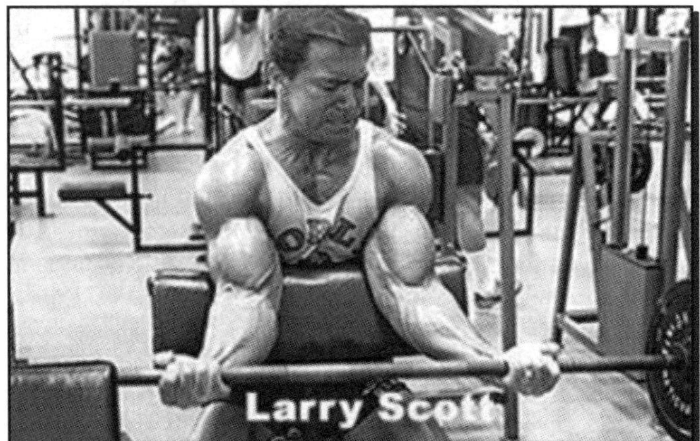

Figure 10-10

In reality, however, Larry Scott's biceps were shaped exactly as his genetics had predetermined. Regardless of which exercises he had chosen to do, his biceps would have had the exact same shape, notwithstanding fluctuations in overall size.

Of course, some people might ask, "How do you know that Larry Scott's biceps would have looked the same, if he had NOT done those curls?" Very simply, it has never been duplicated again, despite thousands of people—if not millions—having done the exact same exercise. No one has ever developed arms like those of Larry Scott.

That is not the only reason you can be assured that it was not "*preacher curls*" that produced those arms. From a physics' perspective, there is simply no way that any part of a continuous muscle fiber—anywhere between its origin and its insertion—can be made to experience more tension than the rest of the muscle fiber.

*Preacher curls* have a resistance curve that is different than that of the *standing barbell curl. Preacher curls* cause the biceps to experience more resistance at the beginning of the range of motion (when the elbow is mostly extended, and the arms are nearly straight), than does the *standing barbell curl.* This factor, however, does not influence the shape of the biceps. It simply causes there to be more resistance earlier in the range of motion, and less resistance toward the end of the range of motion.

Did Mr. Scott believe that "*preacher curls*" influenced the shape of his biceps? Unless he was familiar with physics and biomechanics, he may have actually believed that. On the other hand, he might have also been aware of how many others had used that same exercise, trying to get the same result, but failed. That would have been his first clue that "it was not the exercise" that created the shape of those arms.

Subsequently, Mr. Scott DID try to capitalize on people believing that this exercise would make their biceps more "full." After all, people were willing to pay him money for the "secret" to his extraordinarily full biceps. As such, just like Charles Atlas, who was discussed in the previous chapter, business does not require that an individual be either truthful or accurate. In general, the fitness industry has a long history of untruthful (or misinformed) marketers, as well as products that are actively promoted by way of unsubstantiated or exaggerated claims.

## Folklore Regarding Changing Muscle Shape

Normally, when someone speaks of the "all or nothing principle of muscle contraction," they are referring to "ends" of a muscle fiber—the fact that the entire length of a fiber contracts, if it contracts at all. The "all or nothing" principle, however, could also be used to mean that a muscle that has multiple "heads" (parts), which all contribute to one single function in unison, cannot have its parts emphasized separately by way of exercise, as the following examples illustrate:

- The biceps is comprised of two "heads," but both produce the same primary function: elbow flexion. The two heads converge on the one single tendon, before crossing the elbow.
- The triceps is comprised of three "heads," but all three parts produce the same primary function: elbow extension. All three heads converge on the one single tendon, before crossing the elbow.

- The quadriceps is comprised of four "heads," but all four parts produce the same primary function: knee extension. All four heads converge on the one single tendon, before crossing the knee. It should be noted that one part of the quadriceps also assists in a secondary function, but that secondary function is not primary.
- The calf muscle is comprised of two "heads," but both produce the same primary function: plantar flexion. Both heads converge on the one single tendon, before attaching to the heel bone.

Many people have long believed that the aforementioned muscles can be "shaped"—suggesting that one "head" (part) of the muscle can be emphasized more during a particular exercise, than another other part. Because the function of these muscle groups is singular (producing only one primary movement), however, causing one part of a muscle to be preferentially emphasized is physiologically impossible.

This factor will be further discussed in Chapter 17, as well as in each chapter dealing with the individual muscle groups. Muscles operate on an "all or nothing" basis, both in terms of the ends (origins and insertions), as well as in terms of their separate "heads." When muscles perform their respective functions, the entire muscle (all parts of it) participate in the movement, in unison. The only exceptions to this are the pectorals and the trapezius. These two muscles are unique in the sense that because their fibers run in different directions, they can produce movement in different directions.

*Note: The aforementioned muscles, with the possible exception of the calves, have at least one other function in which they assist. This does not negate the fact that these muscles have a "primary" function, which is the function that most contributes to hypertrophy. The "assist" function of these muscles is not primary enough to cause significant hypertrophy in those particular muscles.*

Your individual genetics determines the shape of your muscles. If your triceps are "short" (i.e., they do not appear to sweep all the way down to the elbow), there is no exercise that can cause the muscle to be, or appear to be, longer. No exercise will change its genetically determined shape. By the same token, if your lats are "high" (i.e., they do not sweep all the way down to the waistline), there is no exercise that will cause the lats to change how they attach to the spine and the pelvis. This factor is also genetically determined. Furthermore, if your quadriceps have a "boxy" appearance to them, and you would like for them to have a more graceful "sweep," there is no exercise you can do that will produce that shape. When your quadriceps contract, they do so in the one-and-only manner they can (knee extension), regardless of the exercise that causes its activation. That activation, then, results in the quadriceps shape that your unique genetics has predetermined.

Again, there are two exceptions to the aforementioned, as noted previously. When you work the pectorals, you can select a direction of humeral movement, using a directly opposing resistance, which allows you to "favor" some fibers more than others. For example, you can direct your arms more toward the sternum (for the sternal fibers); you can also direct your arms more toward the ribs (for the costal fibers); and you can move your arms more toward the clavicle (for the clavicular fibers). This factor will be discussed further in the pectoral section of this book. Still, you cannot preferentially affect the "inner" or "outer parts" of your pectorals.

The second exception is the trapezius. When you work the trapezius, similar to the pectorals, you can select a direction of scapular movement, using a directly opposing resistance, which enables you to favor some fibers more than others. For example, you can move your scapula straight upward (for the upper trapezius fibers), or you can move your scapula in various degrees of "backward," thereby activating the middle or lower trapezius fibers. You cannot, however, preferentially affect either the outer or the inner ends of those fibers.

All other muscles typically move their corresponding lever/limb in one primary direction. This factor not only hints at the fact that that particular muscle cannot be "shaped," according to a person's wishes, but also suggests that there is one "best" direction of anatomical movement for those muscles.

## Summary

As with any endeavor whose followers are very passionate (if not obsessed), there is often a great deal of myth and folklore. This scenario is certainly true in bodybuilding and the pursuit of physique development. These myths and folklore have lead many people to believe that there are "secret" exercises that can produce the exact muscle shape they desire. Unfortunately, there is no truth or science behind these beliefs. In fact, on occasion, the beliefs are entirely illogical.

Weight lifting, bodybuilding, calisthenics, and yoga all have passionate followers. Each of these endeavors has its share of pseudo-experts (gurus), who claim to have an understanding of that undertaking beyond that of others. In many cases, these "leaders" have demonstrated apparent success within that field, even if that success was achieved more by chance than by scientific knowledge. More often than not, that success is a result of exceptional genetics, a great deal of effort, and doing a sufficient amount of "very productive" exercises to offset the exercises that are less productive.

The aforementioned is not to suggest that these "experts," gurus, and champions do not deserve any credit at all. More than likely, they have made positive contributions in their respective fields, even if they inadvertently perpetuated some false beliefs. Furthermore, it is highly likely that they are correct about some aspects of their field, but are wrong about other aspects. Even medical doctors have been wrong about certain beliefs.

Over the years, many of these champions have appeared in magazines, where they are seen demonstrating exercises, which, in fact, are less than optimally productive. The accompanying article may state that "*This exercise works one part of (a muscle), and this other exercise works (a different part) of that muscle.*" To most individuals, such a scenario may seem accurate, or at least innocent enough, even if it's not accurate. It's not that these champions have deliberately intended to mislead readers. Nevertheless, their false statements have contributed to the massive degree of misinformation that currently exists in the field of resistance exercise.

Suggesting that exercises are all equally productive, or that a muscle's shape can be altered by way of certain exercises, is simply incorrect and misleading. In fact, a muscle that contracts against an opposing resistance does so from origin to insertion. It is not possible to preferentially contract one end of a muscle, more than the other end of a muscle.

As such, a muscle's shape is genetically determined. It cannot be influence or altered by using specific exercises.

# CHAPTER 11

# RECIPROCAL INNERVATION AND ACTIVE AND PASSIVE INSUFFICIENCY

- *Human skeletal muscles are often arranged in antagonistic pairs, which produce a contractile force in opposite directions. These pairs are referred to as "agonist/antagonist" muscles.*
- *The central nervous system is designed to inhibit the contraction of an antagonist muscle, while the contraction of the agonist muscle is occurring. For example, it is impossible to contract the biceps, while simultaneously contracting the triceps.*
- *This inhibition is called "reciprocal innervation," which is the automatic relaxation of an antagonist muscle, while the agonist muscle is activated, in order to preclude the body from engaging in self-defeating efforts.*

French philosopher, mathematician and scientist Rene Descartes (1596 – 1650), shown in Figure 11-1, was the first individual to hypothesize "*reciprocal innervation*" in 1626. Subsequently, Charles Scott Sherrington (1857 – 1952), English neurophysiologist, bacteriologist, pathologist, and Nobel laureate—Figure 11-2—established "Sherrington's Law of Reciprocal Innervation" (also known as "Sherrington's Law II"). He gave a more formal explanation of how a muscle relaxes, when its opposing muscle is activated.

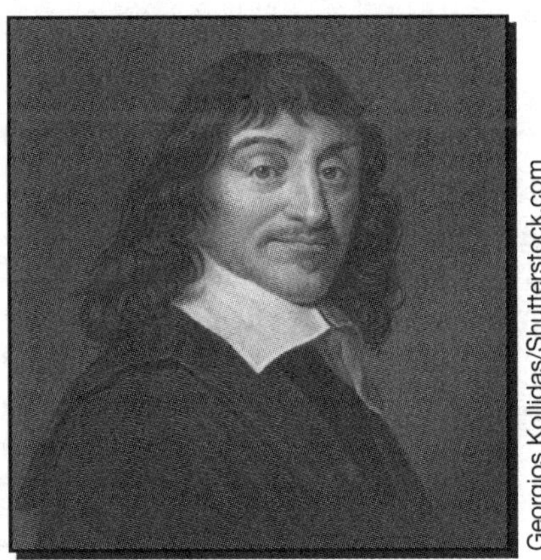

Georgios Kollidas/Shutterstock.com

Figure 11-1

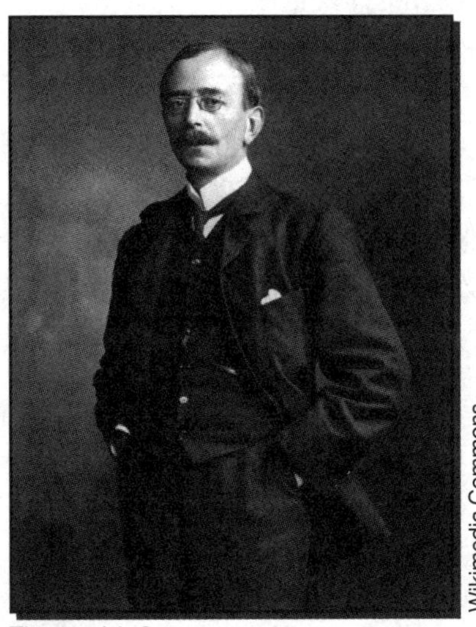

Wikimedia Commons

Figure 11-2

## What Is Reciprocal Innervation?

If you were to pick up a heavy box off a table, with your elbows bent, your biceps would become activated as they resist the downward pull of gravity on the box. The activation of your biceps is immediately registered and processed by your brain and central nervous system, which then send an "inhibitory synapse" to your triceps, causing it to relax—thereby preventing any opposing contraction. This action is nature's way of blocking any interference that would be caused by the *opposing* muscle, if it were to contract at the same time. Figure 11-3 (left side) illustrates the biceps relaxing as the triceps contracts, and the triceps relaxing as the biceps contracts (Figure 11-3, right side).

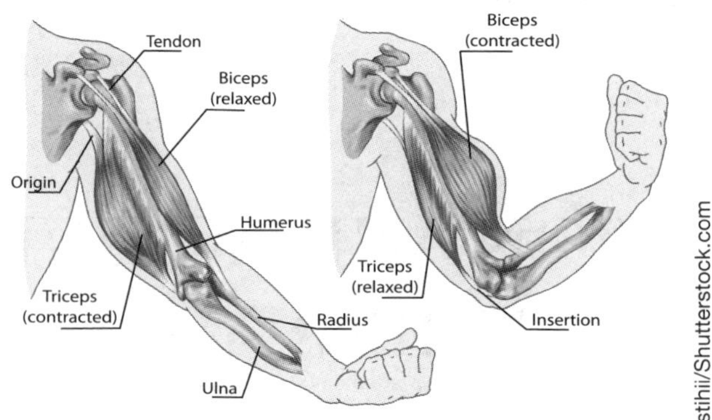


stihii/Shutterstock.com

Figure 11-3

In turn, Figure 11-4 provides a more technical diagram, showing the feedback loop that involves the central nervous system. Here, you can see how the activation of the biceps causes an "excitatory synapse" to be registered by the interneurons of the spinal cord, which then sends an "inhibitory synapse" to the triceps.

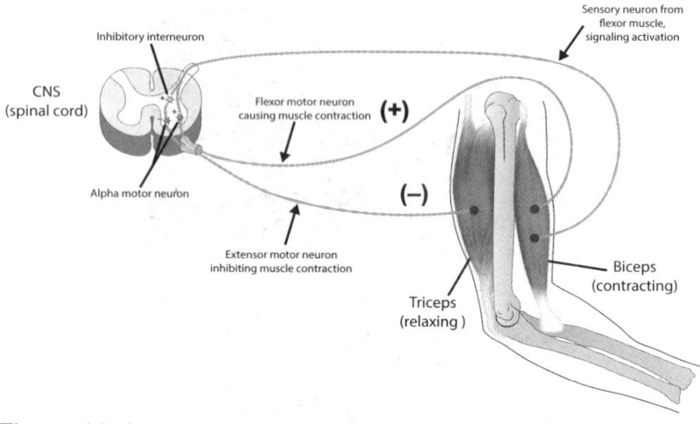


Figure 11-4

## The Relationship Between Reciprocal Innervation and the Apex/Base

In Chapter 4 ("The Apex and the Base"), an overview was presented concerning what happens when a person performs an exercise, during which a muscle's operating lever (limb) crosses over to the other side of the apex or base. The load transfers to whichever muscle is on the opposite side of that "limb." That transfer causes the antagonist muscle to become loaded, which "shuts off" the muscle that was first working (the agonist muscle), due to "*reciprocal innervation.*"

Specifically, that chapter addressed the triceps kickback exercise. When the forearm crosses over to the other side of the base (toward the shoulder), it activates the biceps. The activation of the biceps automatically relaxes (inhibits) the triceps, which is one reason why that exercise is so inefficient with regard to the development of the triceps.

In Figure 11-5, you can see that this person's left forearm has crossed past the vertical position (moving toward her shoulder), after returning from the triceps contraction. This crossing over past the base (the vertical line) activates the biceps (although for only half its range of motion), and causes the triceps to *deactivate*. Since this is meant to be a triceps exercise, the deactivation of the triceps during the execution of the exercise is entirely counterproductive. While this is not the only reason why the kickback is not a "good" triceps exercise, it clearly demonstrates the principle of reciprocal innervation.

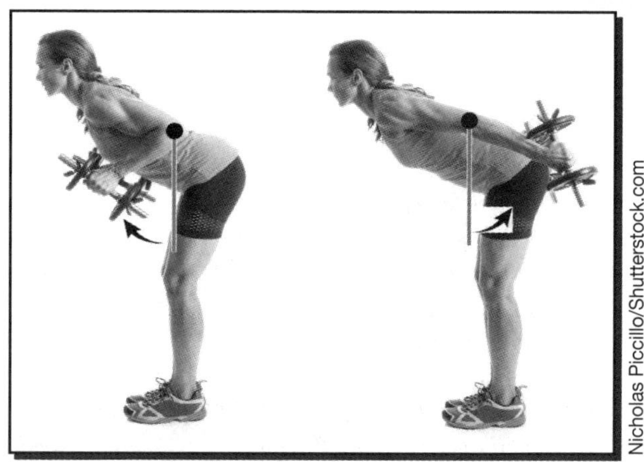

Nicholas Piccillo/Shutterstock.com

Figure 11-5

A list of the major agonist/antagonist muscles of the body is presented in Table 11-1. All of the muscle combinations listed produce movement in opposite directions.

Table 11-1. The major agonist/antagonist muscles of the body

| | |
|---|---|
| Biceps | Triceps |
| Pectorals | Middle trapezius |
| Upper trapezius | Lower trapezius |
| Abdominals | Lower back/erector spinae |
| Quadriceps | Hamstrings |
| Calves | Tibialis anterior |
| Forearm flexors | Forearm extensors |
| Anterior deltoids | Posterior deltoids |
| Gluteus maximus/ hamstrings | Hip flexors |
| Lateral deltoids | Latissimus dorsi |
| Internal shoulder rotators | External shoulder rotators |

The "agonist" is the muscle being activated at the moment; the antagonist is the muscle the muscle that opposes that movement. In other words, the muscle that would move that same limb in the opposite direction. Each muscle assumes the opposite role, whenever the opposing muscle is activated. When one muscle is activated (loaded/contracting/activated), the other relaxes.

You might think that this factor doesn't matter much, since you typically don't deliberately try to work your quadriceps and hamstrings at the same time. However, this is precisely what happens, when you perform a compound movement, such as a *barbell squat* or a *45-degree leg press*. When you perform this type of movement, you load the gluteus. That activation causes a relaxation synapse to be sent to the hip flexors, which includes the rectus femoris, which is one of the four quadriceps muscles. In other words, while you're attempting to optimally load your quadriceps with squats or leg presses, a significant portion of your quadriceps is being inhibited by reciprocal innervation.

In addition, the secondary function of the hamstring is to assist in hip extension, which obviously occurs (with load), while squatting. As a result of this activation of the hamstrings, there is further inhibition/interference of the quadriceps. The opposite is also true. Activation of the quadriceps, while squatting, inhibits/interferes with the optimal loading of the gluteus, caused by the effort to load the rectus femoris (of the quadriceps). The rectus femoris is one of the hip flexors, in addition to being a knee extensor. Accordingly, loading the rectus femoris (as part of the knee extension mechanism) sends a relaxation synapse to the antagonist muscles, which include the gluteus, hamstrings, and adductors—i.e., the hip extensors. As such, for optimal benefit to the knee extensors (quadriceps), the hip extensors (glutes, adductors, and hamstrings), and the hip flexors, each muscle group should be worked separately in order to avoid this interference. This step would constitute performing the movements individually—knee extension, hip extension, and hip flexion.

## What Is Active and Passive Insufficiency?

Separate from the "conflict of interest" that occurs from reciprocal innervation, there are two additional types of interference that sometimes occur when a muscle tries to contract from a disadvantaged position: passive insufficiency and active insufficiency.

Passive insufficiency relates to the contraction of a muscle that is compromised by the excessive stretch of the antagonist muscle. Typically, this type of interference occurs in the arms and legs—e.g., the biceps and triceps, and the quadriceps and hamstrings.

If you attempt to contract your biceps, during an exercise that causes excessive stretching of the triceps, the potential force of the biceps will be compromised, as the body tries to prevent the over-stretching of the antagonist muscle. Two examples of this situation are an *overhead cable curl* and *a prone (flat) leg curl*, which will be discussed shortly.

Active insufficiency relates to the contraction of a muscle that is compromised by its excessive shortening, caused by bringing its insertion too close to its origin. Again, this type of interference typically occurs in muscles that cross two joints, like the biceps and triceps, and the quadriceps and hamstrings. For example, since the biceps crosses the elbow and shoulder joints, biceps force is compromised when the elbow is flexed, while the shoulder is also flexed. Again, the example of an overhead cable curl, as well as the prone (flat) leg curl illustrates this type of interference. Having the shoulder flexed (i.e., the upper arm raised) causes the biceps insertion to get closer to the biceps origin, and results in the biceps becoming disadvantaged by being over-shortened. This situation results in biceps weakness, because the muscle fibers do not have sufficient length for optimal strength.

This factor also occurs during a *lying leg curl* (i.e., "*prone leg curl*"). That hip angle (i.e., having the femur mostly parallel to the torso) causes the hamstrings insertion of the hamstrings to move closer to the hamstrings origin, resulting in the hamstrings having insufficient length for optimal power.

Yet another example of this would be glute bridges, which cause the hip joint to be fully extended, while the knee joint is also flexed. This situation often causes the hamstrings to cramp—caused by the excessive shortening of the hamstrings.

In Chapter 4, we discussed the need to have the resistance curve of an exercise match the strength curve of the target muscle. The point was made that a muscle is stronger when it is elongated, and weaker (i.e., less strength potential) when it is shortened. The compromise of strength potential is caused by the muscle's overlapping of actin filaments. As such, a muscle's greatest strength potential occurs when the muscle is mostly elongated.

For this reason, it is best to perform exercises for the biceps, triceps, quadriceps, and hamstrings that avoid excessive shortening of the agonist muscle and excessive stretching of the antagonist muscle, caused by the simultaneous flexion or extension of the secondary joint. This strategy would prevent the loss of optimal muscle power caused by active insufficiency, as well as passive insufficiency.

In the 60s and 70s, when individuals worked their hamstrings, they did so on a machine like the one illustrated in Figure 11-6. It was a FLAT leg curl machine (...usually a combination leg extension/leg curl machine, which more often than not, was manufactured by "*Universal Gym*"). Subsequently, it was discovered that almost everyone had a tendency to raise their tailbones up, as they performed this leg curl.

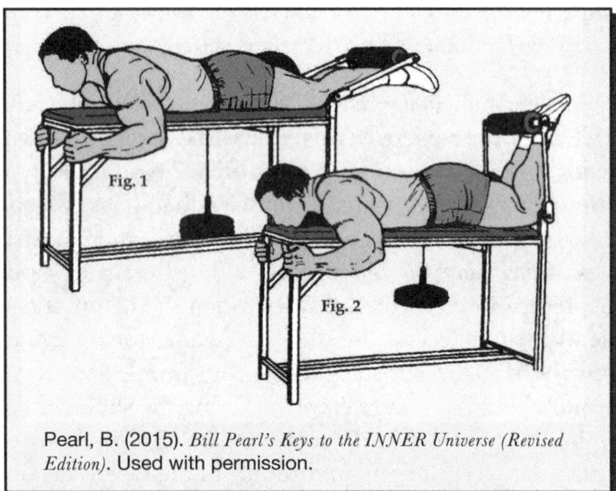


Pearl, B. (2015). *Bill Pearl's Keys to the INNER Universe (Revised Edition)*. Used with permission.

Figure 11-6

*Note: The illustration in Figure 11-6 is not of the machine manufactured by Universal Gym Equipment. Rather, it is that of an older "plate-loaded" version.*

By the late 80s, equipment manufacturers began making "dedicated" leg curl machines (without the leg extension function) and with an elevated section under the hips to compensate for the tendency of raising up the tailbone.

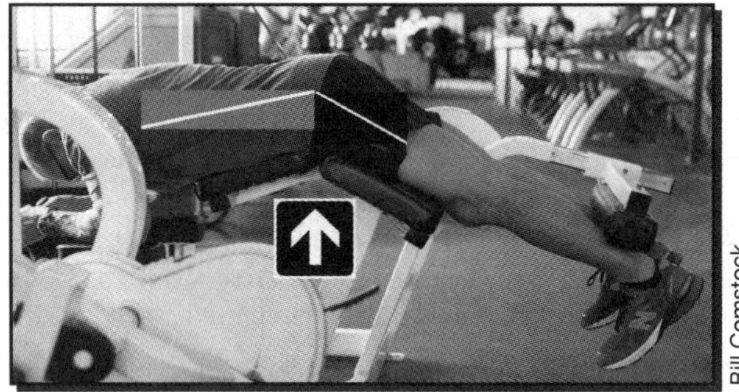

Bill Comstock

Figure 11-7

While raising the tailbone up makes the *lying leg curl* "easier," it still does not provide the optimal amount of hip bend. A person using this type of machine would still find themselves excessively arching their lumbar spine (thereby causing lower back discomfort), in their subconscious effort to create more hip bend. Ironically, some people believe that allowing the tailbone to rise is a type of "cheating." Occasionally, some trainers can be seen pushing down on their client's tailbone to prevent it from lifting up. This technique is entirely misguided.

There's a legitimate reason why the tailbone tends to rise up during *prone leg curls*. The body is merely trying to avoid passive insufficiency caused by the over-stretching of the quadriceps, and active insufficiency caused by the over-shortening of the hamstrings.

In fact, you could conduct an experiment (right now—right where you are) that can help clarify and reinforce this point. While standing on one leg (holding onto the back of a chair for balance), you should do a "knee flexion" (leg curl) with the other leg. While doing this, you should try to keep the femur of the leg that's "flexing" behind the femur of the leg on which you're standing.

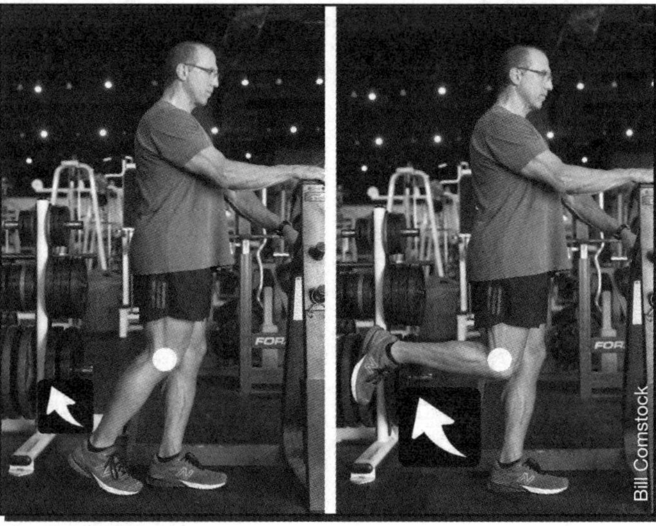

Bill Comstock

Figure 11-8

What you'll discover is that the task is pretty difficult—even though you're not using any added weight. It may even feel as though your hamstring is cramping, the more you bend your knee. In fact, what you're experiencing is active and passive insufficiency—both of which are inhibiting the ability of the hamstrings to optimally contract.

Conversely, if you were to flex your knee with a bend in that hip (on that same side), you will not feel your hamstrings cramping. In this scenario, the hamstrings would not be excessively shortened and the quadriceps would not be excessively stretching, once your hip is bent to about a 90-degree angle (femur to torso).

For this reason, the *prone (lying face down) leg curl* machine is a compromised way of working the hamstrings. Using a *seated leg curl* machine is a much better strategy, because it allows the hip joint to be bent at approximately 90 degrees to the torso, a position that eliminates both of these interferences. You'll also find that using a *seated leg curl* machine also allows a better stretch of the hamstrings (at the beginning of the range of motion), which is good, when it's the agonist muscle (Figure 11-9).

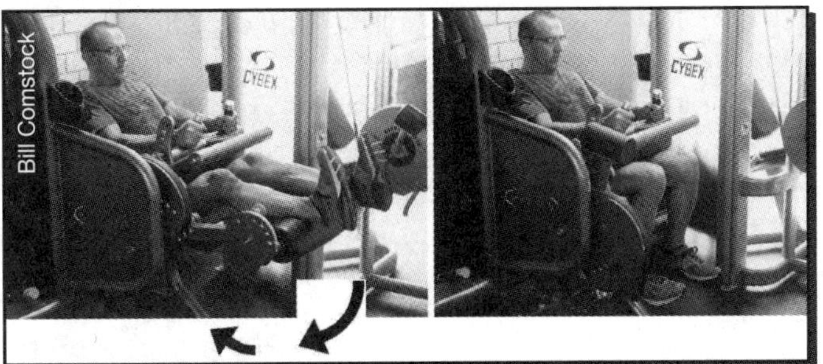

Figure 11-9

Compared with a *lying leg curl* machine, using a *seated leg curl* machine requires a little more adjustment. On the other hand, once you've made the correct adjustments for your individual femur length (i.e., the seat back), lower leg length (i.e., the ankle pad/roller), fulcrum point (having your knee aligned with the machine's pivot point), and preferred range of motion, you'll be doing the very best exercise for your hamstrings. You will have eliminated the interference caused by active and passive insufficiency, which occurs during *prone leg curls*.

A similar situation occurs when you try to load/contract the biceps, while simultaneously stretching the triceps. You may have even discovered that same weakness in your biceps, sometimes even cramping, which occurred in the previous experiment with your hamstrings. The biceps is excessively shortened when "*curls*" are performed with the humerus too far forward or overhead, leading to active insufficiency of the biceps. In addition, the triceps is excessively stretched when the elbow is fully bent and the shoulder/upper arm is in the "overhead" position, leading to passive insufficiency of the biceps.

The higher you raise your elbows, the more the biceps is shortened, the more the triceps is stretched, and the more the biceps is compromised. In fact, even a moderate elevation of the arms shortens the biceps and stretches the triceps, to some degree, thereby triggering both of these interferences, although to a lesser degree. This factor makes it more difficult to *curl* a weight that would be considered fairly "light," if *curled* when your upper arms are positioned down alongside your torso.

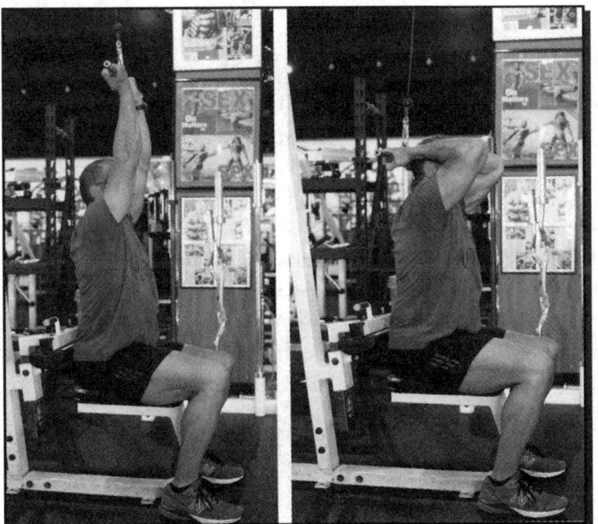

Figure 11-10

During the biceps exercise depicted in Figure 11-10, the insertion of the biceps (on the upper end of the forearm) is brought closer to the origin of the biceps (on the scapula), due to the arms being elevated as shown. Thus, bending the elbow further shortens the biceps, to the point where they become actively insufficient. The biceps are further compromised by the excessive stretching of the triceps, which also occurs with the shoulder joint in this position, thereby also triggering passive insufficiency.

Interestingly, most of the Internet sites on which you'll find this exercise being demonstrated, will say that it helps develop the "peak" of your biceps. Furthermore, these sites sometimes claim that the cramping feeling you experience in the biceps is "proof" of that "peak building." Obviously, that claim is entirely inaccurate. In reality, what you're feeling is the interference caused by active and passive insufficiency, caused by the less-than-optimal shoulder angle. Incidentally, nothing can change the shape of your biceps, nor improve its "peak."

## Using Reciprocal Innervation to Structure Workouts

Because of the fact that relaxation occurs in a muscle when its opposing muscle is contracting, combining *opposing* muscles in a single workout is a good strategy. In fact, you could even do "super-sets" (alternating sets) with those opposing muscles.

Alternating between two opposing muscles ("super-sets") takes advantage of the fact that while an agonist muscle is working (e.g., the biceps), the antagonist muscle (e.g., the triceps) is fully relaxing and recovering. Alternatively, you could do all the sets targeting one body part (e.g., pectorals), followed by all the sets targeting the opposing body part (e.g., back/lats), in the same workout, without any compromise to either muscle group.

Ironically, one of the most *common* muscle grouping strategies is known as "push/pull," but it's very misguided. This strategy is where the (so-called) "pushing muscles" are done on one day, and the (so-called) "pulling muscles" are exercised on a different day. The qualifier is "so-called," because all muscles actually PULL. No muscles "push." When muscles contract, they shorten—pulling the ends together—which then either flexes or extends a joint. Nevertheless, the "pushing muscles" are thought to be the pecs and the triceps, while the "pulling muscles" are thought to be the back and the biceps.

*Note: Obviously "push" and "pull" were so named ONLY because the weight being moved is getting farther away from the body, or closer to the body, during concentric contraction. In reality, this is an absurd method of categorizing muscles, because a muscle has no "idea" whether the weight that is moving is getting closer to the body or farther away from it.*

The rationale underlying this type of grouping is the belief that while the pecs are working, the triceps are assisting. Therefore, you "*might as well*" finish off the triceps at that time. Similarly, when the back muscles (lats, middle traps, teres major, etc.) are working, the biceps are assisting, and, therefore, you "*might as well*" finish off the biceps at that time.

There are several inherent problems with this philosophy. In reality, if you perform the optimal pectoral exercises, there would actually be very little triceps participation. Likewise, if you perform the optimal "back" exercises, there would be very little biceps participation.

If a person experienced considerable triceps or biceps fatigue, while doing their pectoral or "back" workouts (respectively), those workouts could be considered "compromised," if the goal is optimal muscle-building. In reality, an individual would not feel much biceps nor triceps fatigue during highly efficient chest or back workouts, during which they kept the secondary lever (the forearm) mostly neutral during those exercises.

Furthermore, it would be better to work the biceps and the triceps when they are fresh (on a different day), not after having been pre-fatigued by poorly executed chest or back exercises. All factors considered, there is very little wisdom in the "push/pull" muscle-grouping strategy.

## A More Sensible Approach

What makes more sense, in terms of body part grouping, is to combine *opposing* movements in the same workout. In other words, using "reciprocal innervation"—the fact that working an agonist muscles facilitates relaxation of the antagonist muscle—is the better strategy for grouping muscles in a given workout.

Instead of working two muscles that *may* be working simultaneously (e.g., chest and triceps), it's more sensible to work two muscles that DO NOT work simultaneously (e.g., chest and back). When the pectorals work, the back muscles are fully relaxing, and vice versa. This factor ensures that each muscle is *fresh* (recovered) each time you perform a set for that muscle.

The following are a few of the "opposing muscles" that would make for good muscle groupings in a given workout:

- Chest and back
- Front deltoids and rear deltoids
- Biceps and triceps
- Quadriceps and hamstrings
- Abdominals (rectus abdominis) and "lower back" (erector spinae)
- Forearm flexor and forearm extensor
- Glutes (hip extensors) and hip flexors

*Note: Not all movements require an opposing exercise. For example, calves (plantar flexion) does not automatically require that the tibialis anterior be worked. The antagonist muscle of the medial deltoids is the lats, but it's better to alternate between the right side and left side medial deltoids, than it is to alternate deltoids with lats.*

## Creating a Workout Structure

First, you need to decide whether you want to work the entire body during one workout, or divide your workouts into a *two-way* split, a *three-way* split, or a *four-way* split. This decision would be based on your current age and health status, how advanced you currently are, your goals, your time constraints, and your level of discipline.

Personally, I prefer a four-way split program (which could be considered "advanced"), which means doing four separate workouts to work all the muscle groups one time. It allows me to complete each of the four workouts in a reasonable amount of time (approximately 90 minutes), and yet still spend enough time (i.e., 8 to 15 sets) on each muscle group.

The next issue to consider is the frequency with which you would work each physique muscle. Ideally, a muscle should not be worked more frequently than three times per week (with significant intensity), nor less frequently than one time per week.

There are 14 muscle groups that "should" be worked, including the following: pectorals, latissimus, middle trapezius, upper trapezius, medial deltoids, posterior deltoids, anterior deltoids, triceps, biceps, quadriceps, hamstrings, glutes, calves and abs. An individual could also add a few more muscle groups to their workout regimen, including hip flexors, obliques, forearms (flexors and extensors), neck (front, back, and sides), erector spinae, shoulder rotators, etc. Deciding to work these additional muscle groups depends on a person's degree of ambition, and the amount of time that they're able to spend in the gym.

It is important to note that this book is not intended as a "workout guide." It is meant to explain the mechanics of the body, as they relate to resistance. Accordingly, not too much time will be devoted to this subject.

Nevertheless, as a general guideline, I usually recommend that a person who only wants to exercise three days per week should do a full-body workout, performing three sets of one exercise per muscle group, per workout. That regimen would entail approximately 42 total sets—assuming a person works all 14 primary physique muscles. In this instance, a 90-minute workout would allow an average of two minutes per exercise.

A person who is willing to exercise four times per week could split their body parts into two groups (a two-way split), and perform five or six sets per muscle group. This scenario results in each muscle getting worked a little harder, but with a little less frequency—twice per week instead of three times per week.

A three-way split (dividing all the muscle groups into three separate workouts) can be employed by a person who is able to work out four to six days per week. With this grouping, an individual could either do five or six sets per muscle group, and simply have a shorter workout, or he could do 8 to 12 sets per muscle group. This latter option would allow more intensity (i.e., more "volume") in the workout.

A four-way split is useful if a person is doing more body parts than the 14 primary muscles previously mentioned, or wants to do more volume (sets) per muscle group, or wants a shorter workout. This option, however, would ideally require a minimum of five or six workout days per week in order to get enough frequency of workouts per muscle group. The four workouts would simply be rotated around the five or six days of the week that you select as your "exercise days."

The typical workout structure I personally use encompasses the following:

- Day #1: Chest and Back—pecs, lats, and middle traps (aka the "upper back")
- Day #2: Shoulders and Upper Traps—side deltoids, posterior and anterior deltoids, plus the upper trapezius
- Day #3: Arms, Forearms, and Mid-Section—biceps, triceps, forearm flexors, rectus abdominis (abs), erector spinae ("lower back"), and obliques
- Day #4: Legs—quadriceps, hamstrings, glutes/adductors, calves, and hip flexors

The schedule in Figure 11-11 is one of three ways to execute this plan. These same four workouts could be spread out over five days per week (providing two "off" days each week), or the four workouts could be spread out over the seven days of the week (providing no days "off" per week). This latter option, however, generally cannot be sustained indefinitely. This particular workout schedule would allow you to work each muscle group once every four or five days.

## Intensity, Recovery, and Adaptation

Any discussion concerning "how to structure your workout" would be remiss, if the issues of intensity and recovery were not addressed. Again, it is important to note that this book is primarily intended as a guide for the biomechanics of resistance training. Workout frequency and intensity are issues related to muscle physiology, which is another subject altogether—and a complex one at that. Nevertheless, a review of a few of the basic points can be helpful.

In general, a muscle needs one to three days of recovery after a workout, assuming a moderately high level of intensity is used. On the other hand, if you train very intensely, three to five days of "rest" may be required, before that same muscle can be worked again.

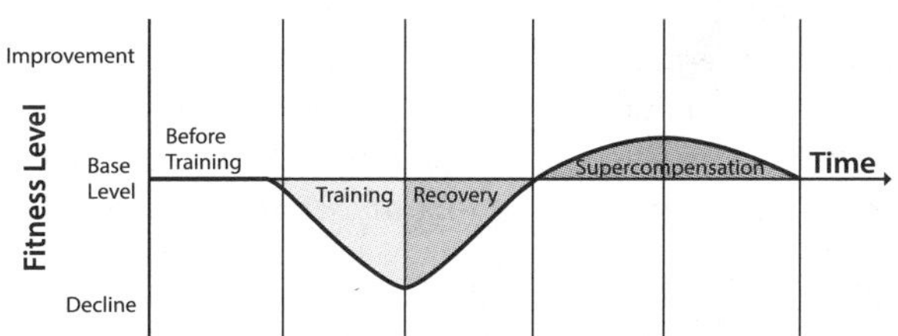


Figure 11-12

Figure 11-12 shows that, after a resistance workout, there is a recovery phase—generally lasting a day or two. During this phase the muscle recovers back to its baseline. Next, the muscle transitions into the "*supercompensation*" phase—generally lasting another day or two. During this phase, the muscle is adapting (improving its performance capacity), preparing itself for the next such encounter.

Ideally, you should work each muscle again when the muscle is at the peak of its "supercompensation" phase. This factor is important, because this phase begins to decline after the peak. If you wait until this phase has completely ended, you return to the baseline, almost as if no previous workout had occurred.

| Sunday | Monday | Tuesday | Wednesday | Thursday | Friday | Saturday |
|---|---|---|---|---|---|---|
| Day 1 | Day 2 | Day 3 | Day 4 | Day 1 | Day 2 | |
| Day 3 | Day 4 | Day 1 | Day 2 | Day 3 | Day 4 | |

Figure 11-11

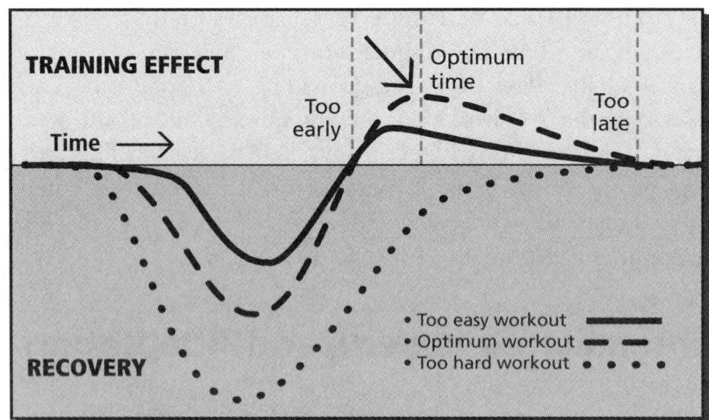

Figure 11-13

Working a muscle again when it is at the peak of its "supercompensation" phase will theoretically push it up to a higher level of strength/growth. This process is how "muscle accumulation" (growth) occurs. It builds on previous "highs," like adding small amounts of sand to a pile, which eventually becomes a "hill." This factor is why workouts that are too *in*frequent (i.e., performed after the "supercompensation" phase has passed) is like starting over again at the baseline each time.

Conversely, if the next workout (for that particular muscle) occurs *too soon* after the previous workout, "overtraining" can occur. "Too soon" would be a scenario in which the workout would be undertaken before the recovery phase is complete; the muscle would not have had the chance to experience even the earliest part of supercompensation. When this happens, progress (muscle growth) for that muscle is impeded.

Of course, the issue of exercise intensity factors into how long the recovery phase needs to be. Employing less workout intensity theoretically warrants *less* recovery time, and using more workout intensity theoretically warrants *more* recovery time—but only up to a point. There is such a thing as an "ideal intensity" for optimal results (Figure 11-13). The intensity should not be too low nor too high, regardless of the subsequent recovery time. The "right" amount of intensity yields the greatest results.

Some individuals believe that annihilating a muscle during a workout (leaving it absolutely limp with fatigue) will lead to maximum muscle gains, but this assumption is not supported by the research. In fact, the research suggests otherwise.

Shorter or longer recovery time is not the absolute equalizer of the intensity level used. You cannot make up for insufficient workout intensity, simply by taking less time between workouts. Nor can you make up for excessive workout intensity, simply by taking an extra day or two of rest, between workouts. Too much exercise intensity results in muscle damage, from which a muscle cannot easily recover. Of course, as you progress in your training, muscle tolerance increases, and a higher intensity workout is possible. In reality, however, there is always a point of "too much" for everyone.

The most extreme form of muscle damage caused by overly intense exercise is called "exertional rhabdomyolysis." When this condition occurs, the muscle severely breaks down. Its byproducts (which enter into the bloodstream) are harmful to the kidneys, possibly leading to kidney failure. Of course, this degree of "overtraining" is extremely rare, especially with advanced athletes who are already highly trained. It can still occur, however, even in advanced athletes.

In fact, there are several stages of overtraining that occur long before the onset of exertional rhabdomyolysis. In other words, you do not need to get to that extreme point, before overly-intense workouts become counterproductive for you.

The "right amount" of workout intensity is required, and this varies from person to person, based on a number of factors. These include your individual health, enough sleep, sufficient caloric intake, adequate endocrine levels, other daily activities (caloric demands), and your current level of muscular strength and endurance. In reality, each person should experiment to find their own optimal level of workout intensity, and then balance that level with the right amount of exercise frequency.

## Relieve Muscle Cramping With Reciprocal Innervation

Because a relaxation synapse (signal) is sent to a particular muscle when its opposing muscle (its "antagonist") is activated, one of the best ways to relieve a muscle cramp is by flexing or tensing its antagonist muscle. For example, if your calf muscle (gastrocnemius) is cramping, as often happens, it is helpful to flex your tibialis anterior (Figure 11-14). By causing the tibialis to pull upward on the forefoot (known as "dorsi flexion"), the calf muscle is sent a "*relaxation* synapse" by the central nervous system (Figure 11-15).

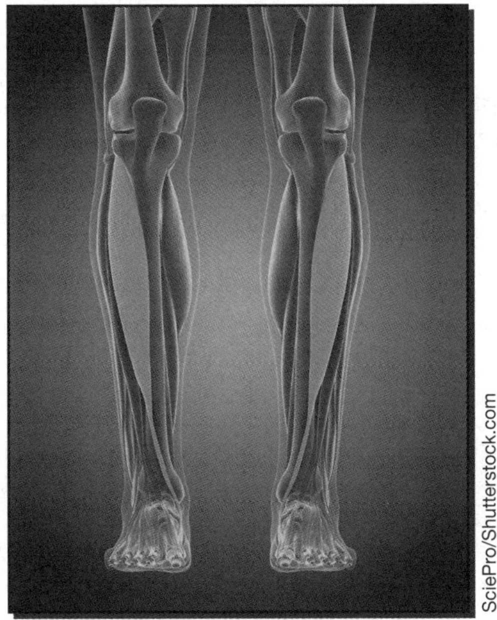

Figure 11-14

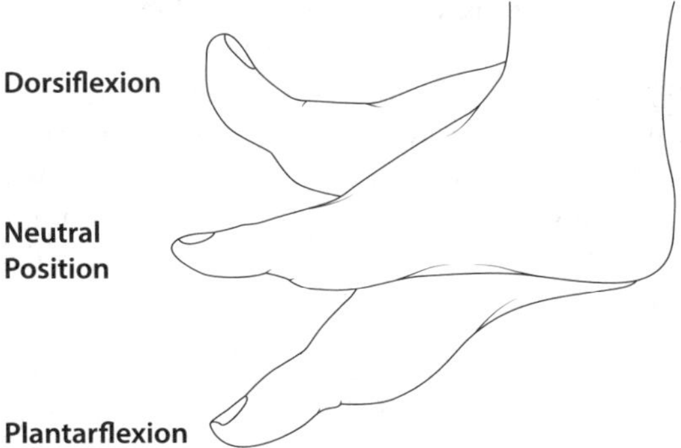

Figure 11-15

Technically, the antagonist of the tibialis anterior is the tibialis posterior. It is impossible, however, for the calf muscle to contract, while simultaneously flexing the tibialis anterior. The tibialis anterior and the calf muscle are on opposite sides of the lower leg, and they produce ankle (foot) movement in opposing directions. They cannot be activated at the same time, due to reciprocal innervation.

A reasonable argument could be made that frequent calf cramps may be caused (in part) by the imbalance of strength between the calves and the tibialis anterior. Therefore, a possible solution for frequent calf cramps could be to regularly exercise the tibialis anterior. On the other hand, the factor for causing a person's frequent calf cramps could be biochemical. If this were the case, exercising the tibialis anterior would NOT help alleviate calf cramps. However, it's worth exploring the possibility of reducing the tendency of calf cramping, by doing the exercise illustrated in Figure 11-16.

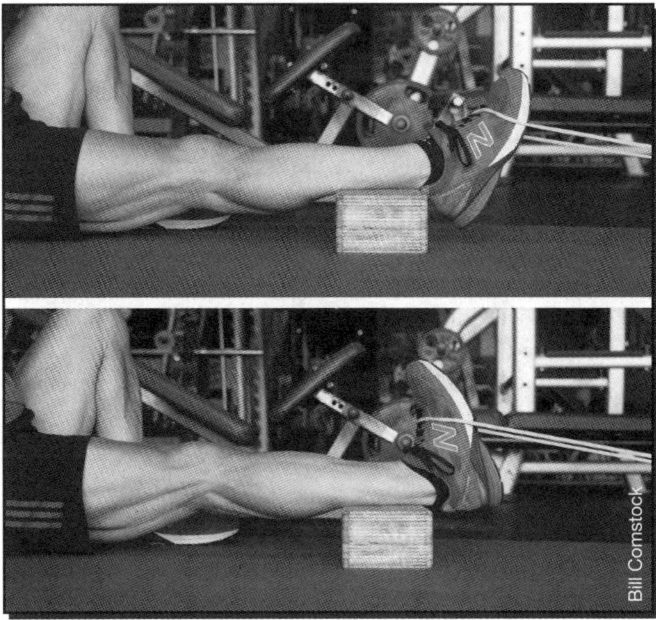

Figure 11-16

This same technique of flexing the antagonist muscle can be used when you are experiencing cramping on the bottoms of your feet. By pulling the toes upward, thereby activating some of the antagonist muscles to those on the bottoms of the feet, a relaxation signal could be sent to the muscles on the bottom of the feet, which might result in them releasing their tension.

Similarly, flexing (or working) the rectus abdominis (the abs) could help relieve cramping in the erector spinae (the "lower back"). This step would not be helpful, however, if the back pain is being caused by a herniated disc pushing against a nerve. This type of scenario is best addressed with medical intervention.

## Summary

Reciprocal innervation is part of the amazing natural design of the human body.

Understanding the role it plays in resistance exercise allows us the opportunity to avoid compromised efforts, caused by a relaxation synapse being sent to your target muscle, precisely when you're trying to optimally load that muscle.

Of course, this factor means rethinking some of the traditional exercises that everyone has been led to believe are "foundational," such as barbell squats and leg presses. Clearly, reciprocal innervation occurs during these exercises, as a result of the simultaneous loading of the hip extension muscles (the glutes) and one of the hip flexors (the rectus femoris), which is a significant portion of the quadriceps. These two muscles cannot optimally contract, simultaneously. Yet, that is what many people typically expect when they perform squats and leg presses.

Furthermore, the hamstrings' participation in hip extension is also in conflict with the activation of the quadriceps (all four parts), due to reciprocal innervation. Again, the point should be emphasized that the hamstrings and the quadriceps cannot be optimally contracted, simultaneously.

Reciprocal innervation—the fact a muscle's function is compromised when its antagonist muscle is also loaded—suggests that muscles should be exercised in a particular order or in specific combinations. As such, grouping opposing muscles together is a very good strategy, for this very reason.

As the last eight chapters in this book point out, some traditional ways of exercising certain muscles ignore this fact. As a result, those muscles are not stimulated as effectively as they could be, compared with using exercises that avoid that interference.

Almost any kind of muscle-group combination will produce some degree of benefit (muscle growth), even if the conventional "push/pull" method (chest and triceps/lats and biceps) is employed. Grouping muscles that produce movement in opposite directions during the same workout, however, is arguably more productive than grouping muscles that produce movement in a similar direction.

In fact, it is very sensible to set up your workout plan in a way that creates as little "conflict of interest" as possible. There are advantages to working a muscle group without it having any pre-exhaustion from a previous exercise, or interference from its opposing muscle.

In addition to avoiding the LOADING of antagonist (opposing) muscles, it is wise to also avoid excessively shortening a target muscle, by positioning its secondary joint in a way that brings the muscle insertion too close to the muscle origin. This situation causes active insufficiency—the excessive overlapping of the muscles' actin filaments, to the point where it loses strength potential. Of course, this factor assumes the goal of optimally loading and stimulating a given muscle, for the purpose of maximum development of that muscle. An example of this is *lying (prone) leg curls*, in which the hip joint is "straight" (i.e, the femur is in line with the torso, or close to it), thereby causing the hamstrings' insertion to be brought excessively close to its origin, while simultaneously bending the knee.

It is also wise to avoid excessively stretching the antagonist muscle of your target muscle, during a given exercise. This situation causes passive insufficiency—the conflict of having the opposing muscle of your target muscle, over-stretching to the point where it interferes/prohibits the freedom of your target muscle to contract with full force. Again, an example of this scenario is *lying (prone) leg curls*, because this "hip straight" position causes the quadriceps to excessively stretch, as the knee is being bent. This excessive stretch of the quadriceps interferes with the optimal contraction of the hamstrings.

For the same reasoning, it's wise to lean back (as far as possible) when doing *leg extensions*. Rather than adjusting the seat back so that it's perfectly upright, it's better to move it as far back as possible, and allow yourself to recline. This positioning lessens the degree of hip bend, which reduces the potential hamstring stretch that could occur when the knees are fully extended, and the torso is upright. This factor is especially beneficial for people who lack flexibility in the hamstrings.

Active and passive insufficiency are also the reasons why it's so much more difficult to raise your leg with your knee straight, as compared with raising your leg with your knee bent. Raising your leg (i.e., hip flexion) with your knee straight causes the hamstrings to stretch beyond the point that the hip flexor's range of motion could otherwise allow. This scenario creates passive insufficiency. In addition, the rectus femoris is over-shortened, because the knee-straight position requires quadriceps contraction, simultaneous to having its insertion brought closer to its origin. This circumstance creates active insufficiency.

CHAPTER 12

# "COMPOUND" VS. "ISOLATION"—THE ORIGINS OF THE DEBATE

- *There has been a pervasive belief, for decades, if not centuries, that "compound" exercises (multi-joint/multi-muscle) are better than "isolation" exercises (single or duo-joint), for every muscle-building, sports conditioning, or fitness training-related goal.*
- *As can be seen in the next chapter, biomechanical analysis proves this belief to be incorrect. Isolation exercises are actually better than compound exercises, for a number of purposes.*
- *The subject of compound versus isolation exercise has been misunderstood. Even the distinction between the two types of exercise is much less clear than many assume.*
- *This chapter discusses how these erroneous beliefs came into being, and lays the foundation for a better understanding of these exercises.*

Physical strength has been revered since the origins of man. According to Greek legend, Herakles (aka "Hercules" in Roman literature)—who is believed to have been born in the year 1276 B.C.—was idolized for his "legendary strength." Milo of Creton—a 6th century wrestler—was also credited with many stories of amazing strength, including that he carried a live bull on his shoulders for daily exercise. By the 1800s, "Amazing Feats of Strength" had become a popular form of entertainment, and a number of early "strong men" grew to prominence in this pursuit, including the following:

- *Arthur Saxon* (1878 - 1921) was a "strongman" and circus entertainer. He became famous for performing one particular lift called "the bent press." This exercise (Figure 12-1) is a one-arm overhead lift, with the torso bent sideways. Subsequently, he set a world record of 370 pounds in this lift.

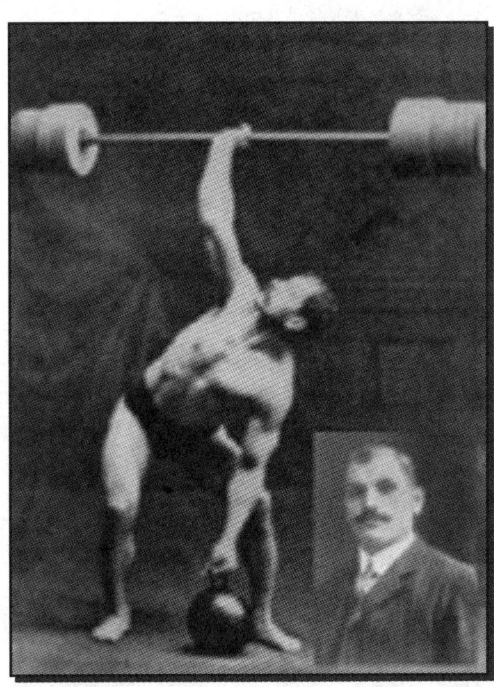

Figure 12-1

- *Louis Cyr* (1863 - 1912, Figures 12-2 and 12-3) performed a variety of strength "acts," including lifting a horse off the ground and holding a platform stacked with 18 men on his back.

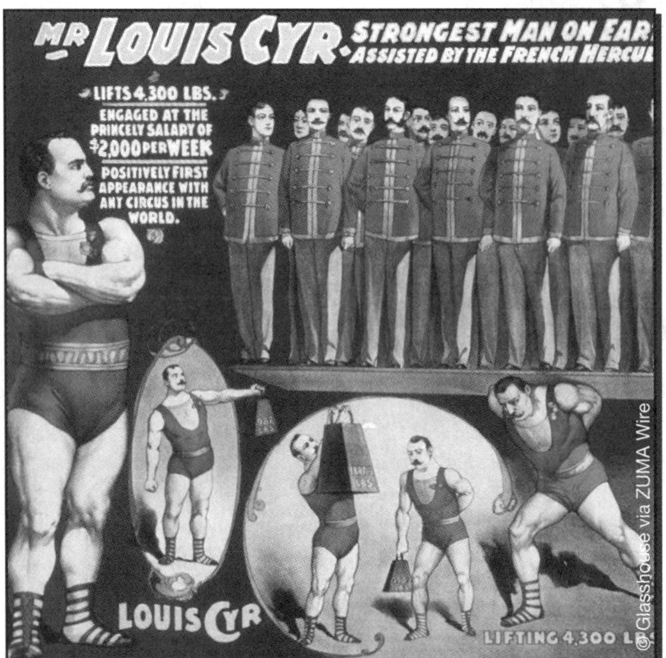

Figure 12-2

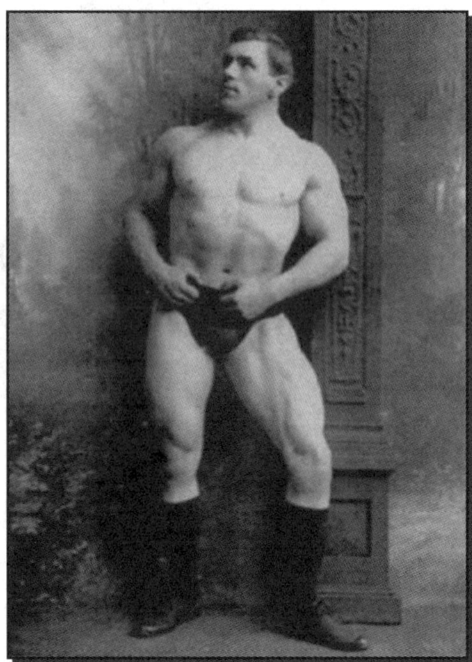
Figure 12-4

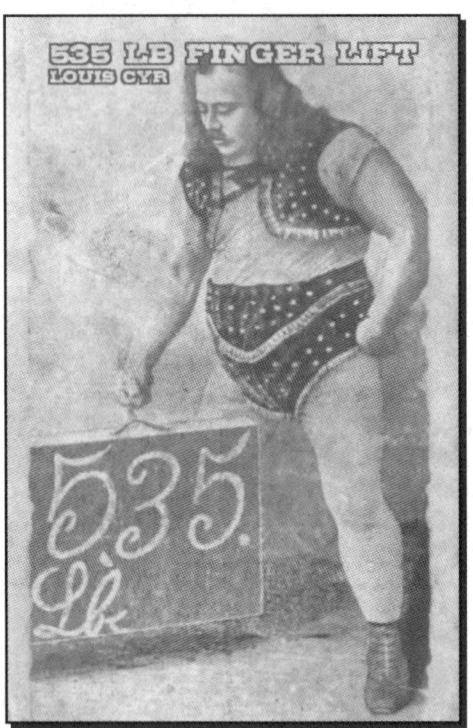

Figure 12-3

- *George Hackenshmidt* (1877 - 1968, Figure 12-4) was a professional wrestler, as well as a "strongman." In 1899, at the age of 18, he performed a "floor press" with 361 pounds. In this lift (Figure 12-5), the barbell is suspended a short distance off the floor by two wooden blocks, providing just enough room for a person to slide

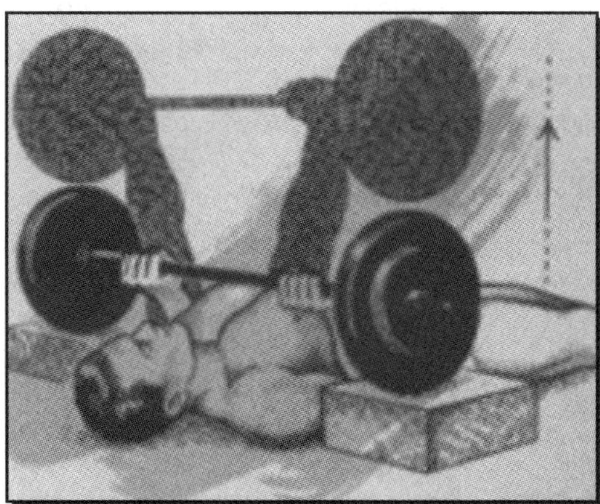
Figure 12-5

underneath the bar. The bar is then pressed upward. Obviously, this "test of strength" was the beginning of what would later be known as the "bench press."

- *Eugene Sandow* (1867 - 1925, Figures 12-6 and 12-7) is often referred to today as the Father of Modern Bodybuilding, because he was one of the first individuals to combine acts of strength, with classic poses displaying a muscular physique.

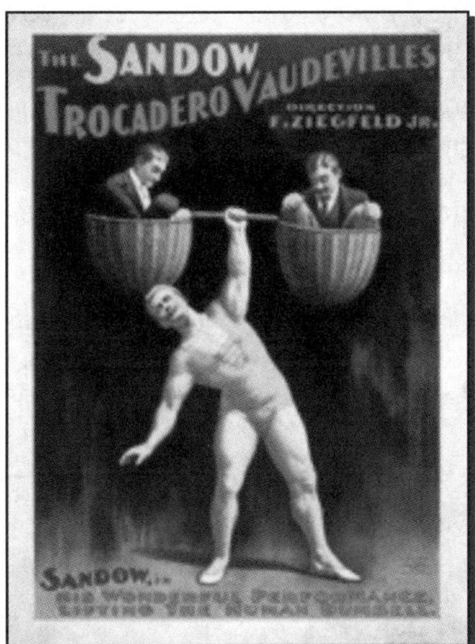

Figure 12-6

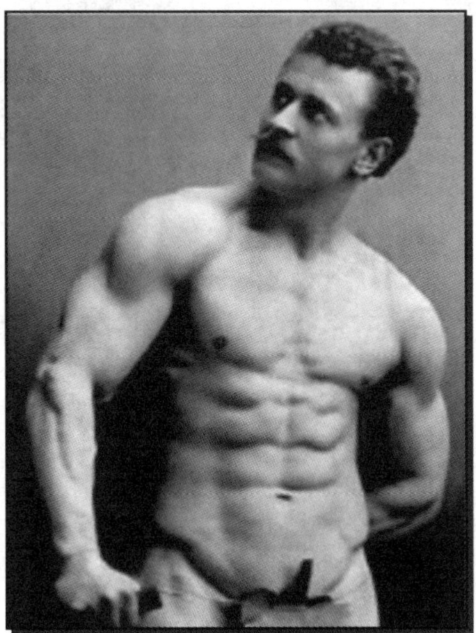
Figure 12-7

## The Birth of "Physical Culture"

In the early 1900s, "physical culture" had become a form of athleticism that was associated with morality. On the magazine cover illustrated in Figure 12-8, the banner below the photo reads "*Weakness a Crime—Don't Be a Criminal.*" This tagline suggested that it was unethical to be "weak." As such, superior physical strength was associated with superior ethics.

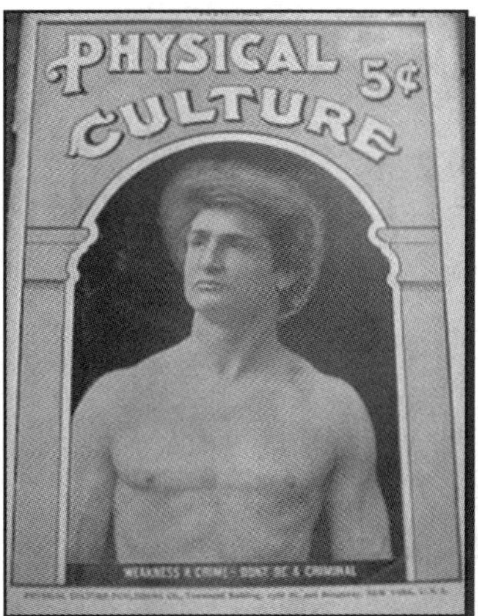

Figure 12-8

The 1907 magazine cover shown in Figure 12-9 displays another demonstration of strength—a man lifting another man on a bicycle. It should be noted that there is no mention of "physique." Physical strength and health were valued above all else. The pursuit of a well-developed physique, as a goal unto itself, was likely considered dishonorable at the time.

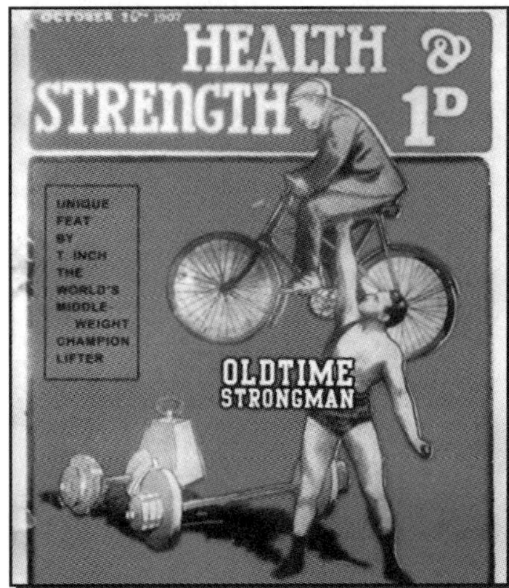

Figure 12-9

By the 1950s, however, the notion of developing the physique began gaining popularity, although it was not to be admitted publicly. On the cover of the 1953 "*Health and Strength*" magazine shown (Figures 12-10 and 12-11), the words "*HEALTH,*" "*STRENGTH,*" and "*STRONG,*" are in bold, uppercase letters. Then, in small, cursive letters—almost like being whispered—it quietly reads "*See Bodybuilder's Forum— inside.*" The concept of physique development was catching on, but it was regarded as a less-worthy goal than the pursuit of strength.

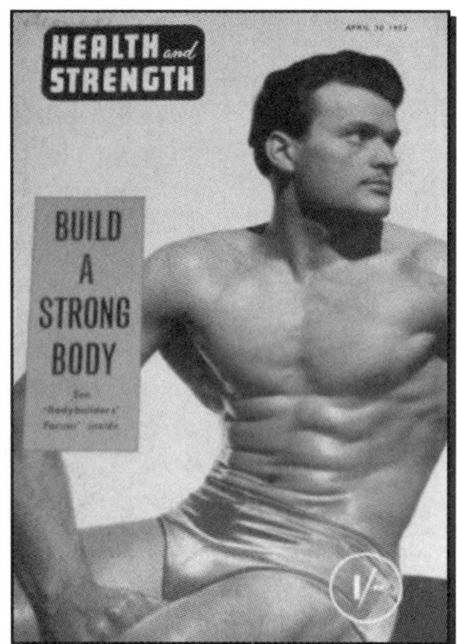

Figure 12-10

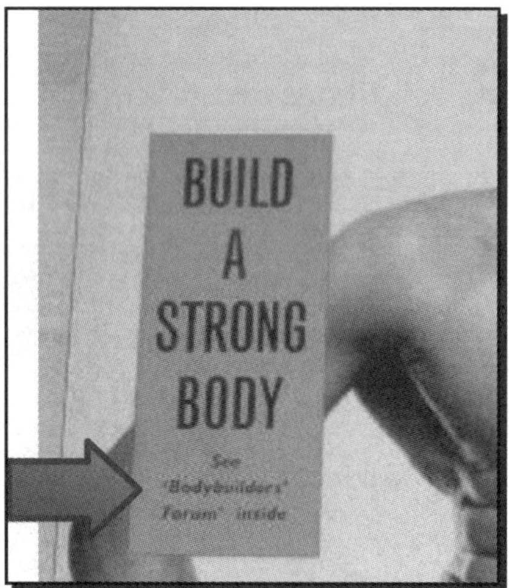

Figure 12-11

It is worth noting that the apparent stigma then associated with the pursuit of physique development was irrational. It was naively believed that physique development was purely "cosmetic"—as if a muscle could be enlarged without its strength increasing. This premise is entirely false. A muscle can only be made larger by challenging it with resistance, and that undertaking naturally results in strength increases.

Not only did a bias exist against the pursuit of "physique development," this bias also extended to the exercises that seemed to be targeting physique development. Exercises that isolated a specific muscle would not allow as much total weight to be lifted, as compared with exercises that involved multiple muscles working simultaneously. Thus, "compound" exercises were glorified, and "isolation" exercises were discredited. In fact, however, "isolation" exercises increase individual muscle strength just as well—if not better—than exercises which involve multiple muscles, even though a lesser amount of weight is used.

In 1920, a sport known as "Olympic lifting" became officially recognized as an Olympic sport. It is comprised of two lifts—"the clean and jerk" (Figure 12-12) and the "the snatch" (Figure 12-13). These lifts are meant to test an individual's strength, balance, speed, coordination and skill.

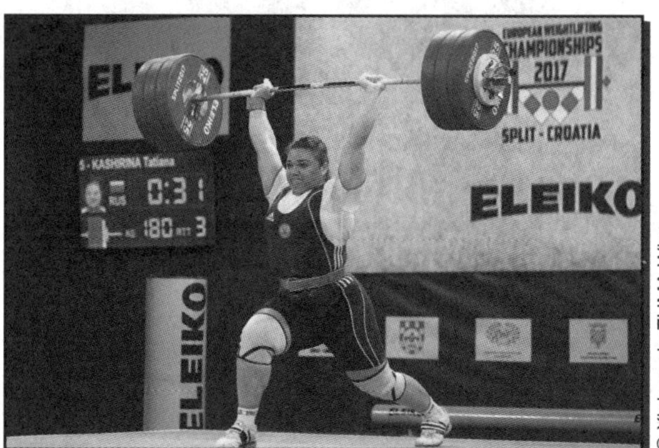

© Xinhua via ZUMA Wire

Figure 12-12

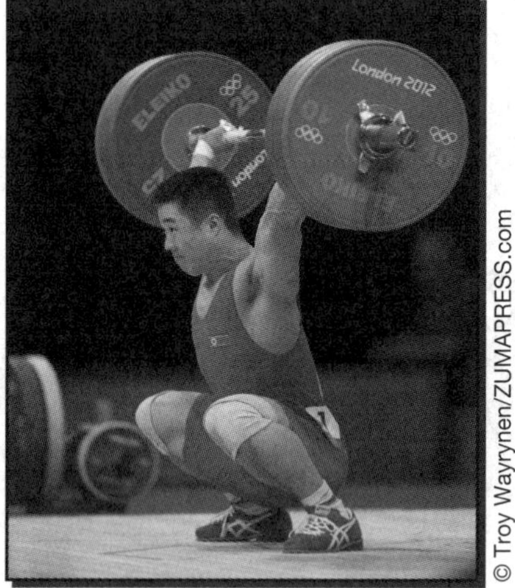

© Troy Wayrynen/ZUMAPRESS.com

Figure 12-13

In the 1950s, a sport known as "Powerlifting" was established. In Powerlifting competition, the goal is to have the highest sum total lifted of the three distinct lifts—the bench press, the squat and the deadlift (Figures 12-14 to 12-16).

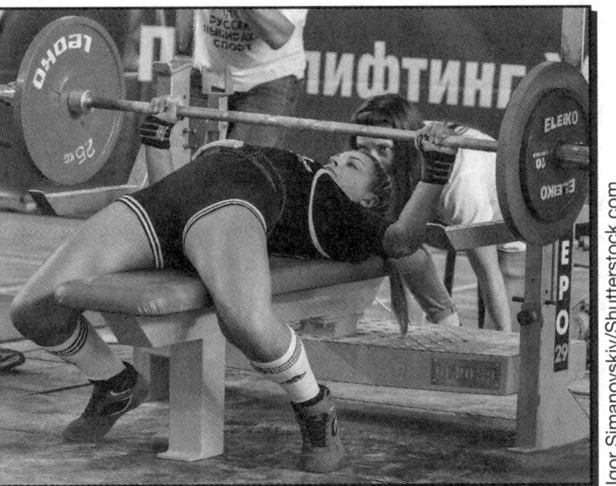
Igor Simanovskiy/Shutterstock.com

Figure 12-14

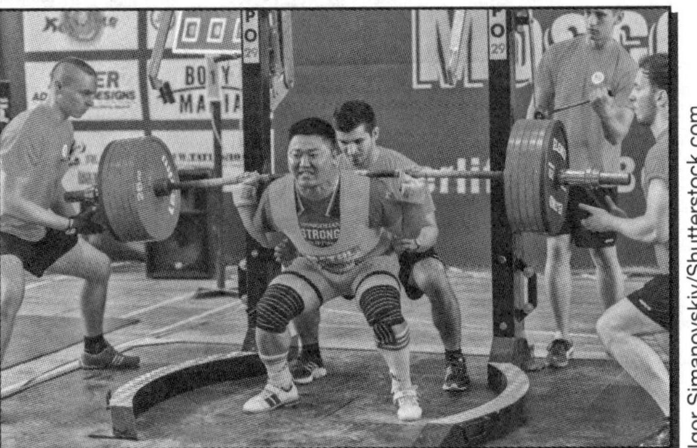
Igor Simanovskiy/Shutterstock.com

Figure 12-15

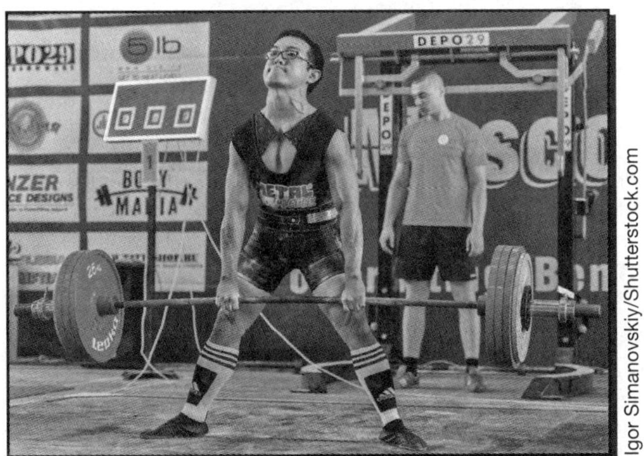
Igor Simanovskiy/Shutterstock.com

Figure 12-16

As such, early bodybuilding was heavily influenced by the preoccupation with "power," as well as the mistaken belief that a well-developed physique *required* a so-called "foundation" in the power lifts. At the root of this misguided belief, however, was a morality-based adulation of "strength." At the time, there appears to have been a misguided notion that doing exercises that were not intended to demonstrate strength (by way of performing a heavy lift) was equivalent to an absence of strength. Since the pursuit of strength—expressed by way of heavy compound lifts—was regarded as honorable, exercise that did not emphasize the use of heavy compound lifts was silently regarded as not honorable.

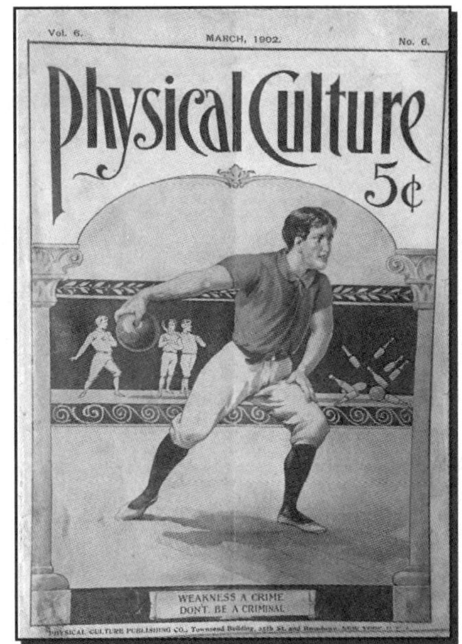


Figure 12-17

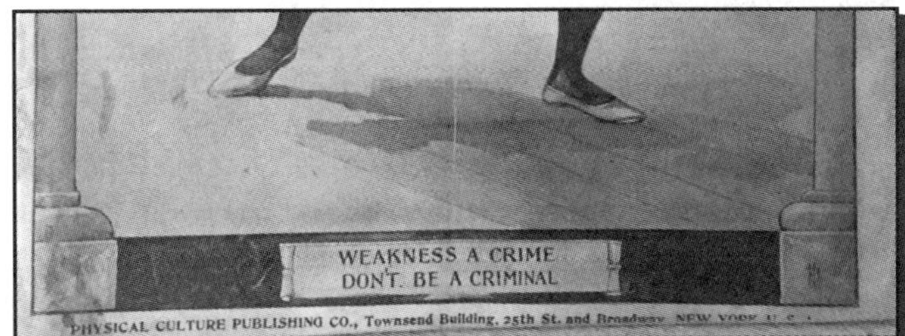


Figure 12-18

If a person elected to perform exercises that isolated specific muscles, it was equated with "neglecting" strength development, even if the individual used maximum effort in those isolated lifts. Of course, this premise is absurd. These two concepts (compound and isolation exercise) are *not* mutually exclusive. An individual muscle increases its strength during any resistance exercise, whether that muscle is made to work alone, or as a unified effort with other muscles working simultaneously.

Other exercises—not involving the use of weights—were also revered as demonstrations of physical prowess. These included gymnastic- and acrobatic-type of exercises, including chin-ups, push-ups, parallel bar dips, hanging leg raises, etc.—and were utilized on a competitive level. As such, people would challenge each other, concerning who could do the most chin-ups, push-ups, parallel bar dips, etc.

Like the power lifts, these exercises were also used as tests of physical superiority or dominance, demonstrating strength and endurance prowess. The focus—the obsession, in fact—was always on exhibiting strength. A person's strength and endurance was always compared to the performance of other people—almost as if exercise had no other value, aside from being used to rate an individual's level of physical prowess.

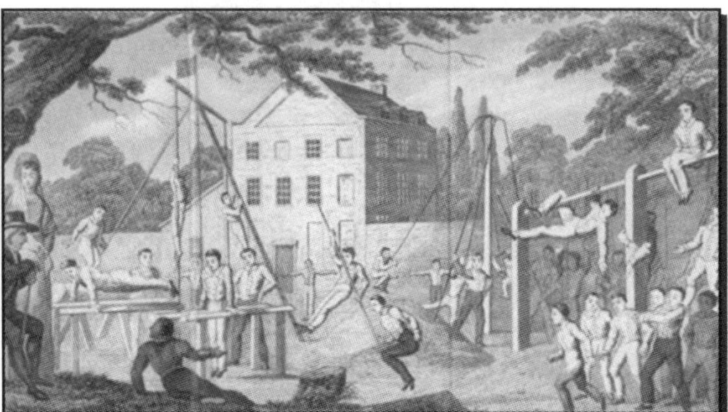

Figure 12-19

The idea of utilizing exercise, *without* comparing a person's performance of that exercise, to that of other people, apparently seemed pointless at the time. Only how a person compared with other individuals, in terms of physical strength and endurance, during specific exercises and "lifts," seemed to have any importance.

Thus, *power lifts* and *calisthenics* became the accepted standard for exercise. These exercises, however, are not necessarily the most productive, nor the most energy efficient, nor the safest way to develop the muscles of the body. They're also not the best way to optimally develop the strength of each individual muscle.

Isolation exercises increase muscle strength, without the injury risks associated with the powerlifts. The fact that isolation exercises are not typically used as a metric for comparison with others does not mean that isolation exercises produce less muscle strength than compound exercises.

## Comparing "Compound" vs. "Isolation" Exercises for Muscle Loading

An individual who is unfamiliar with biomechanics might naturally assume that exercises which allow them to lift a heavier weight would produce more "mass" (i.e., larger muscles). This assumption, however, is incorrect. A muscle that is participating in a compound exercise is being assisted by other muscles, in the lifting of that weight. A unified effort (multiple muscles participating simultaneously in one lift) will naturally allow a heavier weight to be lifted, as compared with only one muscle doing the work. Each participating muscle, however, may not be working at its individual maximum capacity during a compound lift.

In Figure 12-20, a group of men can be seen "lifting" (carrying) a log. Should the assumption be made that each of these men is working as hard as he would alone, but with a lighter log? Of course not. Furthermore, should an assumption be made that all of the participating men are making an equal contribution to the effort? Of course not. A unified effort—a group of men, or a group of muscles—does not automatically cause each man or each muscle to work more intensely than would a single man or lone muscle, lifting a lighter load.

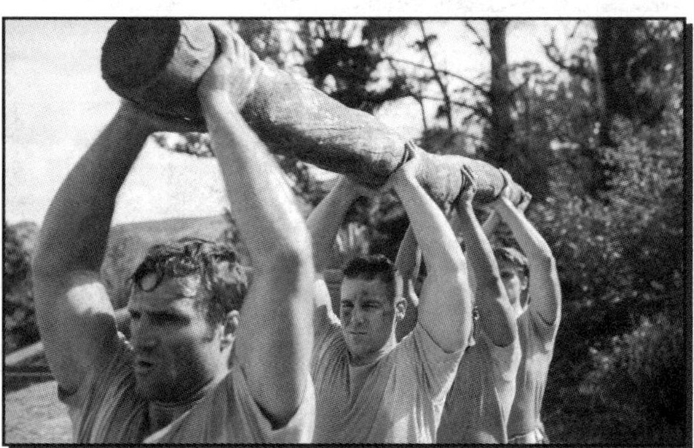

wavebreakmedia/Shutterstock.com

Figure 12-20

In fact, during a "compound exercise," some muscles may be working at 90 percent of their maximum capacity, while others may only be working at 70 percent or even 50 percent of their maximum capacity. This proportion is determined by the mechanics of each exercise—not by the person's choice.

Oftentimes, during a compound exercise, a muscle a person most wants to prioritize is less loaded than a muscle that the person does not want to prioritize, due to the mechanics of that particular exercise. Each muscle, however, could be fully loaded, and be worked with 100 percent efficiency, using an isolation exercise—even though the amount of weight used would be lighter than the weight used during a compound exercise.

It's important to understand the difference between "lifting heavy weights" and "optimally loading a given muscle." Depending upon the circumstances, an individual muscle can be loaded MORE, even though a lighter weight is being lifted, if it is not assisted by other muscles, if the exercise has better alignment, if the resistance curve of the exercise matches the strength curve of the muscle, or if a longer lever is being used. Conversely, an individual muscle could be loaded LESS during a compound exercise—even though a heavier weight is being lifted—because those aforementioned variables are less advantageous.

## Is a Critical Evaluation of a Compound Exercise "Immoral"?

In 2010, I wrote an article entitled "*The Case Against Overhead Presses*," for *Iron Man Magazine*, in which I explained the five biomechanical problems associated with *overhead presses*. Some of the problems with the overhead press relate to its compromised mechanical efficiency, while others relate to the unnatural joint movement and its high risk of injury.

As a rebuttal to my article, an individual named Bill Star wrote an article, which he called, "*In Defense of the Overhead Press*." In his first paragraph, he said he felt "morally obligated" to defend the exercise. Again, this concept of "morality" is brought up in defense of the perceived sanctity of a power lift. He called my explanation "scientific jargon" and a "smoke screen," yet offered no science-based counterpoint. In fact, his article included no physics or anatomy references, whatsoever. His response demonstrated an emotional bias in favor of compound exercises/power lifts, without consideration for the actual physics involved, and also without consideration as to how closely the exercise mimics—or fails to mimic—natural anatomical motion.

Bill Star was a "strength coach," with no background in either biomechanics or physics. His university degree was in sociology, he played college football, and he competed in powerlifting. Strength coaching has historically been focused on the preparation of athletes for power sports, such as football. While on the "grid iron" (the American Football field), there may be some justification for the use of compound exercises. Moving a large amount of weight in a single lift simulates the type of force that will be encountered in the game.

Football players must be prepared for brutal collisions with opposing players, who often weigh as much as 300 pounds. Thus, the high degree of injury risk incurred during a heavy compound exercise is simply part of that preparation. On the other hand, it's certainly not necessary—neither productive nor safe—for a person who is pursuing physique development or striving to simply improve his physical well-being.

Strength coaches often have a bias in favor of compound exercises, such that they consider it practically sacrilegious either to abstain from using them, or to criticize them. To many such individuals, these exercises are the "sacred cows," which are not to be questioned under any circumstances. In contrast, biomechanics involves physics and anatomy, and seeks to evaluate exercises from an engineering standpoint—as opposed to from a philosophical standpoint.

## Survival and Heroism

Men's historical obsession with "super" strength was partly rooted in the irrational belief that the absence of superior strength was immoral. It is also based on the illogical assumption that each muscle that participates in a unified effort (i.e., a compound exercise), benefits more than each of those muscles would if they worked without the assistance of other muscles (i.e., an isolated exercise). Lastly, the obsession with superior strength was also based—originally—on an actual need for survival.

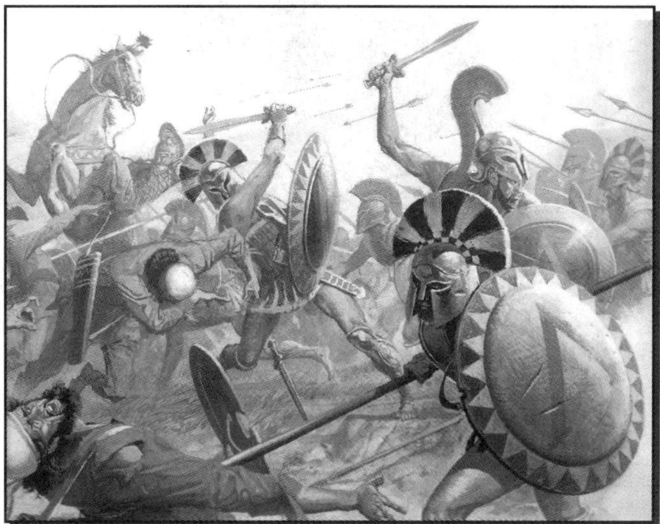

Figure 12-21

During prehistoric times, and for centuries thereafter, men needed to be strong for the sake of survival. Battle was an integral part of life. Civilizations were built and conquered by way of physical labor and hand-to-hand combat. "Exercise" was required preparation for battle among the Babylonians, early Persians, Egyptians, Romans, and Greeks. Accordingly, it is understandable that "exercise" focused on maximizing physical strength, fighting skills, flexibility, and endurance, given that each of these attributes could be demonstrated and compared with that of other individuals, and were often put to the test.

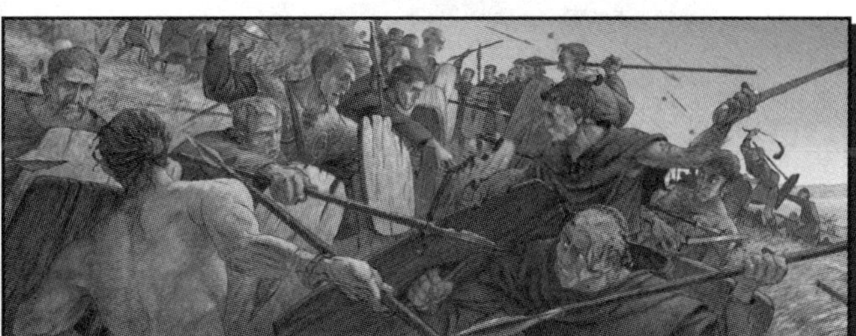

Figure 12-22

Although it's archaic today, the original underlying concept of "fitness" was preparedness for battle or for labor. *"The strongest shall survive"* was not just rhetoric. It was a fact of life. People were selected for battle or labor, based largely on their physicality. Individuals who were weak were a liability. As such, they had a higher risk of injury, were less able to fight, survive and provide, were less admired or dismissed entirely.

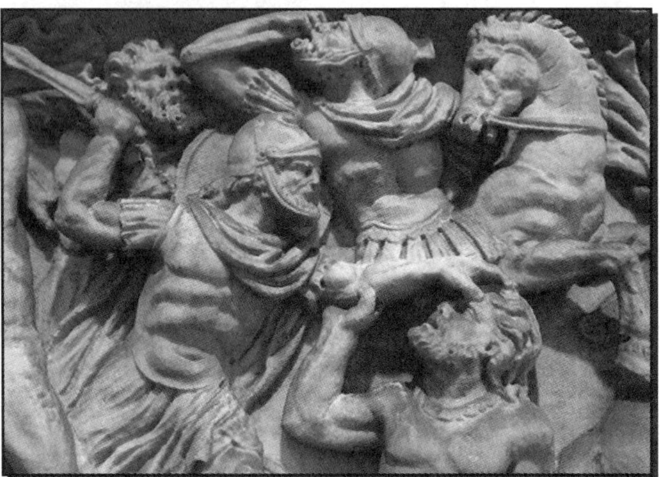

Figure 12-23

Women selected their mates, based primarily on their physicality. The safety and security that a stronger man could provide was essential. A strong male counterpart also meant strong offspring. Women with strong male mates were more likely to have food, shelter, safety, and healthy children. In a harsh world, where "productivity" meant farming, construction, fishing, and hunting (as opposed to a desk job), as well as the protection of the family against invaders, women depended on a strong man. As a result, there was the added value of being able to attract a woman (or women—plural), which further perpetuated men's obsession with "super" strength.

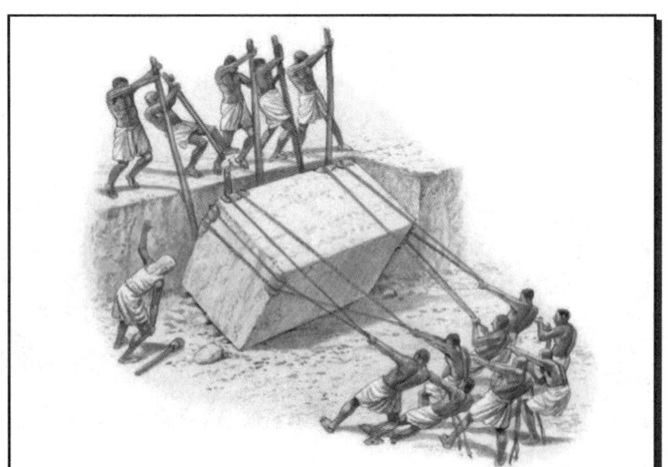

Figure 12-24

It follows, then, that stronger men were admired to the point of being idolized. This situation led to legendary stories of powerful warriors and heroes—real or embellished—who inspired legions with hopes of achieving similar status.

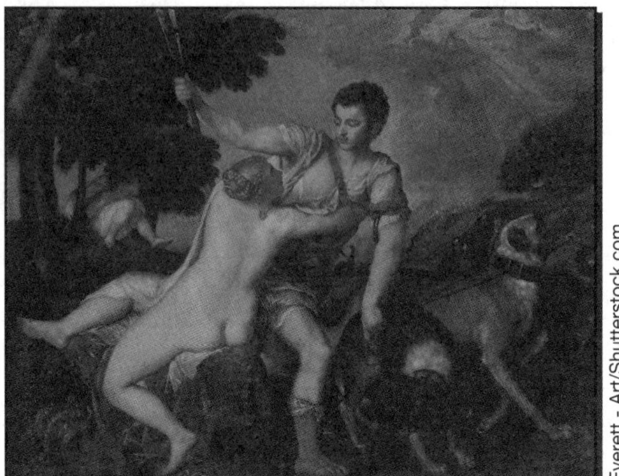

Everett - Art/Shutterstock.com

Figure 12-25

## Comic Books and Mythology

It should come as no surprise that many of today's comic book heroes are based on Greek mythology. A wonderful thesis paper written by Andrew S. Latham*, entitled "*Comic Books vs. Greek Mythology: The Ultimate Crossover for the Classic Scholar*," beautifully outlines this relationship. In fact, many of today's comic book superheroes were inspired by the legends of Hercules, Zeus, Poseidon, Neptune, Triton, and Perseus—among others. This factor further reinforces the notion that extraordinary physical strength has been revered to an obsessive degree by many individuals. Being "heroic" (i.e., super strong) is, and has been for centuries, the ultimate fantasy for millions of men.

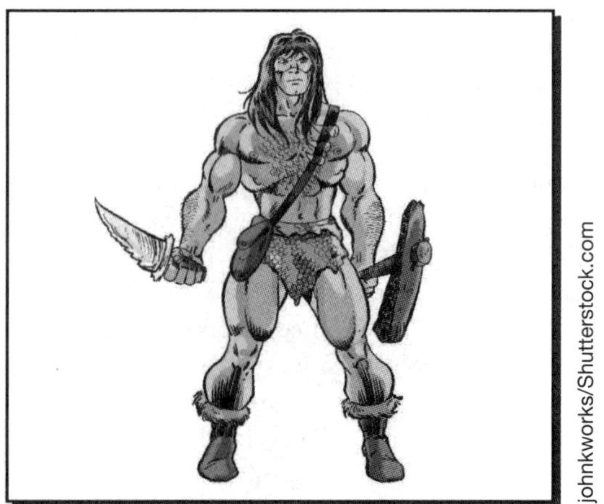

johnkworks/Shutterstock.com

Figure 12-26

*Master of Arts in English/The University of Texas at Tyler, May 2012

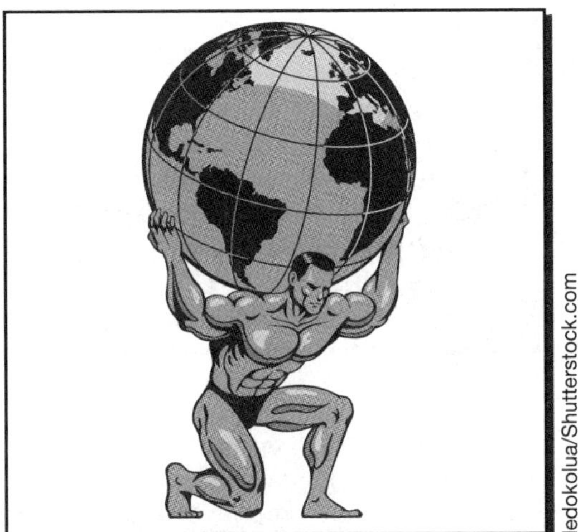
ledokolua/Shutterstock.com

Figure 12-27

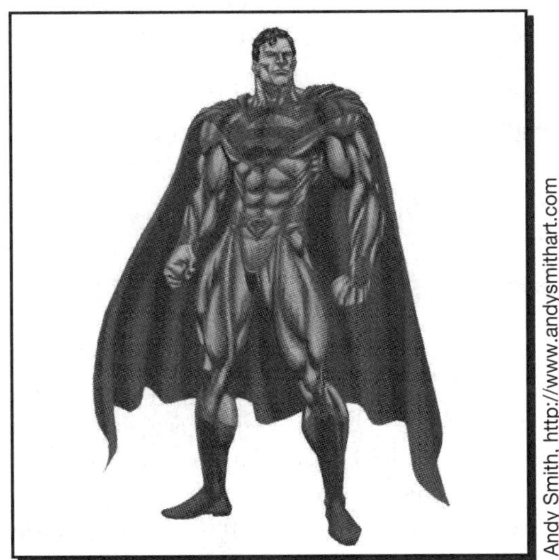
Andy Smith, http://www.andysmithart.com

Figure 12-28

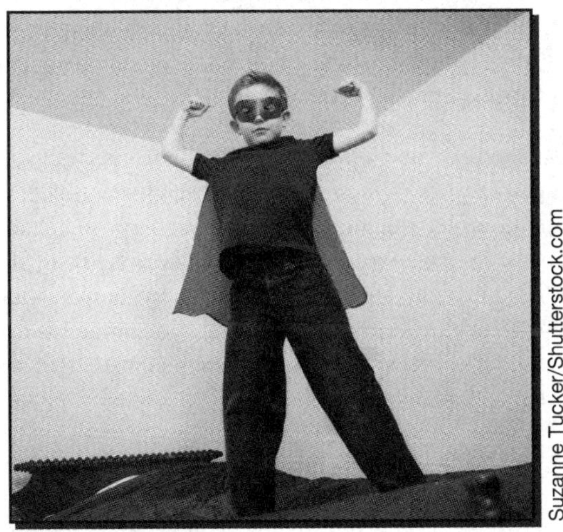
Suzanne Tucker/Shutterstock.com

Figure 12-29

What logical reason could explain an adolescent boy's fascination with comic book superheroes? An eight-year-old boy could not possibly know from personal experience that, once upon a time, great physical strength translated to better safety, better survival, better success in battle, better mating opportunities, and the admiration of his peers.

Why are modern-day sports stars, as well as sports coaches, held in such extremely high regard—often more so than brain surgeons? Why do so many athletes risk their health and their lives—boxing, fighting in mixed martial arts, and playing American football—even as unpaid amateurs?

Most individuals, who live in developed countries in the 21st century, do *not* live in constant fear that an army of sword-wielding warriors on horseback will suddenly invade their village. Generally speaking, no one has to prepare for that type of battle in modern society. People also do not have to go out and plow their fields for food. They simply drive to the grocery store. Furthermore, at the present time, all factors considered, the ability to attract a mate is related more to a person's ability to earn a decent income, than to their ability to slay a dragon.

The underlying point is that many individuals have naively allowed themselves to believe that lifting a large amount of weight in a single compound "exercise," such as *squats* or *dead lifts*, is essential. They have bought into the notion that strength cannot be gained during lifts that load only one or two muscles at a time, and that only the multi-joint/multi-muscle exercises build strength. To reiterate, this notion stems from the misguided belief that if a large amount of weight is not being lifted at one time, then strength is not being developed.

In reality, people have conflated two concepts—lifting a large amount of weight during a *squat* or a *dead lift* and the concept of being strong with well-developed muscles. They are not the same. You do not have to *squat* or *dead lift* heavy weights in order to be strong and have well-developed muscles.

Furthermore, no one should be so naive as to believe that their obsession with performing a heavy *squat, dead lift,* or *bench press* is really about developing strength. In fact, their obsession with that is based largely on "measuring up"—about meeting expectation or exceeding it. In other words, many individuals are irrationally concerned about whether or not their physical strength—as measured by those particular lifts—is adequate, superior, or below "standard." That's a fool's game. The only things that matters are that your strength be improved, that you have more than sufficient strength to do normal activities, that you are healthy and free of injury, and that your physique has the shape you want. How your strength "compares" with that of others is mostly irrelevant.

## The Folly of Impressing Observers

Consciously or subconsciously, individuals often "perform" in the gym. As such, people (usually men) often tailor their gym activities toward that which would be impressive to watch, rather than that which would be the wisest training strategy for achieving optimal fitness/physique development goals.

These "observer-oriented" activities typically include jumping up to a four-foot platform, double- or triple-speed jump-roping, acrobatic-type of chin-ups, one-arm push-ups, handstands, etc. Needless to say, these abilities have very little usefulness in normal, day-to-day life. In reality, they improve your ability to do those specific "displays," more than they improve your overall fitness level. People doing these exhibitions may even know that the benefit and usefulness of what they are doing is extremely limited. Unfortunately, the subconscious desire to demonstrate impressive acts of strength often overrides a more logical/sensible approach to exercise.

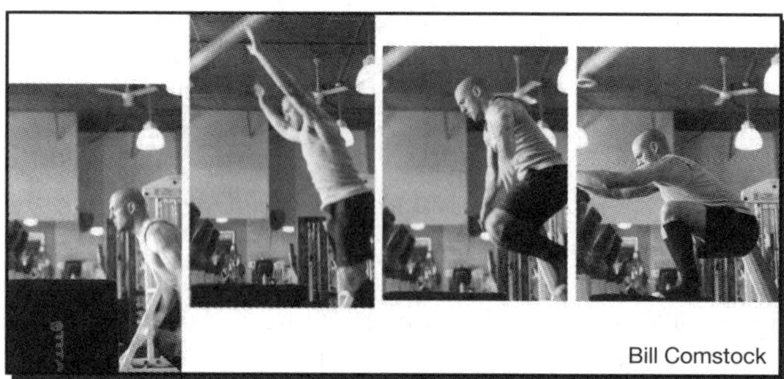
Bill Comstock

Figure 12-30

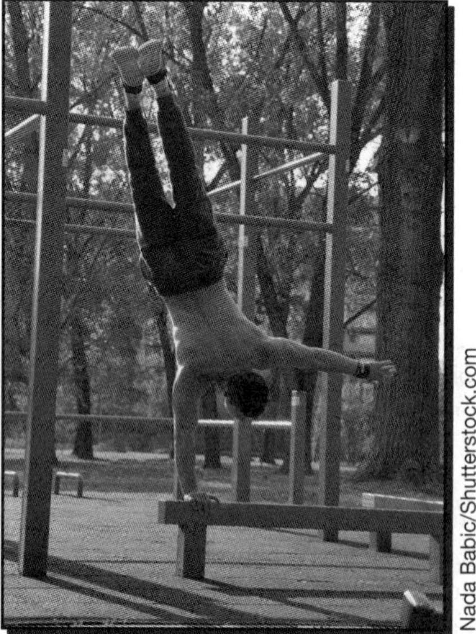
Nada Babic/Shutterstock.com

Figure 12-31

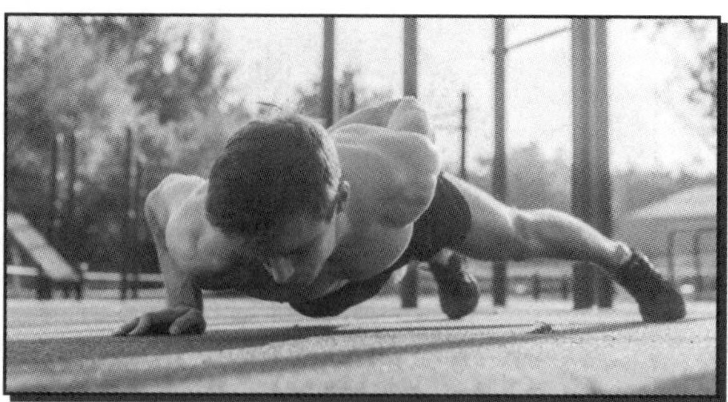
Undrey/Shutterstock.com

Figure 12-32

Given the aforementioned, you should ask yourself, "Is your typical daily workout for the purpose of impressing observers in the gym, or is it for the purpose of getting closer to your goal of having optimal health and an exceptional physique?" This query is not a judgment on those individuals who place a high value on displaying extraordinary athleticism—although it may be worth questioning the need to do so.

One of the primary points of this chapter is to recognize that people's obsessive fascination with extraordinary feats of strength has distorted, and continues to distort, their ability to accurately evaluate certain exercises.

## Departures From Logic

An example that can help clarify how illogical this issue has become entails a look at a type of exercise called "closed chain." Some people (i.e., trainers, physical therapists, and even orthopedic physicians) use the terms "compound exercise" and "closed chain" almost interchangeably. Technically, "closed chain" exercise refers to exercises that have a "grounded" (i.e., fixed) resistance source—for example, push-ups, chin-ups, parallel bar dips, squats, etc. In these cases, either the hands or the feet are in constant contact with the ground, or on some other fixed, immovable surface. Then, the person's body weight (plus, possibly some additional resistance) is pushed or pulled from that fixed surface.

Conversely, an "open chain" exercise is described as an exercise where a person moves a weighted object (barbell, dumbbell, cable, machine, etc.) through space. Examples of this type of exercise would be a barbell bench press (the barbell is moving), a cable triceps pushdown (the hands, attached to the handle, are moving), and a leg extension machine (the tibia is moving through space, as it pushes against the machine's lever arm).

Proponents of "compound exercise" often favor "closed chain" over "open chain" exercises because they were "taught" to favor them. They may try to argue that a "closed chain" exercise more closely resembles the types of activity found in the real world. In fact, they often say that "closed chain" is more "functional" than are exercises that employ some type of hand-held weight or machine.

In reality, however, a working muscle has no "idea" what is happening outside of its individual function. For example, a latissimus muscle pulling on a humerus (upper arm bone) could not possibly "know" what is making the humerus challenging to pull. It might be a chin-up bar and the exerciser's body weight hanging from it … or it could be a lat pulldown bar, against which a cable is pulling upward. Yet, a proponent of the closed-chain theory of exercise would regard the chin-up as "good," and the lat pulldown as "bad." As such, the chin-up would be encouraged, and the pulldown would be discouraged—even though there is essentially no difference between the two, as far as the latissimus is concerned (assuming a comparable amount of weight is being used).

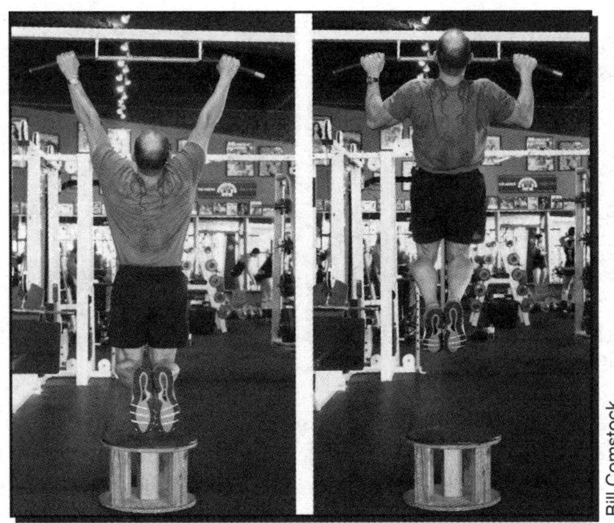
Bill Comstock

Figure 12-33

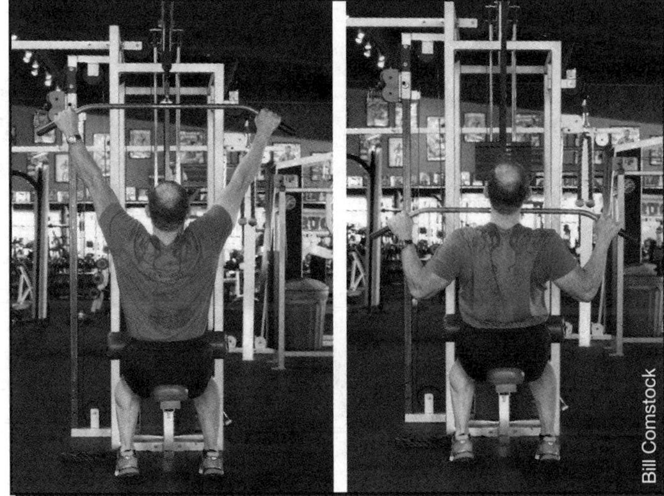
Bill Comstock

Figure 12-34

The same factor is true for squats. A proponent of the closed-chain theory would claim that "*squats* are good because they are 'closed-chain,' and *leg presses* are bad because they are 'open-chain'." In reality, however, the quadriceps muscles (as well as the knee) could not possibly "know" against which type of resistance they are having to work.

In fact, it could be that the exerciser's body weight is being pulled downward by gravity, while the tibia is pushing against gravity—moving the body away from the ground (i.e., when doing a squat). It could also be that the weighted platform of a leg press machine is pushing toward the individual's torso, while the tibia is pushing the platform away from the torso. Either way, the quadriceps is doing the one-and-only thing it CAN do, which is to extend the knee. In both cases, something is stationary (fixed)—either the ground or the seat of the leg press. Whichever is not stationary is moving away from that which is stationary. Either way, the muscle function is the same.

*Note: While foot placement on the leg press does alter the percentage of the resistance that is loaded onto the quadriceps, the mechanism of the knee and quadriceps are still the same.*

Likewise, the pectorals would not "know" whether a push-up is being done or a barbell bench press is being performed. In the first instance, the pectorals are pulling the humerus toward the sternum, which causes the hands to push downward against the ground, which causes the body to rise. In the second case, the Pectorals are pulling the humerus toward the sternum, which causes the hands to push upward against a barbell, which causes the barbell to rise. But, in both cases, the pectorals are doing the exact same thing: pulling the humerus toward the sternum (which is where the origin of the pectorals are situated). In either instance, the humerus is "adducted" in a forward direction. There is absolutely no difference between the two—assuming the weight of the barbell is equal to the percentage of body weight that occurs during a push-up.

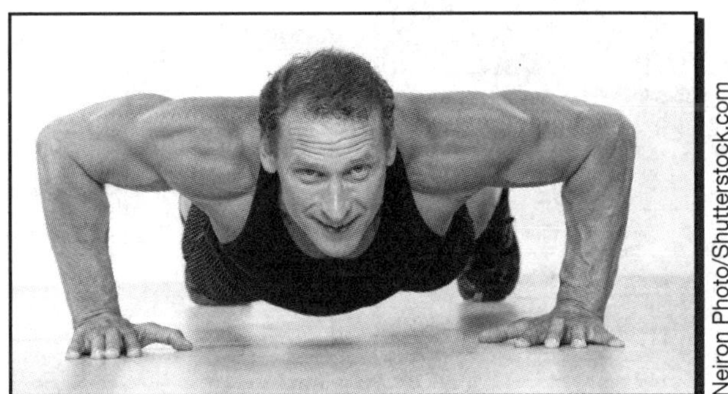
Nejron Photo/Shutterstock.com

Figure 12-35

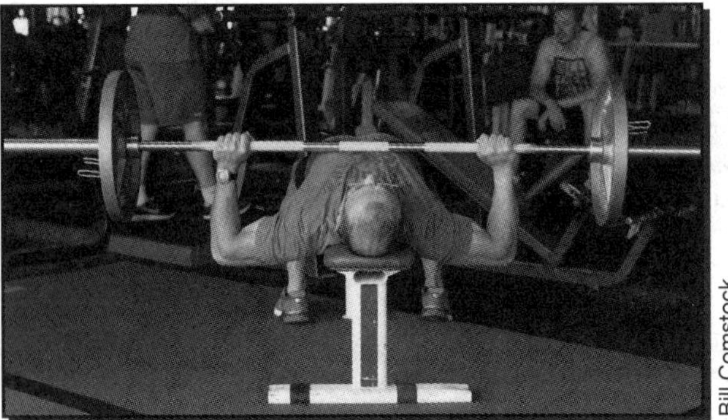

Figure 12-36

*Note: A push-up requires some isometric work to be done by the abs, hip flexors, and quadriceps, in order to prevent the torso from collapsing. During a bench press, this element is not required. As such, they are different in that sense. In terms of the pectorals, however, there is essentially no difference.*

## Leg Extension "Shearing"

Proponents of "compound exercise" typically recommend squats over the use of a "leg extension" machine (Figure 12-37, left image). Part of their rationale is that the perpendicular force applied to the ankle, during a *leg extension*, has a "shearing effect on the knee."

In order to illustrate this factor, they usually use the graphic in Figure 12-37, right image, which shows two vertical rectangles—one stacked above the other. The upper rectangle represents an upper leg (the femur), while the lower rectangle represents a lower leg (the tibia). They also show two horizontal

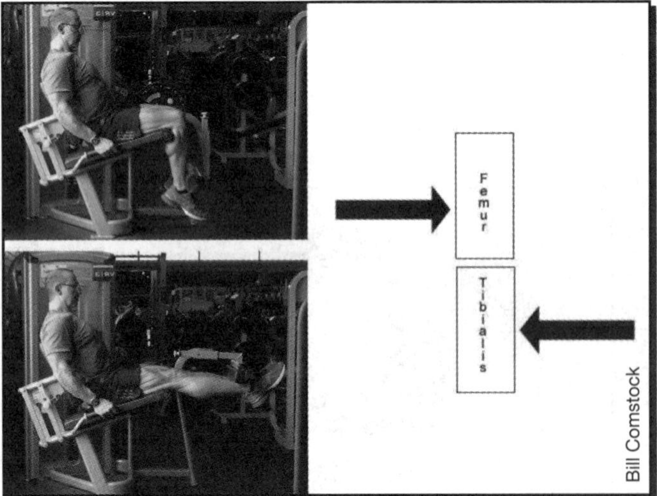

Figure 12-37

arrows: one pointing to the right on the upper "bone" and one pointing to the left on the lower "bone." The suggestion in this instance is that a perpendicular force placed against the tibia would cause the entire tibia to shift inward, and separate from the knee.

This assertion is absurd. First, there are countless similar situations that occur during other exercises, with other joints and other muscles, yet no such concern exists with any other exercise. For example, a *supine triceps extension* (Figure 12-38, right image) operates in the exact same way—the extension of a hinge joint. A perpendicular resistance acts upon the forearm lever, thereby loading the triceps. Yet, no one has ever expressed concern that "elbow shearing" might occur during *supine triceps extension*. That's because there is essentially no risk at all.

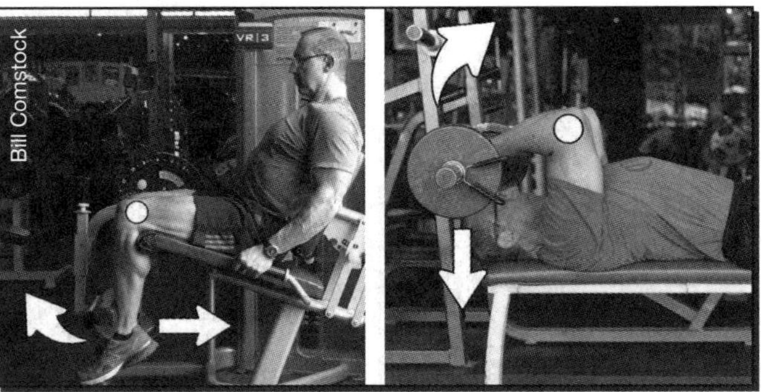

Figure 12-38

In fact, all of the exercises that individuals perform in the gym require that a perpendicular force act against the operating lever (limb) of their target muscle. Were it not for perpendicular forces against a limb, there would be no resistance to work against. As you know, a lever that is not perpendicular with resistance (at least to some degree) is a *neutral* lever.

The most obvious reason that "shearing" does not occur (*with any significance*) during the use of a "leg extension" machine, however, is that in order for the quadriceps to extend the knee, it has to produce a force that is approximately 20 times greater than that which is pushing against the ankle. This factor is due primarily to the magnification caused by the length of the tibia. The force produced by the quadriceps is pulling the tibia upward. This action produces an anchoring effect that is approximately 20 times greater than the force pushing perpendicularly on the ankle. There is simply no way that the tibia could shift inward, while it's being so firmly anchored. This factor can be easily demonstrated with an anatomical model.

In Figure 12-39, the horizontal arrow at the ankle represents what might be a 30-pound (per leg) resistance, pushing perpendicularly against the "distal end" of the tibia, provided by a *leg extension* machine. The arrows above represent the (approximately) 600 pounds of force required and produced by the quadriceps (by way of the patella tendon) pulling upward on the tibia, to extend the knee.

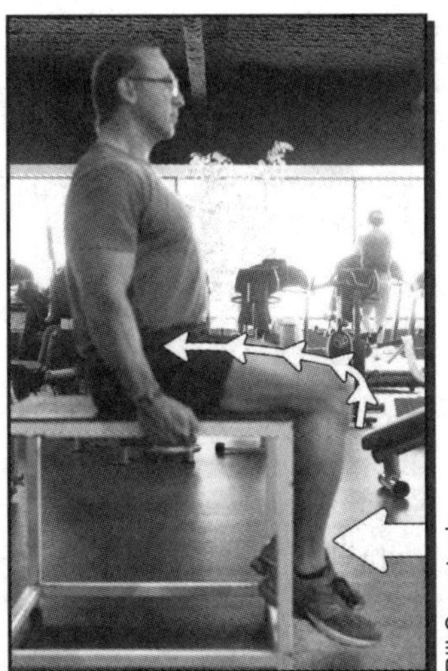

Figure 12-39

> *Note: For a full explanation of the fallacy of this "shearing" issue, please refer to:*
> *http://www.labrada.com/blog/workouts/is-the-open-chain-closed-chain-exercise-philosophy-shear-non-sense/*

It is impossible for a "leg extension" machine to cause any significant amount of knee shearing, and this is very easy to prove. Yet, "educated people" warn against the danger of "knee shearing," when using a *leg extension* machine. Then, these same "educated people" recommend *planks,* which place the same kind of perpendicular force against the lower leg (by way of "ground reaction force"). This situation demonstrates an obvious lack of understanding of physics, as well as an irrational bias in favor of "compound" movements, and against "isolated" movements.

Worse yet, these same "educated people" also recommend *side planks. Side planks* create a perpendicular force against the tibia (by way of "ground reaction force" against the side of the foot)—and this force is trying to bend the knee sideways. Knees are not meant to bend sideways. Any sideways force against the lower leg will certainly load the knee tendons, and NOT the muscle—because no muscle bends/extends the knee sideways. Why would this exercise be acceptable (even recommended), while "*leg extensions*" are not acceptable?

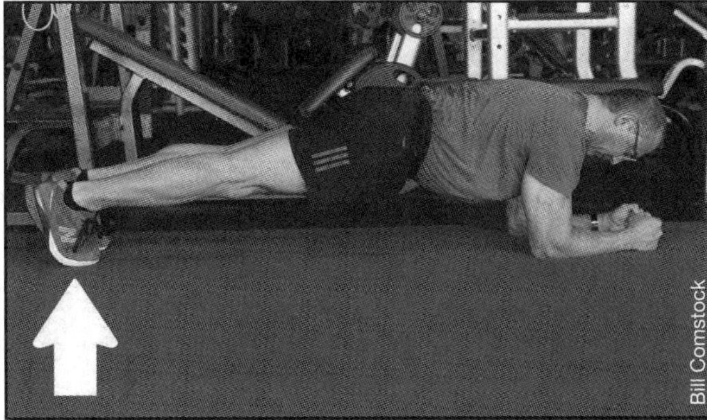

Figure 12-40

It can be helpful to examine this exercise a little more closely. Assume the person in Figure 12-41 weighs 150 pounds. Since she is suspending herself on two points, she's loading each of the two points (elbow and foot) with approximately 75 pounds.

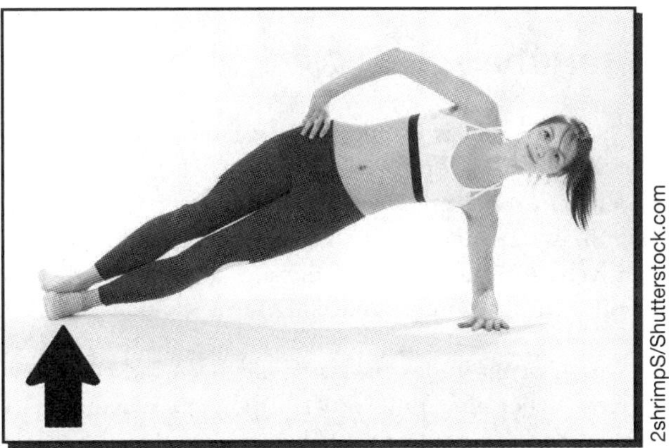

Figure 12-41

As such, 75 pounds of ground reaction force is pressing upward on the lateral aspect of her right foot. Because the average length of an adult female tibia is approximately 13 inches, the magnification of that 75 pounds would be at approximately 13-fold by the time it gets to the knee (i.e., a 13/1 ratio). Therefore, this *side plank* would produce approximately 975 pounds of sideways force on the knee, "trying" to bend it in a direction in which it is NOT designed to bend. Furthermore, there is no quadriceps involvement in this instance, which could produce an anchoring effect. In reality, only the knee tendons and ligaments are preventing the knee from bending sideways during *side planks*.

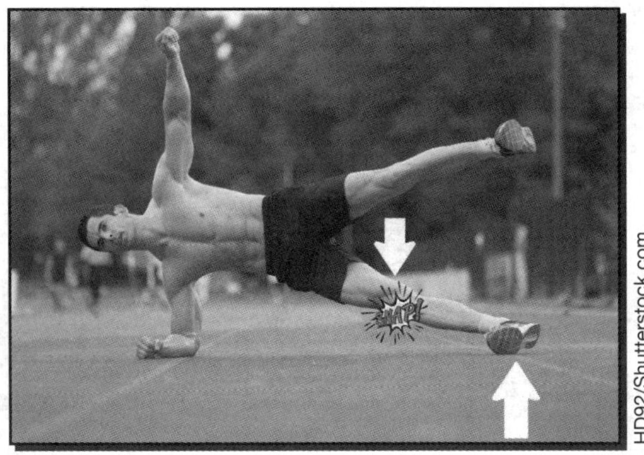


Figure 12-42

Yet, educated people (certified trainers and licensed physical therapists) consider the *side plank "safe,"* but consider the *leg extension "unsafe."* This is absolutely illogical. There are dozens of other examples that could be reviewed, but the point has been made.

## Summary

The human body is essentially a machine that is made up of levers (bones), "pulleys" (muscles), and pivots (joints). Therefore, every movement and every force placed upon this human machine is quantifiable, and should be evaluated exclusively on the basis of physics and "natural human motion"—using biomechanical analysis.

Much of the fitness industry has been biased for years, in favor of certain "power"/"compound" movements that have been revered through the ages, but these movements can easily be discredited by way of biomechanical analysis. The fitness industry has also been biased, for years, against isolation exercises, even though those movements allow each joint and muscle to operate in a perfectly "natural" way, often utilizing more efficient mechanics. They allow more efficient loading of individual target muscles, as compared with compound exercises.

When all skeletal muscles are *individually* strengthened, a person's *"total body strength"* is every bit as useful and "functional" as it would be if those muscles were strengthened by way of compound exercises. The sum is the total of its parts.

Isolation exercises also allow the user to avoid loading non-targeted muscles, which allows exercisers to avoid straining those muscles. Isolation exercises also enable an individual to avoid a "weak link in the chain" (a smaller, weaker muscle) from compromising the loading of the larger target muscle. Furthermore, isolation exercises are more efficient, allowing a target muscle to be loaded more, while using less weight—thereby producing less joint and skeletal strain.

In order to properly evaluate an exercise, each component of an exercise needs to be examined, including each participating bone, joint, and muscle, before declaring the exercise as either "good" or "not good." An exercise should also be compared to alternative exercises.

It is naive to assume that all muscles that participate in a compound exercise are optimally loaded, simply because the total weight that is being lifted is "heavy." The angle of each limb relative to the direction of resistance, the alignment of the participating limbs with the direction of resistance, and the participation of secondary levers all play a role in the amount of load and risk that each muscle and joint experiences during a given exercise.

The reverence that many individuals have for "compound" exercises is not based on either physics or logic, nor on an ideal human joint movement. Rather, it has been based on tradition, on archaic beliefs about morality, and on a mistaken assumption that lifting a large amount of weight by using multiple muscles, somehow benefits each participating muscle better than each muscle could benefit by working alone.

While power lifts certainly have a place in sports, they are generally not the better option for people whose goal is general fitness and physique development. When an exercise is evaluated using a set of standards that are physics-based, it is easy to determine approximately how much load is on a given muscle, and where the risks are. In reality, if a person's goal is the pursuit of optimally efficient muscle stimulation and minimal injury risk, the use of isolation exercises is the best strategy.

Every culture in every society has been influenced by beliefs and biases that are NOT rooted in truth or logic. The fitness industry is no exception. Individuals must recognize that their long-standing biases (positive and negative) have influenced their assessment of exercises, such that certain exercises have been given more credit than they deserve, and other exercises have been afforded less credit than they deserve.

It is necessary for people to be aware that they are largely influenced by a fitness industry that introduces "new" recommendations every year. In reality, many of these recommendations are based on the commercial benefit of the industry—*not* on an accurate (or truthful) analysis of the exercises themselves.

In the next chapter, quite a few side-by-side comparisons of "compound" and "isolation" exercises will be reviewed. These comparisons will demonstrate what is "good" or "bad" with each type of exercise, from a biomechanical perspective.

# CHAPTER 13

# PERIPHERAL RECRUITMENT—COMPARING COMPOUND AND ISOLATION EXERCISES

- *For decades, the conventional wisdom among many individuals in the fitness and bodybuilding communities has been that compound exercises build power and mass, while isolation exercises are only for "shaping." This perception is completely false.*
- *Many trainers and physical therapists believe that compound exercises are more "functional" than isolation exercises. The underlying premise of their beliefs is that strength gained from compound exercises is more useful in day-to-day life, than strength attained from isolation exercises. This belief is also completely false.*
- *Some individuals have even suggested that isolation exercises are "dysfunctional"—meaning that they have a higher risk of injury, or lead to a loss of coordination. This observation is also false.*
- *Some people believe that compound exercises "save time," because they work three or four muscle groups at one time, as compared with isolation exercises, which only work one or two muscles at a time. Indeed, compound exercises do work several muscles at a time, but the quality of benefit each muscle receives is significantly less, compared to that which can be achieved with (biomechanically good) isolation exercises.*

In the previous chapter, we established that a "compound exercise" is defined as an exercise that involves multiple joints and muscles (typically three or more) simultaneously. In turn, an isolation exercise is defined as an exercise that typically involves one or two muscles and usually one joint. An exercise that involves two joints could go either way, depending on the complexity of the movement. As you'll see, however, these definitions could be considered rather meaningless.

Exercises that are commonly referred to as compound exercises include *squats, deadlifts, parallel bar dips, chin-ups, push-ups, bench press, "dead hang cleans," bent-over barbell rows,* etc. Among the exercises that are typically categorized as isolation exercises are *standing barbell curls, supine dumbbell triceps extensions, leg extensions* (on a machine), *standing side dumbbell raises,* etc.

## Assertions in Favor of Compound Exercise

The four primary *assertions* that are typically stated in support of compound exercises are the following:

- Compound exercises develop more power and build more muscle mass, as compared with isolation exercises.
- Compound exercises are more "functional," producing strength that is more useful (applicable) in day-to-day life than isolation exercises.
- Isolation exercises are "dysfunctional," suggesting that they do not produce strength that is useful in day-to-day life, and that they have a higher risk of injury. The supposed justification for these beliefs is that the body was "not designed to function in isolation."
- Compound exercises (theoretically) save time, because they work multiple muscles during a single exercise, while isolation exercises only work one or two muscles during a single exercise.

## Reality Check: Compound Exercise Fallacies

In brief, the "short answer" response to each of the aforementioned assertions is the following:

- Each muscle that participates during a compound exercise works in its "own world." It performs its unique function, "unaware" of whether it is working alone, or as one of several muscles working simultaneously. If a muscle is working at maximum capacity, with full range of motion, it will derive full benefit from that effort, whether that muscle is working alone (during an isolation exercise), or in unison with other muscles (during a compound exercise)

The factors that determine how good the "muscle stimulation" is during an exercise include the following: full range of motion; how similar the movement mimics that muscle's ideal anatomical function; whether the load is providing an "ideal resistance curve" for that muscle; and whether that muscle is getting a sufficient load/fatigue.

In reality, how much total weight is being moved during a compound exercise—as a unified effort provided by several participating muscles—is irrelevant. This factor is especially true when you consider the fact that most compound exercises often utilize inefficient levers (i.e., levers that are not fully perpendicular with resistance, and/or levers that are reduced in their effective length by a secondary lever).

Furthermore, during a compound exercise, not all muscles that contribute effort are working at their maximum capacity. Some muscles work more, and some work less—as a percentage of their maximum ability. In reality, the degree to which each participating muscle works—during a compound exercise—does not necessarily coincide with the exerciser's goals. In other words, a muscle that is working MOST during a compound exercise may NOT be the muscle the individual most wants to prioritize. In addition, a muscle that is most prioritized by that person, may actually be the muscle that is working the LEAST.

There is no such thing as "mass building" exercises and "shaping" exercises. A muscle grows larger when it is worked with sufficient load and intensity, regardless of which "type" of exercise provides that load. An individual muscle can be loaded more during an isolation exercise, than it could be from a compound exercise. Accordingly, the belief that compound exercises build mass, while isolation exercises build "shape," is absolute nonsense.

- Proponents of compound exercise often argue that "life is not an isolated exercise," which is why compound exercises are "better." On the other hand, the fact that tasks in life often involve multiple muscles working simultaneously does not require that muscles be strengthened in "groups." In fact, the strength that is gained by individual muscles, by way of isolation exercises can certainly be used in day-to-day tasks.

It is true that a person who consistently performs a compound exercise will improve their coordination in *that particular exercise.* This factor is sometimes confused as "functional strength." The coordination that is gained from a particular exercise would be useful during motions that are similar to the particular compound exercise, thereby utilizing the coordination gained from that exercise. That should not be confused with the fact that the strength gained by individual muscles, during a compound exercise, is somehow greater—or more useful—than strength gained by isolation exercises.

For example, the coordination that is gained during "*dead hang cleans*" (Figure 13-1) would not be useful during daily activities, unless those daily activities resemble *dead hang cleans.* Furthermore, the strength acquired by performing *dead hang cleans* can easily be gained by doing other exercises involving the same muscles that are engaged during *dead hang cleans*—with less risk of injury.

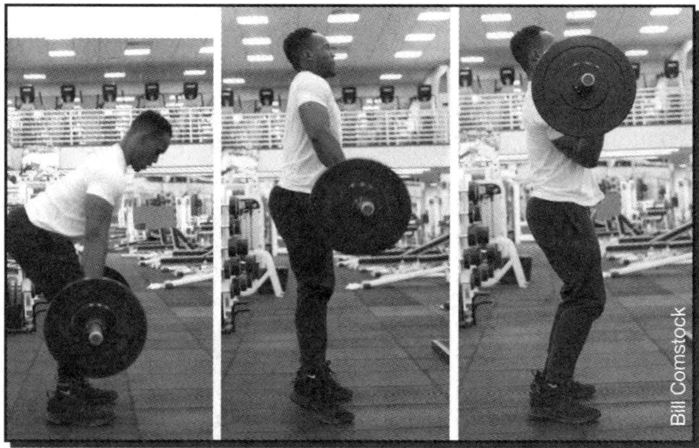

Figure 13-1

Suggesting that a person who does mostly compound exercises will be more capable of handling day-to-day activities, as compared with a person who does mostly isolation exercises, is illogical. The body can easily coordinate the strength of all its muscles, during daily activities, regardless of how that strength was gained.

- The assertions that isolation exercises may "cause" dysfunction (the loss of coordination) and that isolation exercises pose a higher risk of injury are both false. With regard to the risk of injury, the opposite is more likely to be true. A movement that has more moving parts, such as a compound exercise, and which often requires the use of an individual's body weight (i.e., does not offer the option of using a resistance level that is less than body weight) would naturally have the higher injury risk.

Isolation exercises, by definition, are exercises that are designed to follow the exact motion of a particular muscle and its joint. As a result, it would, therefore, produce a more natural movement for that particular muscle and joint. Conversely, an exercise that involves the participation of several muscles and joints may be safe for one or two muscles and joints, but not necessarily for all participating muscles and joints.

There is no evidence—not even empirical evidence—that isolation exercises result in a loss of coordination. In my 40 years "in the trenches," I have yet to see anyone become less coordinated because they used isolation exercises. What exactly is meant by this assertion? The belief that a person may become "spastic" (i.e., experience a loss of motor skills/loss of muscle control), because—although they exercised all of their muscles—they did so "one muscle at a time," is ridiculous.

Personally, I have used mostly isolation exercises my entire career (40+ years), and have gotten only positive results. Conversely, many of my contemporaries (who relied heavily on compound exercises) have had numerous orthopedic surgeries, including shoulder reconstruction, hip and knee replacements, spinal fusion, etc. I am still competing in bodybuilding at the age of 59 (43 years of training and competing), without any injuries or joint pain. I can also still play basketball, dance, swim, and do any of the other activities I did when I was younger.

- In terms of saving time, the assertion that compound exercises are more time-efficient would be true if (and only if) each muscle participating in a compound exercise receives the same quality of muscle stimulation as could be achieved with separate isolation exercises. If that were the case, it would eliminate the need to do any additional exercises for those participating muscles. In reality, that is absolutely NOT the case.

  Most bodybuilders who perform compound exercises ALSO do separate exercises for those individual muscles. In other words, while multiple muscles may be participating in a compound exercise, the participation of each of those muscles is generally not "good enough" to qualify as the only exercise necessary for those individual muscles. Those muscles still require another (better) exercise.

  On the other hand, a person who does one "good" isolation exercise for each primary skeletal muscle does NOT need to do an additional exercise for those particular muscles. Therefore, the person saving time is the individual who does only the isolation exercises.

  Of course, if a person is content with only getting 40 percent, 50 percent, or 60 percent as good a stimulation per muscle during a compound exercise, as compared with an isolation exercise, then that individual might consider the compound exercise a "timesaver." On the other hand, most bodybuilders want 100 percent benefit for each muscle. Most compound exercises, however, do NOT deliver 100 percent benefit to each participating muscle. As such, for the person who wants optimal results (in terms of muscular development) doing compound exercises would not save time. Instead, it would be the cause of wasted time and effort.

## Comparing Compound Exercise vs. Isolation Exercise

❑ Range of Motion, Natural Joint Function, Target Muscle Loading vs. Stabilizer Muscle Loading, and Load Efficiency (Lever Mechanics)

To be clear, the comparison that is being made in this instance is between compound and isolation exercises, for the primary purpose of muscular development. Training for physique development, however, is not a purely cosmetic pursuit. It is impossible to make a muscle larger, without making it stronger. The process by which a muscle is visibly developed requires the loading of that muscle, and then causing that muscle to stretch and contract against that load. A muscle naturally increases its strength in that process.

Stretching and contracting a muscle against an opposing resistance does not require that a group of muscles be worked simultaneously. In fact, it is easier to focus on the deliberate stretching and contracting of a muscle, against resistance, when the person is able to isolate that one muscle's primary function.

The previous chapters reviewed the fact that a number of physics-related factors influence how much load is placed on a given muscle, regardless of the actual weight being lifted. These factors include lever length, lever position (relative to resistance), the position of a secondary lever, alignment, and mechanical disadvantage. In reality, these factors can cause a muscle to be loaded more, even though the weight being lifted is not "impressive." These factors can also cause a muscle to be less loaded, even though the weight being lifted is "impressive."

For example, it was demonstrated how a triceps can be loaded with only 119 pounds of resistance, when a 180-pound man performs parallel bar dips. It was also shown how a triceps can be loaded with 240 pounds of resistance when a person performs a supine dumbbell triceps extension, using a pair of 20-pound dumbbells (40 pounds total). The key point is that more weight being used does NOT automatically translate to a muscle being loaded more.

So the question you must ask yourself, in order to adequately compare exercises, is *what are the biomechanical factors that most contribute to muscle growth?* These biomechanical factors can then be used as a "checklist" for evaluating the load, efficiency, and productivity of any exercise. Without this knowledge, you would be relegated to judging the productivity of an exercise ONLY by the total amount of weight lifted, which is a grossly inaccurate method of evaluation.

The following are the biomechanical factors that most contribute to muscle growth, efficiency (amount of weight moved versus amount of load on the target muscle), and movement safety:

- *Direction of movement:* Ideally, a muscle should pull its operating lever directly toward its origin. Thus, a "good" exercise would provide a "pathway of movement" that allows the operating lever (i.e., the limb) to move directly away from, and then directly toward, the origin of a target muscle. This sequence produces maximum muscle lengthening (stretch) and muscle shortening (contraction). The more the movement of an exercise resembles a given muscle's primary action, the more stimulation that muscle will experience.
- *Range of motion:* Ideally, an exercise should provide a mostly full "range of motion" for the target muscle. Full range of motion is more productive than an "isometric" contraction, and also more productive than a partial range of motion. This has been well documented.
- *Alignment and opposite position loading:* The ideal direction of resistance for a given muscle should be directly opposite the direction of anatomical movement. The resistance should originate from a point that is directly opposite the target muscle's origin. The target muscle's origin and insertion should be on the same plane as the direction of movement and the direction of resistance. This factor would provide the most efficient delivery of the load to the target muscle (i.e., the least amount of misdirected resistance). It would also minimize the risk of injury.
- *Resistance curve:* Ideally, the direction of resistance would provide "early phase loading" to the target muscle—"heavier" at the beginning of the motion and "lighter" at the end of the range of motion. The presence of any mechanical disadvantage must be factored into the resistance curve.
- Ideally, an exercise would utilize a mostly "active" lever (the limb interacting perpendicularly with the direction of resistance) during the range of motion. This factor would load the greatest percentage of the resistance being used onto the target muscle, requiring less wasted effort.
- Ideally, an exercise would allow for natural joint motion, without any unnecessary joint contortion, spinal compression, or tendon/bursa impingement.
- Ideally, an exercise should provide relief from any "mechanical disadvantage," wherever it may present. In other words, during an exercise (an anatomical movement) in which a mechanical disadvantage occurs, a direction of resistance should be selected that is less perpendicular with your operating lever (limb) at the point of mechanical disadvantage.
- Ideally, an exercise should be performed with deliberate muscle force, rather than with momentum ("swinging"/"cheating").

The amount of weight being lifted during an exercise matters, but not at the exclusion of the aforementioned criteria. Lifting weights that are very heavy, while not complying with the aforementioned factors, may lead to some muscle loading and growth, but not in the most efficient manner possible, and with a much higher injury risk. The "cost" of the exercise (i.e., the energy it requires and the risk of injury it creates) will be higher, and the benefit is likely to be lower.

When evaluating a compound exercise, every lever (limb), muscle and joint that is involved in the movement should be assessed. You can readily see which limbs interact perpendicularly with gravity and to what degree they do so. You can then determine whether the priority muscles are most loaded, or the non-priority muscles are more loaded. You'll have a better undemanding of this factor once you are familiar with the musculoskeletal system—Chapters 18 through 25.

Very often, during a compound exercise, a muscle that you do *not* want to emphasize is more loaded than is your target muscle. For example, when doing *parallel bar dips*, the anterior deltoids are most loaded—more so than the pecs or triceps. Yet, no one does parallel bar dips with the primary goal of working their anterior deltoids.

Another example of this situation occurs during (any kind of) *leg raises*, when the hip flexors are working much harder than are the abs. Yet another example of this factor arises when a person performs a *bent-over barbell row*. The lower back and posterior deltoids are more loaded than are either the lats or the middle trapezius. During these (and other) compound exercises, the benefit is compromised, while the injury risk and the energy cost are elevated.

When evaluating an exercise, whether it's a compound exercise or an isolation exercise, you should do so without any bias. You should be like a jury in a courtroom that looks only at the facts (i.e., the physics and physiological principles). You should ignore any preconceived notions or traditional beliefs that exist about a particular exercise. You can then evaluate what each lever (limb) and joint is doing, and determine whether the mechanics of that exercise are favorable or not, or to what degree they are favorable.

## The Bias in Favor of Compound Exercise

Peripheral recruitment refers to the participation of muscles, during a given exercise, that are not the primary "target" of that exercise. Peripheral recruitment happens during all compound exercises, but it also occurs—to some degree—during most isolation exercises. Sometimes, the peripheral recruitment that occurs during an exercise is acceptable, while other times, it is problematic.

For example, consider the *standing barbell curl.* It is generally considered an "isolation exercise" for the biceps. The biceps, however, are not the only muscles that are working during this exercise. The lower back (erector spinae) is also working, because it is preventing the person from falling forward, while the biceps bend the elbows. The erector spinae are working isometrically, while the biceps are working dynamically. In addition, the glutes and hamstrings are also participating—"peripherally"—helping maintain the person's posture during the exercise. All of this is acceptable.

When a person does a *hanging leg raise*, however, the circumstances are not acceptable. During this exercise, a person typically holds onto a chinning bar, with their arms straight. Then, both knees are brought up toward the chest (Figure 13-2), or the legs are raised with the knees straight (Figure 13-3).

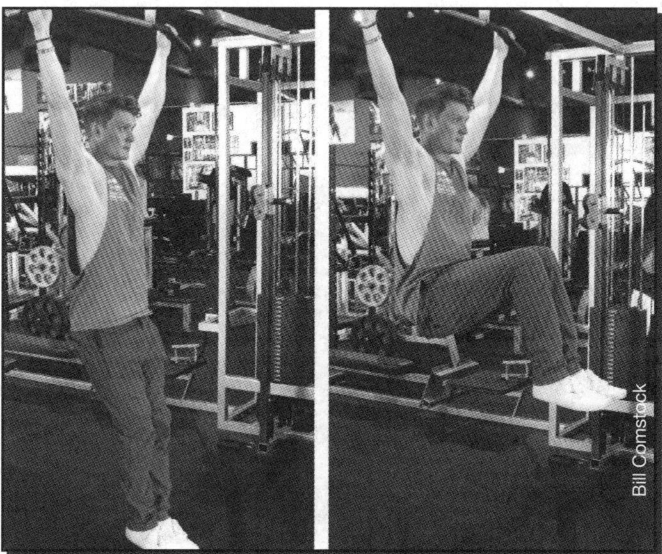

Figure 13-2

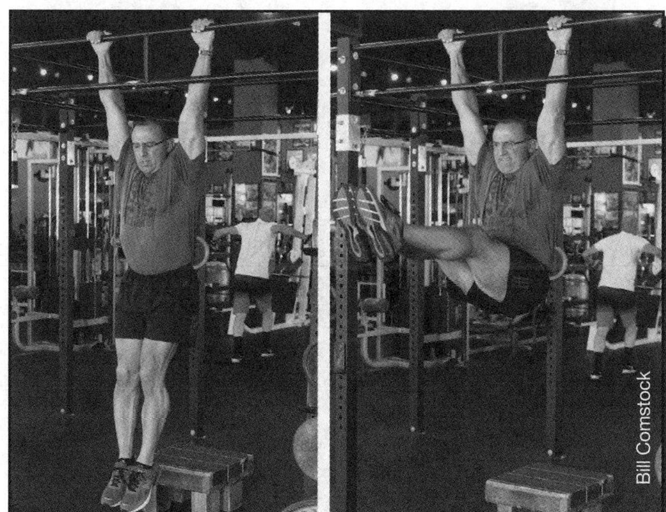

Figure 13-3

The intended "target" of this exercise is the abs (the rectus abdominus), but quite a few other muscles are "peripherally recruited." For example, the muscles of the hands and of the forearms are working isometrically, holding tension without movement. The hip flexors are working quite a lot—dynamically. The quadriceps are also working to a degree (more so when the legs are straight)—in this instance, isometrically. In addition to these muscles participating, there may also be a degree of strain to the shoulder joint.

A proponent of compound exercise would argue that a *hanging leg raise* is "good," because it is working a number of different muscles. These advocates would suggest that this exercise saves time, as well as creates a greater caloric demand, when compared with doing an isolated abdominal exercise. While that may SOUND appealing, upon closer inspection, you can see that the *hanging leg raise* has serious issues.

For example, the muscle that is working the most, during *hanging leg raises*, is the hip flexor group, which is likely not the muscle you want to prioritize. The muscles of the hands and forearms are working very hard (i.e., straining), but not necessarily in a way that is productive. If your objective is to visibly develop the forearm muscles, you will need to do dynamic "wrist flexion" and "wrist extension" exercises. The abs are mostly producing isometric tension, which causes fatigue (i.e., a burning sensation), but is not nearly as productive as dynamic abdominal contraction (i.e., "crunches") would be. As a result, the "cost" is very high, but the benefit is very low.

When analyzing any exercise, one of the primary questions you should ask yourself is: *"Is the insertion of your target muscle being moved toward the origin of that muscle?"* With regard to *hanging leg raises,* the question could be asked more specifically: *"Is the distance between the pubic bone and the ribcage maximally decreasing (upon contraction) and maximally increasing (upon muscle elongation)?"* That action would produce "spinal flexion," which is the primary function of the abs. Clearly, however, there is far less spinal flexion occurring during this exercise, than there is hip flexion. On occasion, there is no spinal flexion occurring, because it is extremely difficult to cause spinal flexion, while the hip flexors are lifting the weight of the legs.

Yes, the "hanging leg raise" is a compound exercise, and it causes a high caloric demand. It is, however, mostly a waste of time and energy as an exercise for the development of the abs.

*Note: The use of straps (attached to the chin-up bar, by which a person can then support their body weight without the use of their hands) eliminates the potential strain on the hands and forearms. These straps, however, do not change the fact that the hip flexors are working significantly more than are the abs.*

Conversely, a standard ab crunch (Figure 13-4) is considered an isolation exercise. Yet, it's much more effective for developing the rectus abdominis (the abs). It dynamically loads the abs better, without straining the shoulders, hands, fingers, and forearms. Furthermore, it does not waste energy unproductively by engaging the hip flexors, and does not produce "abs interference," which is caused by engaging the hip flexors at the same time as you are trying to contract the abs (a factor that will be explained in Chapters 23 and 24).

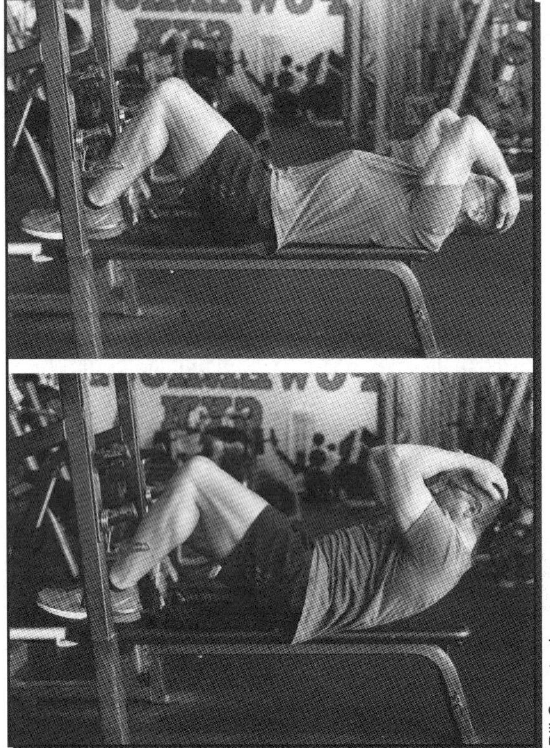

Bill Comstock

Figure 13-4

Proponents of compound exercise also often recommend *planks* (Figure 13-5) as a "better" alternative to *ab crunches.* They claim that a *plank* is a "compound exercise," and that it's good because it involves the hip flexors and quadriceps, as well as the abs. Again, this may sound good, but it's not quite accurate, and not very productive.

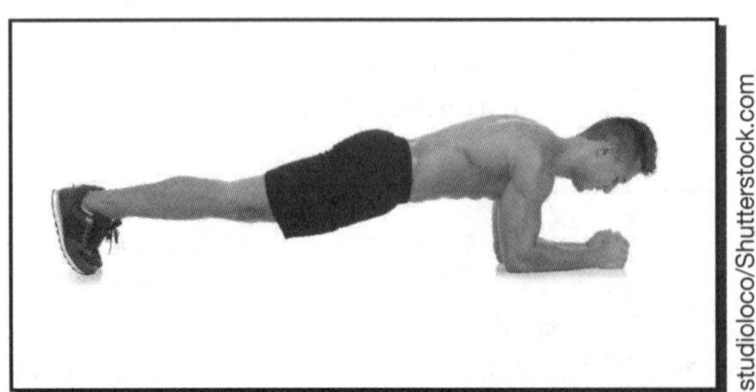

studioloco/Shutterstock.com

Figure 13-5

Yes, *planks* "peripherally recruit" the hip flexors and quadriceps, in addition to engaging the abs, but none of these are optimally beneficial. Muscle tension without movement is "isometric," which has been proven to be less productive (for most goals) as compared with dynamic muscle tension (i.e., with movement). Therefore, none of the muscles that are participating in *planks* are getting as much benefit as they would get if you were to work each of those muscles separately, using dynamic exercises—like knee extensions for the quads, spinal flexion for the abs, and hip flexion for the hip flexors.

Barbell squats (Figure 13-6) is a compound exercise, however, it is very compromised. In Chapter 2, the topic of "active levers and neutral levers" was discussed. This discussion looked at how the standard *barbell squat* causes the tibia to barely arrive at an angle that is approximately 30 degrees from the "neutral" (vertical) position. Therefore, only about 30 percent of the "available resistance" is loading the quadriceps, while 100 percent of the weight that is on your back is compressing your spine.

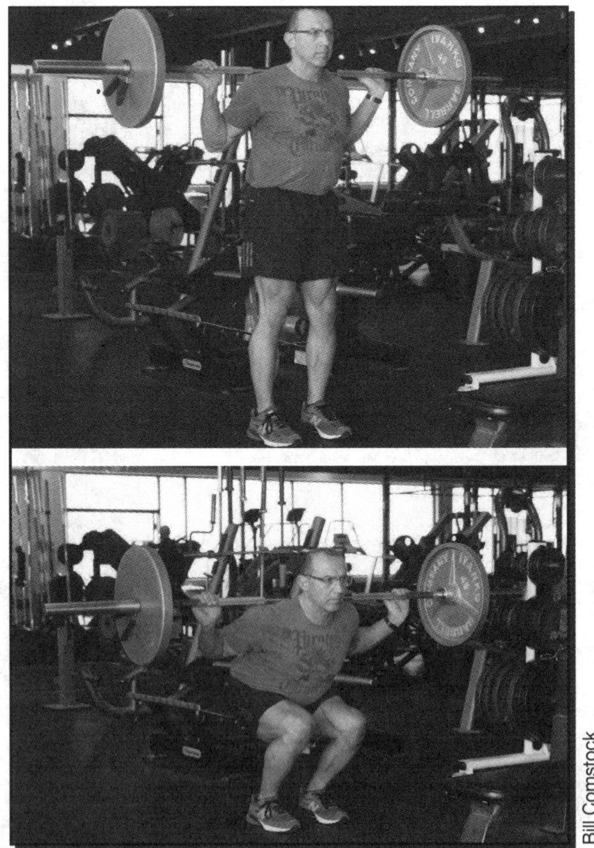

Bill Comstock

Figure 13-6

Conversely, you could do *cable squats* (Figure 13-7) using *half as much weight* as you'd use when doing standard barbell squats, and get as much load on your quadriceps—or more—without having a metal bar pressing downward on your spine.

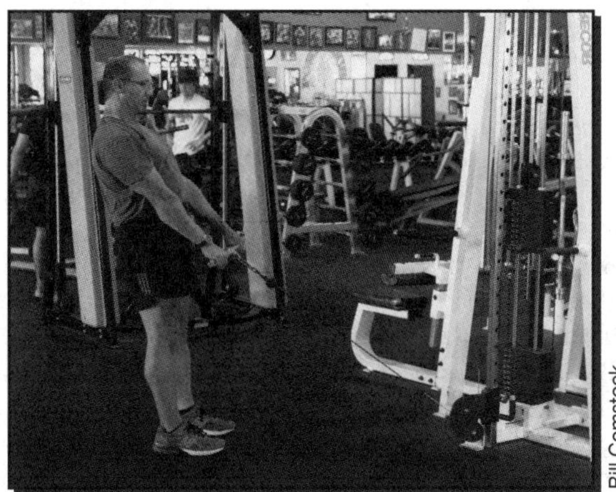

Figure 13-7

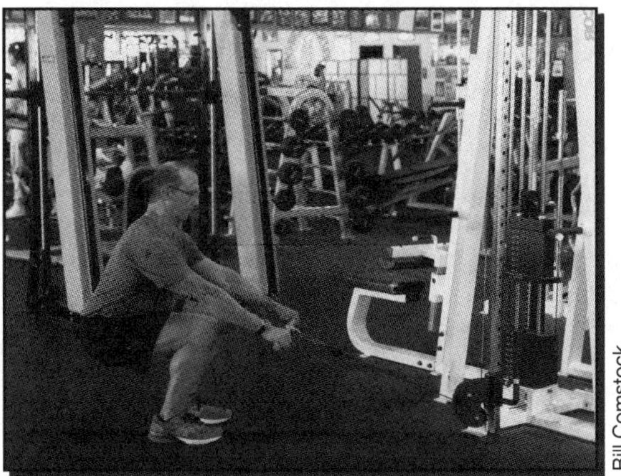

Figure 13-8

Both of these "*squats*" are compound exercises, because they both involve the same joints and the same muscles. The average bodybuilder, however, is more likely to choose *barbell squats,* over *cable squats,* because they can use a heavier weight.

What this scenario tells you, is that individuals often conflate the concept of a "compound exercise" with an exercise that allows them to perform an exercise using heavy weight. People seem to favor compound exercises, in part, because they associate the use of heavy weight with more muscle growth. This thinking is misguided.

The two versions of *squats*—depicted in Figure 13-6 and in Figures 13-7 and 13-8—require the exact same motion and involve the same joints and muscles. The primary difference is the direction of resistance, which alters the percentage of resistance that loads the quads, the glutes, and the erector spinae. Yet, because *cable squats* force individuals to use a lighter weight, people question whether it's a "compound exercise." In fact, it is a better (and safer) compound exercise, for the purpose of working the quadriceps, glutes and adductors, as compared with barbell squats.

In fact, it's a mistake to regard ALL compound exercises as either "good" or "bad." It depends entirely on the mechanics of each individual exercise. For example, *regular squats* without the addition of holding a barbell on your shoulders, is generally a very good compound exercise. The fact that the tibia only interacts with gravity at an angle of about 30 degrees from neutral is acceptable, especially if "body weight" *squats* is challenging enough. On the other hand, once the user finds it necessary to add resistance, the strategy of loading additional weight onto the spine is not particularly wise.

The better strategy is to perform squats with a slightly frontward/downward-pulling cable resistance. This does not convert *squats* into an isolation exercise. It is still a compound exercise, but with a more productive, more efficient and more safe direction of additional resistance.

The ability to use a heavier weight should NOT be the deciding factor with regard to exercise selection, when the goal is muscle building or general fitness. The better choice would be the exercise that provides the same "net" load to the target muscles, but with less "cost"—less energy spent, less load on non-target muscles, and less skeletal strain.

## The Mechanical Inefficiency of Most Compound Exercises and the Folly of Prioritizing the Lifting of "Heavy" Weight

As noted previously, people often justify their preference for compound exercises by making the claim that they are able to use more weight. From a mechanical perspective, however, lifting a heavy weight does not guarantee that the participating muscles are any more loaded than they would be if other exercises with better mechanics were used—even with a lighter weight.

In Figure 13-9, you can see a rock slab being lifted, with the help of a pry bar. Clearly, this man is not extraordinarily muscular, so it's reasonable to assume that he's not exceptionally

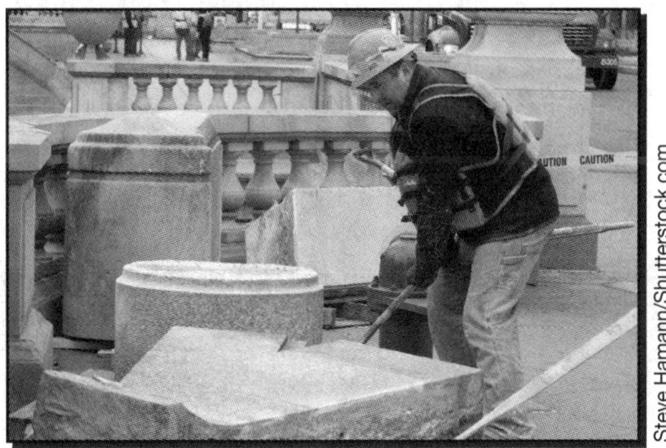

Figure 13-9

strong. In fact, it's safe to assume that he would not be able to move that heavy slab WITHOUT the pry bar. It would be foolish for this individual to believe that the advantage gained by using the pry bar is benefitting his muscles more, than it would be if he tried to lift a lighter object, without the advantage of a pry bar.

The same factor applies with exercise mechanics. Lifting a very heavy weight with inefficient levers, allows you to appear stronger (allowing you to lift a heavier weight), than lifting a lighter weight with efficient levers. Lifting a heavy weight by using inefficient mechanics does NOT mean that the participating muscles are working any harder than they would, if they lifted a lighter weight, with more efficient levers.

When you perform *barbell squats* and *leg presses*, the levers involved are magnifying the resistance LESS, because of the angle of the tibia in relation to the direction of resistance. That angle allows more weight to be moved. Moving more weight, however, does NOT automatically translate to loading the target muscles more.

As was discussed in the previous chapter, most individuals have a subconscious bias in favor of choosing exercises that allow them to use a heavy weight, because it leads them into believing that they are "very strong." How many people have had a friend take a photo while they're doing a set of very heavy squats, or a set of very heavy leg presses, and then posted the photo to Facebook or Instagram? This scenario is a byproduct of self-deception. In fact, you can load your quadriceps and your gluteus with as much (or more) resistance, USING LESS WEIGHT, but using more efficient mechanics (better exercises).

In reality, you should not fool yourself into thinking that you are "super strong," nor concern yourself with how strong you are perceived to be. You should only concern yourself with training efficiently (i.e., maximum muscle load) while avoiding the unnecessary risk of using more weight than is necessary.

When you challenge your muscles with resistance, they become significantly stronger. Using an amount of resistance that forces you to use near-maximum effort—during an isolation exercise—will produce the same (or more) stimulation for increases of individual muscle strength as would occur using a similar effort during a compound exercise.

You should not assume that avoiding compound exercises (which allow you to use a "heavy weight" during a single lift) will stifle your ability to gain strength. Strength is gained whenever the demands on a muscle cause it to be challenged beyond its existing capability, regardless of how much weight is actually being used. This factor is known as the "Stress Adaptation Principle," which was advocated by the noted endocrinologist Hans Selye, in the 1930s.

Another factor that must be considered, when evaluating the muscle-building value of a compound exercise, is whether or not each participating muscle is doing precisely what it is designed to do. As noted previously, one of the eight biomechanical factors that most contributes to muscle growth is how closely an exercise's movement resembles a target muscle's ideal anatomical motion. For example, the pectoralis major moves the humerus toward its various points of origin, which are located mostly on the sternum. A small percentage are located on the ribs (the "costal" fibers), while another small percentage is located on the medial (closest to the center) part of the clavicles (the "clavicular" fibers). For this reason, a "good" pectoral exercise would produce a movement that moves the humerus parallel to those fibers, as well as toward those muscle fiber origins (Figure 13-10).

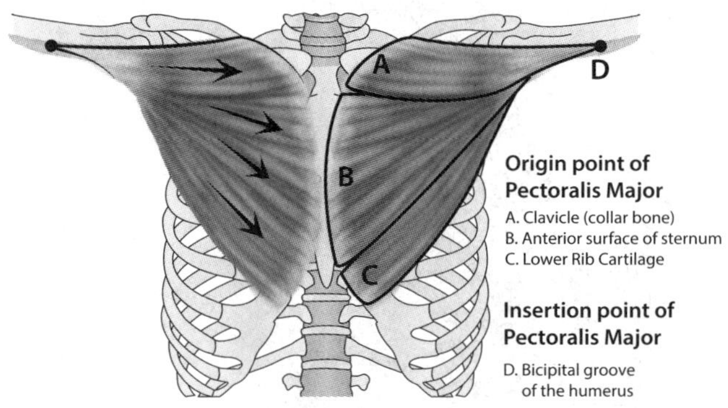


Figure 13-10

Keeping this factor in mind, let's compare *parallel bar dips* and *decline cable press*—and ascertain which one allows a better anatomical movement for the "sternal" and "costal" pectoral fibers. In Figures 13-11 and 13-12, compare the concluding point of both exercises (*parallel bar dips* versus *decline cable press*). Then compare the beginning point of both exercises. You can clearly see which exercise provides the more ideal anatomical motion for the pectorals.

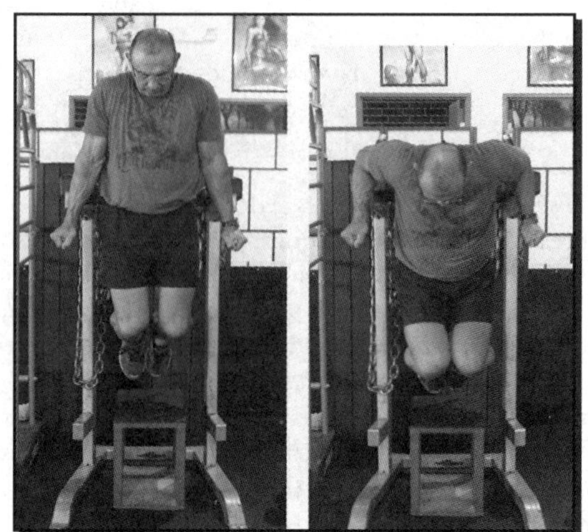


Figure 13-11

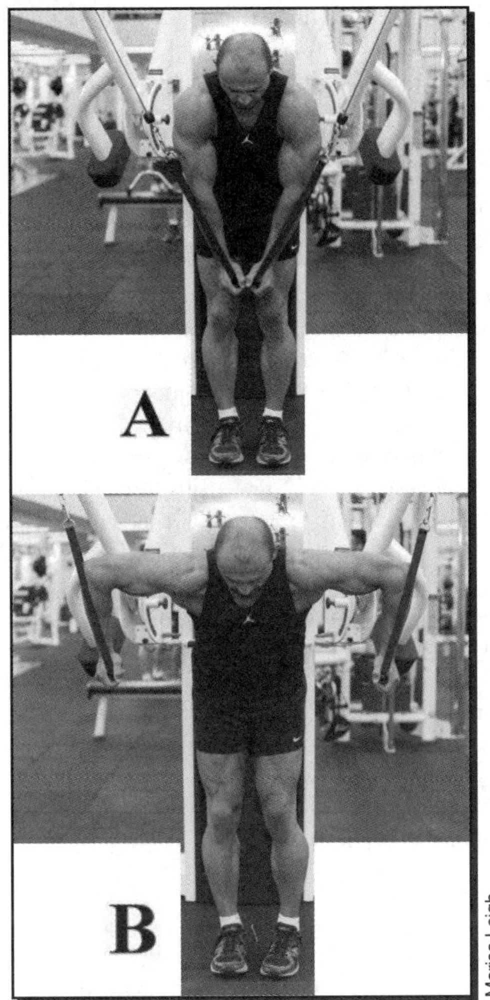


Figure 13-12

Note that the *decline cable press* provides a direction of resistance that moves parallel with the pectoral fibers. This aspect allows a movement (of the humerus) that starts from an "outside" angle, and moves INWARD, toward the center—toward the pectoral origins. In contrast, the movement of the humerus during *parallel bar dips* runs vertical—in a straight downward direction, a movement that is NOT toward the pectoral origins. Therefore, although the pectorals participate during *parallel bar dips*, the movement does not mimic the ideal humeral motion of the pectorals, which is more inward, toward the pectoral origins.

Of course, "traditionalists" favor *parallel bar dips* over the cable exercise because *parallel bar dips* are regarded as a compound exercise. You can clearly see, however, that *parallel bar dips* do not produce an ideal anatomical motion for contracting the pectorals.

Yes, *parallel bar dips* involve "other" muscles, but not very productively. They load the triceps, but with only about half as much resistance as a simple supine dumbbell triceps extension would (due to the mostly vertical forearm). *Parallel bar dips* also load the anterior deltoid, too much, actually, and with excessive stretch and insufficient range of motion on the contraction end.

Is it logical to favor *parallel bar dips* because the exercise works multiple muscles, even though none of the three muscles involved are working as well as they each could work, while doing other, more isolated exercises? Should you accept the inadequate pectoral contraction, the inefficient loading of the triceps, and the risk of anterior deltoid injury (and its compromised benefit to the anterior deltoids), and also ignore the fact that it forces you to use body weight (possibly too much)—JUST because it's a "compound exercise?" Logically speaking, there are more "negatives" than "positives" associated with *parallel bar dips*.

Let's examine the *bench press*. It's considered a "foundational" exercise by many people, and it is one of the most popular compound exercises. It mostly engages the pectorals, along with some involvement of the triceps and the anterior deltoids. In addition to being used for the purpose of muscular development, it is also considered a "strength builder." The question is, how does it compare with other pectoral/triceps exercises, in terms of effectiveness, efficiency, and safety?

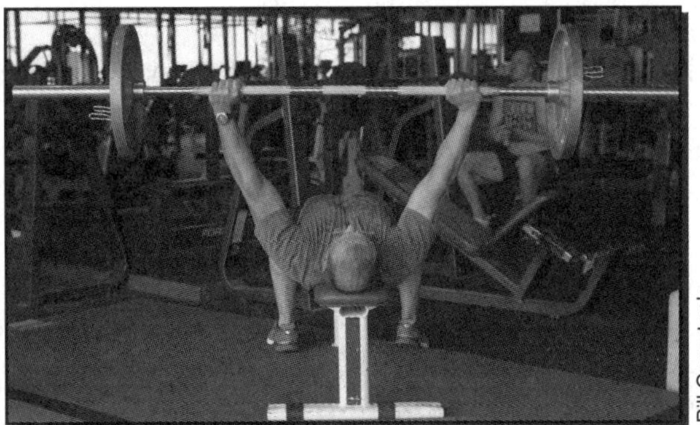


Figure 13-13

From the standpoint of developing the pectoral muscles, the range of motion is obviously shorter, as compared with an exercise that allows the hands to come together in the center (above the chest). Bringing the hands all the way together would allow for a more complete contraction of the pecs—a full range of motion. Furthermore, since both arms are sharing the same instrument, each arm is not working independently. As a result, there is a loss of "crossover" benefit as well.

We sometimes see individuals with well-developed pectorals and triceps performing this exercise, but that is not necessarily "evidence" that the *bench press* is an excellent exercise for the pectorals and triceps, as compared with other exercises. The lack of complete pectoral contraction and the insufficient range of motion for the triceps cannot be ignored. Although the pectorals and triceps are stimulated by performing *bench press*, the stimulation is compromised by the insufficient range of motion.

Most people with notable muscular physiques typically do other pectoral exercises, in addition to bench presses. They also perform other triceps exercises. Therefore, their pectoral and triceps development cannot be attributed solely to the *bench press*. Unfortunately, an incorrect assumption is often made, that the *bench press* is primarily responsible for superior pectoral development. The mechanics of the bench press fail to meet the criteria necessary for optimal muscle stimulation.

Imagine, if you will, conducting an experiment which involved two people with the exact same genetics. "Person #1" does only the *bench press*, while "person #2" does only the *flat bench dumbbell press* (for the pectorals) and *supine dumbbell triceps extensions* (for the triceps). What you would discover is that person #2 achieved better pectoral development and triceps development, as compared with person #1. In fact, there is no muscular benefit that is attained by doing the *bench press* that cannot be achieved more successfully with other exercises.

Now, let's examine the *bench press* from a biomechanical perspective, as well as from a philosophical perspective. Many people assume that the *barbell bench press* builds more "power" than exercises using dumbbells. In fact, the *barbell bench press* has—for many years—been regarded as a "foundational strength building exercise," as well as the standard "barometer" of strength—neither of which is quite accurate.

The following statistics (Figure 13-14)—provided by the American College of Sports Medicine—reference how much weight men "should" be able to *bench press*. As the chart suggests, the amount of weight that can be used during any exercise depends on several factors, including the person's age, their level of fitness, and their body weight. In this chart, the 50th percentile is considered "average," while the 70th percentile is considered "very good." The 90th percentile is considered "excellent." These stats are based on a ONE-REP MAX, which entails exerting an all-out effort, for only one repetition.

According to this chart, the average 50- to 59-year-old man "should" be able to *bench press* 150 pounds, if his body weight is 200 pounds. The average 20- to 29-year-old man "should" be able to *bench press* 296 pounds, if his body weight is 200 pounds. As noted in the previous chapter, people seem to care quite a lot (far more than they should, in my opinion) about how their strength in this one lift, compares with the strength of others.

I question whether it is entirely prudent for the American College of Sports Medicine to be making recommendations about how much weight a man "should" be able to *bench press* for a ONE-REP MAX. It would be more reasonable to expect this sort of recommendation from the National Strength & Conditioning Association, given that they tend to be more focused on the power lifts and the power sports, like football. I feel that for a sports medicine institution to be recommending people perform a ONE-REP MAX *bench press* at all—given its potential injury risk, when a heavy weight is used—is somewhat irresponsible. Furthermore, suggesting that individuals strive for a heavier *bench press*, so they can qualify as "acceptable" (meeting expectations) is also irresponsible. "Exercise"—for most everyone, except powerlifters and football players—should *not* be about the maximum amount of weight lifted, as much as it should be about optimal health, optimal development, reasonable strength gains, and joint safety.

It's not as common now as it was in years past, but the standard question to ask someone who apparently "lifted weights" was "*How much do you bench press?*" or more simply "*How much do you bench?*" I always thought that was such a ridiculous question, because it's only one exercise, which mostly involves only two muscles—the pectorals and the triceps. Why would that one exercise be used as a measure of anyone's "total strength?" Furthermore, since I was a bodybuilder, "*Why would it matter how much I lift during any of my exercises? What matters is how well my physique is developed.*"

In addition to placing too much importance on a ONE-REP MAX of a particular exercise (assuming an individual's goal is physique development, optimal health, and overall fitness), it's also extremely difficult to account for different anatomical structures. Taller people with longer arms will

| Men Age | 50th Percentile | 70th Percentile | 90th Percentile |
|---|---|---|---|
| 20-29 | 106% of bodyweight | 122% of bodyweight | 148% of bodyweight |
| 30-39 | 93% of bodyweight | 104% of bodyweight | 124% of bodyweight |
| 40-49 | 88% of bodyweight | 93% of bodyweight | 110% of bodyweight |
| 50-59 | 75% of bodyweight | 84% of bodyweight | 97% of bodyweight |

Figure 13-14

have more difficulty lifting "heavy," as compared to shorter people with shorter arms. This factor is due to the increased magnification effect of longer levers (limbs).

There are also several categories of "somatotypes" (bone thickness and ratio of muscle type—"fast twitch"/explosive versus "slow twitch"/endurance). In addition, people's natural endocrine (hormone) levels also influence the amount of weight they are able to lift. In other words, concerning yourself with whether you are able to meet a certain "strength standard" (i.e., amount of weight lifted, as a ONE-REP MAX), is rather foolish, unless you are competing in powerlifting.

If your goal is muscular development, you never need to perform a ONE-REPETITION MAXIMUM lift, of any kind. It's completely unproductive for the goal of muscular development. The lowest number of reps that is likely to be "productive" for muscle growth is four, although—realistically—it's probably closer to six. Performing fewer reps than that, with heavier weight, produces less muscular growth, with a much higher risk of injury.

As discussed in Chapter 3, there is a tremendous mechanical disadvantage that occurs in the fully descended position of the *bench press*. That mechanical disadvantage is made much more dangerous by the effort to lift the heaviest weight possible for one repetition. Realistically speaking, what advantage does a person think they'll gain by taking that risk? Gaining the admiration of a few friends in the gym is hardly worth the possibility of a life-altering injury.

One potential consequence of doing a very heavy *bench press* is illustrated in Figure 13-15. This injury is called "anterior dislocation of the humerus." A normal shoulder joint is illustrated in Figure 13-15, left image. As you can see, the humeral head sits comfortably in the glenoid socket. Figure 13-15, right image, shows the humeral head pulled forward, out of the glenoid socket.

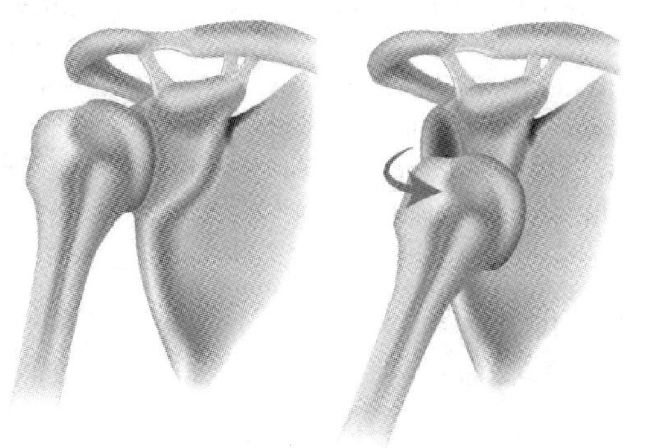


Figure 13-15

When performing a *bench press*, when the barbell is at the level of the chest (or close to it), the pectoral muscle is pulling the humerus mostly "inward"—toward the sternum—because that is where the pectoral origins are situated. As you can see in Figure 13-16, this factor causes the pectoral muscle to pull on the humerus from an almost completely parallel angle. This mechanical disadvantage dramatically increases the muscle force required, such that the pectoral muscle can actually pull the humeral head forward—out of the glenoid socket.

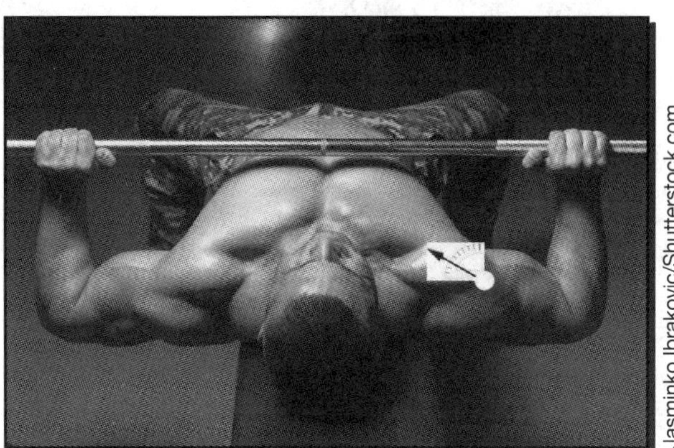


Figure 13-16

If the humeral head is pulled forward, the muscle tendons that are attached to the humerus—the infraspinatus, teres major, latissimus, posterior deltoid, and lateral deltoid—all get pulled forward as well. Some of these tendons may rupture, as a result of being pulled beyond their stretch capacity. As such, the remedy for this type of injury may not be simply putting the humeral head back in place. Needless to say, this type of injury would be extremely painful, and would likely result in some degree of permanent shoulder pain and dysfunction, for the rest of that person's life, even after surgical repair.

The *bench press* can be used safely, with some degree of benefit, when using moderate weight. On the other hand, it is still not an especially "good" exercise for physique development. There are better pectoral exercises, as well as better triceps exercises. This statement is not meant as an indictment, per se, of the *bench press*. Rather, the *bench press* is simply another example of a popular compound exercise, which is not as "good" as everyone has been led to believe. As such, biomechanical analysis allows us to see why that is so.

The exercise shown in Figure 13-17, known as the *deadlift*, is perhaps the most revered of all the compound exercises. It has often been referred to as a "foundational" exercise. It's likely that you've performed this exercise at some point in the past, using "heavy" weight (i.e., limiting you to fewer than three repetitions). It would be understandable if you have, since the exercise has been so enthusiastically promoted. The question is, how productive is it—actually—for the purpose of muscular development, and how much injury risk does performing heavy *deadlifts* create?

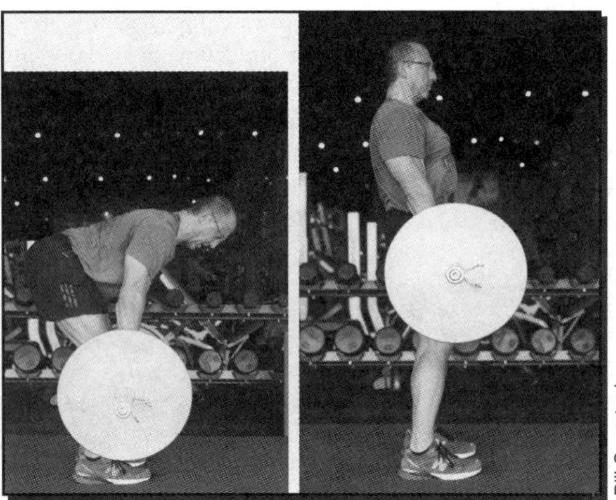


Figure 13-17

In the starting position for the *deadlift* (Figure 13-17, left image), you can see that the torso is in a mostly horizontal position—perpendicular to gravity. Therefore, the torso (as a lever) is mostly "active" when the weight is lifted off the floor. Therefore, the muscles that "operate" the torso-lever would be fully loaded. By "operate," I mean "produce hip extension" and "prevent the spine from folding forward." These muscles would include the gluteus, hamstring, adductors (for hip extension), and the erector spinae (preventing the spine from folding forward). The femur is at an angle that is between vertical and horizontal, which contributes to the hip extension component. The lower leg (the tibia) is mostly vertical (i.e., mostly "neutral")—mostly parallel with gravity. As a result, the quadriceps do not play as much of a role in this lift, as do the hip extensor muscles and the erector spinae.

The dynamic movement in this exercise is mostly a hip extension. The hip joint is the primary "pivot"—the joint that moves the most—during *deadlifts*. Accordingly, it is the muscles that produce hip extension—the gluteus maximus, hamstrings, and adductors—that are working dynamically. This does not necessarily mean, however, that those are the muscles that are most "loaded." "Load"—as you will recall—is comprised of weight, plus lever length, plus the angle of the lever, relative to resistance.

Furthermore, what constitutes "heavy" for one muscle is not always the same as what constitutes "heavy" for another muscle. This factor is relative to the strength capacity of each muscle. A reasonable argument could be made that the erector spinae (although working isometrically) is more loaded (relative to capacity) than are the gluteus, the hamstrings, and the adductors. This factor would explain why we so often see the spine folding forward (failing to be kept arched), when people perform "heavy" deadlifts.

Accordingly, when evaluating the *deadlift,* we would ask the following questions: "How productive is this movement for the gluteus, hamstrings, and adductors? How productive (and safe) is this movement for the erector spinae? Are there better alternatives for working (loading) the gluteus, hamstrings, and adductors, without the risk of overloading the erector spinae and the potential injury risk to the spine (i.e., disc herniation), which is created by that overload, as well as the spinal compression created when the weight is held at the top of the movement? Is there a more productive and more safe exercise for the erector spinae?."

The fact is that the gluteus, hamstrings and adductors (i.e., the hip extension/"posterior chain" muscles) can be worked more productively (loaded more) by isolating hip extension with the multi-hip machine. This would also avoid overloading the erector spinae, as well as eliminate the risk of herniating an intervertebral disc of the spine. The erector spinae could be worked more productively, as well as more safely, by performing a dynamic spinal extension exercise (i.e., better than isometrically contracting the erector spinae), with significantly less weight.

The *deadlift* is primarily a power lifting movement, plain and simple. The only individuals who should perform this movement *with heavy weight* should be people who are seriously pursuing competitive power lifting. It has very limited value either as a "fitness exercise" or as a "physique development" exercise. In order to adequately challenge the hip extension muscles one would have to use a weight that overloads the erector spinae and risks spinal injury. On the other hand, if a lighter weight is used—thereby protecting the erector spinae and the intervertebral discs—the hip extension muscles will not be sufficiently challenged.

It simply is not sensible to consider the deadlift a good "fitness" or "bodybuilding" exercise. The adulation that this exercise is typically given illustrates how the line has gotten blurred between "power lifting" and "physique development"/"general fitness." It also illustrates how the overcommercialization of fitness has led to what could be considered "imprudent" recommendations. In an article in a somewhat recent issue of *Men's Journal* magazine, the author encouraged the use of *deadlifts*, and provided the following rating system (for men). This "evaluation" would be for a ONE-REP MAX (as heavy as possible, for one repetition)— *deadlift.**

Less than your body weight = "you're a novice"

1.25 x your body weight = "you're average"

1.5 x your body weight = "you're pretty strong"

2.0 x your body weight = "you're a beast"

**Men's Journal: "Deadlift: Test Your Strength,"* by C.J. Murphy

It's absurd for a person who is mostly interested in developing a muscular physique, or improving their physical fitness, to be performing a ONE-REP MAX of any exercise—especially an exercise with such a high degree of spinal injury risk.

Most men are wired to believe that "fitness" means being tough, strong, and "beastly." Accordingly, it's rather easy to convince a reader that lifting a large amount of weight is "good," even if the exercise has a very high risk and very little reward. From the perspective of physique development and general fitness, however, heavy *deadlifts* are a very bad investment.

The only sensible way of doing this exercise is with a moderate weight (e.g., not more than 100 pounds for men) and with absolutely perfect form (i.e., a perfectly arched/rigid spine). Even then, the value of this exercise, as compared with other (better) exercises, can be questioned. Regrettably, however, what is most frequently seen is people doing *deadlifts* like the person pictured in Figure 13-18.

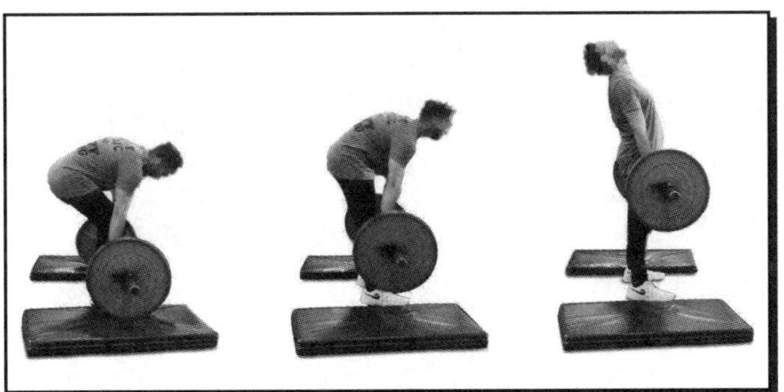

Figure 13-18

Notice the degree of torso forward flexion (curling forward of the spine) in Figure 13-18. This situation is very dangerous. He is failing to use his erector spinae to keep his posture straight and protect his spine. The result of this is a "squeezing" together of the inner edges of his vertebrae and a subsequent "opening" of the outer edges of his vertebrae, which could easily cause a posterior rupture of an intervertebral disc.

Some weight lifting veterans might say that using bad form during a *deadlift* is a "rookie mistake." They might claim that it's easy enough to keep the spine straight. Yet, veteran bodybuilders and weight lifters are often seen using similarly bad form. In fact, it is very common to see people using this kind of bad form in the gym. I see it all the time and I cringe whenever it happens. I also see those people showing signs of having back discomfort, after performing a strenuous set with bad form. It's not my place to correct everyone I see doing it, but I believe those people will regret it later. Furthermore, there is very little reward for jeopardizing their spine this way.

As mentioned previously, the reason excessive forward flexion of the spine happens is because the hip extension muscles have a greater capacity for power, as compared to the erector spinae. Because the erector spinae is the weak link in the chain, it naturally fails before the hip extension muscles do. Unfortunately, people are often more concerned with the amount of weight they are lifting, than anything else. They believe they need to lift an "impressive" amount of weight, even though it has very little to do with muscular development and general fitness.

Spinal compression and herniated discs are prolific problems, especially as individuals get older. There are millions of people who struggle with back pain, who never pulled a 300 barbell during a *deadlift*. The last thing we need is an additional potential cause of spinal compression and herniated disc problems. The less spinal compression and hyper-flexing of the spine (while loaded) we experience in our lifetime, the better.

The belief that doing *deadlifts* is necessary for everyone who uses weights as part of their exercise program simply does not make logical sense. Not only is the *deadlift* not "foundational," it can hardly be regarded as even "moderately beneficial," when its mechanics are carefully evaluated.

## Summary

The concept that compound exercises are always better than are isolation exercises, regardless of the individual's goal, is simply illogical. If the goal is physique development and general fitness, the objective should be to load specific target muscles as efficiently as possible. This step requires precise anatomical movements that mimic each muscle's most natural motions, as identified by their origins, attachments, and joint design.

Most compound exercises fail to mimic the precise movements of the various muscles and joints involved. They also fail in providing proper alignment, the ideal resistance curve, or a proper range of motion for each of the muscles and joints involved.

The belief that lifting a heavy weight, by way of engaging multiple muscles at one time, and using inefficient levers, is somehow more beneficial than having those same muscles working individually, using more efficient levers, is nonsense. In fact, a muscle can be loaded as much, or more, using a lighter weight during an isolation exercise, than it can be as one of several participating muscles in a compound exercise.

A compound exercise that allows a very heavy weight to be used typically involves the use of inefficient levers (reduced length limbs and non-perpendicular limbs), which minimize the magnification to the muscles involved. This situation has an effect that is similar to using a pry bar to lift a heavy object. It allows more weight to be lifted, but without loading the muscles involved any more than a lighter weight would, using more efficient levers. The heavier weight, however, still strains the skeleton, as well as the smaller, non-target muscles.

Every exercise, whether it's a compound exercise or an isolation exercise, has its own individual set of biomechanical circumstances. Understanding how to identify them allows you to see what the benefit is (or isn't), and what the degree of risk is. You can then compare that information to the benefit and risk of other exercises, and select the exercises that have higher benefit and lower energy cost and lower injury risk.

Engaging several muscles with one single exercise virtually guarantees that each participating muscle will NOT be getting the most productive stimulation, as compared with working those same muscles separately. In other words, the argument of "saving time" is misguided. If saving time is your primary objective, and you don't mind a compromised benefit for each participating muscle, and you are willing to accept a higher risk of injury, then selecting compound exercises makes sense. On the other hand, if your primary objective is getting the optimal degree of benefit for each muscle, then isolation exercises are the better choice.

Strengthening each individual muscle separately is at least as "functional" (useful and productive)—if not more so—than working a group of muscles with one exercise. Furthermore, it would be wise for people to stop thinking of certain exercises as "foundational," which is how many people regard compound exercises. Rather, every exercise should be regarded as a particular set of biomechanical circumstances, which can be—and should be—evaluated logically, mathematically, and with an awareness of "natural" anatomical motions.

# CHAPTER 14

# MOMENTUM AND THE USE OF "GOOD FORM"

- *When exercising for muscular development, the objective is to load a muscle with resistance, and then cause the muscle to deliberately contract against that resistance, until it is fatigued. This process leads to muscle adaptation—increased strength, size, and endurance.*
- *Momentum is a type of force that is typically produced by "throwing" a weight. It usually reduces the load on a working muscle, when used during resistance exercise. People often initiate momentum, in an effort to use a heavier weight than deliberate muscle contraction would allow. For this reason, it is often referred to as "cheating," and is considered "bad form."*
- *Using a weight that is technically "too heavy" for a particular muscle, and then using MOMENTUM (swinging/cheating) to lessen the resistance to that working muscle, is both impractical and inefficient.*
- *The use of momentum, during muscular development training, usually reduces the benefit of the exercise. It also increases the risk of injury, and results in wasted effort.*

## The Difference Between Good Form vs. Bad Form: Momentum

The two images in Figure 14-1 show a man doing a *standing barbell curl*, using fairly good form. He keeps his torso upright and stationary the entire time, from the beginning of the movement until the end. The weight is being "lifted" (elbow flexion) almost exclusively by way of biceps contraction. This technique is very efficient. Since he is not "swinging" the weight up, there is no need to use more weight than the biceps can handle.

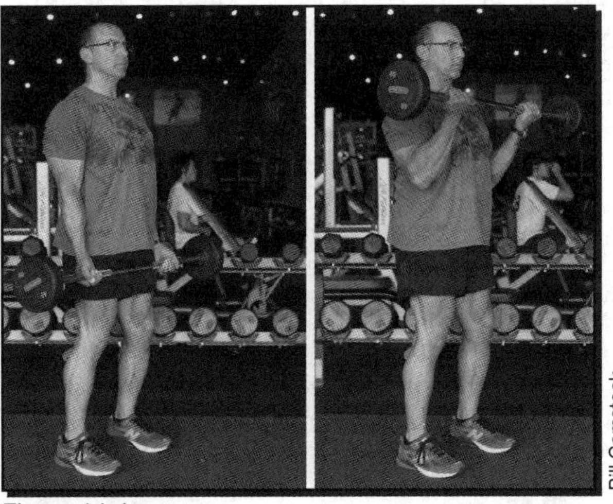
Bill Comstock

Figure 14-1

## Momentum Example #1

Figure 14-2 shows an illustration of a man performing a *standing barbell curl* with very bad "form." This character is using a weight that is "too heavy" to allow good form, because it's far more than his biceps are capable of handling. So, he uses momentum (swinging the weight) to reduce the load on the biceps.

A lifter like this typically heaves his torso backward, thereby propelling the weighted barbell upward. The result of this approach is that the biceps get a lesser percentage of the load than is actually on the bar, and his "lower back" (unproductively) gets a greater percentage of the weight, as well as a significant level of strain. This technique—whoever uses it—is very foolish.

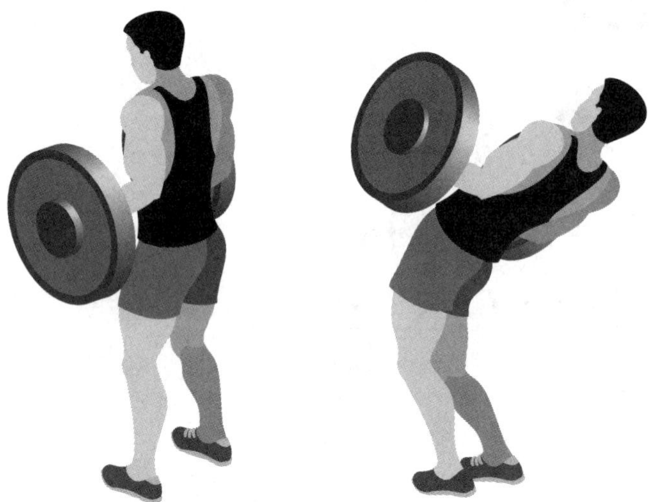

Figure 14-2

The aforementioned example is unusually dramatic. We don't often see people in the gym using quite so much momentum during *standing barbell curls*, although we often see slightly lesser versions of this type of "cheating." This particular example, however, dramatically illustrates what the use of momentum in resistance exercise looks like. Performing a *barbell curl* like this is very inefficient, because the biceps are not working any harder than they would be if the person were using less weight, without the momentum. Extra energy is being spent, even though the net load on the biceps is the same. It results in wasted effort, and also leads to an increased potential risk for injury.

To fully understand the folly of using momentum during an exercise, consider the following. Hypothetically, say that a person uses *maximum effort* for eight repetitions during a set of strict (no cheating) *standing barbell curls*, using 100 pounds. If this person adds another 20 pounds to the barbell, and uses momentum (cheating) to help accomplish eight reps, how is that more load on their biceps than the previous set of "maximum effort?" Maximum effort cannot be improved upon. The decision of whether to add more weight or not should be decided by the ability of the biceps—not by a person refusing to accept what their biceps are "telling" them, nor by an arbitrary decision to use "as much weight as their training partner is using"—whether it's sensible or not.

In Chapter 5 ("The Apex and the Base"), I explained how—when a weight is moving through the lower half of the sphere—there is a tendency for a person to "swing" the weight upward. *Standing barbell curls* are one example of that inclination. During this exercise, the barbell starts at the base position (forearm parallel with resistance, below the pivot point)—which is neutral.

Whenever the starting point of an exercise's range of motion is neutral (zero resistance), it is very easy to begin the movement with a big swing. The temptation to initiate a heavy *curl* with a nudge is ever-present, because most individuals sense that the resistance will get "heavier" as the forearms move upward (i.e., as they become more "active"). Subconsciously, people want to get a "running start," so to speak.

There are two very interesting aspects about this situation: first, the degree to which even a slight "nudge" can significantly reduce resistance, and second, how subconscious it is for individuals to initiate any kind of *standing* free-weight *curl* (barbell or dumbbell) with a "nudge/swing." Both of these concepts can be tested, by initially performing a "normal" *standing barbell* or *dumbbell curl*, and then doing it with your back up against a wall, which prevents any degree of torso swing. The comparison between these two techniques—in terms of the weight that can be used—is dramatic.

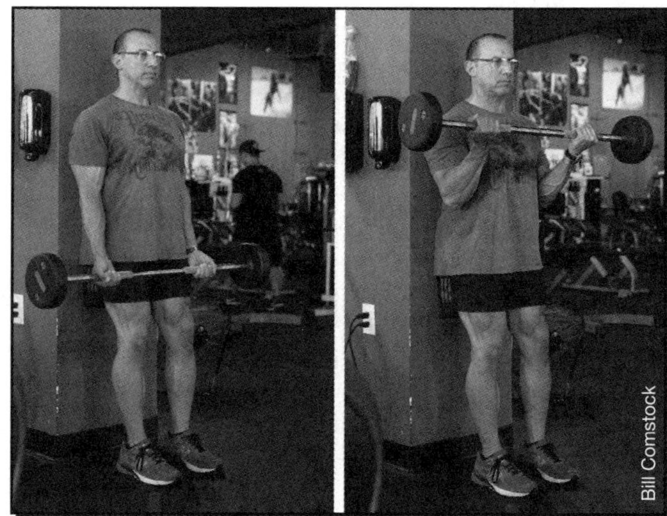


Figure 14-3

While I am not necessarily recommending that *curls* always be done with your back against a wall, it is a good way to identify the tendency to initiate a *standing curl* with a torso swing. This technique also enables you to realize how much of a difference it makes in terms of load reduction. Almost everyone swings their torso, when performing this exercise, to some degree. In reality, a strict *dumbbell* or *barbell curl* is much more efficient, on a cost/benefit basis.

Using good form on *standing biceps curls* can be done without leaning against a wall, but it requires careful attention, on every single repetition, to ensure you are not swinging on the initiation of the reps. If the biceps are working to maximum capacity, they are getting the full benefit, even if less weight is being used than the addition of momentum would otherwise allow.

Since using "good form" limits how much weight you can use, it might create the illusion that the weight you use when you CHEAT is the correct representation of your biceps strength. It is not. It just proves that "cheating" (while doing *standing dumbbell* or *barbell curls*) has become so "normal" that you don't realize you're doing it, nor how it misrepresents what your actual biceps strength is.

## Momentum Example #2

Chapter 5 included an example of the *dumbbell triceps kickback.* This exercise is also typically performed—by most people—using momentum, but a bit differently than is typically used during the *standing barbell curl.* Using momentum with the *standing barbell curl* requires a sudden thrust of the torso, in order to initiate the propelling of the weight from the starting position. With a *triceps kickback*, the weight is able to swing both ways, almost entirely by itself. This type of momentum is like kids swinging in the park—back and forth—past the base, each way.

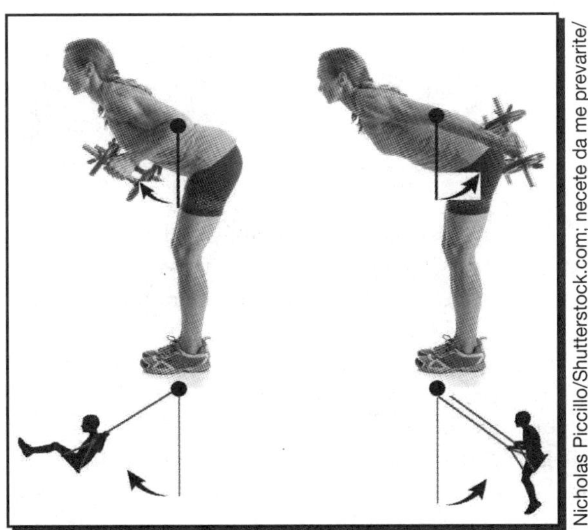

Figure 14-4

Nicholas Piccillo/Shutterstock.com; necete da me prevarite/ Shutterstock.com

The movement being produced, when doing *triceps kickbacks* this way, is usually due more to the "swing," than to deliberate muscle force. It could be as much as 60 percent "swing" (momentum) and only 40 percent deliberate muscle contraction. Furthermore, since the forearm crosses the base in the middle of the range of motion (i.e., when the forearm is vertical), neither the triceps nor the biceps can be loaded at that point, because the forearm is in the neutral position. That midpoint in the range of motion (for both the triceps and the biceps) is arguably the most important phase for either muscle to be optimally loaded—yet they both get zero load at that point. This exercise has very little value, even when done without the swinging. With the swinging, it's essentially useless.

## Momentum Example #3

In both of the images in Figure 14-5, you can see what a *supine triceps extension* looks like, when using good form. You should notice that the elbows hardly move, from beginning to end. In contrast, the two images in Figure 14-6 show the exerciser winding up, so that he can "propel" the barbell upward, by way of a latissimus thrust. Even if this person had more weight on the bar, his triceps would likely be getting less load than the person in Figure 14-5, who could be using less weight. It is foolish to add "extra" weight onto a bar, only to then reduce the triceps load by "throwing" the bar upward with the lats. Incidentally, this technique is not productive latissimus work either, because it's not a full range of motion for the lats. It's just extra energy being spent, without providing any additional benefit to the triceps.

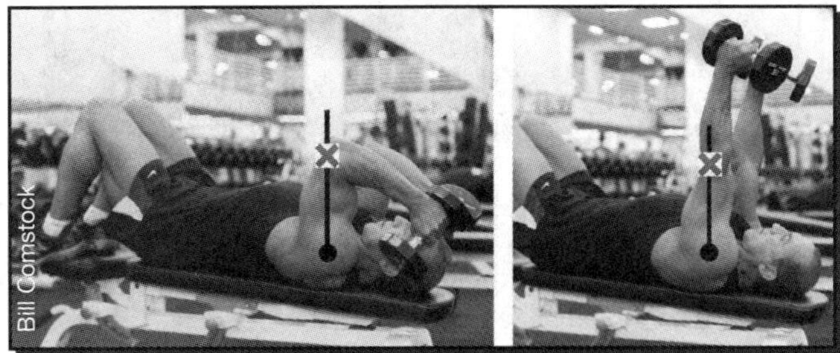

Bill Comstock

Figure 14-5

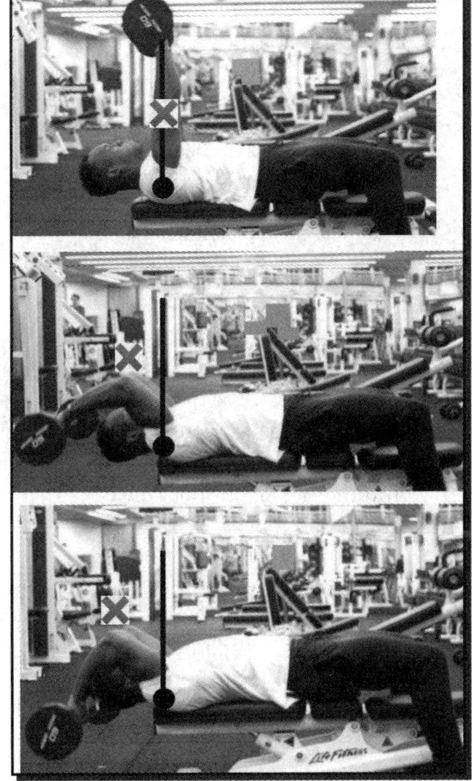

Figure 14-6

Bill Comstock

## Momentum Example #4

In Figure 14-7, you can see a series of photos of a man doing a heavy "*bent-over barbell row*," using quite a bit of momentum. The individual starts with an explosive upward "thrust" as soon as the bar leaves the ground (notice the immediate elevation of the torso), using mostly his glutes and erector spinae. The bar then "travels" upward—largely by way of the initial propulsion—until gravity begins to slow down its trajectory. At that moment, the man quickly lowers his torso, so that his chest touches the bar. Notice the level of the torso in the last two images, as well as the height of the bar in the same two photos. Clearly, his torso drops more than the bar rises up.

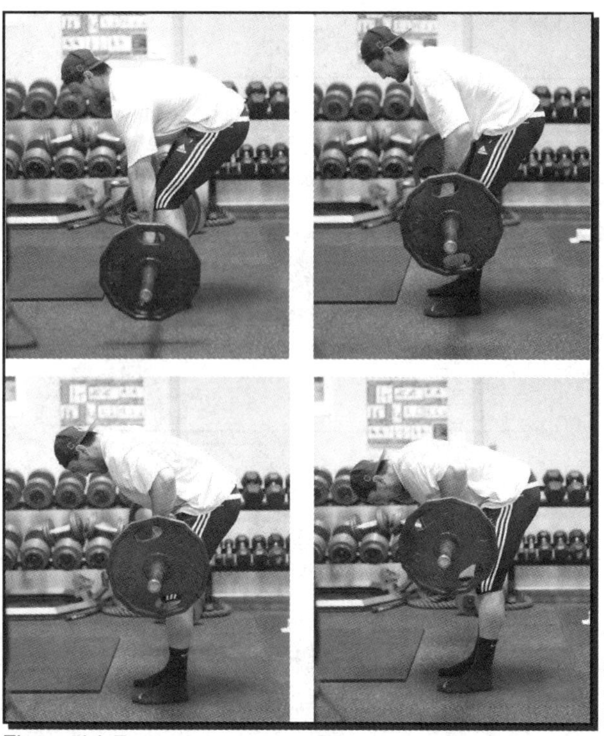

Figure 14-7

Of course, this technique is ridiculous as a muscle-building effort. The exercise itself (*bent-over barbell row*) has other biomechanical problems, even if the weight being used doesn't require momentum (a point that is explained further in Chapter 19). On the other hand, the concept of "propelling" the bar upward, and then quickly dropping the torso, in order to touch the bar with his chest, is nonsense. In essence, he is pretending that he used deliberate muscular force to pull the bar up to his chest, when—in fact—he "faked" it. Does he think his upper back muscles would be fooled by this?

## "Cheating" in Two Ways

*Note: In this context, "cheating" simply refers to the deprivation of benefit, caused by poor mechanics. It is not meant as a person's intentional effort to avoid working hard.*

The exercise in Figure 14-8 is commonly referred to as "*reverse crunches*." This example enables you to see how a person can use two different types of momentum in one exercise. In the left image in Figure 14-8 (the starting position), a dot has been placed on the man's hip joint (#1) and another on his mid-spine area (#2). The hip joint (#1) is the pivot which is operated by the hip flexors, while the mid-spine is the pivot (#2) which is operated by the abs.

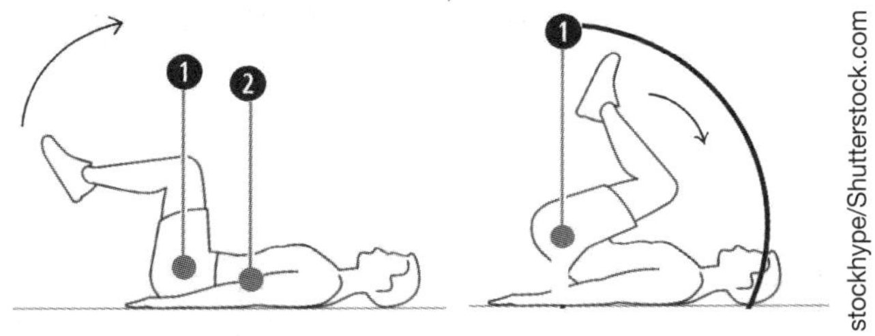

Figure 14-8

The exercise begins with a semi-circular upward "throw" of the legs. This "leg throw," which is produced mostly by the hip flexors, initiates the first type of momentum (i.e., the abs do not produce this upward leg thrust). Then, after the weight of the legs passes over to the right side of the apex (the midline of the half circle above-right), the legs begin to FALL in that direction—without requiring any muscular force at all. If you recall, in Chapter 2, a discussion was presented concerning what happens when the cart being pushed up the hill, goes over the top, and then begins free-falling down the other side of the hill.

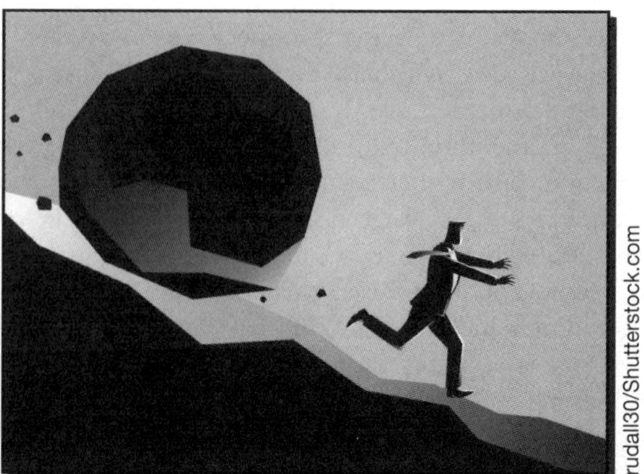

Figure 14-9

After the legs cross the apex, the weight of the legs falling in that direction PULLS the pelvis (hips) farther upward. This action creates the illusion that the abs are doing the work, but they are not. In addition, the arms—which are pushing downward against the ground—also help to push the tailbone upward, further perpetuating the illusion that the abs are working. This downward "free fall" of the legs is the second type of momentum—movement that is not being produced by the deliberate contraction of the target muscle.

Some people then PUSH their legs upward, toward the ceiling, once their spine is fully "coiled." Again, this action is NOT produced by the abdominal muscle. Rather, it is mostly the glutes that are pushing the femurs upward, by way of hip extension. Furthermore, before you start thinking that this technique might be beneficial for the glutes, the weight of the legs is hardly a challenge for the glutes. This scenario just adds another layer of illusion to this "exercise," which some people mistakenly believe is a "good" abdominal exercise.

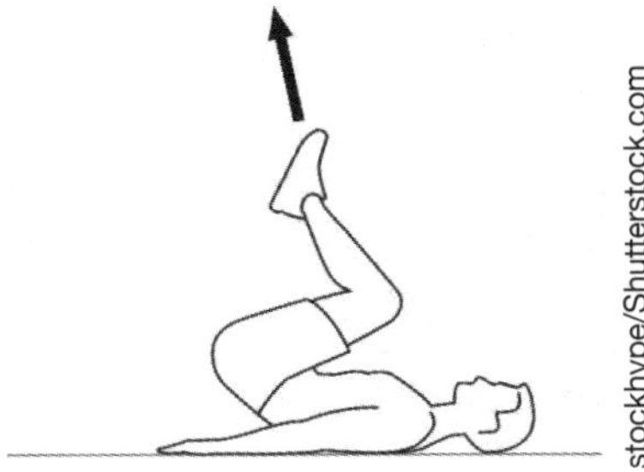

Figure 14-10

The abs do not participate much during any kind of *leg raise* movement, because the abs do not connect to the femurs (thigh bones), nor do they cross the hip joint. Rather, during a *leg raise* (when the legs are rising, before they reach the apex), the abs mainly just stabilize the spine, while the hip flexors do the actual "lifting."

This elaborate movement spends energy, but without much benefit to the abs. "Throwing" the legs upward and then allowing them to "free fall" down the other side, both produce momentum (non-deliberate movement), which deprives the muscles that should be working deliberately of having to work at all.

## "Bouncing" on a Stability Ball

Another kind of momentum that occurs with some regularity is "bouncing" on a stability ball, while doing *ab crunches*. Of course, this momentum does not happen all the time. Some people perform this exercise with good form, as shown in Figure 14-11. When it is performed correctly, it's a good exercise.

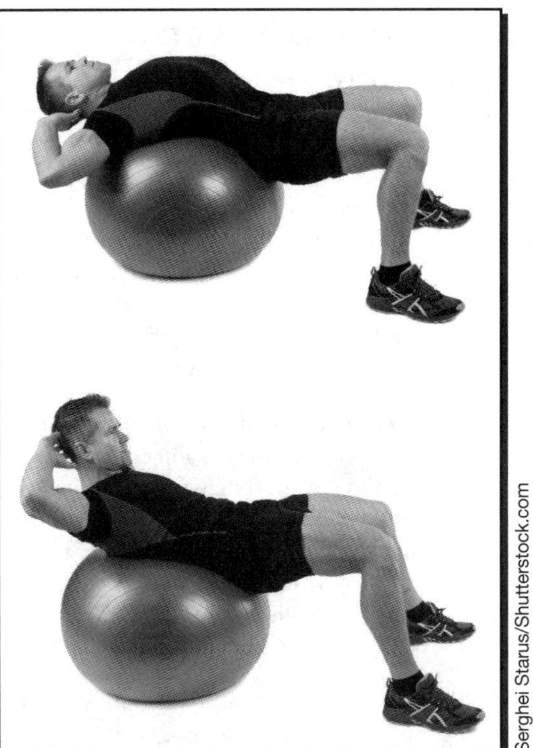

Figure 14-11

Occasionally, however, you see people who drop their torso back so quickly that they literally bounce off the ball, which then propels him forward—thereby reducing the need for the rectus abdominis to produce the force. It's almost as if they are bouncing off of a trampoline, which launches their torso upward, thereby minimizing the amount of work the abs must do. Instead of allowing their abs to do 100 percent of the work, this momentum reduces that need by 30 to 50 percent, depending on the degree of bounce.

Needless to say, this technique is counterproductive. This approach could qualify as being "foolish," except for the fact that some people unintentionally seek the easiest way to do an exercise, without even being aware they're doing it. In fact, some individuals, upon "discovering" that bouncing off the ball makes it easier, might even think (ironically) that they've figured out how to do them "correctly." Of course, they're wrong.

All of the aforementioned aberrations result in the same outcome. They all produce momentum, which then reduces the load against which the target muscle must work. This "technique" defeats the purpose of resistance exercise, which is to make a muscle work more—not less.

## Acceptable Applications of Momentum*

*(*although still not useful for physique development training)*

Olympic lifting is a sport that requires the use of momentum. The endeavor is a test of strength combined with coordination, speed, and timing. There are two "lifts" involved. The two lifts involved in Olympic lifting—the "*clean and jerk*" and the "*snatch*"—utilize an explosive "heave" to propel the bar up to a particular height, either to shoulder height or directly overhead.

In the "*clean and jerk*," the lifter begins by pulling the weight from the floor, by way of deliberate force produced mostly by the quads, glutes, and erector spinae. Then, at the point where the barbell is just past the knees, the torso is forcefully thrown up and back, and the legs are fully extended. This sequence results in the barbell being "propelled" upward—creating momentum—to a height that then allows the lifter to drop under the barbell, into a squatting position.

The lifter then stands, using deliberate quadriceps and gluteus force. Next, the lifter semi-squats (the "wind-up"), and again "launches" the barbell upward (producing more momentum, by using the quads, glutes, and deltoids) to a height that allows him to drop under the barbell with arms straight. Finally, he brings both feet together, while holding the barbell overhead, until the indicator acknowledges the lift is "good."

Although it might appear that he's using his arms to "push" the barbell over his head, the arms play a minor role compared to the quads and glutes. Ultimately, the lifter drops under the "propelled" barbell twice—once to get it to his shoulders, and again to get his straight arms underneath it.

The "*snatch*" lift begins with an explosive upward "heave" of the bar (from the floor), which is produced primarily by the quads, glutes, and erector spinae. This initial explosive thrust propels the barbell up to a height, which then allows the lifter to drop entirely underneath it, with his arms straight and wide on the bar, into a squatting position. This movement is undertaken in one fluid motion. He then squats upward, while holding the barbell overhead (using mostly glutes, quads, and adductors), and holds that position until the indicator signals that the lift is "good."

Both of these "lifts" involve the use of momentum. This type of weight lifting, however, is not suitable for physique development. In fact, it is a method of lifting that is completely opposite that which is required for physique development training. Olympic lifting seeks to maximize output (the amount of weight lifted), by using momentum and technique to minimize the need of relying on muscle contraction. Conversely, training for muscular development is most efficiently done by relying purely on muscle contraction. In this sense, these two endeavors could not be more opposite.

It should also be noted that because the goal of Olympic lifting is to lift the heaviest amount of weight, there is always a relatively high risk of injury. These injuries could occur either in the gym, while training, or during a competition.

Some people mistakenly assume that any endeavor that involves the lifting of weights leads to similar results. This assumption is entirely incorrect. Although the same principles of physics apply, the goals are drastically different. Therefore, it's a completely different application of the principles.

Magazines and other commercial enterprises often encourage people to combine the various uses of weights (barbells), which tends to blur the distinction between "fitness," "powerlifting" and "Olympic lifting" in the minds of consumers. This blurred distinction benefits gym owners, magazine publishers, manufacturers, and retailers—economically speaking.

On the other hand, "powerlifting" and "Olympic lifting" have significantly less benefit and higher risk for the person whose goal is muscular development and general fitness. Suggesting that all activities, which involve the use of weights produce similar results, as well as have similar degrees of risk, is extremely misleading and unfair to consumers.

## Kettlebell Training and Momentum

Some kettlebell exercises utilize momentum as part of the method. The exercise pictured in Figure 14-12, known as the "*kettlebell swing*," is an example of this. This exercise is not necessarily "bad," if your goal is primarily to burn calories and improve cardiovascular endurance. This exercise, however, would not be good for the purpose of muscle-building, as compared with other exercises, which require deliberate

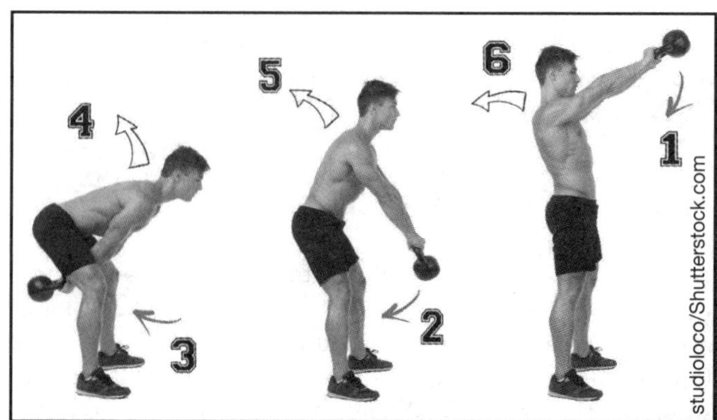


Figure 14-12

muscle contraction. This exercise also has a degree of spinal injury risk, if it is not done correctly. It's critically important that the spine be held in the arched position throughout the exercise, and that the movement be performed smoothly.

As an analysis of the forces involved during the *kettlebell swing*, the kettlebell is propelled upward from the bottom position by way of a thrust (momentum) initiated primarily by the glutes, quads, and erector spinae. Once the kettlebell is at its highest point, it then begins its downward "fall." This downward trajectory is coordinated (timed) with the person's descent into a squat position. The kettlebell picks up some additional downward "centrifugal force" as it falls, which is synchronized with the eccentric phase of the squat.

Since the swinging action pivots at the level of the shoulder, there is very little deliberate muscular force required by the deltoids. The kettlebell's upward swing is produced mostly by way of the momentum created by the legs and back. The force required (by the legs and back) to produce the upward propulsion of the kettlebell (from the bottom of the movement) is slightly greater than the weight of the kettlebell. This additional force is the result reversing the downward centrifugal force.

As a result, the eccentric deceleration, combined with the concentric reversal of the kettlebell's downward trajectory, increases the load to the quadriceps and glutes beyond the weight of just the kettlebell. This loading results in a fairly good legs and cardio workout, even if it isn't the best exercise for actually developing the quads and glutes. Again, good form is critically important with this exercise (e.g., not rounding the back), in order to not injure the erector spinae or intervertebral discs.

## Summary

During resistance exercise, momentum is sometimes produced by an explosive "heave" at the initiation of a repetition. This scenario essentially "throws" a weight through a portion of the range of motion, reducing the need for the target muscle to use deliberate muscle contraction.

This "heaving" is usually done subconsciously, in order to handle a weight that is heavier than the muscle can handle by way of its own deliberate force. Arguably, the subconscious "reason" it's done is because of an unrealistic expectation that a person might have with regard to the amount of weight they think they "should" be using.

This expectation could be called unrealistically ambitious. Nevertheless, it is unproductive. Adding momentum to a resistance exercise increases the energy cost, without providing additional benefit to the target muscle. It also increases the risk of injury.

Momentum can also be produced by swinging the weight, back and forth, from one side of the base to the other side, or by bouncing off a BOSU or stability ball. Again, this action reduces the productivity and efficiency of the exercise, by reducing the amount of force the target muscle would otherwise have to produce.

Subconsciously adding momentum to a resistance exercise often creates the illusion (false belief) that the muscle is "stronger" (can handle more weight) than is actually the case. Extra energy is thus required in order to handle the additional weight, but that extra energy does not necessarily cause the target muscle to work harder. The additional weight is only needed in order to compensate for the reduction caused by using momentum. Adding momentum to a resistance exercise is very inefficient. The definition of "efficiency" is "more load with less energy expended"—not "less load with more energy expended."

# CHAPTER 15

# BALANCE/CORE EXERCISES IN PHYSIQUE DEVELOPMENT TRAINING

- *One of the most prolific trends these days is people combining resistance exercises with instability. The purpose of this approach, in theory, is to improve "balance" and to strengthen "the core." However, these concepts are not well understood by most participants, including most trainers.*
- *This method of exercise is not as productive as it might seem.*
- *This chapter explores the following questions:*
    - *Do "unstable exercises" actually produce improvements in balance?*
    - *Does adding "instability" to a resistance exercise compromise the physique development benefits of that exercise?*
    - *Does the average person need to improve their balance?*
    - *What is the "core" and is "instability" the best way to strengthen it?*

One of the most common things that can be seen in gyms these days is people doing exercises while standing on one leg (instead of two legs), while sitting on a stability ball (instead of on a bench), or while standing on an unstable surface, like a wobble board (instead of solid ground). In other words, people are doing resistance exercises, while unstable. Examples of this approach to training would include *one-legged dumbbell curls* (Figure 15-1) and *squats on a BOSU ball* (Figure 15-2).

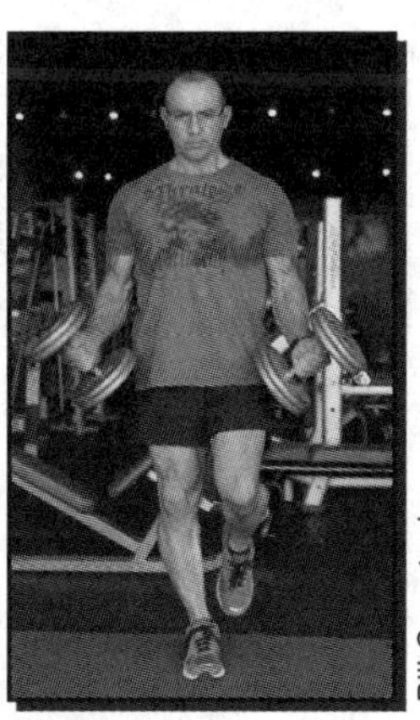
Bill Comstock

Figure 15-1

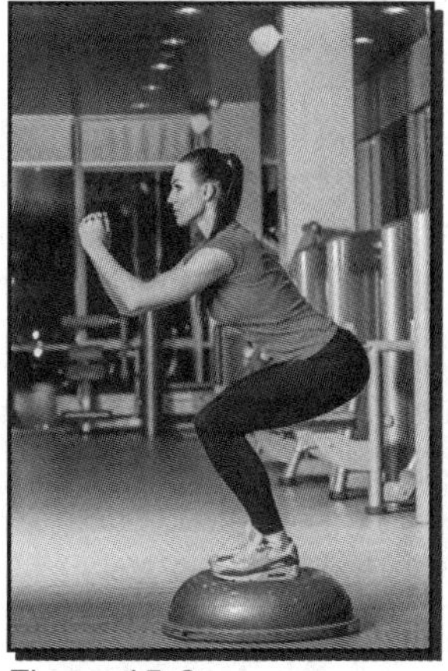
Satyrenko/Shutterstock.com

Figure 15-2

This type of modification is, ostensibly, intended to improve balance, while simultaneously developing the physique and strengthening the body. As such, it can be helpful to ascertain where this trend fits in with traditional fitness goals.

Historically, the following goals have been the primary objectives associated with physical fitness for the last 50 to 100 years:

- Leanness (lower percentage of body fat)
- Muscular development (visible hypertrophy)
- Muscular strength
- Muscular endurance
- Cardiovascular endurance (heart and lung capacity/ $\dot{V}O_2max$)
- Flexibility
- Improved health (reduced risk of cardiovascular disease, etc.)

The vast majority of people are usually quite content making progress toward one or more of these seven goals. The methods by which these objectives are achieved are generally straightforward, including the following:

- Individuals do higher reps with lower weight for muscular endurance, and lower reps with heavier weight for muscle strength—both of which contribute to muscle growth.
- People engage in aerobic exercise for cardiovascular endurance, and, together with the anaerobic exercise and dietary modifications, they achieve leanness.
- For flexibility, individuals stretch and do full range of motion resistance exercise.
- For their health and personal enjoyment, some people play a sport periodically, such as tennis, golf, basketball, soccer, etc.
- All the aforementioned activities provide a variety of health-related benefits, such as improving a person's insulin sensitivity, reducing their risk of diabetes, lowering their blood pressure, enhancing their $\dot{V}O_2$max (ability to utilize oxygen), increasing their bone density, and boosting their coordination.

Since the early 1900s, millions of people have developed exceptional levels of physical condition, using these types of activities. Even world class athletes have trained for their respective sports, using these methods.

Sometime around the late 1990s, however, so-called "balance" training started becoming popular. Due to prolific marketing, many people have been convinced that "balance" training is absolutely essential. This mindset, however, begs the question: If it is "essential," how could people have gotten into such good condition before this type of exercise became so commonplace?

Does "essential" refer to its effects on general conditioning (body fat loss, muscular development, cardiovascular enhancement, and metabolic benefits), or to its improvement of people's balance. A brief examination of each of these issues can lend clarity to the matter.

The chart detailed in Figure 15-3 shows that since 1960, obesity rates in the United States have been steadily rising. As of the date of this study (2010), nearly 36 percent of all Americans qualified as "obese" (i.e., defined as > 30 pounds overweight). Currently, obesity is more prevalent than ever before, and is projected to reach the 50 percent mark by the year 2030.

**Prevalence of Obesity Among U.S. Adults Aged 20-74**

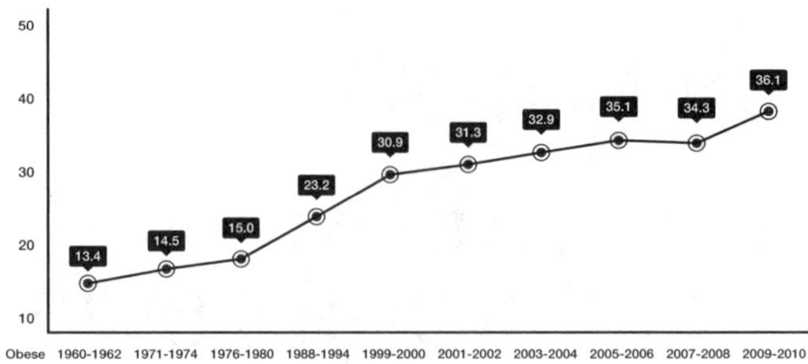


Sources: CDC/NCHS, NHES, NHANES

Figure 15-3

It is interesting to note that revenues spent on "fitness club memberships" have also been rising at approximately the same rate (Figure 15-4). In fact, there are now more dollars being spent annually on fitness products and services than ever before (Figure 15-5).

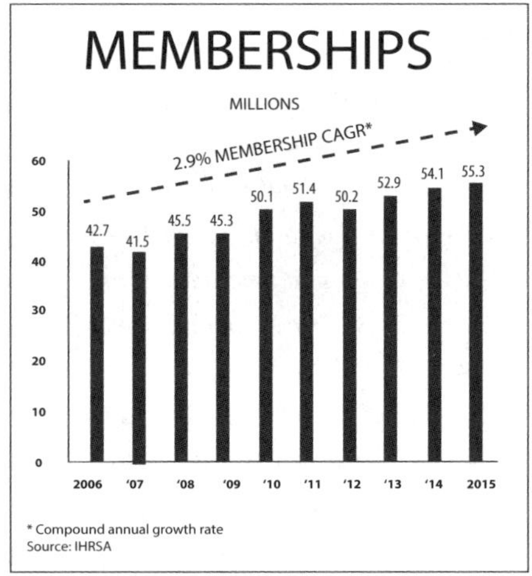


Figure 15-4

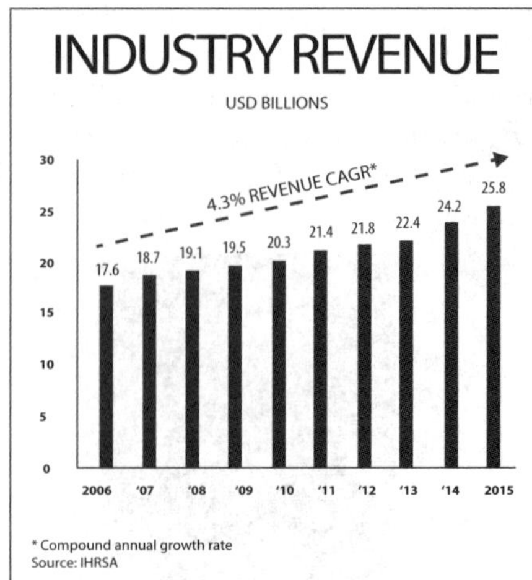


Figure 15-5

Despite the increasing amounts of money being spent on "new products and services" (which includes "balance/stability" products and instruction), it does not appear that these increases are translating to fewer people being overweight. Furthermore, those individuals who are participating in fitness programs today are not necessarily in "better" shape than people who participated in fitness programs 20 or 30 years ago, as defined by traditional measures (body fat level, muscular development, cardiovascular risk factors, etc.).

Therefore—given that overall fitness has not improved since "balance exercise" became popular—it would appear that "balance exercise" is not essential for the goal of general fitness. Should the assumption be made, then, that "essential" refers to the improvement of balance?

If that is the context, the initial step would be to establish that "balance" was a problem for most people, before the advent of this type of exercise. Then it would be necessary to demonstrate that "balance exercise" has made a significant improvement on this "problem." Only then, can we legitimately conclude that this type of exercise is "essential." Did the majority of people, before, have a real problem with "balance," and has it now been dramatically improved? Unfortunately, there is no evidence that either of these factors being true. The claims are theoretical.

With the exception of people over the age of 70, few people ever site "improved balance" as one of their fitness goals. The idea of "improving balance" appeals to most people, even when they don't actually have a problem with balance. In reality, however, people under the age of 50 generally do not complain of "falling down frequently."

## The Origin of "Balance Training"

It is interesting to note that the advent of "balance exercise" coincides with the use of "proprioception" training, which top-level athletes and physical therapists began using and advocating in the late 90s. Around that time, a number of high-profile athletes—tennis players, basketball players, golfers, martial artists, boxers, etc.—began employing proprioceptive (unstable) exercises in their training regimens, for the purpose of improving their particular sports performance requirements.

Then, fitness magazines began writing stories about these competitive athletes and how they train for their respective sports. Publishers (marketers) were well aware that consumers love the idea of using the same training program used by their favorite celebrity or professional athlete. After all, since the primary goal of magazine publishers is to sell magazines, anything that appeals to readers—whether it's actually useful to those readers or not—is fair game.

Of course, the performance requirements of a high-level tennis player or boxer are very different than the goals of the average fitness consumer. They're also very different than the goal of a person pursuing physique development. Nevertheless, "sports star/celebrity" workouts became massively appealing, and the marketing opportunities became instantly apparent to the fitness industry.

Suddenly, a multitude of new "balance" products and programs began popping up, targeting fitness consumers. These products were marketed as vital to either "*performance*" training or "*remedial balance*" training. Since this type of marketing was so catchy, an entirely new category of "fitness" was created (Figures 15-6 to 15-11).

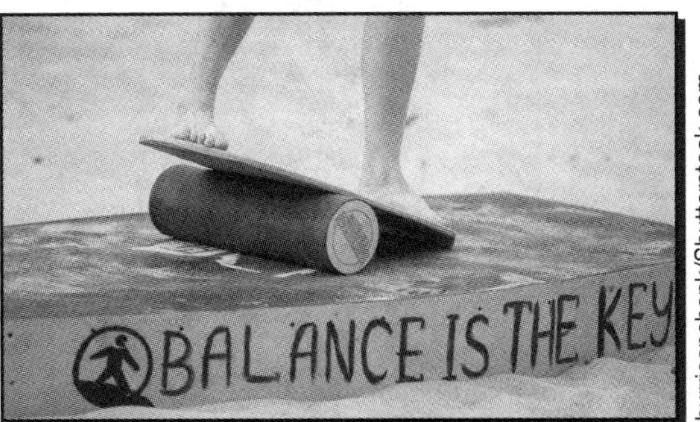


hurricanehank/Shutterstock.com

Figure 15-6

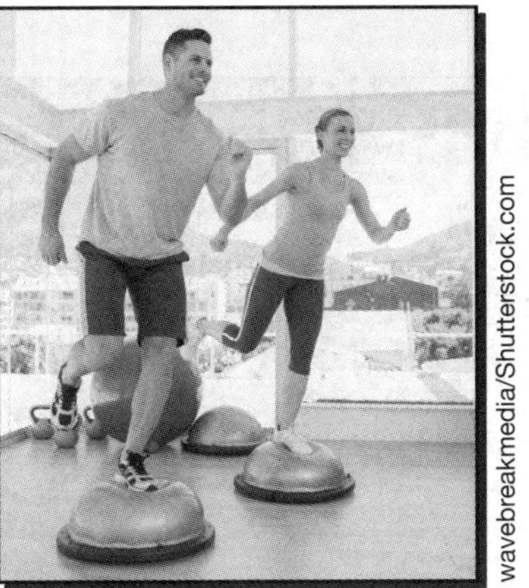

wavebreakmedia/Shutterstock.com

Figure 15-7

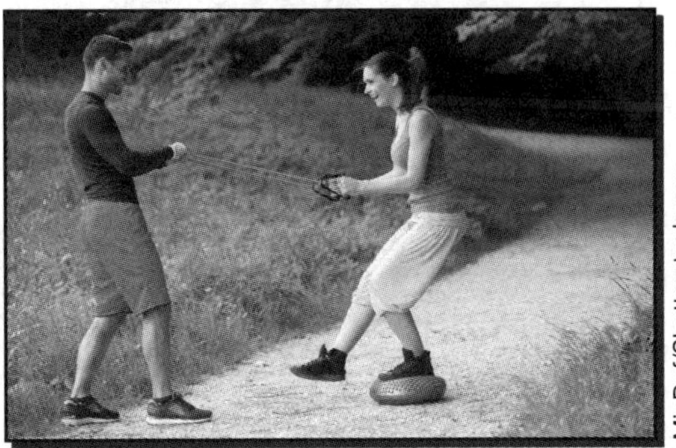

MinDof/Shutterstock.com

Figure 15-8

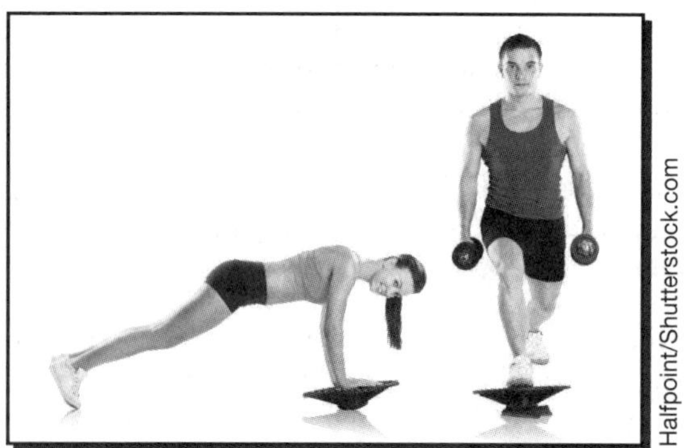

Figure 15-9

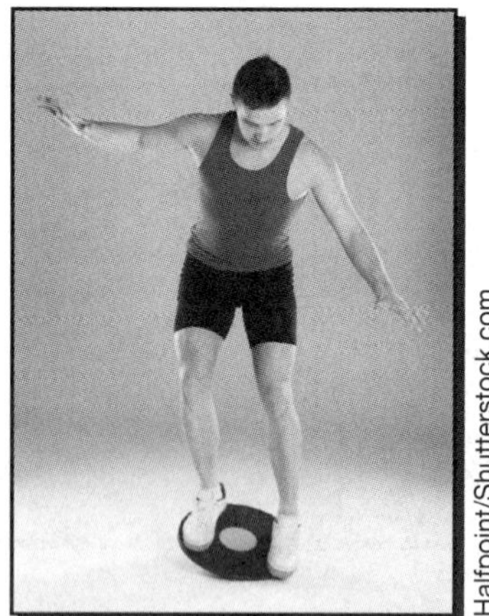

Figure 15-10

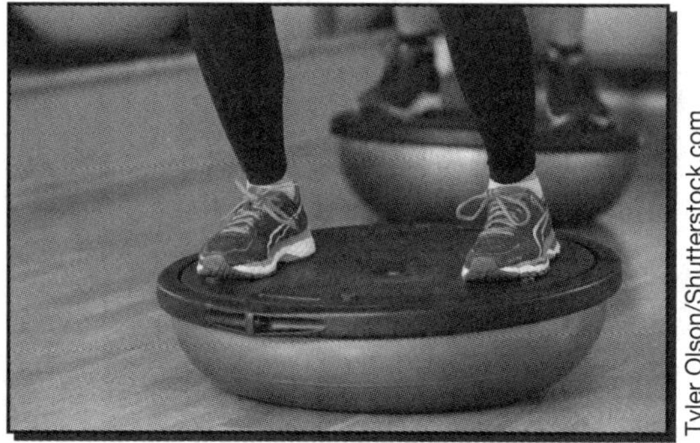

Figure 15-11

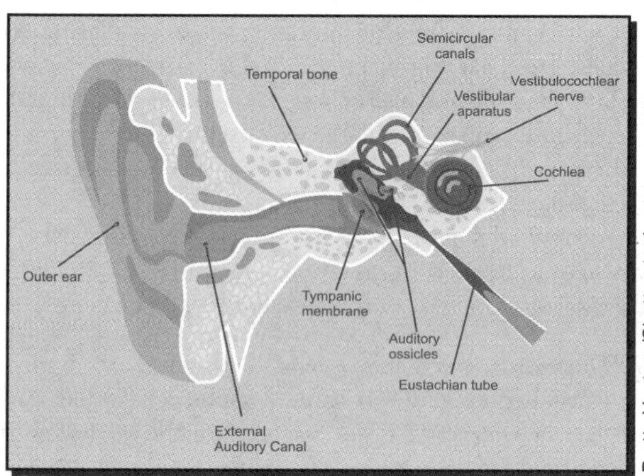

Figure 15-12

## What Is Balance and Equilibrium?

Technically speaking, balance is known as "spatial orientation." In essence, it is your ability to sense the position of your body, relative to gravity. It allows you to know if you are leaning to the right or to the left ... forward or backward. It allows you to sense whether you are standing on a flat surface or on one that is slightly inclined. Everyone is born with this sense of balance, because the mechanisms are built into the anatomy. It involves the brain's innate ability to receive and process information from the various balance sensors throughout the body—primarily the inner ears, as well as the eyes, feet, and joints.

The "vestibular system" in your inner ears is your primary balance sensor. It is made up of tiny fluid-filled canals that are lined with microscopic hairs, plus a network of nerves and calcium crystals. This inner-ear system, together with your eyes, as well as the sensors on the bottoms of your feet and in your joints, inform your brain whether you are stable or off-balance.

Older people (usually over the age of 70) who begin having difficulty with their spatial orientation typically experience a degradation of these balance sensors. This situation causes a person to feel as if they are about to fall, when they are actually stable—or to feel as if they are stable, when they are actually leaning too far in one direction or the other. On occasion, this faulty perception is accompanied by dizziness (i.e., "vertigo").

"Disequilibrium" (compromised spatial orientation) can be caused by a variety of factors, including dysfunction in the inner ear, vision problems (cataracts, macular degeneration, glaucoma, etc.), "peripheral neuropathy" (numbness in the legs and/or feet), or some other neurological disorder. These are medical issues that need to be addressed by a neurologist or "otolaryngologist" (i.e., ear, nose and throat doctor)—not by a personal trainer.

## What Is Proprioception?

Proprioception is a type of coordination. It is a learned ability to execute movement with your limbs and torso, "automatically"—without much thought or focus. For example, when you drive a car, you can maneuver the brake and gas pedal, without consciously thinking about them. You are able to apply just the right amount of pressure on each pedal, at precisely the appropriate time, without much conscious thought, just as an experienced pianist or guitarist is able to play their instrument without much conscious thought of what their fingers are doing. Proprioception is ONLY similar to "spatial orientation" in the sense that the brain receives signals from various sensors. On the other hand, proprioception training is NOT a remedy for "disequilibrium."

Proprioception is the subconscious learning of physical skills, so they become "second nature"—like juggling or punching a speed bag. Improving your ability to *squat,* while on a BOSU ball (without falling off), is a learned skill, in which your central nervous system and muscles become increasingly familiar with the feeling of standing on a surface that is not solid.

Specifically, the body is learning to respond to the pliable surface on which the person is standing. As such, the learned skill of squatting, while on a *BOSU ball,* is useful primarily for occasions which resemble that situation. It is relatively useless, when that person stands on a solid surface, and there is no "floor pliability" to which the body has to adjust. Standing on a solid floor does not require "pliable floor" skills.

This factor explains why people who spend a considerable amount of time doing this type of exercise, do not notice much difference in their day-to-day "balance" (i.e., coordination)—even though they may have gotten very good at stabilizing themselves on unstable surfaces. Their body has learned how to compensate for a "wobbly" foundation, but that is only useful when the foundation wobbles.

In fact, calling a "*dumbbell curl, while standing on one leg,*" or a "*BOSU ball squat,*" "balance training" is a misnomer. Rather, it should be called "proprioceptive training." This definition is not just semantics. In fact, referring to it as "balance training" is borderline marketing deception. You are learning a specific skill—the coordination of performing that specific task. You are not, however, improving your equilibrium.

Referring to unstable exercises as "balance" training suggests individuals are correcting an essential part of their physicality, which might be failing. This mindset naturally makes people feel obligated to do it. They might even think it is "essential," and would likely feel irresponsible, if they "neglect" it. Interestingly, some people may call that "good marketing."

On the other hand, referring to unstable exercises as "skill learning" would likely make people think twice about whether or not they want to spend time and energy learning that particular skill. In fact, it might make them wonder if it's wise to MIX that type of activity with normal resistance exercise. The truth is that it does, in fact, compromise the effectiveness of resistance exercise.

That is the trade-off. Learning to balance yourself on a stability ball will only manifest its value when attempting to perform daily activities that are very similar to that particular skill, which is not likely to happen very often. Meanwhile, the resistance exercise to which you have added instability will be less productive than it would be if you performed it while stable. Thus, even if you think there is a value in learning how to coordinate yourself on unstable surfaces, should you simultaneously combine that effort with resistance exercise? The answer is "no."

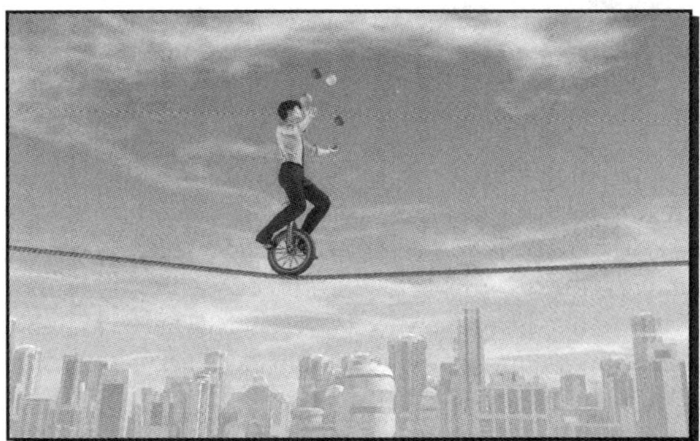
Orla/Shutterstock.com

Figure 15-13

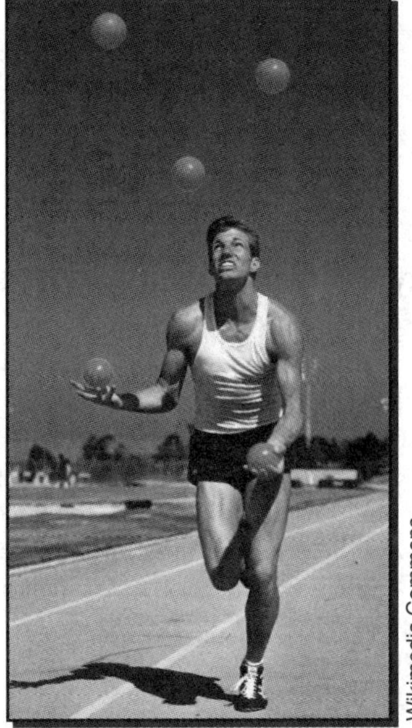
Wikimedia Commons

Figure 15-14

## Who Needs Proprioceptive Exercise?

There are individuals with special circumstances who could benefit from learning proprioception of the feet and legs—for example, anyone who participates (competes) in a sport that requires exceptional reactive coordination of the legs. It might also include people with a neurological disorder, or people over the age of 70, who have lost some of their coordination due to inactivity. In those cases, standing or *squatting* on unstable surfaces—as an exercise—might be useful, although dancing and various coordination drills would likely produce a better result.

As such, proprioceptive training is a specialized activity that is appropriate mainly for people with coordination/proprioception problems, or with sport-specific needs. Proprioceptive exercise is not "necessary," nor useful, for everyone.

Proprioceptive exercise is tedious and time-consuming. For best results, it should be done frequently. Thirty minutes per week is not enough to make a significant difference, assuming a "difference" (i.e., an improvement) is required. Any type of learning—especially tactile learning—requires frequency, so that the activity produces an automatic response. Like learning to play the piano or to dance, proprioception exercise requires frequency and consistency. Ultimately, individuals need to be aware of precisely what it is that they are "learning," and how they might be able to benefit from that learned skill—if at all.

Unfortunately, the fitness industry is promoting this type of activity to everyone—even to individuals who are not experiencing a neurological disorder, and to people who are under the age of 50 who have NOT expressed any concern with a lack of coordination. People with basic fitness goals are often treated as if they have a coordination "problem" that needs correcting. In fact, proprioceptive training has become "standard prescription" for the masses now.

## The Folly of Combining Instability With Strength Training

Consider the following hypothetical situation. An overweight man in his 40s joins a gym. He's been neglecting the need to exercise for a while, in part, because he feels embarrassed about his current condition. He assumes that most people in the gym will be more fit than him, and thinks that he'll stand out as "the fat guy." Now, he has finally mustered up the courage to join a gym, and is eager to get "lean, strong, and healthy." For discussion purposes, let's call him "Joe."

One day, when Joe is at the gym, he starts doing a set of *supine dumbbell presses* (Figure 15-15) for his pectoral muscles, with a pair of 30-pound dumbbells. Joe is not entirely sure what his fitness goals are, but he knows that this exercise is good for his pectorals, and figures it's a good place to start.

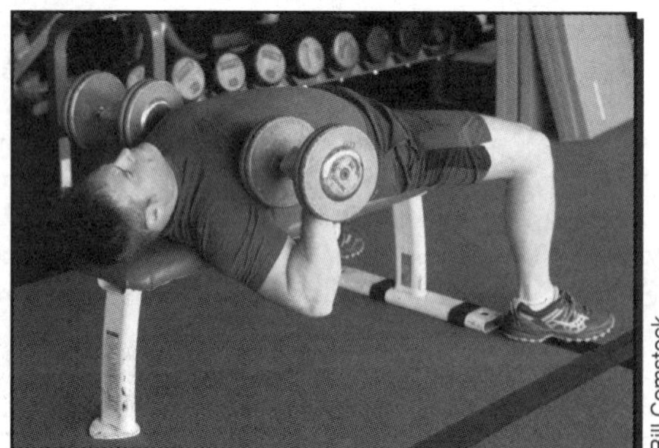

Figure 15-15

Along comes a trainer, who is employed by this particular gym. The trainer sees this "overweight man in his 40s," and correctly assumes that this individual may be a little unsure about what he's doing. Accordingly, the trainer approaches Joe and says, "*Would you like me to show you a better way of doing that?*"

Joe is delighted that this trainer is offering to help him, and automatically assumes that this trainer will honestly show him a "better way." Joe replies, "Yes, thanks!"

The trainer leads Joe to an area where the large "stability balls" are kept. The trainer asks Joe to lie on the ball, with the same 30-pound dumbbells he was previously using. Joe complies, lies back on the ball (Figure 15-16), and places both feet securely on the ground, with a wide foot stance. He then begins doing the same movement he was doing on the bench. Naturally, it feels a little less stable than it did when he was on the solid bench. The ball is a little bouncy and less solid than the flat bench, but it's not entirely uncomfortable. It's still within Joe's ability to do the exercise with the same weights.

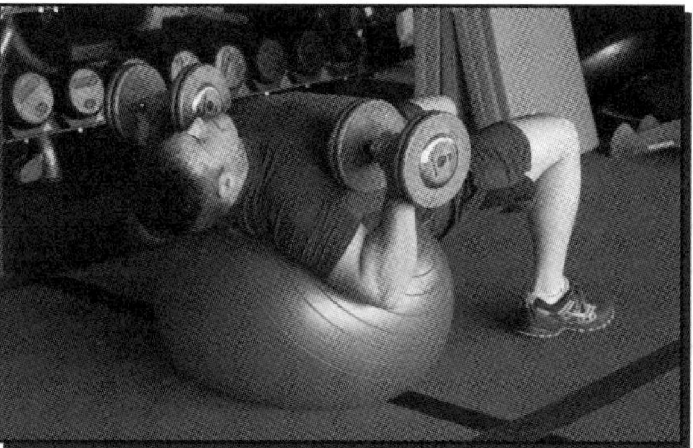

Figure 15-16

The trainer, however, stops Joe, and tells him that he wants him to do it a bit differently. He asks Joe to raise one foot off the ground (with his leg straight), and place the other foot in the center, on the floor. Joe follows this instruction, and quickly realizes that it's much less stable than it was with both

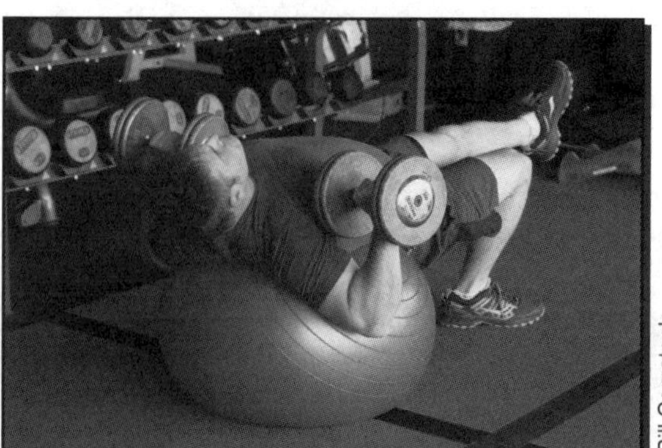

Figure 15-17

feet on the ground. Before, because there were three points of contact with the ground, it was a "tripod." Now, there are only two points of contact with the ground, so it is a "bi-pod."

As such, Joe realizes that in order to stay balanced, he needs to keep both dumbbells equally distant from the center of his torso, as he brings them down. This requirement is similar to a situation that involves a person walking a tightrope. That individual would have to keep his balance-bar equally balanced on both sides.

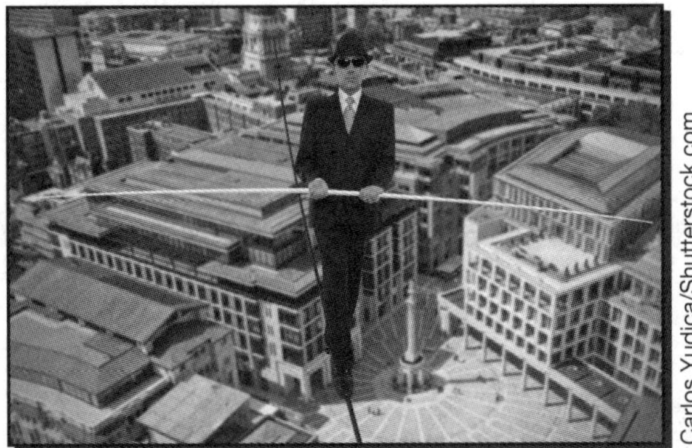
Carlos Yudica/Shutterstock.com

Figure 15-18

Then, the trainer makes an additional request. He wants Joe to bring the dumbbells down "alternately"—first only the right arm, while keeping the left arm up ... and then only the left arm, while keeping the right arm up. Not knowing what to expect, and assuming the trainer is the "expert," Joe complies with the instruction.

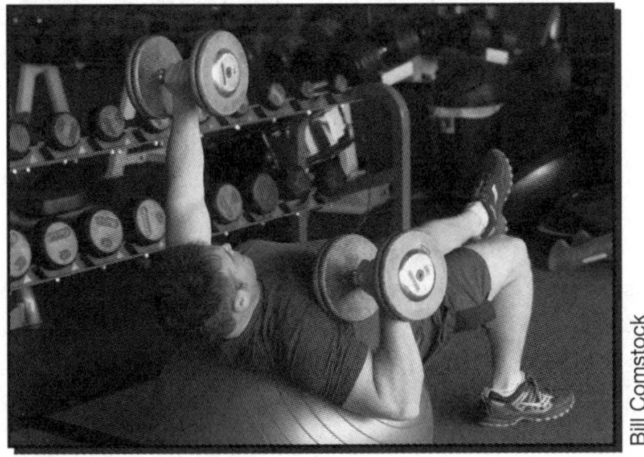
Bill Comstock

Figure 15-19

Almost immediately, Joe falls to the right side of the ball, because he had extended more weight to the right side of his body, than to the left side of his body. In essence, it would be the same as if the tightrope walker had extended his balance bar too far to the right, creating "imbalance."

Joe is now on the floor, feeling embarrassed that he was not able to stay on the ball. He thinks he's clumsy and blames himself entirely for not being able to stay on the ball. The trainer looks at Joe, with an amused smirk, suggesting, "*It looks like we've found a 'problem' with your BALANCE.*"

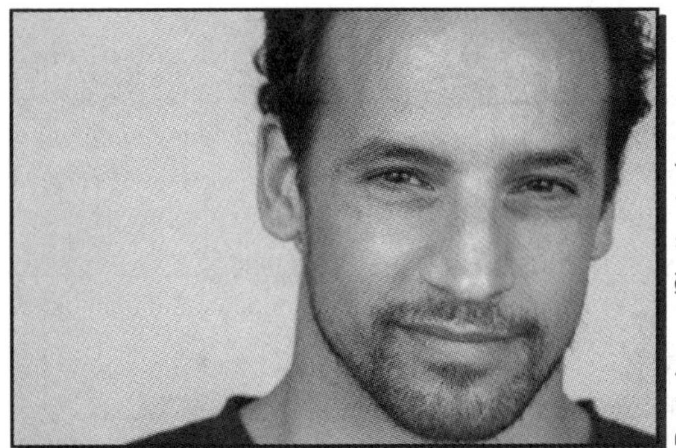
Ranta Images/Shutterstock.com

Figure 15-20

Joe is now concerned that he has a more serious issue to worry about, other than the fact that he's overweight and has very little muscle tone. Apparently, he has a "balance problem," or so he is being led to believe.

The trainer helps Joe stand up and tells him to try again. Joe is determined to NOT fall off the ball, and will try his best to prevent that from happening. He exchanges his 30-pound dumbbells for 20-pound dumbbells, knowing this switch will reduce the odds of him falling off.

At that point, he gets back on the ball with the lighter weights. It is a bit easier to keep his balance by using the lighter weight, but still not quite easy enough to be certain he won't fall off again.

Accordingly, he brings the weight (the dumbbell) closer to his side as he lowers it, rather than so far out to the side. This alteration creates LESS imbalance, because it reduces the magnification of the weight (due to a shorter lever) that is extended out to the sides. This factor helps Joe stay on the ball.

After a few sets of this, Joe asks the trainer what the difference is between him doing the exercise on a solid bench, using both arms simultaneously, versus doing it on a stability ball with one leg off the ground, and using only one arm at a time. The trainer—with complete confidence—replies, "*Core.*"

While many people have heard of this concept, they are not exactly sure what it means. So Joe asks the trainer what it's all about. The trainer tells Joe that the "core" is the "*center of your body.*" He tells Joe that it "*stabilizes your lower back and abdomen, and helps you coordinate all your movements—including balance.*" Of course, this is the standard statement that is taught to trainers by the industry.

The trainer further explains that "*without a strong core, you have nothing.*" He then asks Joe the (standard) rhetorical question, "*You wouldn't build a house on a weak foundation, would you?*"—all the while, exhibiting a smug expression of "common sense."

> *Note: This is a ridiculous comparison. An architectural foundation is a flat slab of concrete, on which the weight of an entire house SITS. The muscles of the midsection are important, but they do not serve the same function as an architectural slab of concrete.*

"Wow," says Joe, thinking how lucky he is to have had this trainer help him discover this glaring "balance" problem he has. Almost immediately, Joe asks the trainer if he has any openings in his schedule for some "training sessions." Bingo—the trainer has a new client.

## Bait and Switch: "Balance" Training Being Sold as Fitness Training

It's important to examine what actually occurred in this hypothetical situation involving Joe. When Joe was doing his *supine dumbbell press* on the flat bench, he was effectively working his pectorals. He was using a pair of 30-pound dumbbells, employing "good form." During the exercise, he brought his humerus (upper arm bone) laterally out to the side, with a vertical (neutral) forearm, so that the humerus maintained a normal lever length. This technique is the proper mechanics for getting the most benefit to the pectorals.

Later, when Joe experienced difficulty staying on the stability ball while using the 30-pound weights, he reduced the resistance to 20 pounds. He also brought the weight in closer to his torso, which shortened the effective lever length of the humerus. Both of these "adjustments" reduced the level of resistance to his pectorals.

Joe was then told that doing this unstable version of a *supine dumbbell press* would improve his "core." In essence, Joe was told that the "trade-off" for him getting less pectoral benefit was that he would be rewarded with benefits to his CORE, plus an improvement in his balance. These assertions, however, are not true.

In fact, both of the "exercises" being simultaneously attempted on the Swiss ball (the *dumbbell press* and the *static torso rotation*) are compromised. Not only is the pectoral stimulation significantly reduced, his "core" stimulation is half as effective as it could be. The reason why both exercises are compromised is entirely due to the instability involved.

If Joe had continued doing his normal, flat bench *supine dumbbell press*, using the 30-pound weights that he was originally using, and maintained the "normal" arm length (90-degree elbow bend), he would have been able to work his pectorals much more effectively. Furthermore, although Joe wasn't entirely aware of it, the instability of being on the ball forced him to perform the "core" part of the exercise with half the resistance he'd be able to use, if he had been in a more stable situation.

If Joe stood securely on the ground and performed a *standing torso rotation*, with a cable (Figure 15-21), he'd be able to load his torso-rotation muscles with twice as much resistance. As a result, he would be working his "core" muscles much more effectively, as compared with lying on the stability ball.

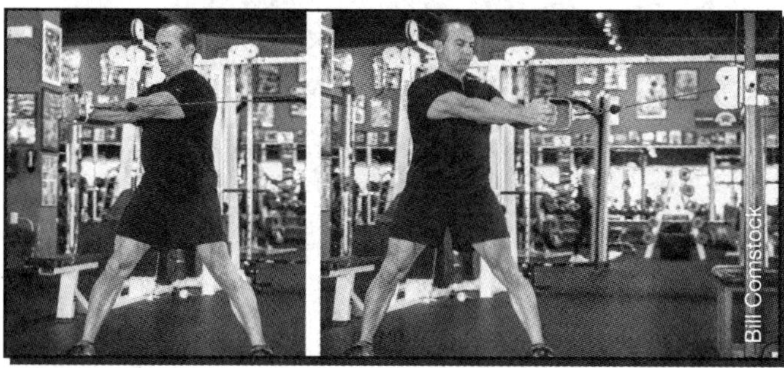


Figure 15-21

Imagine trying to do the *standing torso rotation*, if the ground was covered with oil, making it "unstable." The oil would prevent a firm footing on the ground, and would force the person to use a lighter weight in order to prevent sliding. The instability, and the required use of a lighter weight, would then compromise the loading of the target muscles. The key point to remember is that instability always limits the amount of weight that can be used, which then compromises the strengthening/development of the target muscles.

Attempting to work both muscle functions—the pectoral contraction and the isometric torso rotation—simultaneously, compromises both. Some people may think it's a clever way to exercise, because they assume it allows both muscle groups to be worked simultaneously. This assumption would only have merit, however, if both muscle groups were able to work as well together, as they could be if each was worked independently. In reality, however, combining these two movements FAILS to work each muscle as well as each could be worked separately.

Would there be a proprioceptive benefit of performing *alternating dumbbell press on a Swiss ball*, with only one foot on the ground? Yes, Joe would learn how to coordinate himself on the Swiss ball, such that he would eventually get pretty good at not falling off the ball while performing this "stunt."

On the other hand, that would only be optimally useful, if he encounters situations exactly like this in his day-to-day life. Otherwise, it's just a compromised version of both exercises (i.e., pectoral press and torso rotation).

Some people may consider it "fun"—trying to avoid falling off the ball, while doing this exercise. It may feel like a game that tests their skill. That's fine—some individuals perceive juggling as "fun" and "challenging" as well. No one, however, should delude themselves into thinking that they're gaining some enhanced fitness benefit by doing an exercise that compromises their power by adding instability. In terms of strength gains and muscle development, what this trainer instructed Joe to do was mostly counterproductive.

In retrospect, it should be clear to you that the trainer did not show Joe a "better way" to do that exercise. Instead, he led Joe to believe that Joe had a problem with his balance, which needed to be corrected. In fact, Joe did not have a balance problem that needed "fixing." Instead of showing Joe a better way of building muscle, losing fat, developing endurance, and becoming healthier, the trainer actually impeded Joe's efforts and led him in an entirely different direction. It almost could be viewed as a "bait-and-switch," except that not even the trainer is aware that the "advice" he's giving Joe is counterproductive to Joe's actual fitness-related goals.

It's not that the trainer is corrupt, deceptive, or unscrupulous. A trainer simply wants to earn a living, and wants to do his job well. The problem is that the fitness industry has convinced trainers that doing their job "well" (these days) requires focusing on "balance" and "core." The industry has taught trainers that this emphasis creates more business opportunities, more activities, more services, more equipment, and more gadgets. Unfortunately, trainers teaching "balance" and "core" exercise is usually perceived by consumers as "good." In addition, it makes the trainer seem more knowledgeable. Neither presumption, however, is quite true.

Teaching exercise that is marketed as "balance" and "core" is lucrative for health clubs; it's lucrative for the fitness associations that host workshops and conventions; it's lucrative for manufacturers of products; it's lucrative for publishers of magazines; it's lucrative for presenters and for trainers. On the other hand, it is not very beneficial for most consumers, as demonstrated by industry statistics.

There is an inverse relationship between a person's ability to use a significant amount of weight during an exercise and the degree of instability during that exercise. The more unstable the exercise, the more the ability to generate power is compromised. In addition, the heavier the weight that is used, while unstable, the greater the potential for injury. Instability limits the amount of weight a person can use during an exercise, and that naturally compromises the muscular development benefit of that exercise.

❑ Instability Example #1

You may have noticed that some people take this "instability" training to an absurd level. For example, in Figure 15-22, you can see a man performing a *barbell squat*, with a fairly heavy weight on his back, while on a Swiss ball. Obviously, this scenario is extremely dangerous. If one of his feet slips off the ball (which could easily happen), he could experience a spinal injury, a twisted knee, a dislocated shoulder, a broken ankle, a torn muscle, a ruptured tendon, or any number of other possible injuries. Furthermore, what could the benefit of doing this exercise, in this ridiculous way, possibly be?

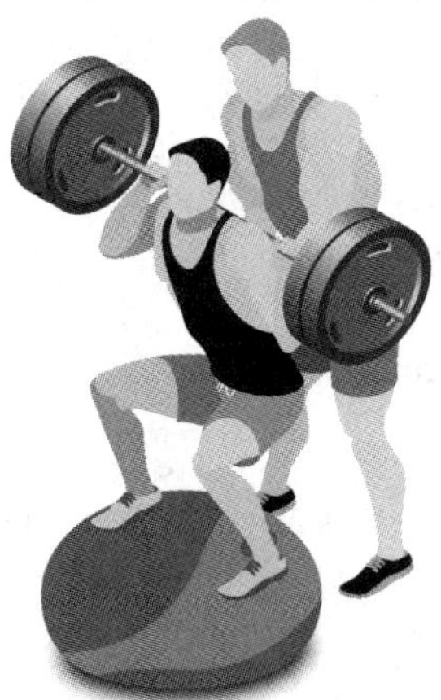

Figure 15-22

He is not gaining any improvement in coordination that can be applied in day-to-day life. Since it's highly unlikely that he'll ever encounter a similar set of circumstances in daily life, this "skill" is essentially worthless. In addition, his ability to use a heavier weight is greatly limited by the instability, which then compromises his ability to stimulate muscle development.

While it's true that this particular "exercise" (Figure 15-22) is not seen very often, exercises that are less extreme—such as "*squats on a BOSU ball*" with no additional weight (Figure 15-34)—are very common. Although the "risk/benefit" ratio of a *BOSU ball squat* is less dramatic, the same questions should

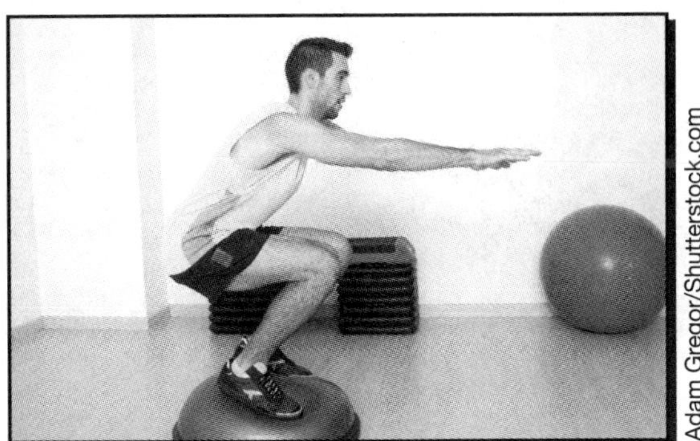

Adam Gregor/Shutterstock.com

Figure 15-23

be asked: What is the actual benefit? What is the risk? To what degree are the potential benefits compromised by the instability?

In virtually all cases, the potential muscle-building benefit of an exercise is significantly compromised by the addition of instability. Furthermore, the learned proprioceptive skill (i.e., not falling, despite the "wobbly" foundation) has very little "real world" application. Unless an individual surfs regularly or rides a skateboard, it's unlikely that a similar "wobbly" foundation will be encountered in day-to-day life.

If you have any doubt about this lack of benefit, simply turn the question around—"What is the disadvantage of not performing unstable exercise?" Do we ever see people showing signs of that "disadvantage," because they failed to do unstable exercise? Do we later see them having "cured" that disadvantage, because they began doing unstable exercise? In fact, there is no disadvantage that a person would experience, if they abstain from doing "unstable" exercise.

❑ Instability Example #2

Standing on one leg, while curling a pair of dumbbells, may seem innocuous, but it has some degree of risk. This potential injury risk is in addition to the compromised ability to generate as much power, and the subsequent limitation of target-muscle stimulation that would result from that. In order to compensate for the fact that only one leg is supporting the bodyweight, you must shift the center of your body mass directly over the one foot that is on the ground. This causes the supporting leg to not be vertical.

In Figure 15-24, you can see the angle change of the left leg (femur) supporting the weight of the body, because the right foot has been lifted off the ground. The arrow shows how the foot has been placed directly under the center of the body mass, to prevent falling. If this "automatic" shift is not done, the person would fall toward the side of the elevated leg. Unfortunately, this shift increases the "Q angle" at the hip joint that is bearing the weight.

The "Q angle" is the variance between the line that follows upward from the tibia (the lower leg bone), and the line that follows from the knee toward the origin of the quadriceps. The wider the hips, the more severe the "Q angle" is, even when standing on both legs. Since women tend to have wider hips than men, they tend to have a slightly more dramatic Q angle. A small degree of Q angle is somewhat inevitable, but it's not good to exacerbate it. The greater the Q angle, the more strain there is in the hip joint.

When you stand on one leg, you exacerbate the Q angle. Then, if the quadriceps contracts, it naturally pulls the quadriceps insertion toward its origin, which pulls the patella (knee cap) laterally, because of this variance. This shift and compensation then causes a degree of knee strain.

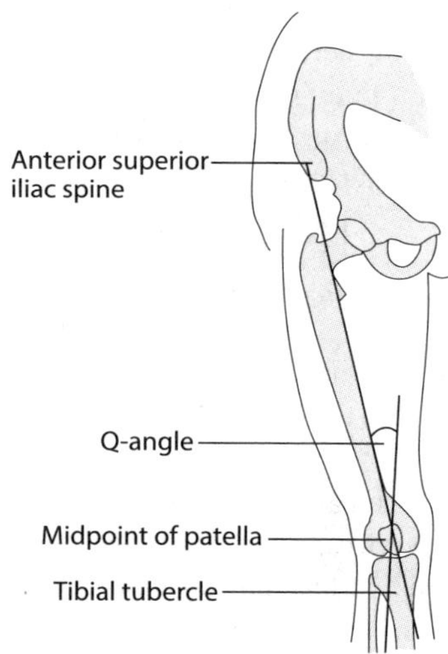


Figure 15-25

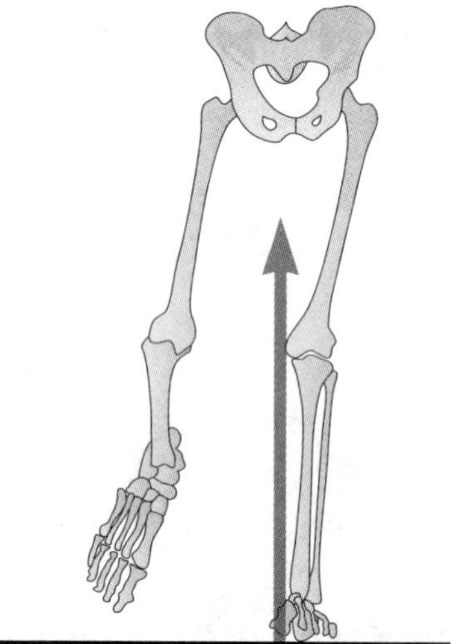

Figure 15-24

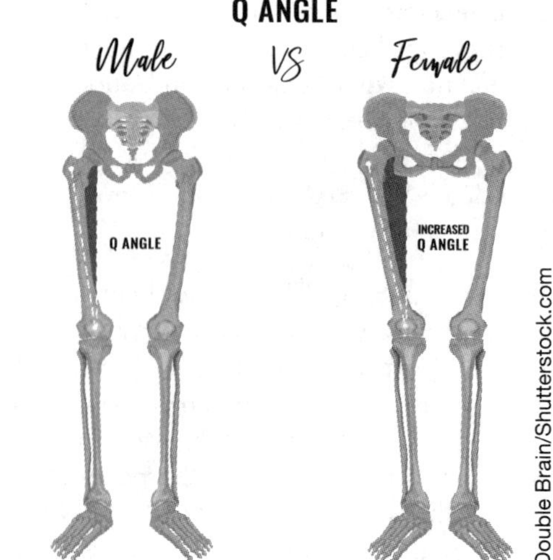


Figure 15-26

Increasing the Q angle also tends to create a compensatory shifting of the lower leg—medially (inwardly), which strains the knee to some degree. This displacement is called "valgus" (Figure 15-27). Some people have "genu valgus" (genetically caused), even when they stand on both legs. In either case (genetic or not), it is exacerbated, when you stand on only one leg.

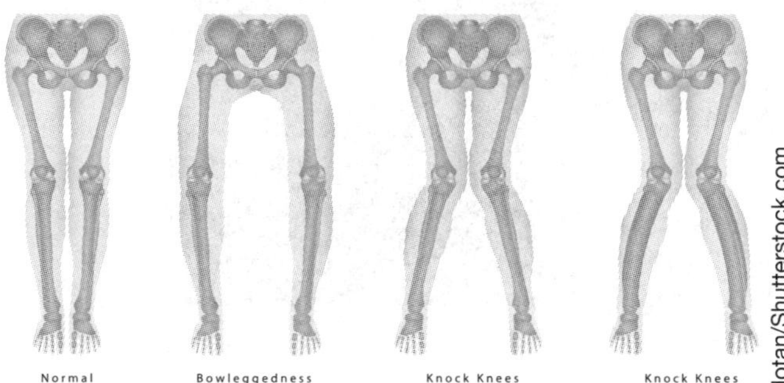

lotan/Shutterstock.com

Figure 15-27

Accordingly, regularly standing on one leg, while performing a weighted exercise, could eventually lead to hip and knee pain. Furthermore, this risk is not offset by any kind of extraordinary benefit. "Spatial orientation" will not improve, as a result of standing on one leg on a regular basis. The coordination to do this particular "exercise" (proprioception) will improve, but that has little value in daily life. In addition, the muscular benefit that could otherwise be experienced will be compromised by the instability.

In Figure 15-28, you can see a man standing on one leg, on a surface that's unstable, while pressing a single dumbbell overhead. Or, to put it another way, "This man is creating a degree of hip strain due to a compensating Q angle, as well as causing a degree of knee strain due to his lower leg's valgus. He is also possibly distorting his right ankle by pronating it, and possibly impinging his supraspinatus tendon (of his left shoulder) by pressing a weight overhead. He considers this a 'balance/core' exercise." In reality, the only benefit he'll gain from it is the improved ability to perform this one exercise—the proprioceptive skill of doing this one maneuver.

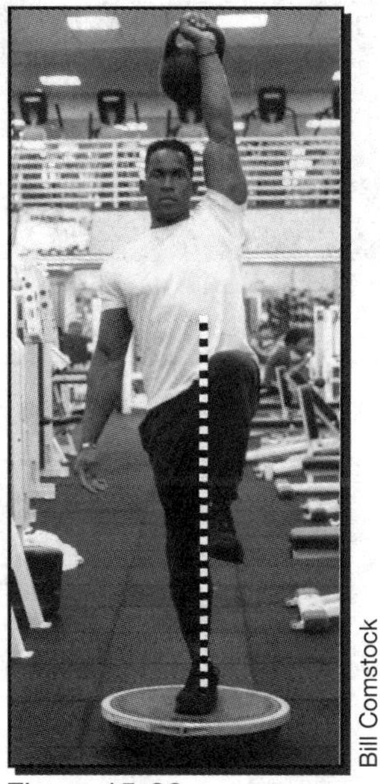
Bill Comstock

Figure 15-28

Any of the muscles involved in this maneuver could be better activated, and better loaded, using exercises that are stable, with minimal injury risk—assuming the goal is to have stronger muscles that are visibly developed. Either way, spatial orientation (i.e., equilibrium/balance) is not affected.

## The Compromises of Training While Unstable

It is very common to see people performing this type of *squat* in the gym these days. Many people believe that the difference between doing a *one-legged squat*, versus a *two-legged squat* is that the one-legged version improves their balance and their "core." Let's see if that is accurate.

It obviously doubles the load on the one working leg, as compared with two legs—that much is clear. Some people simply like the challenge of seeing whether or not they are able to do it. They feel gratified when they discover they can—or eventually can, and may even revel in the fact that others cannot.

An examination of the "pros" and "cons" of doing this type of *squat* can help clarify the issue. For example, it is known that standing on one leg does not actually improve a person's balance, as per the technical definition of balance ("spatial orientation"). It is just another form of proprioceptive training—a skill. In fact, regularly performing *one-legged squats* familiarizes a person with that movement, thereby allowing them to "learn" how to coordinate it. Thus, individuals improve their ability to do the exercise, in addition to challenging (i.e., strengthening) the muscles of the working leg.

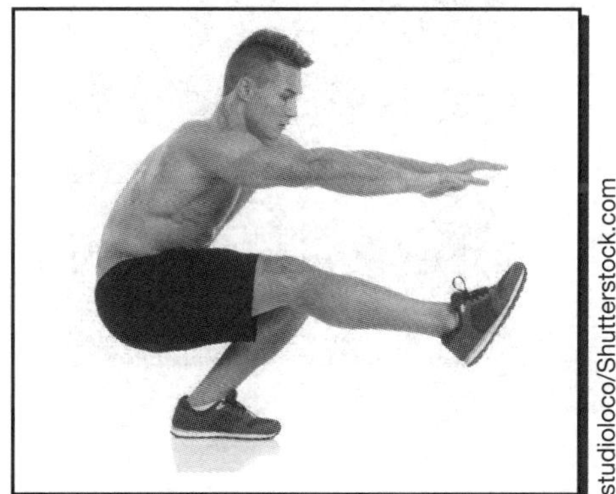
studioloco/Shutterstock.com

Figure 15-29

Unfortunately, this exercise does not improve a skill that has much practical application in daily life. An individual could easily do a *two-legged squat*, holding a pair of dumbbells, and achieve the same amount of load per leg, as using one leg with only bodyweight. That leaves the question of risk. What is the potential consequence to doing this exercise?

Figures 15-30 to 15-32 show two front views and one back view of a *one-legged squat*. As you can see, the lower you descend, the more drastic the Q angle becomes. As a result the tendency to create valgus with the knee and tibia also increases.

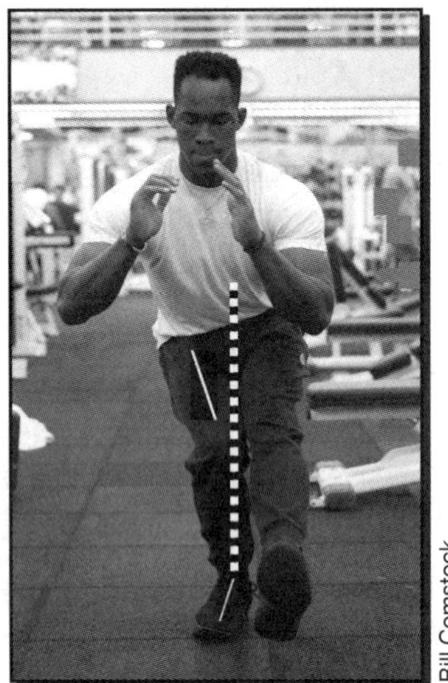
Bill Comstock

Figure 15-30

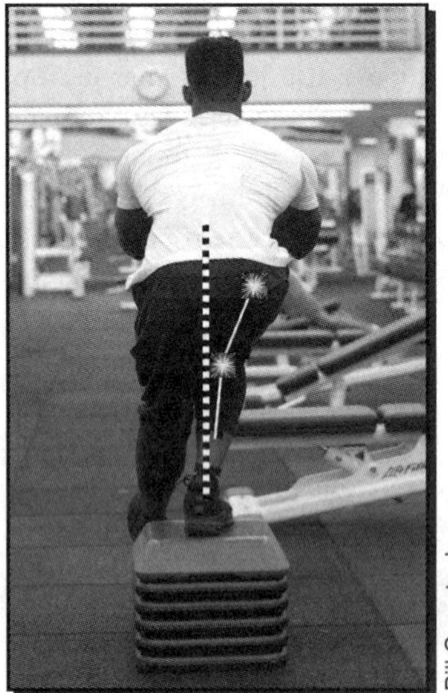
Bill Comstock

Figure 15-31

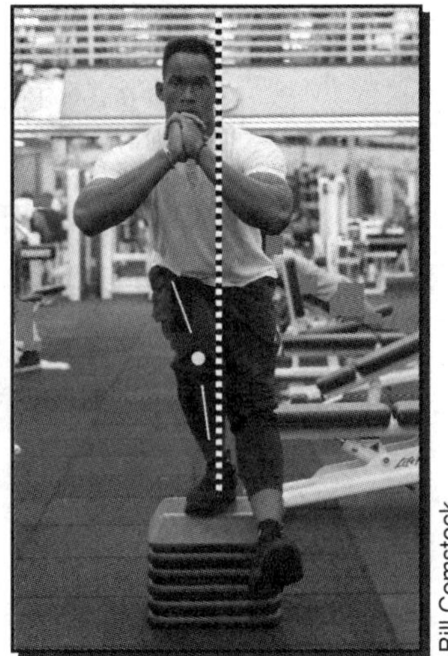
Bill Comstock

Figure 15-32

In addition to the Q angle and valgus compensation that occurs, there is also the issue of the spine. While it's fairly easy to keep a neutral spine when doing *two-legged squats* (Figure 15-33), it is virtually impossible to do so when performing *one-legged squats* (Figure 15-34). This factor adds a third skeletal stress to this exercise—the possibility of intervertebral disc damage, in addition to possibly straining the erector spinae or the quadratus lumborum.

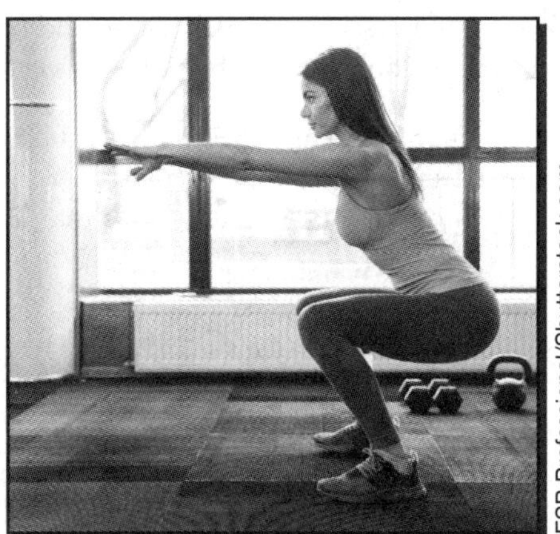
ESB Professional/Shutterstock.com

Figure 15-33

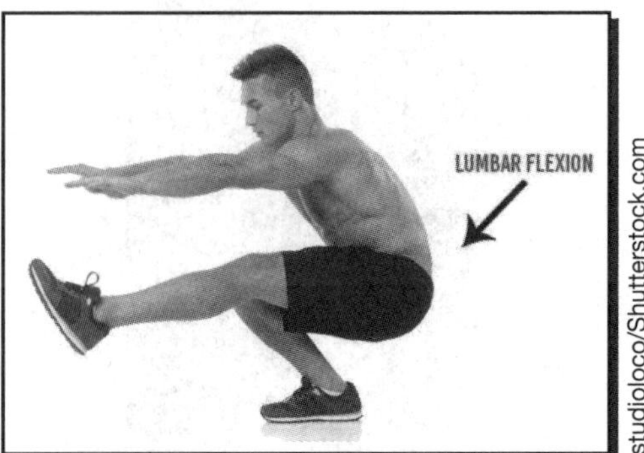

studioloco/Shutterstock.com

Figure 15-34

It is impossible to descend to the bottom of a *one-legged squat*, without the tailbone tucking under, thereby rounding the spine. The reason this "rounding of the spine" happens is because the hamstring of the leg that is held out in front is required to stretch beyond its capacity, if the tailbone is held back (spine arched). Stretching the hamstrings creates "passive insufficiency" which inhibits the ability of the hip flexors and quadriceps to hold the leg up high enough to clear the ground. In order to elevate the front leg high enough, the hamstrings stretch must be reduced, and this is accomplished by rounding the spine. This compensation increases the risk of spine injury.

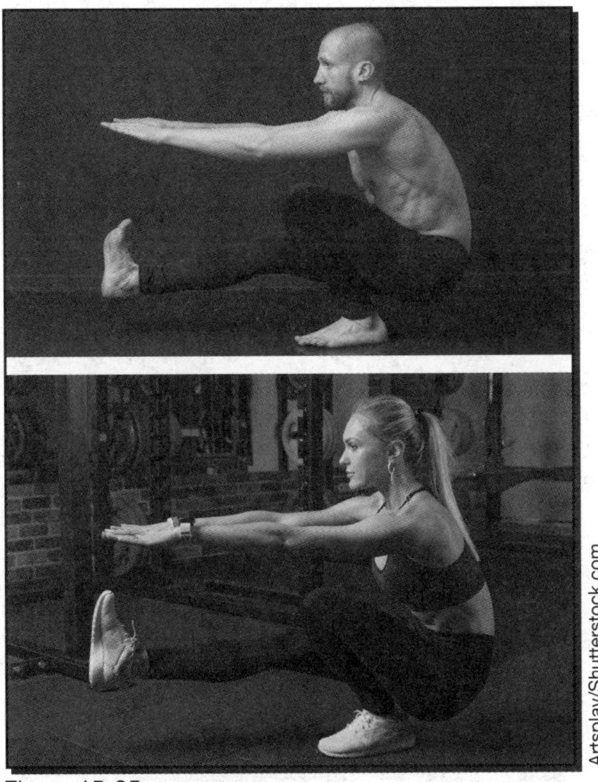
Artsplav/Shutterstock.com

Figure 15-35

A better result could be achieved—in terms of actual fitness benefits—by doing a standard *two-legged squat* (Figure 15-36), with higher reps or the addition of hand-held weights (dumbbells). You could also use a slightly forward pulling cable with weight, or you could do "jump squats" (Figure 15-37). In all of these instances, the demand on the working muscles is increased, WITHOUT creating the skeletal distortion that occurs with *one-legged squats*.

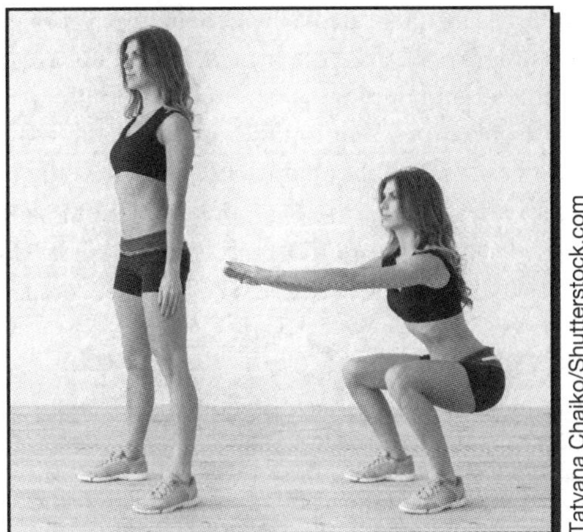
Tatyana Chaiko/Shutterstock.com

Figure 15-36

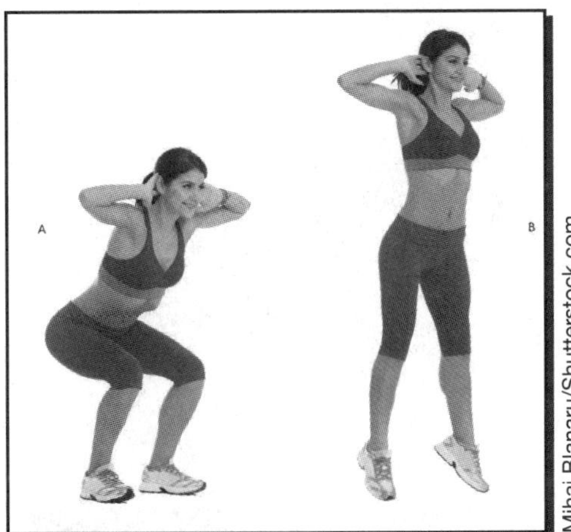

Mihai Blanaru/Shutterstock.com

Figure 15-37

*Note: Jump squats should not be done while holding weights.*

## What Is the "Core," and How to Train the Core Correctly?

The "core" refers to the group of muscles that surround your midsection. This group includes the rectus abdominis, the erector spinae, the internal and external obliques, the transverse abdominis, and the quadratus lumborum. These are the muscles that bend your torso forward, backward, side-to-side, rotate the torso, pull your abdomen inward, and assist in breathing. They are also important for posture and spinal support, and they participate in most whole-body movements, like dancing, tennis, basketball, etc.

Figure 15-38 illustrates a front view of a torso, showing the "abs." Figure 15-39 provides a rear view of the torso, showing the erector spinae (aka "spinal erectors") and the quadratus lumborum. The images in Figure 15-40 show the internal and external oblique muscles, as well as the transverse abdominis. These six muscle groups constitute your "core" and will be discussed more thoroughly in Chapters 23 and 24.

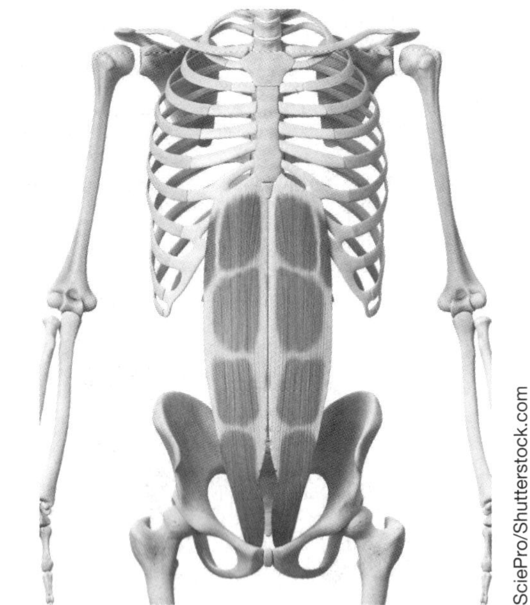
SciePro/Shutterstock.com

Figure 15-38

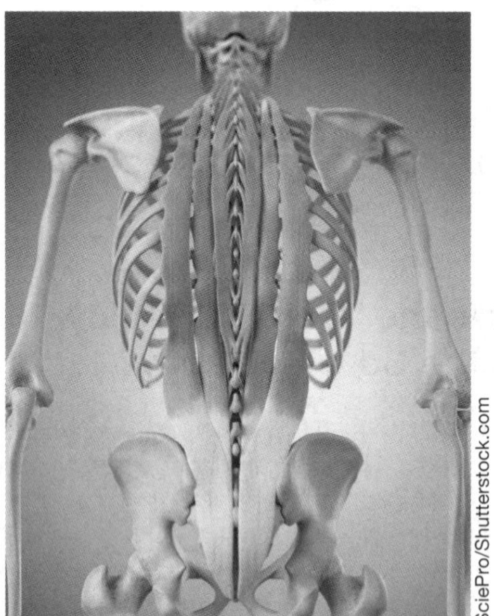
SciePro/Shutterstock.com

Figure 15-39

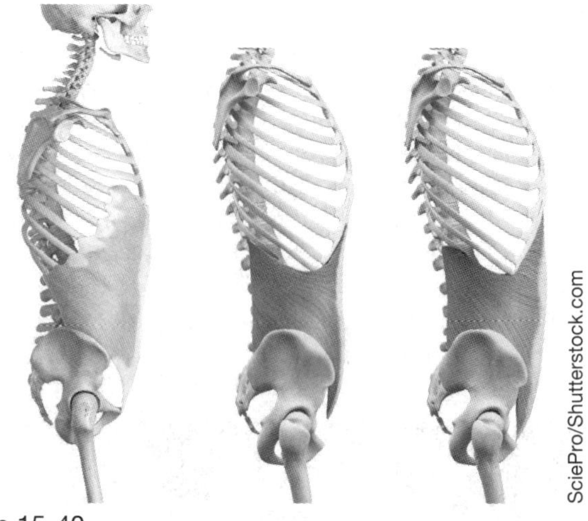
SciePro/Shutterstock.com

Figure 15-40

A discussion of the "core" is included in this chapter, primarily because it is frequently included in the conversation about "balance"—although somewhat inappropriately. In fact, the term "core" itself is overused. It is usually referred to in very ambiguous terms, and often incorrectly.

In the aforementioned theoretical "scenario" involving "Joe" and his trainer, the trainer's rationale for recommending *dumbbell presses* on the stability ball, while keeping one leg off the ground and using one arm at a time, included the terms "core" and "balance," as the justification. In addition, people are often heard making statements such as, "*tightrope-walking (or on a narrow board) is good for the core;*" "*standing on one leg is good for the core;*" "*kneeling on a Swiss ball is good for the core,*" etc. Unfortunately, many people hear and embrace this mentality, without questioning its validity. They then pass along this misinformation, as if it were a fact. In reality, however, it's not quite true.

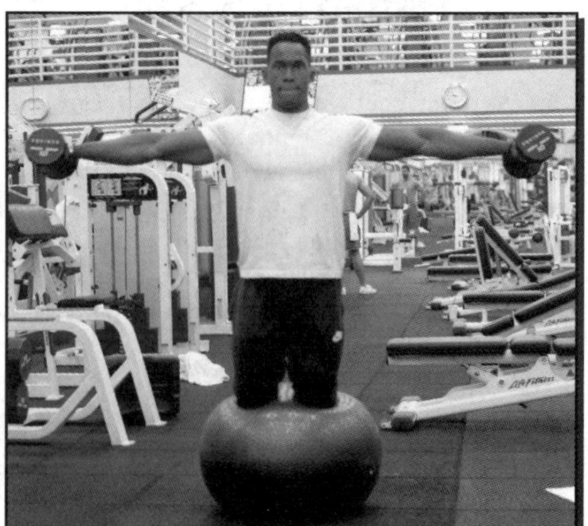
Bill Comstock

Figure 15-41

Because these exercises do NOT (and cannot) affect a person's "spatial orientation," they do not improve balance, in that sense. What they do, however, is to improve the learned coordination of that one activity, which is technically called "proprioception." On the other hand, those learned skills are not applicable in situations that are much different than those specific "exercises."

Do they affect an individual's "core"—the muscles that surround the waistline, as shown in Figures 15-38 through 15-40? The answer is "perhaps a tiny bit," although not nearly as much as playing basketball or dancing would, and certainly not as much as doing resistance exercises that directly target those muscles.

Exercises that are truly good for the "core" are those that deliberately work (load, extend, and contract) the abs, the obliques, and the spinal erectors. Athletic activities and sports typically involve the core muscles, but more from the perspective of coordination—rather than strengthening.

If a person regularly performs exercises for the abs, the obliques and the spinal erectors, they will have a strong core. As such, there is no need to do off-balance/unstable exercise, in order to have a strong core.

Tennis, basketball, dancing, and other similar activities will "proprioceptively" coordinate the muscles of the body, including the core muscles. All in all, the more you do those types of activities, the better you get at doing them, and the more "athletic" (coordinated) you become. On the other hand, playing basketball and dancing are not a replacement for directly "working" the core muscles—the abs, the obliques, and the spinal erectors.

## Summary

Because people who have a legitimate problem with balance ("spatial orientation") likely have a problem with their inner ear, eyes, feet and/or neurological system, they should seek help from a qualified medical professional. Performing exercise while standing, lying, or sitting on an unstable foundation will not resolve a balance problem that is caused by an inner ear, eye, feet and/or neurological system dysfunction.

In fact, exercises performed on an unstable foundation will improve the "proprioceptive" skills required of that specific activity, and—to a degree—other activities which also involve an unstable foundation. Performing an exercise on an unstable foundation, however, compromises your ability to simultaneously optimally perform resistance exercise, as compared to performing those exercises on a stable foundation. This situation leads to compromised strength and muscular development benefits.

Unstable exercises generally have a higher degree of injury risk, when compared with stable exercises. When unstable exercises are performed with additional weight (beyond body weight), the injury risk increases. The more weight that is added, the more the injury risk increases.

Activities involving movement of the whole body (e.g., dancing, sports, and specific coordination drills) tend to be more productive for the improvement of coordination, than activities in which you simply stand on one leg or try to stabilize yourself on a wobble board. In fact, as people get older, they tend to engage in fewer activities that are "physical/athletic" which require moving the body in multiple directions. As a result, they naturally lose some of the ability to move their body in multiple directions, with coordination. The solution to this loss is not standing on one leg or on an unstable board, but to begin doing activities that require whole-body movement in multiple directions. These could be in the form of dancing or in well-designed "skill drills," supervised by a trainer.

Moving the feet (as in dancing), side-stepping, backward stepping, and stepping over low barriers in all four directions (ideally, while also moving the arms—perhaps even catching and throwing a light ball) all help the body/brain coordination connection. These are "macro" movements, which are far more beneficial for regaining coordination, than are the "micro" adjustments that are required when standing on an unstable foundation.

A good exercise for older adults, which improves coordination of lateral (side-to-side) motion, is one in which a person shuffles two steps to the right, catches a ball, throws it back, and then shuffles two steps to the left, catches a ball, throws it back, etc. This type of activity causes the lateral leg movement to become more "automatic" (i.e., without need of deliberate thought), because the person focuses more on catching the ball, and the feet go into "auto-pilot" mode.

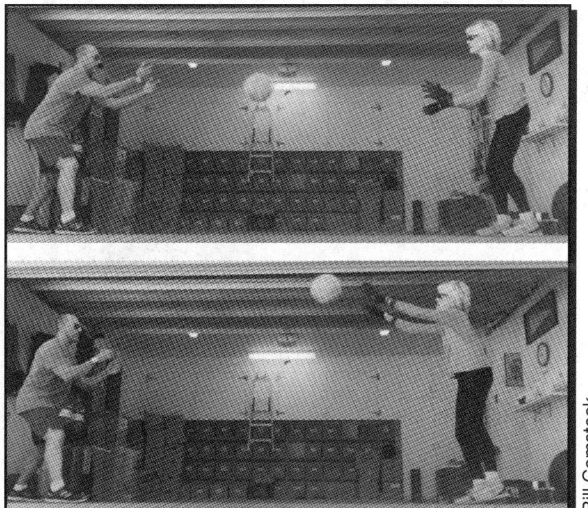

Bill Comstock

Figure 15-42

Furthermore, this type of "proprioceptive" learning allows the feet and legs (as well as the brain) to be better prepared (coordinated) for the possibility of having to suddenly shift or step sideways. For example, if an older person is bumped sideways or backward in a crowded place, the legs and brain need to react automatically by lifting the leg, stepping over an object, and/or repositioning the leg to accommodate a bodyweight shift.

Simply losing strength in the legs (which is common in older people), as a result of inactivity or "under-activity," often results in what feels like a loss of balance. Walking up stairs, walking on unpaved or uneven surfaces, climbing a ladder, etc., will all feel "unstable," if a person's legs are WEAK. Accordingly, simply strengthening the legs by doing leg exercises (squats, leg extensions, leg curls, calf raises, etc.) is the first step in improving an older person's stability.

"Core" exercises should not be considered synonymous with "balance" (proprioception). While the "core" muscles are peripherally involved in many activities, exercises that are truly good for the core should be those that adhere to the same biomechanical principles that are applied to all the other skeletal muscles, including "range of motion" and "opposing resistance."

If you feel that you would benefit from performing proprioceptive exercise, that type of training should ideally be done separately. It is not wise to combine it simultaneously with resistance exercise. In reality, resistance exercise, which is intended for the purpose of muscular development, is compromised by simultaneously incorporating instability.

The notion that combining instability and resistance exercise "saves" time is far from accurate. When performing these types of training simultaneously, the effectiveness of both is compromised, and the risk of injury greatly increases.

# CHAPTER 16

# "CROSS EDUCATION" AND THE BENEFITS OF UNILATERAL EXERCISE

- *"Cross education" is a neurophysiological feature, whereby an adaptive exercise benefit crosses over to an untrained limb following unilateral resistance exercise with the opposite, contralateral limb. The crossover benefits, although only in small percentages, include improvements in muscle strength, muscle size, muscle elasticity, and coordination.*
- *Contralateral benefit caused by unilateral exercise proves that there are neurological adaptations to resistance exercise, in addition to the more obvious muscle growth caused by direct (ipsilateral) resistance exercise.*
- *Performing "unilateral" (independent limb) exercise also provides benefits beyond those achieved with "bilateral" (two limbs sharing a single instrument) exercise.*

In 1894, Edward Wheeler Scripture (1864-1945), an American psychologist, physician, and speech scientist, published a paper in the *Yale Psychology Laboratory*, called "On the Education of Muscular Control and Power," in which he revealed certain interesting phenomenon concerning unilateral exercise. The genesis of his writings was his review of an earlier study conducted by a German scientist named Alfred Wilhelm Volkmann (1801-1877). In that effort, Volkmann had demonstrated that touch sensitivity would improve over time, with repeated training of one hand. More importantly, however, he demonstrated that the untrained hand also improved its touch sensitivity, although to a lesser degree.

Curious about this interesting "crossover" improvement of touch sensitivity training, and aware of other studies demonstrating increases of strength with repeated exposure to exercise, Dr. Scripture conducted his own study, to see if these two types of benefits could be combined.[1] In his study, he had two people perform two different unilateral (single-arm) exercises—one designed to improve strength and the other designed to improve skill (accuracy with speed). The subject performing the strength training increased her strength in the trained arm by 70 percent, but also in the UN-trained arm by 40 percent. The individual performing the skill training improved her dexterity in the trained arm by 45 percent, but also in the UN-trained arm by 25 percent. These were the degrees of crossover benefit he reported, although subsequent studies have found differing degrees of crossover benefits, for example:

- In a 2007 article by Michael Lee and Timothy J. Carroll called "*Cross Education: Possible Mechanisms for Contralateral Effects of Unilateral Resistance Training,*" a 35 percent strength improvement in the ipsilateral (activated) limb and a 7.8 percent (average) strength improvement to the contralateral (not activated) limb, was reported.[2]
- A study conducted in 1997 investigated the concept of "cross education," in which the strength level of both (right and left) quadriceps of volunteers was measured before the experiment. Subsequently, a 12-week program of progressive resistance exercise was undertaken, using only the left leg. At the conclusion of the 12 weeks, the authors reported a "significant" strength increase in the unexercised (right) quadriceps of the volunteers.[3]
- Two other studies, both published in the *Journal of Exercise Science and Fitness,* reported strength gains in untrained limbs that ranged between 5 percent and 15 percent of those achieved in the trained limbs, depending on which limb was "dominant." Furthermore, they found that cross education is typically more pronounced, when the dominant limb is the one that's doing the unilateral exercise.[4a & 4b]
- In addition to strength increases transferring from one limb to the contralateral limb of the opposite side, another study found there is also a crossover enhancement of

endurance. That study demonstrated that there was enhanced activation of the genes that support endurance, in the untrained contralateral limb, for several days after exercising the opposing ipsilateral limb.[5]

- On occasion, "cross education" is referred to by another name—"Neural Integration of Interlimb Coordination." This name was used by researchers Howard and Enoka in their renowned study, which makes more clear the apparent neurological connection between unilateral exercise and coordination/skill learning.[6]
- Most of the research on "crossover benefit" has been done on the contralateral benefit—benefit that is passed from one side of the body to the other side of the body (i.e., to the opposite limb). On the other hand, it appears there may also be some crossover benefit from UPPER BODY to LOWER BODY, and vice versa. This factor suggests a "systemic" benefit. This finding was reported by the authors of a June 2015 article that appeared in the *Journal of Sports Science and Medicine*.[7]

Of course, the amount of benefit an un-exercised (contralateral) muscle receives will always be significantly less than that which is received by the directly exercised (ipsilateral) muscle. Even a 5 percent benefit, however, is extremely interesting and potentially very useful. Several studies, however, report a much greater percentage of crossover benefit.

## What Is Cross Education?

Researchers are not entirely sure of how this crossover benefit happens, but it's clear that "cross education" involves the brain and central nervous system. It's well-documented that there is a neurological component in all resistance exercise, but especially in unilateral exercise.

The two possible hypotheses by which scientists believe this phenomenon might occur were detailed in a July 2011 article that was published in "*Arbeitsphysiologie*" (*European Journal of Applied Physiology*) entitled, "Ipsilateral resistance exercise prevents exercise-induced central sensitization in the contralateral limb: a randomized controlled trial." In this article, the author described two potential neural mechanisms for how "cross education" occurs. Figure 16-1 accompanied the article.

In reality, unless you are planning a career in neurobiology, you do not need to be overly concerned with how "cross education" works. If, however, you are a person pursuing optimal results in resistance exercise or possibly considering a career as a personal trainer, you need to understand that "cross education" actually happens—that there is a percentage of crossover benefit that is transmitted to a limb, when its contralateral limb performs unilateral exercise.

According to evolutionary biologists, every aspect of the human design stems from an evolutionary need for survival. Over the resulting millennia, the survival of individuals has relied on their ability to adapt to environmental conditions. As such, cross education seems likely to have evolved as an evolutionary aid for survival.

No doubt exists that symmetrical functionality is better than asymmetrical functionality—a factor that bolsters the argument that evolutionary survival was the reason for the development of "cross education". It also gives support to the theory that humans (subconsciously) find other humans "attractive," largely on the basis of visible symmetry.

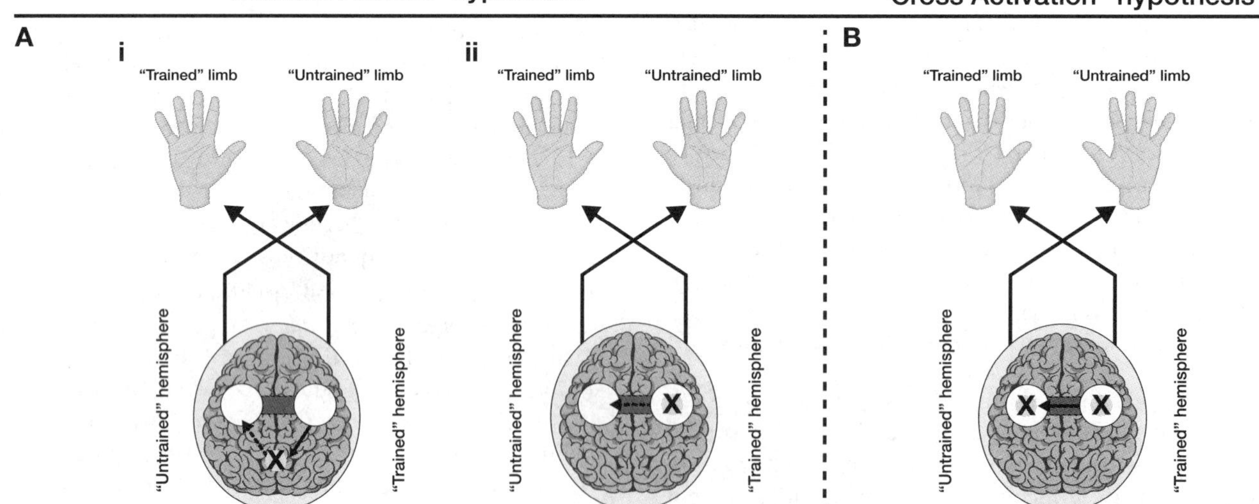


Reprinted by permission from Springer Nature Customer Service Centre GmbH: Springer Nature, *European Journal of Applied Physiology*, Ipsilateral resistance exercise prevents exercise-induced central sensitization in the contralateral limb: a randomized controlled trial, Mahdi Hosseinzadeh et al, 2015.

Figure 16-1

Individuals who are visibly symmetrical are likely more functionally symmetrical, which would translate to a person being better able to survive, to provide shelter and food, and to pass on those genes.

This factor might also explain the discrepancy, concerning the differing percentages of crossover benefits observed by the researchers who conducted the various studies. It's possible that the individuals who experienced a greater percentage of crossover benefit, were those individuals who were more genetically inclined for survival—more robust. Arguably, the individuals who are less genetically inclined to adapt to challenging situations may be the ones who experienced a lesser percentage of crossover benefit. Regardless of this difference, it seems that everyone experiences some degree of contralateral benefit from unilateral exercise.

## The Benefits of Unilateral Resistance Exercise

The most obvious application of this feature, in modern society, would be during the rehabilitation of an injured limb, or rehabilitation from a stroke. After a limb injury or a stroke, a person might be inclined to stop exercising altogether. The better option, however, is to continue—or even start—exercising all the limbs and muscles that are not injured or otherwise disabled.

As such, a person can reasonably expect to get some degree of benefit in a disabled limb by exercising the opposite, still fully-functional limb. Furthermore, exercising the healthy limbs will improve an individual's systemic health, as well as their psychological well-being.

Some people worry that if they continue exercising the stronger limb, while the injured/immobilized limb performs no exercise at all, the stronger limb will get so far ahead of the disabled limb that the disabled limb will never catch up. This concern is inaccurate.

The limb that is stronger will not continue getting stronger and stronger, endlessly. Eventually, it will reach a genetically determined plateau, at which point its progress will either slow considerably or stop entirely. When the weaker side resumes exercising, its progress will be much faster than normal, because it has more strength potential ahead, and its regaining strength it had before (i.e., sometimes referred to as "muscle memory"). From that point forward, it's only a matter of time before the two limbs return to their pre-injury difference. It should be noted that some degree of difference between opposing limbs always exists, even if an injury has never occurred.

The size and strength of an injured limb eventually returns to the size and strength it had before the injury, within 6 to 12 months after resuming exercise with that limb. That's faster than it would be if one did not continue working the uninjured limb. (*Note: This outcome assumes that the surgical repair and/ or healing were completely successful.*) I have experienced this situation myself.

I tore my left biceps tendon in 1998 (not in the gym, by the way), and had it surgically repaired (Figure 16-2). I was not able to use my left arm at all, for approximately six weeks following the surgery. I was instructed to keep it immobilized, in a sling. During that time, I continued working my right arm as normal. I also exercised all the other muscle groups, to the degree that I could—all the while, having my left arm in a sling.

After the initial six-week period, I was able to begin exercising my left arm with very light weight. Initially, I started doing *one-arm dumbbell curls* with only a one-pound weight, and even that was painful. Soon, however, I progressed to three pounds, then five pounds, and so on. Within six months, my left arm had returned to approximately 90 percent of its normal size and strength. Within a year, it was impossible to see any difference whatsoever between my two arms. Eighteen months after the injury, I was competing again (Figure 16-3).

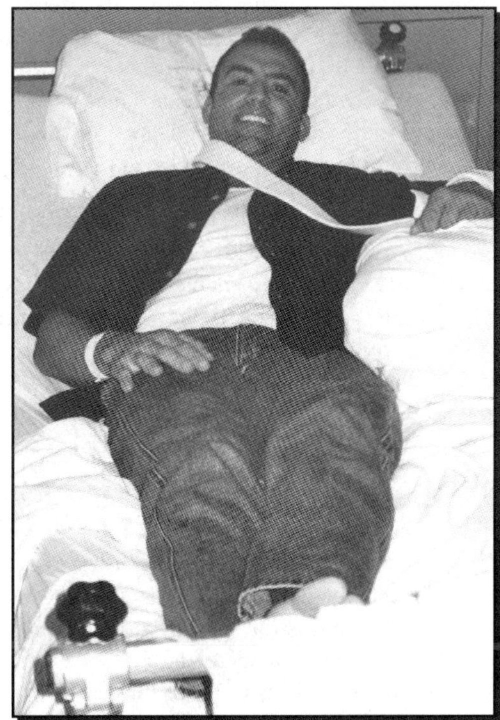

Figure 16-2

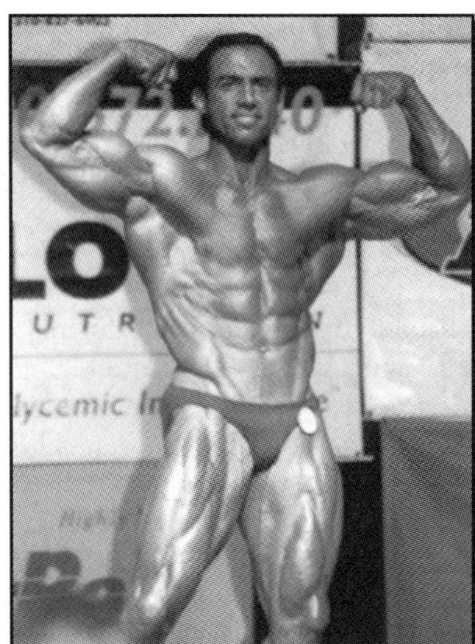
Figure 16-3

## Using Cross Education to Improve Muscular Symmetry

It should be noted that all people have some degree of imbalance of muscular size, strength, and shape, from one side to the other. Curiously, it's not always the dominant side that's stronger or larger. Furthermore, it's also not consistent either. In other words, it is usually not the entire right side—or entirely the left side—that is larger and stronger. For example, you might have a stronger left biceps, but a stronger right triceps. In addition, if you have had a previous injury, there may be a slight, but permanent, weakness in the muscle of that particular side.

The good news is that—with cross education—you can be confident that some of the benefits from the stronger side will cross over to the weaker side. In fact, the research suggests that the percentage of contralateral benefit is usually greater to the weaker limb, when it's the stronger limb doing the work. That would make sense, of course, given the apparent tendency of the human body to seek symmetry.

This feature allows you to use whatever weight is manageable for each side, even if you must use a lighter weight on the weaker side. In fact, this technique is advisable. It would not be wise to use a weight that is "too heavy" for the weaker side, simply because that is the weight you're able to use on your stronger side. People tend to do that, because they're afraid they'll perpetuate or exacerbate the asymmetry. That concern ignores the benefit of "cross education." Furthermore, using a weight that is too heavy for the weaker side will encourage bad form, which increases the risk of injury.

## Redefining "Unilateral" Exercise

The studies that have been undertaken concerning cross education demonstrate that performing an exercise with one limb—independent from the opposite limb—has a benefit beyond that which is only gained by the working limb. Consider the following:

If you are able to get a 5 percent to 10 percent crossover "bonus benefit" to the opposing limb, by working its contralateral limb independently—when you're injured—it is likely that you'll achieve a similar crossover benefit when you're not injured. The degree of benefit might be less, simply because there would be less asymmetry for which to compensate. On the other hand, it's reasonable to assume that there is some degree of crossover benefit anytime unilateral exercise is performed. So, the question that must be asked is, what exactly is "unilateral?"

The cross education studies that were performed involved the use of only one limb, because the basic point of the study was to measure the benefit that could be achieved by the inactive limb. In those studies, this procedure was typically referred to as "unilateral" exercise.

The fitness industry, however, has defined "unilateral exercise" as "one limb working at a time." This description is not quite accurate, because the issue is not "timing"—but rather "independence." The reason "unilateral" exercise has extra value is because that limb is working "independently." If you perform a dumbbell curl with the right arm, it is working independently, even if the left arm is also curling a dumbbell at the same time.

As such, the term "unilateral" should be equated with "independence," instead of with "timing." All exercises, during which a limb is working independently, could (and should) be called "unilateral." In that regard, two dumbbells, being curled simultaneously, would still be "unilateral."

Consider the two bicycle riders, riding side-by-side, in Figure 16-4. Their paths and speed coincide, but each is working separately. This situation is analogous to two arms curling separate weights, simultaneously.

Next, consider the two bicyclists riding "tandem" in Figure 16-5. Because they are sharing the same instrument, they are sharing participation in the movement of that singular instrument. Neither person is solely responsible for the movement of that instrument, and each rider's actions affects the other rider, to a degree. They are not working independently. This scenario would be like a person using two arms, both of which are contributing to the movement of a single barbell.

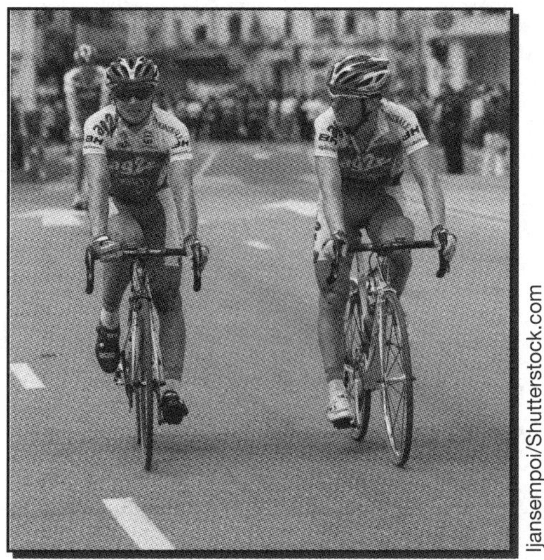
Figure 16-4
ljansempoi/Shutterstock.com

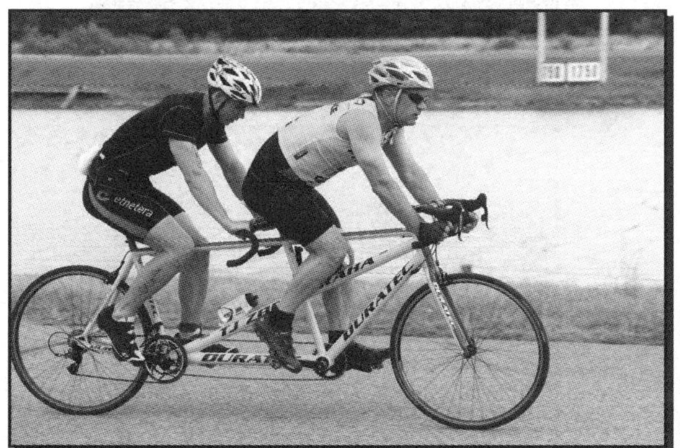
Figure 16-5
Milan Humaj/Shutterstock.com

The term "bilateral" has traditionally been used to describe an exercise in which a person is using two arms simultaneously, even if each arm is lifting its own separate weight. As such, the term "bilateral" should not be used to broadly describe "both arms working simultaneously," because it does not stipulate whether the arms are working independently of each other (e.g., two dumbbells), or are sharing an instrument (e.g., one barbell).

A *standing barbell curl* (Figure 16-6) does not have the exact same mechanical/neurological effect on the biceps, as does a *standing two-arm dumbbell curl* (Figure 16-7). Accordingly, they should not BOTH be called "bilateral." The array of "cross education" studies proves that there is an added benefit to having the limbs work independently. Therefore, the description of an exercise needs to identify whether the limbs are working independently or not. As such, "bilateral" should be defined as "*both limbs contributing simultaneously to the movement of a singular instrument.*"

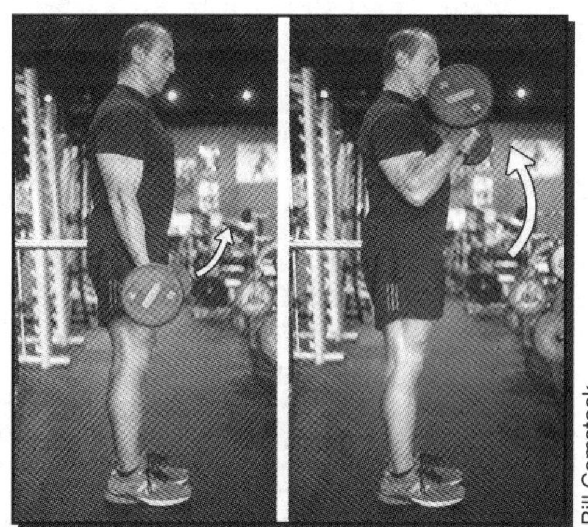
Figure 16-6
Bill Comstock

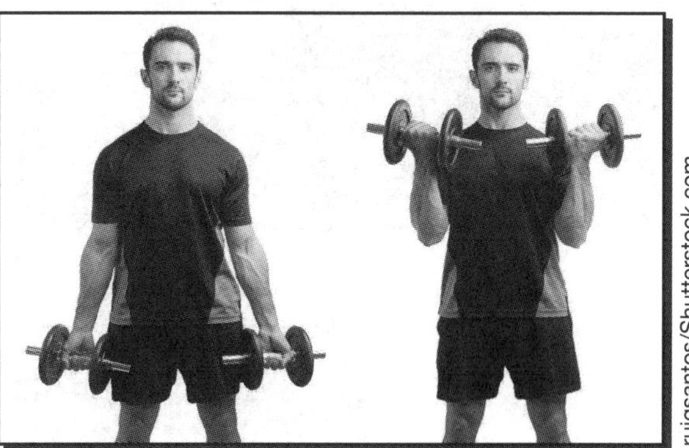
Figure 16-7
ruigsantos/Shutterstock.com

In contrast, "unilateral" should be defined as "*a limb working independently of its opposing limb, regardless of the timing of the two limbs.*" In that regard, "unilateral" (independent limb) exercise can be performed in the following three ways:

- Isolated unilateral exercise: only one limb working
- Alternating unilateral exercise: two limbs working alternately (e.g., left, right, left, right)
- Simultaneous unilateral exercise: two limbs working simultaneously and independently.

All three types of unilateral exercise share in common the fact that the limbs are working independently of the other. The only difference is timing.

## When to Use Isolated Unilateral, Alternating Unilateral, and Simultaneous Unilateral Exercise

There are circumstances (exercises) during which each of the aforementioned versions of "unilateral" is ideal. On occasion, this has to do with the stability of an exercise, while other times, it has more to do with "bilateral deficit"—soon to be explained. In still other instances, it has to do with "unidirectional focus"—also soon to be explained.

For example, in the exercise shown in Figures 16-8 and 16-9, I am doing a "*one-arm side cable raise.*" This is an excellent exercise, and the best way of performing it is using one arm at a time—"Isolated Unilateral"—performing all of the reps of the set with the one arm, and then switching to the other arm, and performing all the reps of the second half of that set.

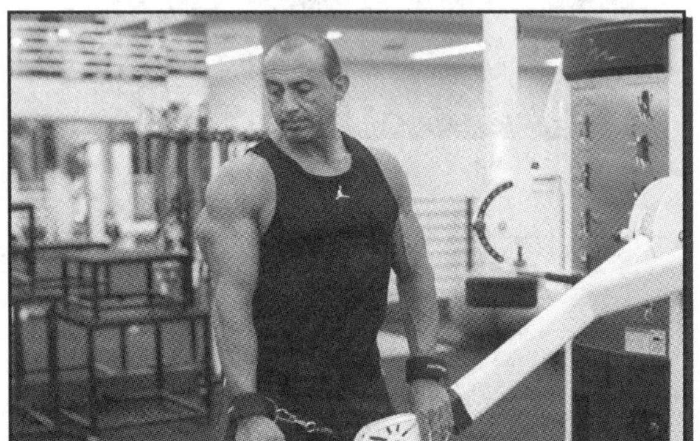
Marisa Leigh

Figure 16-8

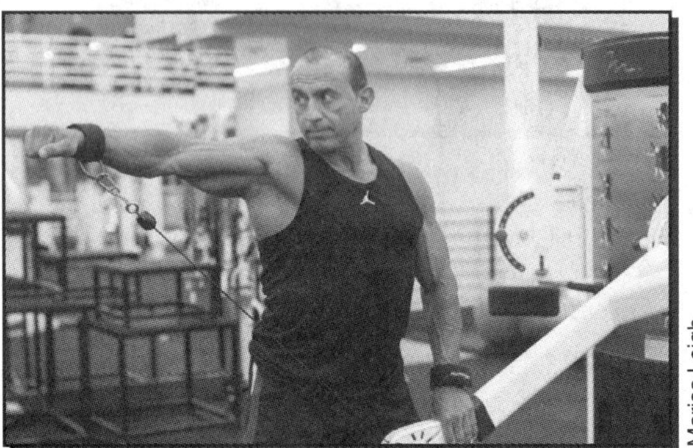
Marisa Leigh

Figure 16-9

There are two reasons why it's best to perform this exercise this way. First, it would be difficult to set up two pulleys at this exact height, but in opposing directions. Although it could be arranged, the cable handles would collide in the middle, which would make it cumbersome. The more important reason, however, is because it's BETTER for an individual to focus ALL of their attention on producing movement toward the right side, or movement toward the left side—rather than trying to divide their focus on producing movement in two OPPOSITE directions. The reason for this will be fully explained, shortly.

In the exercise illustrated in Figures 16-10 and 16-11, "*standing alternating cable curls,*" I am using both arms, in alternating fashion, but independently. This type of unilateral exercise would be considered an "alternating unilateral" exercise. There are two good reasons why this would be the best method of doing this exercise (reasoning which also applies to *alternating dumbbell curls*).

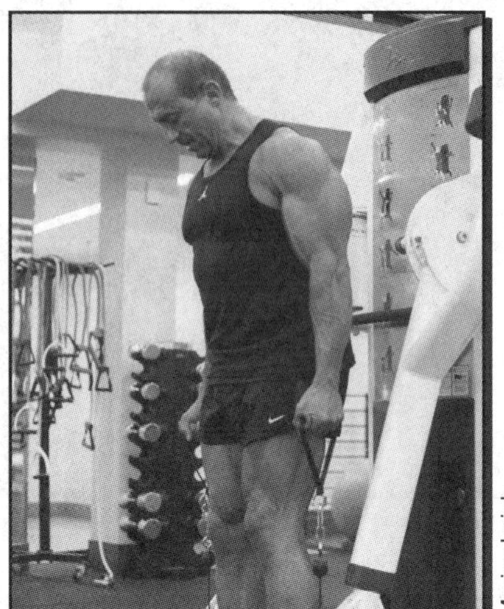
Marisa Leigh

Figure 16-10

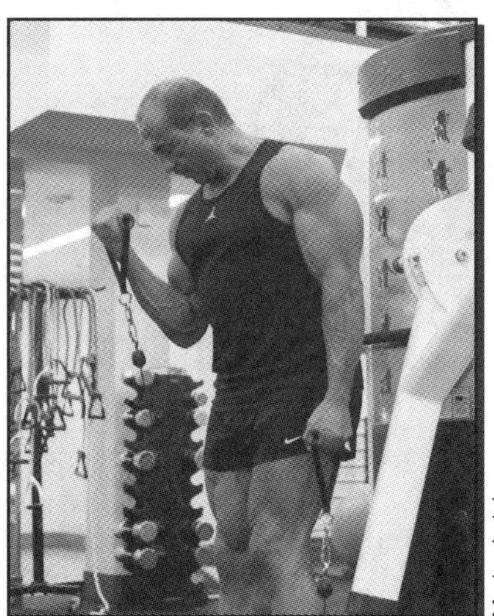
Marisa Leigh

Figure 16-11

Curling one arm at a time reduces the load on the lower back by 50 percent, as compared with curling both arms simultaneously. Of course, the heavier the weight you are using, the more this matters. The more important reason for curling in alternating fashion, however, is because of "*bilateral deficit,*" which is a neurobiological phenomenon that allows more weight to be lifted when using one limb at a time, versus two limbs at a time (i.e., one arm working alone can lift *more* than 50 percent of the weight that could be lifting using both arms simultaneously).

The exercise shown in Figures 16-12 and 16-13—*decline dumbbell press*—would be classified as a "simultaneous unilateral" exercise. Each arm is working independently, but at the same time as the other arm. In this instance, the advantage of using both arms simultaneously is better stability. As was discussed in the previous chapter, using only one arm at a time (especially when using a heavy weight) would pull the user over to one side. Using both arms simultaneously provides stability. Yet, because each arm is still working independently, the crossover (contra-lateral/neurological) benefit is still achieved. Dumbbells also have the advantage of better range of motion, as compared with using a barbell.

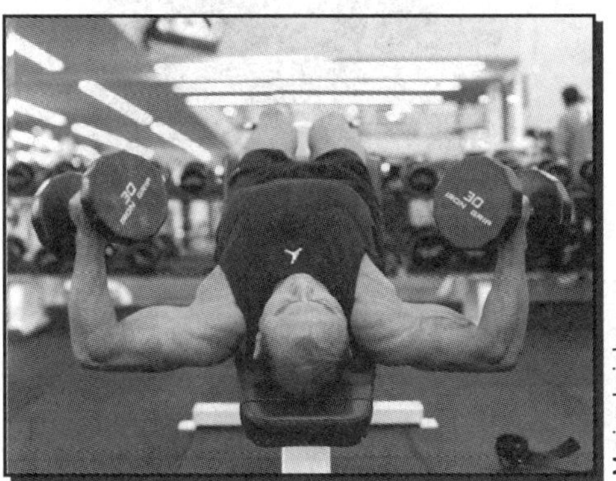
Marisa Leigh

Figure 16-12

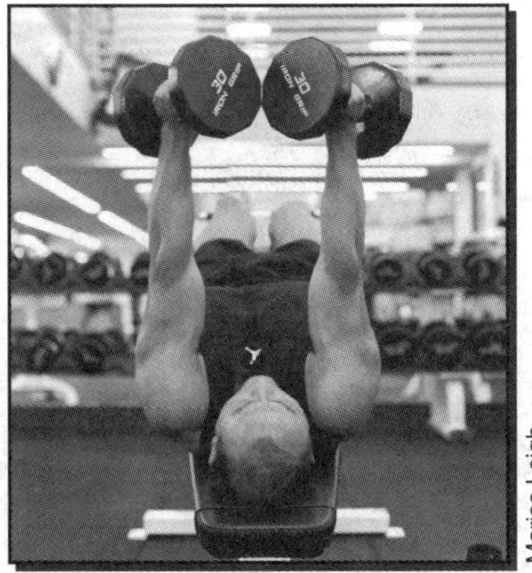
Marisa Leigh

Figure 16-13

In all three of the aforementioned exercises, I am doing a different version of a unilateral exercise. Still, in all three instances, the arms are working independently of each other. The only difference between the three exercises is the timing between the repetitions. In the first exercise, I perform all the repetitions with one arm, and then all the repetitions with the other arm. In the second exercise, the timing is "left/right/left/right" (alternating). In the third exercise, the timing is simultaneous.

There are numerous other exercises in which each of these types of "unilateral" repetitions are best applied. The same logic would be applied in all cases. The goals are to seek stability, the ability to use proper form, the avoidance of straining areas that are not the target (muscles and joints), the ability to optimize your ability to focus on the task at hand, the avoidance of "bilateral deficit" (whenever possible), and the ability to use "uni-directional focus" (explained in the following section), when applicable. Whenever it is practical to do so, it is best to allow the limbs to work independently, even if they are working simultaneously.

## "Unidirectional Focus" and the Avoidance of Moving Limbs in the Opposite Direction During Resistance Exercise

With most skeletal muscles, the direction of movement produced by the muscle on the LEFT side of the body, is the same as the direction of movement produced by that muscle on the RIGHT side of the body. For example, the left and the right biceps BOTH produce movement in the same direction—"forward/upward." The left and the right triceps BOTH produce movement that is "forward/downward." This feature is also true of the quadriceps and hamstrings, as well as most of the other skeletal muscles of the body.

There are a few skeletal muscles (same muscle, right side/left side), however, that produce movement in opposite directions. For example, the right lateral deltoid produces movement toward the right side of the body, while the left lateral deltoid produces movement toward the left side of the body. These are OPPOSITE directions of movement, which is quite different than what occurs with the biceps, triceps, quadriceps, hamstrings, etc.

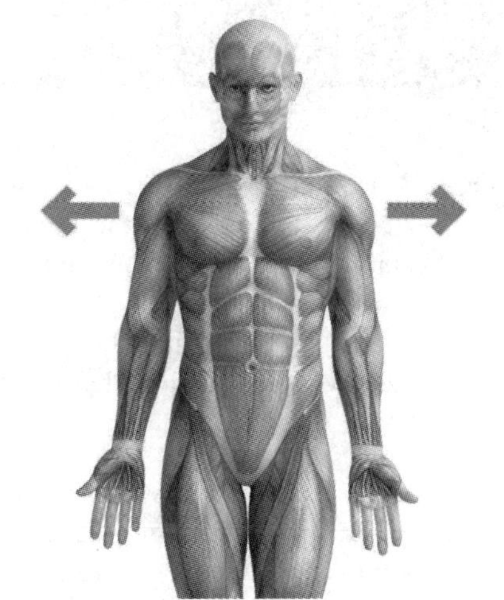
adike/Shutterstock.com

Figure 16-14

Although you may be unaware of it, moving in two different directions requires a type of "split focus" that ultimately compromises the exercise. This compromise does not occur when you do *triceps pushdowns* (using both arms simultaneously), or *standing dumbbell curls* (using both arms simultaneously), because you are able to use "unidirectional focus" during those exercises. You are able to focus the effort of both arms in one, single direction. When working both triceps simultaneously, you focus all of your effort "downward". When working both biceps simultaneously, you focus all of your effort "upward". When you work both lateral deltoids simultaneously, however, you are forced to divide your focus between an effort to the left, and an effort to the right.

As you can see in the exercise shown in Figure 16-15, the motion of the arms is directly opposite each other at the beginning of the movement—one to the left and the other to the right. As the arms move around their respective shoulder axis (pivots), their pathway becomes progressively less "opposite"— but they never quite get to the point where both arms move in the same direction. The movement ends just before the arms arrive at that point, which is the primary reason why the *one-arm side cable raise* exercise shown in Figures 16-8 and 16-9 (as well as any other lateral deltoid exercise) is best done one arm at a time. It allows the user to focus all of their attention on a movement that is in one, single direction.

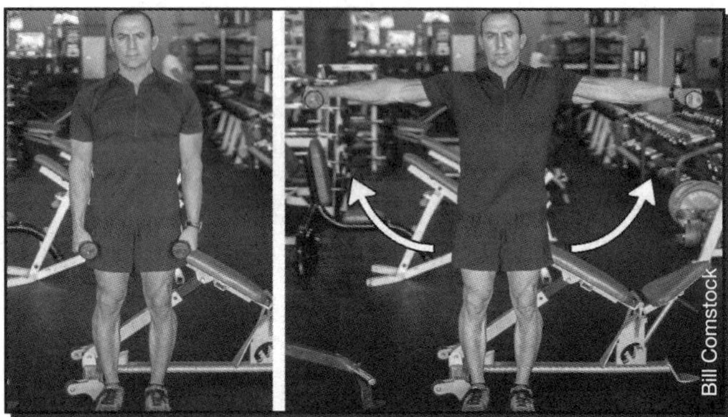

Figure 16-15

The exercise illustrated in Figure 16-16—*one-arm seated side dumbbell raise*—also allows "unidirectional focus." Unfortunately, because this particular exercise is not "early phase" loaded, it's not nearly as productive as the previous cable version. Nevertheless, the principle of "unidirectional focus" still applies, as does the principle that will be discussed next: "bilateral deficit."

To get a sense of what happens when you exert force in two different directions, try this experiment shown in Figure 16-17 the next time you're at the gym. Perform a heavy *triceps pushdown* with one arm, and a heavy *standing cable curl* with your other arm—simultaneously.

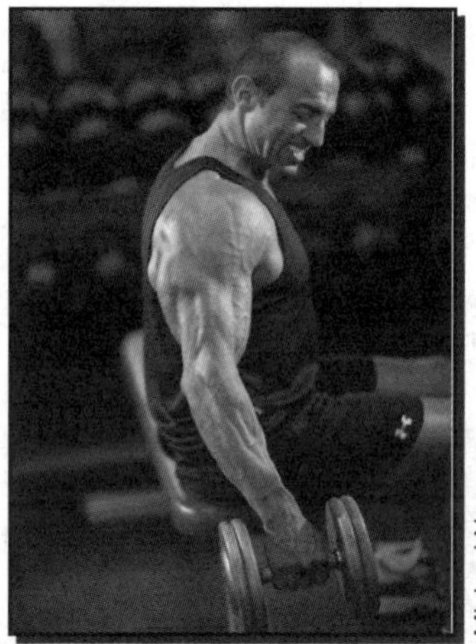

Figure 16-16

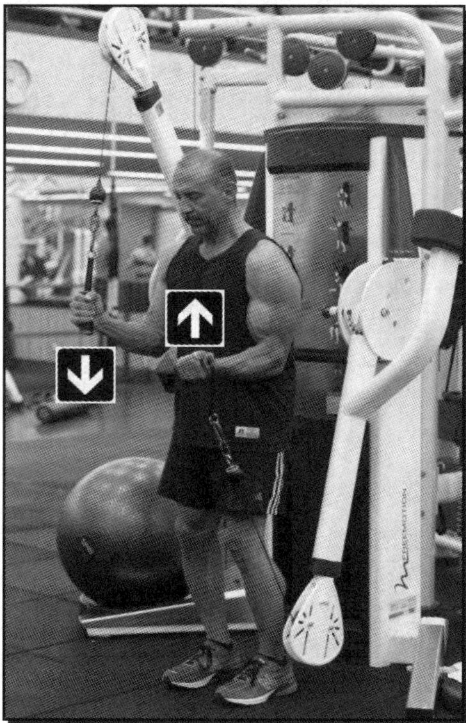

Figure 16-17

Next, perform a *two-arm triceps pushdown* (Figure 16-18) and a *two-arm cable curl* (Figure 16-19). Then, compare the two "exercises"—the one in which you moved both arms in the same direction, with the one in which you moved your arms in two different directions. Take special note how much weight you were able to use with each version, as well as your ability to control and contract the muscle that each movement targeted.

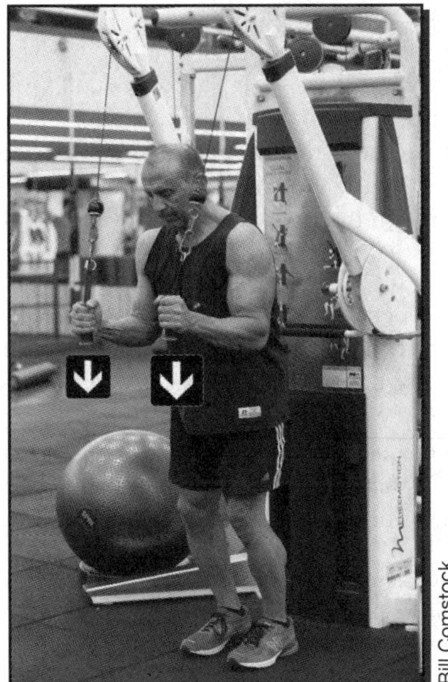

Figure 16-18

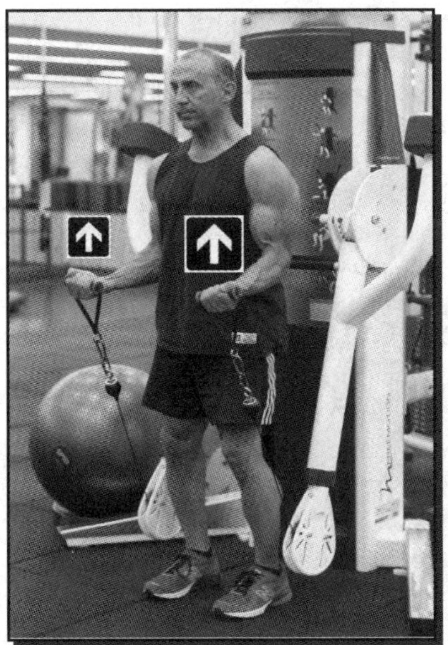

Figure 16-19

What you'll discover is that it is more awkward—and less powerful—to perform two opposing movements at the same time, as compared to doing either one direction or the other. The difference in strength potential between the two versions could be as much as 20 percent. Typically, you are able to move more weight and contract the target muscle better, when your efforts are either entirely upward or entirely downward—entirely to the left or entirely to the right—entirely forward or entirely backward.

Since your objective is to achieve optimal muscular development, it makes sense to perform an exercise using methods that allow you to have the most control, to use the most weight (with good form, of course), and to achieve the best contraction. On the other hand, if your objective is "optimal dexterity," or to challenge brain/body coordination (instead of optimal muscular development), then doing exercises that produce movement in two separate directions would not necessarily be bad. Since this book is intended for individuals who are pursuing optimal physique development, the methods recommended here are with that goal in mind.

The lateral deltoids are the primary muscles that produce movement in opposite directions. The latissimus dorsi is the next most primary muscle, for which this rule applies. Because the origin of the lats is on the spine, the ideal movement for the lats would be inward (toward the spine)—at a slight diagonal. Despite conventional wisdom, the ideal movement for the lats is not "downward" (vertically, as would be the case with *pull-ups*) nor "backward" (posteriorly, as would be the case with *rowing* exercises).

In other words, the left latissimus produces a movement that begins from the left side and moves inward, in a right-bound direction (with a slight downward diagonal). The right latissimus produces a movement that begins from the right side and moves inward, in a left-bound direction (with a slight downward diagonal). These are mostly opposite directions of movement.

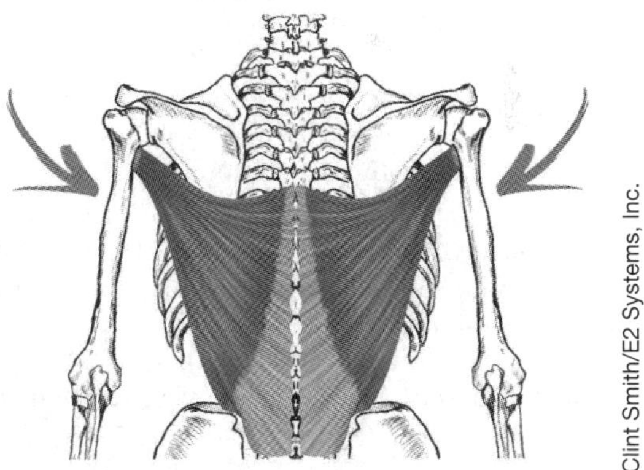

Figure 16-20

Because the lats pull mostly inward—toward the spine—the motion should ideally begin from a mostly lateral/slightly upward origin, and move inward and slightly downward. The lats do participate more during pulldowns and chin-ups (downward movements), than they do in rowing motions, but neither movement is as ideal as a pull-in (diagonal/inward), shown in Figures 16-21 and 16-22. Because the direction of movement, of each side's latissimus, is so opposite, performing the movement "one arm at a time" (isolated unilateral) is significantly better than doing it with both arms simultaneously.

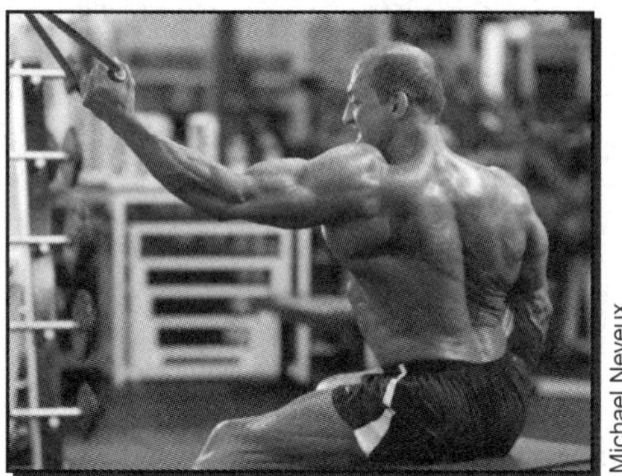

Figure 16-21

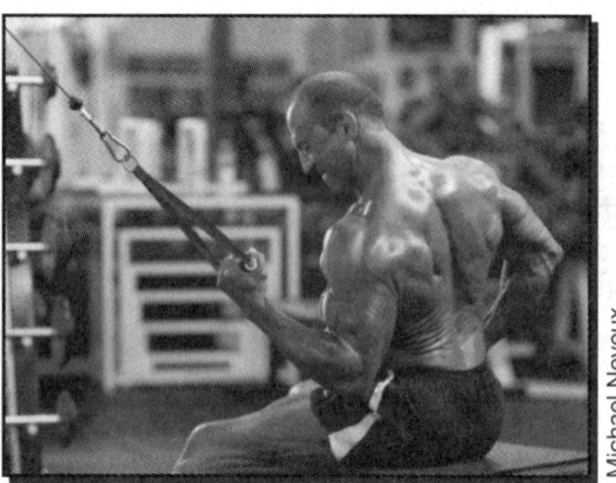

Figure 16-22

It would be impossible to produce this exact motion, using both arms simultaneously. As you'll notice in Figures 16-21 and 16-22, as the arm is pulled inward, there is a natural lean of the torso, toward the resistance, as well as a slight rotation of the torso, toward the resistance. Using both arms at the same time would prevent this natural torso lean and rotation from occurring.

Because it's very easy to brace yourself with your foot against a block—when doing *one-arm pull-ins*—there is no need to "counterbalance" yourself by doing the other side at the same time, the way you would during a *supine dumbbell press*. During a *supine dumbbell press*, there is no way of bracing yourself from falling to one side, if you perform the movement with only one arm. Therefore, counterbalancing (using both arms simultaneously) is required when doing a *supine dumbbell press*. That's not the case, however, with a *one-arm lat pull-in*, provided you find a way to brace your foot.

The (internal and external) obliques also face opposite sides of the body, and perform motion in opposite directions. The oblique muscles MUST be worked "one side at a time" (isolated unilateral)—not only because they move the torso in opposite directions—but also because the obliques fall into the category of "reciprocal innervation." Because they are on opposite sides of the same "limb" (i.e., the torso), they are agonist/antagonist. When one oblique is loaded and activated (laterally), the other side automatically de-activates, to a large degree. This is not the case with the right and left lateral deltoids, nor with the right and left latissimus.

The obliques (both left and right sides, simultaneously) do participate in "forward flexion" of the torso, but neither side works as directly during forward spinal flexion, as they do when performing lateral spinal flexion. In any case, however, the left obliques and the right obliques must also be performed one side at a time. They cannot be worked (loaded) simultaneously. The obliques, therefore, are the third most prominent muscles that produce movement in opposite directions.

The muscles on the sides of the neck (*splenius capitus* and *sternocleidomastoid*) move the head laterally—toward one side or the other. While it's true that both sides CAN participate simultaneously, when flexing the neck posteriorly/toward the back (the *splenius capitus*) and anteriorly/toward the front (the *sternocleidomastoid*)—these muscles do not engage as fully posteriorly and anteriorly, as they do laterally. Therefore, like the obliques, right-side neck flexion and left-side neck flexion must be performed separately, each with its own separate direction of resistance. The muscles on the sides of the neck are also similar to the obliques in the sense that they are agonist/antagonist muscles. When one side is activated, the other side shuts off, due to reciprocal innervation.

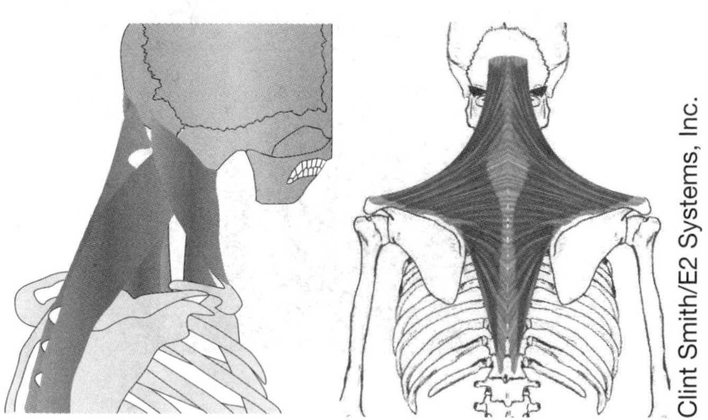

Figure 16-23

The left side and right side of the MIDDLE trapezius (Figure 16-23, right image) are best worked simultaneously, because of the need for stability. Like the lats, each side produces movement in the opposite direction—the left side, toward the right (toward the spine), and the right side, toward the left (toward the spine).

Therefore, each side must have its own, separate direction of resistance. The left-middle trapezius pulls toward the right—toward the spine—so it requires a direction of resistance that comes from the left side (slightly anterior). Given that the right-middle trapezius pulls toward the left—toward the spine, it requires a direction of resistance that comes from the right (slightly anterior).

Despite the left and right sides of the middle trapezius producing movement in opposite directions, it is best to engage them simultaneously, for the sake of stability. Performing a one-sided *scapular retraction* would tend to inadvertently cause (or encourage) torso rotation. Torso rotation (rotating away from the resistance) would cause the origin of the middle trapezius to "retreat" from the approaching muscle insertion—thereby compromising contraction. For this reason, it makes more sense to engage the two sides simultaneously. The best exercise for the middle trapezius is the scapular retraction, which is discussed in Chapter 19.

The gluteus medius (Figure 16-24, left image) and minimus (Figure 16-24, right image) produce femural movement in opposite directions (lateral hip abduction), although not exclusively. These muscles also participate in posterior movement (hip extension). Generally speaking, these small muscles don't "need" dedicated lateral abduction exercise, especially when normal hip extension exercises (e.g., squats, lunges, glute extensions, etc.) are performed. Nevertheless, they can be worked by way of lateral abduction—either one side at a time (lying horizontally on a floor mat) or simultaneously, on a hip abduction ("outer thigh") machine. Because the strength capacity of these small muscles is not great, "unidirectional focus" is not required in this instance.

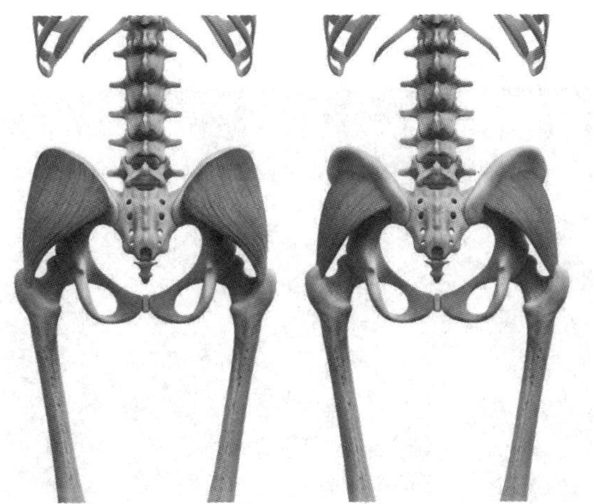
SciePro/Shutterstock.com

Figure 16-24

## "Bilateral Deficit" (BLD)

"Bilateral deficit" is a term that refers to how (often, but not always) the sum of the weight lifted by both limbs individually is greater than that which is lifted with both limbs simultaneously. For example, if you curl a pair of dumbbells with both arms simultaneously, your strength potential is generally less than if you curl a pair of dumbbells alternately—one arm at a time. This is why it's called a "deficit." The sum total of the two dumbbells you curl simultaneously (as a maximum effort) is usually less than the sum total of the two dumbbells you curl alternately.

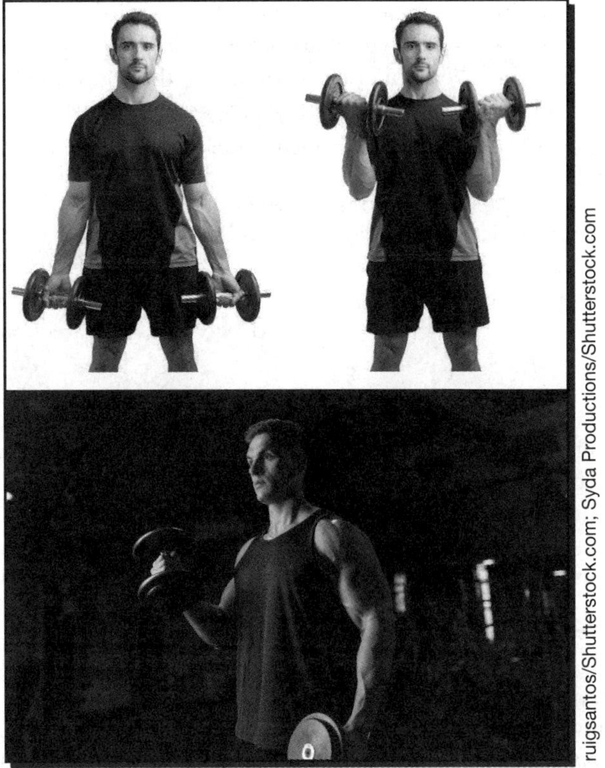
ruigsantos/Shutterstock.com; Syda Productions/Shutterstock.com

Figure 16-25

This feature is true, even if you were to pause longer between repetitions, when curling the two dumbbells simultaneously. In other words, it's NOT the slightly longer pause between repetitions, as would occur when curling alternately, that accounts for the slightly stronger capability that occurs by curling "unilaterally," compared with "bilaterally."

It is interesting to note that the sum total of curling two dumbbells simultaneously would also be less than the weight of a single barbell being curled (even if the percentage of *effort* is equal) with both arms. Of course, using a single instrument reduces the need for as much coordination and stabilization, as compared with simultaneously lifting two separate dumbbells. This is the reason why you can usually move more weight with a barbell, than you can with two dumbbells, during the same type of movement.

"Bilateral deficit" (BLD) is commonly described as follows: *"When the sum of the torque (force) generated by each limb (individually) in the unilateral condition is greater than that generated by both limbs simultaneously (bilateral condition), it is termed the bilateral limb deficit."*[8, 9] On the other hand, scientists/anatomists have not yet reached a consensus as to how BLD occurs. Among the theories that are currently being considered in that regard are the following:

- An increase in electrical activity may cause a greater recruitment/activation of muscle fiber types, while performing an exercise with one limb.
- During BL (bilateral) activity, both brain hemispheres are activated simultaneously, possibly resulting in an interhemispheric inhibition, reducing motor unit (muscle) recruitment and torque generation.
- BLD may be a result of higher muscle-shortening velocities.

The mechanism may be something similar to that which occurs during "unidirectional focus." Your cerebral attention, as well as a greater percentage of your energy, is directed toward one direction of movement—or toward one side—rather than having to be divided between two directions of movements, or two sides.

There is also the issue that on occasion, you employ slightly different mechanics when using both limbs simultaneously, versus only one limb at a time—depending on the exercise. Similar to what occurs during "unidirectional focus," the body may "need" to turn or lean toward the side that's operating, but it cannot turn or lean toward both sides simultaneously.

As such, two of the most commonly cited examples of "BLD" (in the scientific literature) are the *single-legged deadlift* (Figure 16-26) versus the regular *two-legged deadlift*, and the *single-leg jump* (Figure 16-27) versus the *two-legged jump*. Theoretically, a person doing a TWO-LEGGED deadlift while holding a 10-pound kettlebell would find that that action is NOT significantly easier than doing a ONE-LEGGED deadlift, using the same 10-pound kettlebell—as one might expect.

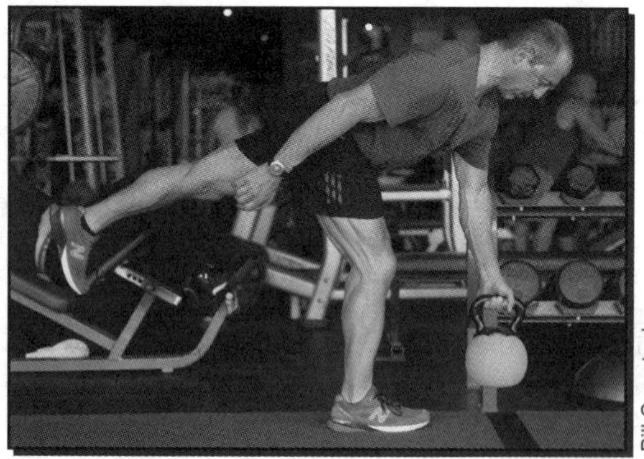


Figure 16-26

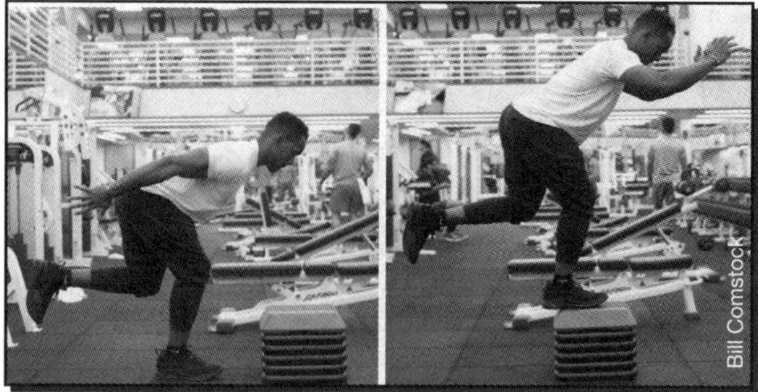


Figure 16-27

Other factors, however, are also at play in this instance, besides "one leg" versus "two legs." The legs are not the only component in a *deadlift*. The erector spinae plays a role in both the one-legged version, and the two-legged version—so there is no diminishment of strength potential in this regard. Furthermore, when the *one-legged deadlift* is performed, the leg that is not on the ground, is raised backward—rather than allowing it to stay alongside the other leg, but without touching the ground. The weight of the raised leg then becomes a counterbalance, which offsets the weight of the kettlebell, on the other side of the torso (Figure 16-28). In essence, it works like a "seesaw" at the park—both sides teetering back and forth, in balance.

This can be easily proven by putting an ankle weight on that back leg, and seeing how much more it actually assists in lifting the front end upward. If you attempted to do a *one-legged deadlift*, while keeping both legs together (even though one foot is not touching the ground), the outcome would be very different.

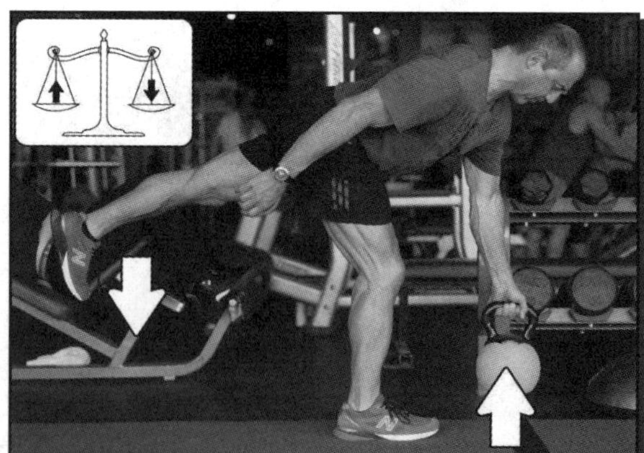


Figure 16-28

Let's examine the mechanics of the *one-legged jump* (Figure 16-29). It would seem that a person could only jump half as high when using one leg, as compared with using both legs. In reality, however, the upward thrust is NOT produced only by the legs. Some of the upward momentum (propulsion) is produced by the erector spinae (lower back) and also by the gyration of the arms. This same momentum is produced in both the one-legged and the two-legged versions.

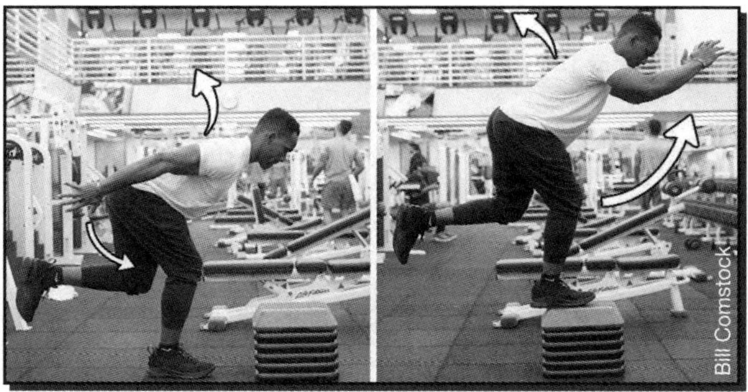


Figure 16-29

Of course, anyone who has *deadlifted* 405 pounds (e.g., an Olympic bar with four 45-pound plates on each side) knows it would be extremely difficult, if not impossible, to *deadlift* 200 pounds, using only one leg, even if one leg was lifted backward with an ankle weight. There would also be a much greater risk of injury in attempting this technique. In other words, "bilateral deficit" does not work in all scenarios. Nevertheless, the principle of "bilateral deficit" can be used productively for physique development and general fitness, as part of the preference for "independent" limb work, whenever stability is not compromised.

## Summary

Cross education is a bioneurological characteristic that allows exercise, which is performed by a limb on one side of the body, to transmit a degree of benefit from that exercise to the contralateral limb on the other side of the body, even though that contralateral limb may not have been exercised at all. This factor is useful in the rehabilitation of an injured limb, as well as for "evening-up" muscular development differences that are on opposite sides of the body.

The studies demonstrating "crossover benefit" to a contralateral limb, caused by the exercising of an ipsilateral limb, suggest that there is a distinct advantage in doing unilateral/independent limb exercise. Therefore, using dumbbells likely provides more muscular/neurological benefits than does using barbells—in addition to its other significant advantages.

The traditional definitions of "unilateral exercise" and "bilateral exercise" have failed to identify "independent" versus "non-independent" limb exercise. The traditional definitions have only accounted for repetitions that are simultaneous (left side and right side) or not, regardless of whether the simultaneity is happening with a single instrument (e.g., a barbell) or with two separate instruments (e.g., dumbbells or cable handles). Whether the repetitions are simultaneous or not matters much less than whether the limbs are working independently of each other.

The timing of the repetitions, whether they are simultaneous or alternating, also matters, as evidenced by the studies on "bilateral deficit." As such, there seems to be an advantage in performing repetitions alternately (left side, right side, etc.) or as an isolated unilateral exercise, whenever doing so does not compromise stability.

Muscles that are on the opposite sides of the body, as well as those that produce movement in opposing directions, are best worked one side at a time. The lateral deltoids and latissimus dorsi are the two muscle groups that benefit most from isolated unilateral exercise (one side at a time), as compared with simultaneous unilateral, or alternating unilateral. Furthermore, opposite direction movements (i.e., movement performed by the same muscle on each side of the body, but which produce movement in opposite directions) seem to function better when using "unidirectional focus."

## Cited References


1. Scripture EW. On the education of muscular control and power. A psychological method of determining the blind-spot. *Studies from the Yale Psychological Laboratory.* 10 volumes. Yale University. 1893-1902.
2. Lee M, Carroll T. Cross education: Possible mechanisms for contralateral effects of unilateral resistance training. School of Medical Sciences, Health and Exercise Science, University of New South Wales, Sydney, New South Wales, Australia. 2007.
3. Hortobagyi T, Lambert NJ, Hill JP. Greater cross education following training with muscle lengthening than shortening. *Med Sci Sports Exerc*. 1997; 29:107-112.

4a. Zhou S. Cross education and neuromuscular adaptations during early stage of strength training. *Journal of Exercise Science and Fitness*. 2003; 1(1):54-60.

4b. Lee M, Carroll T. Cross education: Possible mechanisms for the contralateral effects of unilateral resistance training. *Sports Medicine.* 2007; 37(1):1-14.

5. Milène C, et. al. Pronounced effects of acute endurance exercise on gene expression in resting and exercising human skeletal muscle. *Plos One.* 2012; 7:11.
6. Howard JD, Enoka RM. Maximum bilateral contractions are modified by neurally mediated interlimb effects. *J Appl Physiol.* 1991; 70:306-316.
7. da Silva JJ, et al. Unilateral plantar flexors static-stretching effects on ipsilateral and contralateral jump measures. *J Sports Sci Med.* 2015; (14)2:315-21.
8. Botton CE, et al. Bilateral deficit between concentric and isometric muscle actions. *Isokinetics & Ex Sc.* 2013; 21:161-165.
9. Bobbert MF, et al. Explanation of the bilateral deficit in human vertical squat jumping. *J. Appl Phsiology.* 2006; 100:493-499.

# CHAPTER 17

# ASSESSING AND SELECTING EXERCISES, USING "IDEAL" BIOMECHANICAL PARAMETERS

- *The previous 16 chapters addressed issues that relate to the "ideal" direction of resistance, based on physics, as well as several physiological factors (e.g., the strength curve of a muscle, cross-education, reciprocal innervation, dynamic versus isometric, etc.).*
- *The next eight chapters discuss the ideal direction of anatomical movement for each physique muscle, which can be determined by referencing the origin and insertion of a muscle, the design of the joint over which that muscle crosses, the direction of the target muscle's fibers, and the evolutionary role of that muscle.*
- *Together, these two factors—the direction of resistance and the direction of anatomical movement—allow individuals to identify the exercises that could be considered "best" for each muscle group.*
- *The same criteria that help qualify an exercise as "best" also informs individuals of which exercises qualify as "bad" (i.e., less productive, less efficient, and more risky), as well as those exercises that are in-between. As such, exercises can all be rated from "best" to "worst," in a relatively logical manner.*
- *If your goal is to maximize training efficiency (i.e., optimal muscle stimulation, least wasted effort, least risk of injury), the wisest approach is to use only the "best" exercises, and forego the exercises that rate poorly.*

Chapter 2 ("Active Levers and Neutral Levers") included a discussion of how an exercise like a standard *barbell squat* could be considered "compromised" as a quadriceps exercise, due to the fact that the tibia lever is only about 35 percent active, at best. It was also pointed out how *parallel bar dips* could be considered "compromised" as a triceps exercise, given the fact that the forearm lever is only about 11 percent active, at best.

Chapter 8 ("Opposite Position Loading") presented an overview of how a standard *seated cable rowing* exercise could be considered "compromised," due to the fact that the origins of the target muscles (latissimus and middle trapezius) are not positioned directly opposite the direction of resistance. That chapter also recommended exercises that are more efficient because they provide a better direction of resistance—one that is directly opposite the target muscle's origin.

Many exercises are compromised because they lack "efficiency"—i.e., the target muscle is not getting 100 percent of the available resistance, despite you having to produce 100 percent of the effort required to move that weight. The energy cost is high, and the benefit is less than optimal. Sometimes, the compromise occurs because the operating lever of the target muscle does not encounter a perpendicular angle with the direction of resistance, while other times it's because the direction of resistance is not coming from an angle that is directly opposite the target muscle's origins. These compromises are caused by an "incorrect" (less-than-ideal) direction of resistance, relative to the limbs of the body or the position of the target muscle.

An "incorrect" (less than optimal) direction of resistance can also be the cause of other compromises to an exercise, including misalignment (discussed in Chapter 7), a sub-optimal resistance curve (discussed in Chapter 4), and an incomplete range of motion (discussed in Chapter 9). Clearly, the direction of resistance that is provided by a given exercise has a profound effect on the efficiency and productivity of that exercise.

Separate from the compromises that are caused by an "incorrect" direction of resistance, an exercise could also be compromised because the anatomical motion it requires is not ideal. If an exercise fails to mimic the target muscle's primary movement, or if it distorts and strains a joint, the potential benefits are further compromised and injury risk increases.

It is important to identify the exact primary movement of each physique muscle. Once that motion is identified, you can easily see how departures from that specific motion would result in less efficient loading of a target muscle, and/or joint distortion.

In order for an exercise to be optimally efficient and productive, as well as maximally safe, it should meet the following criteria:

- It should mimic the target muscle's primary motion, allows a mostly full range of that motion, and does not require joint distortion/strain.
- It should utilize a direction of resistance that:
    - Is in alignment with the direction of motion, as well as with the origin and insertion of the target muscle.
    - Provides a productive resistance curve, taking into account "early phase loading" and "mechanical disadvantage."
    - Pulls in a direction that is directly opposite the target muscle's origin, for "opposite position loading."
    - Interacts with the limb(s) being operated by the target muscle, from a mostly perpendicular angle.
- It does not load non-target muscles more than the target muscle.

Exercises that fail to meet these criteria typically do so in gradations. Accordingly, those exercises that meet all these criteria are considered excellent exercises. In turn, exercises that miss one or two of these criteria are less than ideal, but could still deemed fairly good. Finally, exercises that fail to meet most of the aforementioned criteria could be judged as poor exercises.

The key point to keep in mind is that exercises all have a different set of mechanical and anatomical factors, which determine their efficiency (energy cost versus muscle load), level of productivity, and injury risk. As such, people who are in the health/fitness profession, or are competitive bodybuilders, or are otherwise dedicated to optimally efficient resistance exercise, should be familiar with the principles that qualify an exercise as "excellent," "inefficient," or "dangerous." Furthermore, you should know how to distinguish between two exercises for the same muscle—whether they are mostly redundant (i.e., the same mechanics) or not. In reality, you should be able to explain, in terms that are logical and accurate (from a physics standpoint, and from an anatomy standpoint), how each exercise works, mechanically speaking.

## Using Biomechanical Factors to Evaluate the Potential Benefits and Risks of Resistance Exercise

There are several very logical ways of identifying a muscle's primary function. The primary clue, as to any muscle's principle function, is the origin and insertion points of that muscle. When looking at an anatomical illustration of a muscle, you can clearly see where these two points are located. You can also see the joint(s) over which that muscle crosses. When that muscle contracts (i.e., shortens), the muscle insertion moves directly toward its origin, which causes the joint in between those two points to move (e.g., flex, extend, rotate, etc.).

A muscle fiber is like a rope, which pulls its insertion toward its origin. For example, the pectoralis major *participates* in numerous functions, even when you're just washing dishes over the kitchen sink. There are, however, very specific motions that can be designated as the pectoral's "purest" or "ideal" motions. Likewise, there are various motions in which the pectorals participate that can be classified as varying degrees of "NOT ideal."

In some cases, a muscle might "barely participate" in a task, because the motion being performed does not closely mimic that muscle's primary motion. On the other hand, it might be "engaged a little more" in a different task, because that task is slightly more similar to that muscle's primary function. It might "participate substantially" in another movement, because that motion is much more similar to its primary function. Finally, it could be "fully engaged" in yet another motion, because that motion is precisely what that muscle is designed to do.

One of the ways to understand this concept is to imagine yourself holding the end of a rope, which is tied to a heavy box. When you pull that rope, the only direction in which you can pull that heavy box is directly TOWARD you. You cannot pull that heavy box in any direction OTHER than toward you. Muscles operate the same way. Because the origins of a muscle are in a fixed location on the anatomy, they pull their insertion points, which is attached to a limb, directly toward that origin.

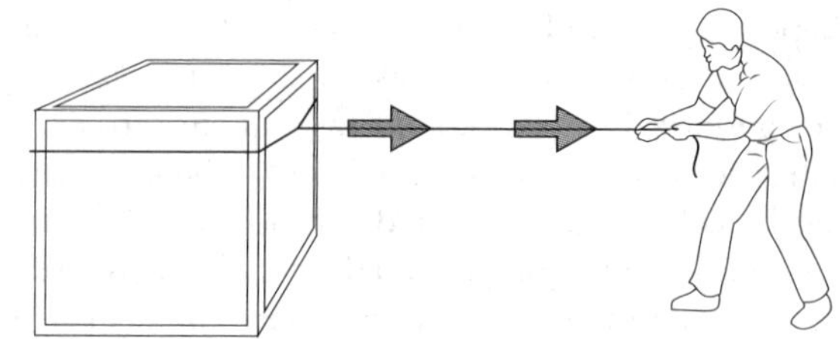

Figure 17-1

In Figure 17-2, you can see this concept applied to the anatomy. The man in this image is "standing" on a human sternum, where most of the pectoral muscle fibers originate. Imagine he is holding a pectoral fiber—like a rope—pulling a loaded humerus. The only direction in which he can pull that humerus is toward him. Of course, given that a number of the other pectoral fibers are also pulling, the humerus moves in the direction of the combined efforts. The combined efforts, however, still move the humerus toward the collective pectoral origins on the sternum (or clavicle or ribs).

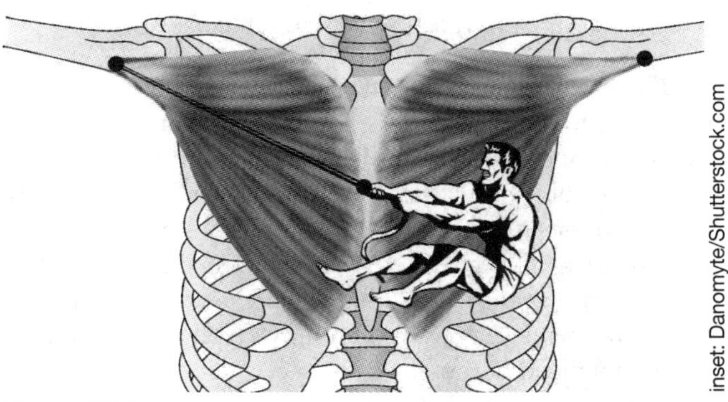


Figure 17-2

Since each muscle fiber's origin pulls directly toward itself (and only toward itself), the first step in knowing "which direction a muscle pulls" (or what motion a muscle ideally produces) is knowing where these origins are. Collectively, all of these muscular origins will be reviewed in the next eight chapters.

It's worth noting, with regard to the pectorals, that once the arms are raised so that they are perpendicular with the torso, ALL of the pectoral fibers are either parallel with the shoulder joint (which is the pivot of the humerus—the joint being moved by the pectorals) or below the shoulder joint. None are above the shoulder joint.

There are NO pectoral fiber origins above the shoulder joints, nor above the clavicles. Accordingly, it is impossible for the pectorals to participate much in pulling the arms (the humerus) in a direction that is above the shoulder joint, or above the clavicle line. Yet, one of the most common exercises performed in the gym is an *incline press*, which moves the arms in a direction where there are NO pectoral fibers.

Figure 17-3 shows the direction from which the pectorals would have to pull in order to produce an "incline" movement. As such, you would have to have pectoral fiber origins on your chin or on your neck (above the shoulder joint, and above the clavicles) in order to be directly engaging any pectoral fibers during an *incline press*. In reality, you do not have pectoral fiber origins on your chin or on your neck. In other words, *incline presses* do NOT work the upper pectorals very well, even though the conventional wisdom, for nearly a century, has been that "*the best exercise for the upper pecs is an incline press.*"

This advice is plainly incorrect. This is not an opinion. It's a physics fact. Any student of physics or an engineer can clearly see that it's impossible for a muscle (or a pulley, or a rope) to pull a lever in a direction toward which it is not located.

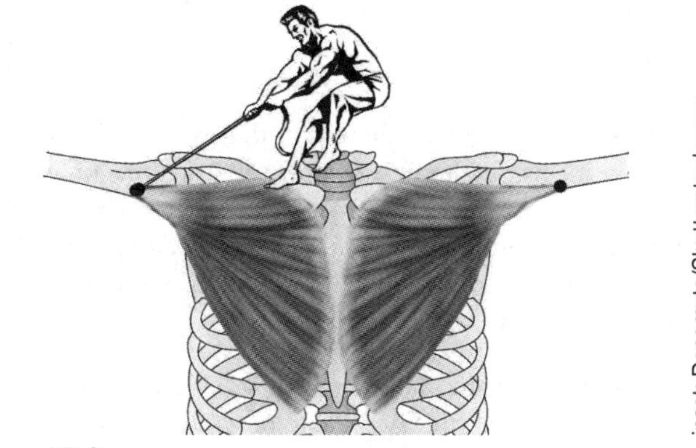


Figure 17-3

The aforementioned is one example of how understanding that "muscles always pull toward their origin" (and knowing where the muscle origin and insertion points are) enable you to determine what the ideal anatomical motion for each muscle might be. It also allows you to see how a decades-long belief (i.e., that *incline presses* "target" the upper pecs) can be demonstrably proven false.

## The Role of Evolution in Determining Natural Human Motion

Although no one currently on the planet was alive a million years ago, we can make reasonable assumptions about the physical tasks that our early ancestors probably needed to do from day to day. It's reasonable to assume that there were no "incline exercise benches" during those days. Any "weights" that were lifted were logs and heavy rocks, and those could not possibly have been moved in a direction that was 45 degrees upward from the torso and opposite gravity (i.e., an "incline" angle)—certainly not on a regular basis, if at all.

We humans evolved from quadrupeds (i.e., arms perpendicular with the torso) and gradually began walking more upright, using the pectoral muscles and shoulder joint in increasingly more downward ("decline") directions. The fact that the pectoral muscle is positioned entirely below the arm line (where the arm connects to the torso), demonstrates that it evolved to push in directions that were straightforward and in various degrees of "downward" (decline), over millions of years.

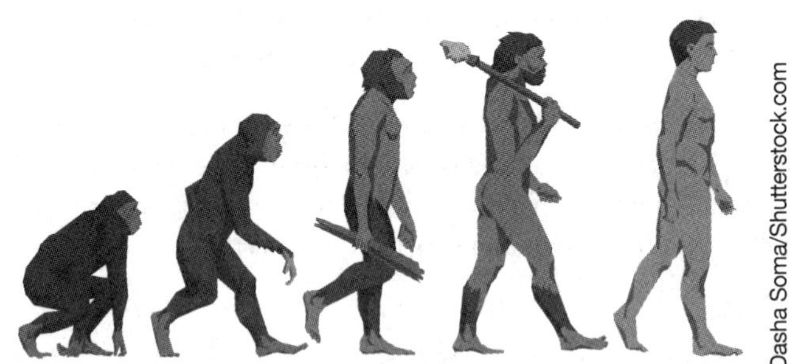

Dasha Soma/Shutterstock.com

Figure 17-4

It is safe to surmise, therefore, that pushing/moving the humerus in an "incline" direction (upward/diagonal to the torso) was not an evolutionary "need" for survival. Neither the shoulder joint, nor the position of the pectorals, in relation to the shoulder joint, have the apparent design of evolving to accommodate that motion.

The fact that the shoulder joint is ABLE to produce that movement (i.e., an "incline" angle press) is not evidence that the pectoral muscles were meant to perform that task, nor that the pectorals will benefit from that task. As another example of this, we are able to put our forearm behind our back, even though there was probably very little evolutionary need for that capability, nor do we attempt to perform *biceps curls* behind our back.

In addition to there being a correlation between the way our muscles perform today and the evolutionary needs of our early ancestors, there is also a correlation between the way our joints operate today and the evolutionary needs of our early ancestors. For example, it is not likely that our early ancestors needed to push a heavy log or rock, directly (straight) over their heads, up and down, repeatedly. What could possibly have been the purpose of that? Of course, that is the movement that today people call an *overhead press*—a motion for which humans had no evolutionary need to adapt.

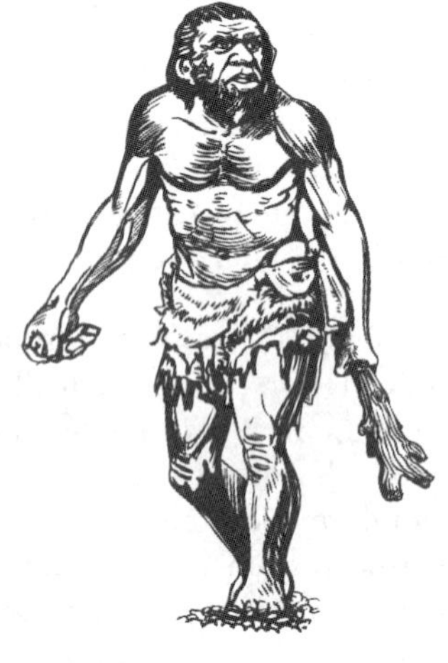

Cimmerian/Shutterstock.com

Figure 17-5

They may have needed to push or throw a heavy log or rock, in a forward direction, in battle, or in labor. Having to push a heavy object in a straight-upward direction (vertically, overhead) or in an "incline" direction—repetitively—however, is extremely unlikely.

The fact that the shoulder joint was not designed for the arms to repeatedly push straight upward is corroborated when the shoulder joint is examined. You can see that "impingement" (pinching) of the supraspinatus tendon, as well as the subacromial bursa, is inevitable when moving the arms directly overhead. It's obvious the shoulder joint did not evolve to allow that motion, repetitively, without consequence.

The following eight chapters review the primary function of each "physique" muscle and its corresponding joint(s), sometimes referencing the likely evolutionary tasks each muscle and joint needed to accommodate. We can then see if those motions mimic the common exercises used today, for those muscles. The goal is to examine whether the motion of common exercises is "ideal," and whether there are other movements (exercises) that more closely resemble each muscle's intended purpose.

## Determining Which Movements Are Most "Natural," Most Productive, and Most Safe

Instead of assuming that a muscle would most benefit most from a complex movement, it's more logical to assume that a simple movement would be most beneficial to a muscle. For example, look at the lateral deltoid (Figure 17-6). Consider the simplicity of the insertion point on the humerus ("A") moving directly toward the origin point on the scapula ("B"), as the muscle contracts. That action would raise the arm to the side—a movement called "lateral abduction" (aka "*side raise*"). It is the purest, most natural function of the lateral deltoid.

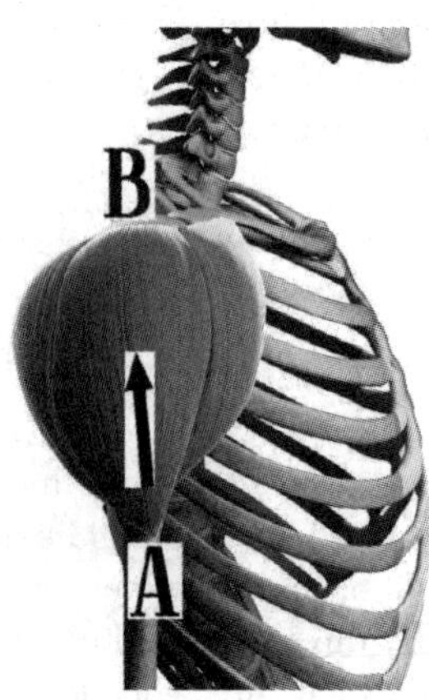


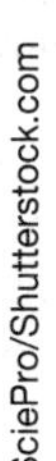


Figure 17-6

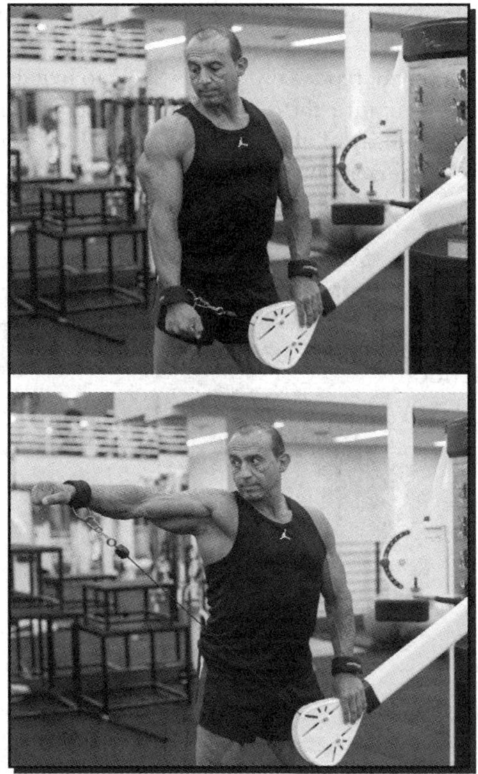

Figure 17-7

Performing this muscle's most natural function—a *side raise*—with the ideal direction of resistance and sufficient load, is all that is required to maximally stimulate muscular development of the lateral deltoids. Nothing more complicated is necessary.

Despite it being obvious, however, that "lateral abduction" is this muscle's most natural movement, and despite it being obvious that moving the arms overhead repeatedly causes shoulder "impingement," many people still believe that the *overhead press* (Figure 17-8) is either a "good" shoulder exercise or "the best" exercise for the lateral deltoids.

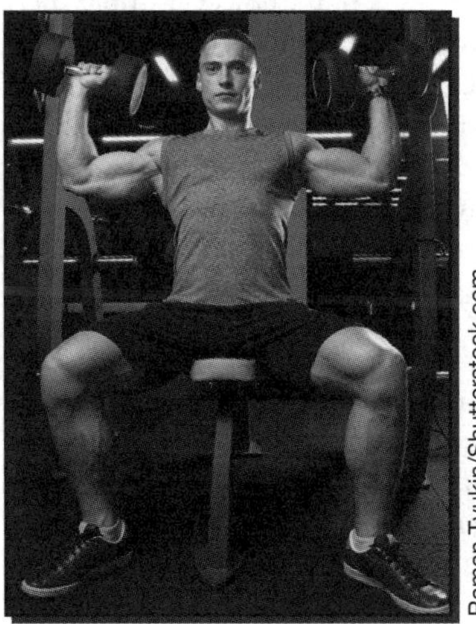

Figure 17-8

In reality, the *overhead press* requires an extreme degree of shoulder joint rotation, just to assume the starting position. In Figure 17-9, you can see the degree of external humeral rotation—a full 90 degrees from its "normal/natural" position—that is required in order to do this exercise correctly. For many individuals, this much external rotation of the humerus is impossible.

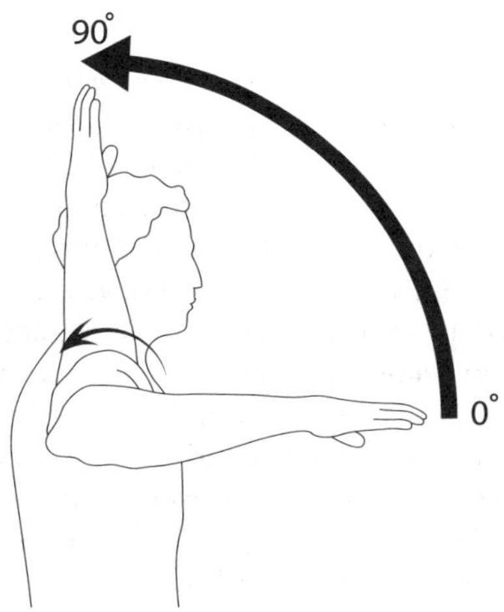

Figure 17-9

For the many people who are unable to position their humerus vertically, the forward slant of their forearm will strain the external rotator cuff muscle (the infraspinatus), when using a heavy weight. In addition, moving the arms directly overhead, repeatedly, with resistance, is the most common cause of impingement syndrome—where the suprasinatus tendon and/or subacromial bursa are squeezed between the humerus and the acromion process (the upper/outer edge of the scapula), causing inflammation and, on occasion, a rupture.

As if these two potential risk factors are not enough to disqualify the *overhead press* as a "good" exercise, there is also the fact that the external rotation of the humerus moves the target muscle (the lateral deltoids) out of alignment with the direction of resistance. As a result, rather than getting 100 percent of the downward resistance, the lateral deltoids only get about 40 percent of the downward resistance.

The point to keep in mind is that the *overhead press* is not "natural" motion—neither for the individual muscles involved, nor for the shoulder joint. It does not mimic any motion for which humans have evolved. As a result, it has a much higher injury risk than does "*side raises*," and it also has a much more compromised benefit.

In fact, the *overhead press* is a movement that was "inherited" from turn-of-the-century circus performers whose primary objective was simply to move an impressive amount of weight, for the entertainment of observers. It was NOT "designed" with proper biomechanics in mind.

*Upright rows* is another exercise that requires an unnatural motion. People often describe this exercise as "uncomfortable," but they do it anyway, because they think the discomfort might be their own unique problem. They also believe that the industry would not mislead them. In fact, *upright rows* force you to bend your wrists sideways, and also forces internal rotation of the shoulder joint. In addition to these two skeletal strains, the exercise then provides the deltoids with less loading than do simple *side raises*.

Yet another unnatural motion is *overhead triceps extensions*. The primary function of the triceps muscle is to extend the elbow, and it does this the same, whether the arms are down alongside the torso or overhead. Having the arms down alongside the torso is the more natural position for the shoulder joint. So, a reasonable question to ask is, "Why would you do a triceps exercise with arms overhead, if the triceps works the same either way, and it's more uncomfortable with the arms overhead?." Of course, there are those individuals who would argue that overhead triceps exercises stimulate the triceps "differently," than do the exercises performed with the arms down. In fact, however, as you'll soon see, there is no logic nor science behind that belief.

Across the board, you'll see that the less contorted an exercise is, and the more its motion resembles the way the body naturally moves and has evolved, the better the exercise. There is no advantage, in terms of muscle-building benefit, in overcomplicating a resistance exercise. Keeping it simple and "natural" is the best strategy for optimizing the benefit and minimizing injury risk.

## Referencing Joint Design in Exercise Evaluation

Another "clue" that informs us of a muscle's "ideal" motion is the design of the joint over which that muscle crosses. By understanding that joint's natural function, we are better able to understand the skeletal motion its corresponding muscle produces. We can also better understand what is NOT an ideal motion—when you identify the limitations of a joint—and the consequence of forcing a joint to move in a direction it was not meant to move.

For example, when you examine the elbow joint, you can easily see that it only moves in one direction—it "opens" and "closes" like a hinge. The biceps, which crosses the elbow joint, is the primary muscle that bends (flexes) the elbow. Since the elbow only bends in ONE direction, and since both biceps "heads" merge into one single tendon, both heads of the biceps must participate simultaneously, anytime "elbow flexion" occurs. There is simply no way you could preferentially activate the "inner head" or the "outer head" of the biceps, because both parts share the same tendon, and the elbow only bends in one direction.

An examination of the shoulder joint is also very revealing. It's very easy to see how "pushing" the humerus directly overhead, repeatedly, is very likely to irritate, inflame, and possibly rupture the supraspinatus tendon (and/or the subacromial bursa) of the shoulder joint. This condition is known as "impingement syndrome" (Figure 17-10).

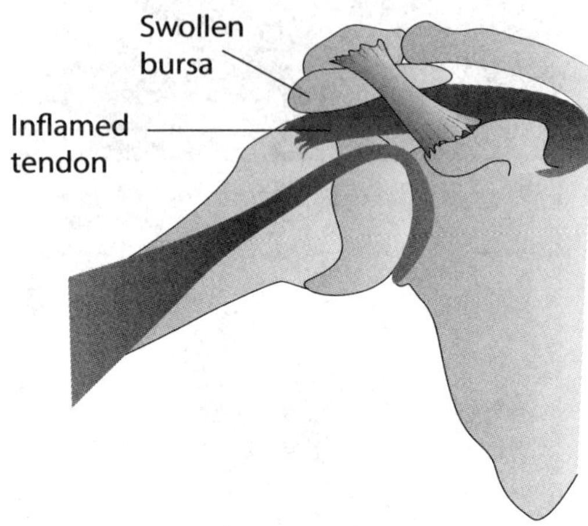


Figure 17-10

Some people are fortunate, and never develop impingement syndrome, despite doing *overhead presses* regularly, for many years. This outcome, however, is like the life-long cigarette smoker who never develops lung cancer. There's plenty of evidence that smoking causes lung cancer, just as there's plenty of evidence that frequent, repeated, weighted, *overhead pressing* movement tends to cause impingement syndrome. The few exceptions to the rule do not prove that overhead pressing is perfectly safe, just as the fact that some smokers never get lung cancer does not prove that cigarette smoking is safe.

Yes, your shoulder joint does allow you to lift and place a heavy box on a high shelf, or hold an object over your head for short periods of time—without consequence. This is considerably different, however, than performing heavy *overhead presses* on a regular basis. More importantly, the deltoids can be developed perfectly well without doing *overhead presses*, and the deltoid strength gained from doing *lateral abduction* (i.e., side raises) can be effectively used for placing a heavy box on a high shelf. As such, the *overhead press* is not a "necessary" exercise for developing the deltoids.

An examination of the scapula (the shoulder blade) reveals something interesting as well. The motion of pulling the arms downward, from an overhead position, is much more safe than pushing a weight upward. This is because the upward pull of resistance (coming from *bodyweight chin-ups* or *cable pulldowns*) pulls the scapula upward, which allows there to be more clearance between the humerus and the acromion process (Figure 17-11).

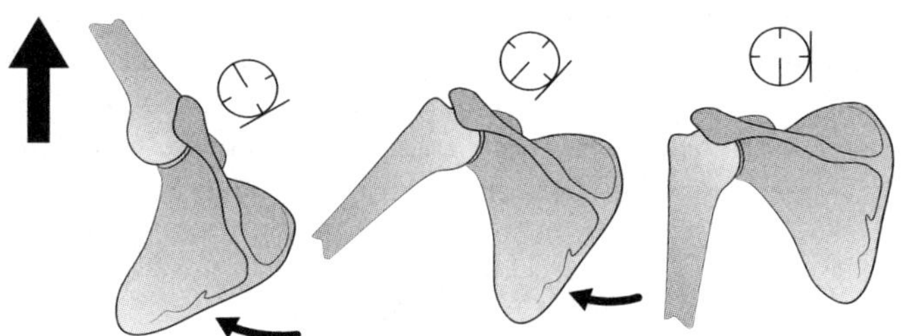

Figure 17-11

Conversely, the downward resistance utilized during *overhead presses* holds the scapula down, while the humerus moves upward underneath it. This factor contributes to the circumstances that lead to the pinching of the supraspinatus tendon and bursa. Again, this fact should not be surprising, in light of the evolution of humans. It's easy to imagine our early ancestors climbing and pulling downward on tree branches, even though the angle of that pulling was slightly different than a "*lat pulldown*" or a "*chin-up.*" It's not so easy to imagine an early human having to push a heavy object straight upward, vertically, on a regular basis. The evolutionary need to pull downward (with frequency) was present, but the evolutionary need to push upward (with frequency) was not.

## Referencing the Direction of a Muscle's Fibers

On occasion, the direction of a muscle's fibers indicates the direction of movement that would constitute the ideal movement for that particular muscle. In those cases, it's obvious that the muscle fibers would be pulling their operating lever (i.e., limb) toward the muscle's origin—a pathway that is parallel to those muscle fibers.

For example, the pectoral fibers essentially "point" in the direction they pull the humerus—toward the pectoral origins located on the sternum, clavicles, and ribs. Clearly, that movement would be parallel to those pectoral fibers. This factor is also true with the latissimus dorsi, as well as the biceps. Not all muscle fibers, however, are "straight," like those of the pecs, lats, and biceps (Figure 17-12).

In fact, there are seven types of "muscle architecture." Three of these have fibers that run in straight lines; another three have fibers that run diagonal to the origin and insertion of the muscle; and one has circular fibers. This last one is irrelevant, in a discussion about skeletal movement and biomechanics.

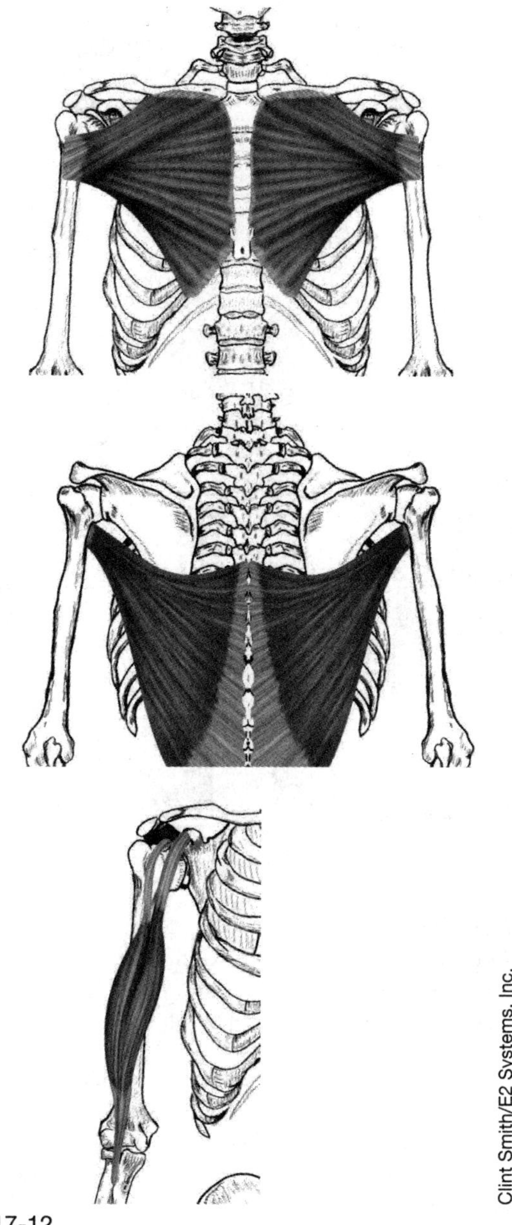



Figure 17-12

Figure 17-13 shows all seven types of muscle architecture. "Convergent," "fusiform," and "parallel" (the top three on the left) all have fibers that could be considered "straight." They run in the same direction as the line that can be drawn between the muscle origin and insertion. The primary difference between these three is the way they converge with their tendon.

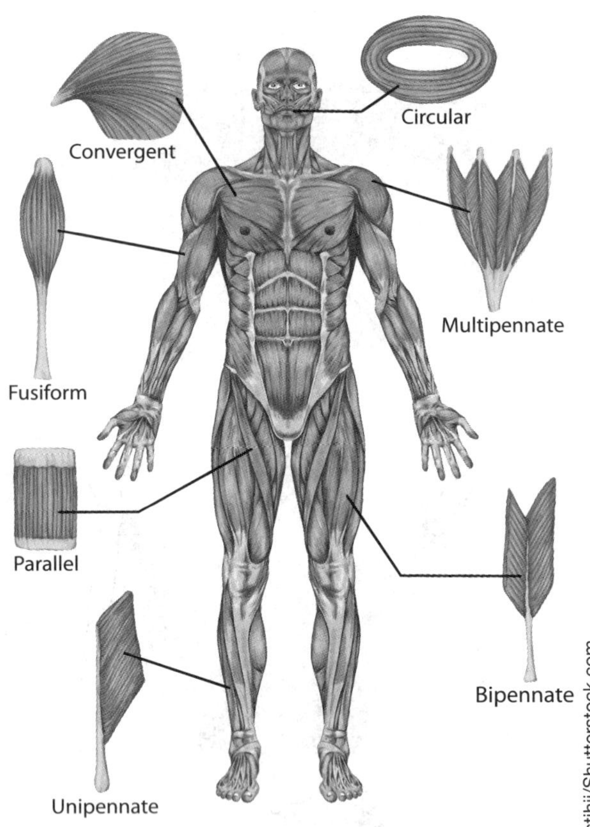

Figure 17-13

The next three (Figure 17-13, moving counterclockwise) have fibers that cross diagonally to the line that can be drawn between the muscle origin and insertion. These are called "unipennate," "bipennate," and "multipennate."

The seventh type of muscle architecture is called "circular" (Figure 17-13, top right), and is only found at the opening of the eyes, mouth, and anus. This factor is why this particular type of muscle architecture is not relevant in a discussion of biomechanics.

"Pennate" muscles have a stronger ability to contract, as compared with straight muscle fibers. This is because pennate fibers pull on their tendon from an angle, so they don't need to move their tendon as far as straight muscle fibers do. This situation is similar to the physics of a bicycle that has a "low gear" for hills and a "high gear" for flats. Pennate muscles are essentially "low gear" muscles. In essence, they trade shorter distance for greater power (torque).

A pennate muscle also packs more muscle fibers into a given space, because they're angled. This factor adds more strength capacity, as compared with a parallel muscle of the same size. The more muscle fibers, the more myofibrils and sarcomeres, which translates to greater power.

You should note that the triceps and the quadriceps have "cross-hatching" striations, while the pecs, lats, biceps, and hamstrings have straight muscle striations. Notice that the triceps and quadriceps are "extension" muscles, while the pecs, lats, biceps, and hamstrings are "flexion" muscles.

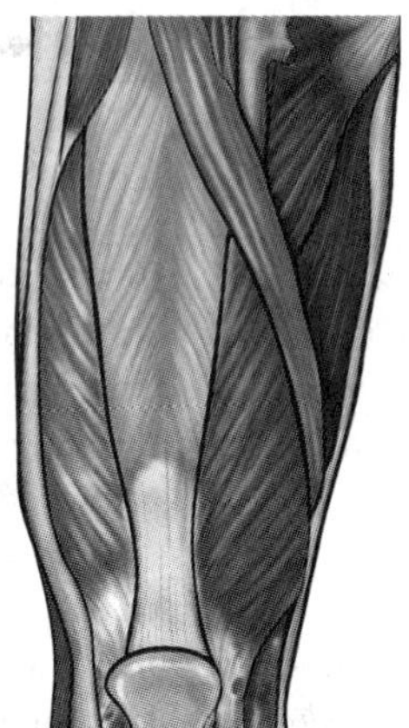
Figure 17-14

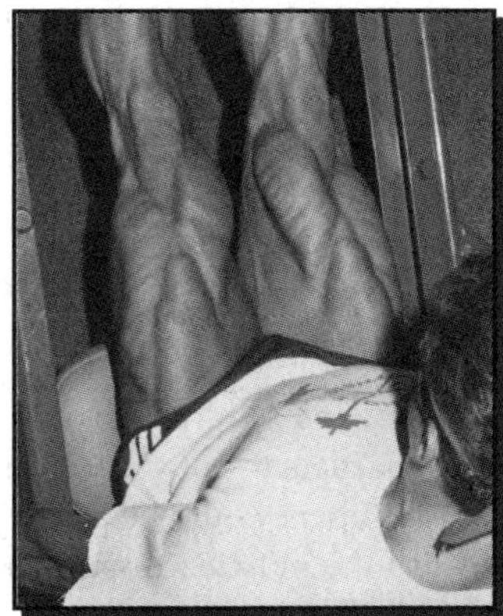
Figure 17-15

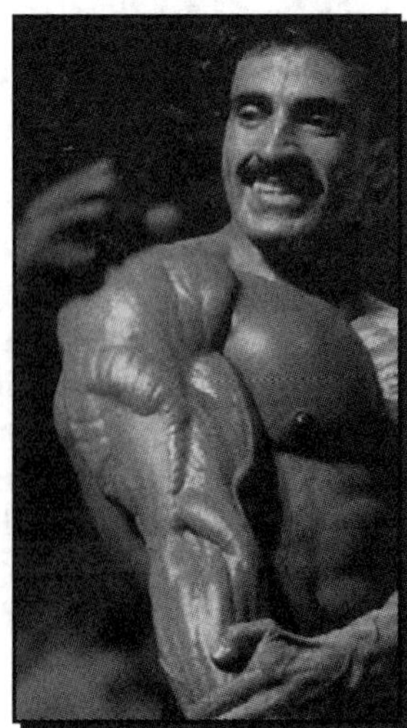
Figure 17-16

In Chapter 3, it was made clear that muscles which "flex" a joint (e.g., pectorals, biceps, hamstrings, etc.) are more vulnerable to rupture, as compared with muscles that "extend" a joint. The apparent reason for this is that muscles which extend a joint have adapted to the fact that they ALWAYS operate with a mechanical disadvantage. As such, they always require more force. Clearly, most extension muscles have evolved as pennate muscles to accommodate that need.

Conversely, muscles which flex a joint have the "advantage" of being able to pull perpendicularly on their respective bones (at least during part of their range of motion), and this allows them to produce anatomical movement with less muscle force. As such, they evolved as straight muscle fibers.

Therefore, you can only use "muscle fiber direction" as an indicator of the "ideal" direction of motion for an exercise, when examining muscles that flex a joint. You cannot use it when examining a muscle that extends a joint. When you are identifying the ideal skeletal motion produced by a pennate muscle (a muscle that extends a joint), you can draw a line between the muscle's origins and insertion, which serves equally well as an indicator of the ideal direction of limb movement for that muscle.

## Recognizing the Difference Between Bad, Good, Better, and Best Exercises

Once the ideal anatomical motion has been identified for a particular muscle, the next step is to identify the ideal direction of resistance for that motion. Combining these two—the ideal anatomical motion and the ideal direction of resistance—reveals the exercises that can be classified as "best"—the most efficient, most productive and least risk of injury.

The ideal direction of resistance provides proper alignment, an optimal resistance curve (early phase loading and relief from mechanical disadvantage if necessary), opposite position loading, and the highest efficiency (the use of mostly "active" operating levers, as per Chapter 2). As you can imagine, this combination of mechanical characteristics greatly narrows down the number of exercises that can be classified as "ideal." It also enables you to have a sense of which exercises are farthest from "ideal," and which ones would fall somewhere in between.

Theoretically, a person could use a "checklist" of these mechanical requirements, and issue each exercise a ranking. This step could be done either on the basis of "first best, second best, third best," etc., or by giving each exercise a rating between 1 and 10, with 10 being best. This undertaking would be a "judgment call," to some degree—although a very well-informed judgment call.

For example, as you have learned, *parallel bar dips* load the triceps with approximately HALF as much resistance as a *supine dumbbell triceps extension* ("DB skull crushers"), even though four times more weight is used during *parallel bar dips*. This factor would qualify *supine dumbbell triceps extensions* as being "better than" *parallel bar dips*—as a triceps exercise. In fact, you could rate *supine dumbbell triceps extensions* as a "9" or "10," and rate *parallel bar dips* as a "4" (as a triceps exercise), although other mechanical factors also must be taken into consideration.

Logically speaking, the following question should arise: "If an individual is truly dedicated to physique development, and wants maximum efficiency (i.e., the most benefit, the least wasted effort, the least injury risk), why would he bother using exercises that rate lower than a 9 or a 10?" I am not necessarily suggesting that an exercise that rates a "5" should never be used. After all, an exercise that rates a "5" is better than nothing. This factor is especially true if you have no idea how to assess an exercise, and don't know which exercises are better.

Ideally speaking, however, a person who selects an exercise that rates a "5" should be aware that they are using a less efficient/less productive exercise. As it is now, most people think that all exercises are relatively equal in "value" (efficiency, productivity and safety). All factors considered, they believe this, because the industry has done a poor job of establishing the parameters by which resistance exercises can be assessed and rated.

Resistance exercises are not all equally productive, equally efficient, and equally safe, in terms of injury risk. If you want to "mix it up" (i.e., use a wide variety of exercises) for the sake of fun or convenience, that's fine, provided you understand that many of those exercises are less productive, less efficient, and less safe.

Of course, doing only the exercises that are rated highest, may make workouts seem more repetitive or monotonous, at least for some people. This prospect is likely to make some people nervous, because they've heard for so long that they need to "change exercises frequently." That assertion, however, is simply not true. It is based entirely on unsubstantiated speculation.

Many people have been led to believe that certain exercises "shape" muscles differently, and that changing exercises frequently provides "necessary variety" to prevent "stagnation." These beliefs are entirely false, as you'll soon see.

Furthermore, some of the exercises that are most exciting to watch are NOT the most productive for muscular development, and exercises that are most productive for muscular development are often not very exciting to watch. Generally speaking, the exercises that are most productive are usually much less dramatic to photograph or video-record.

As an example, it's more "exciting" to see someone *squatting* 500 pounds, than it is to see someone using maximum effort on *sissy squats* or on *glute extensions* (on a multi-hip machine). On the other hand, these "less dramatic, but mechanically superior" exercises produce better results (with much less energy cost and injury risk), even though they are less visually exciting or impressive.

If a person is able to separate their ego from the assessment of an exercise, it is likely they will immediately feel the advantage of using "better" exercises. There is no denying that they'll experience a higher quality of muscle contraction, muscle soreness, muscle gain, and relief from joint pain. Other individuals, however, will be afraid to use only the more highly rated exercises. Instead, they will combine the highly rated exercises with other, less-productive exercises. As a result, they will not know exactly which exercises contributed more or less to their results—perhaps even assuming that the lower-rated exercises contributed more, and the higher-rated exercises contributed less. Thus, they'll continue wasting time and energy using the less-productive exercises, because they're not able to let go of their emotional attachment to the less productive (but more dramatic) exercises.

Some individuals will declare with absolute—but misguided—certainty that, "It is essential for them to change exercises every four to six seeks, so that their muscles don't adapt to the exercises." Yet, despite their commitment to that notion, this theory has never been proven. Be assured, the person making that statement has never personally tested that theory. Furthermore, the individual from whom that person "learned" it (heard it) has also never personally tested it. Everyone just embraces it without either requiring proof or exhibiting an appropriate level of skepticism.

## Is Changing Exercises Regularly Necessary?

While there are some advantages to changing exercises occasionally, achieving a physiological benefit is NOT one of them. Yes, it can be more fun to change exercises, and, on occasion, it may be more convenient. For example, the station or equipment you want to use may not be available. The claim that a muscle benefits from changing exercises, however, is entirely false.

In order to help clarify the issue, consider the following simple question: What does a muscle "sense" from an exercise? For example, imagine that you are a pectoral muscle, for a moment. Imagine that one end of you is holding onto the point of origin (on the sternum), while the other end is holding onto the insertion point (on the humerus). Because you have no eyes, you cannot see anything the person who is exercising is doing. All you can do is feel. As the muscle, you cannot possibly "know" (sense) any of the following:

- You do not know what the resistance source is (e.g., free weight, cable, machine, etc.).
- You do not know the position of the person (standing, sitting, lying supine, facing north, facing south, etc.).
- You do not know whether you (the muscle) are working alone (i.e., "isolated"), or with the help of other muscles ("compound"). You are just performing your function.
- You do not know whether the resistance you feel is comprised of a heavy weight with less magnification (i.e., a short lever, mechanical advantage, and a mostly neutral lever), or a lighter weight with greater magnification (i.e., a longer lever, mechanical disadvantage, and a mostly active lever). All you know is the amount of "net" resistance you're feeling.

On the other hand, you (as the muscle) DO "know" (sense) the following:

- You know whether you're performing a full range of motion, a partial range of motion, or a static contraction (no range of motion).
- You know whether the resistance is greater at the beginning of the range of motion and lighter at the end of the range of motion, or vice versa (i.e., the "resistance curve," "early phase loading" versus late phase loading).
- You know whether the load you are lifting is "heavy," thereby limiting you to to six repetitions ... or whether it's "light," allowing you to perform 20 or 30 repetitions.
- You know whether you are working at near maximum capacity, or not ... whether you're feeling a high degree of fatigue, or not.
- You know whether your insertion is moving directly toward your origin during the concentric phase, or not.

Each of these five ("do-know)" factors are "biomechanical components." As such, each of these characteristics has a "better than" or "worse than" value. As such, any change of exercise that affects the biomechanical components will be perceived by the muscle as either "superior" or "inferior"—relative to the biomechanical components of another exercise. They will not simply be perceived as merely "different."

For example, it is better to use full range of motion, rather than partial range of motion. It is better to use early phase loading, rather than late phase loading. It is better for a muscle to contract dynamically, rather than isometrically. It is better for a muscle to pull its operating lever directly toward its origin, than not. It is better to have the resistance pulling directly away from the muscle's origin, than from a different direction.

As such, it is never advantageous to change from an exercise that has "good biomechanical components" to an exercise that has "inferior biomechanical components." In fact, any change that does not alter the biomechanical components of an exercise will not be perceived by the muscle as a change at all—which is fine, if those components are "good."

## Does the Body Really Adapt to the Same Exercises?

This belief is without logic or common sense, let alone scientific evidence. For perspective, consider the following comparative examples.

Exposure to UV light produces stimulation of pigment in the skin, which results in a TAN. A person's skin gets darker, little by little, until they reach a limit, in terms of skin pigmentation. When that happens, should a person switch to a different type of light? Incandescent? Fluorescent? Infrared? No, because UV light is BEST for the stimulation of pigment. The other types of light are "inferior" options, for the purpose of tanning. Ultimately, the person is better off staying with the "superior" type of light, rather than switching to "inferior" types of light (i.e., for the purpose of tanning). "Variety" does not supersede quality.

Of course, a person can only get so tan. Likewise, a person can only get so muscular. As such, skipping a week of sun exposure can make UV light "new" again. A person will not only resume the tanning process, but may also be susceptible to burning. Likewise, skipping a week of exercise makes all exercise "new" again, even when the same exercises are used. A person will resume the muscle stimulation process, and may even be susceptible to overtraining.

Another example is the food we consume. If you were to eat the 50 most nutritious foodstuffs on a daily basis, would you ever become "accustomed" (adapted) to those foods, such that you would be unable to extract the nutrients from them? Of course not. Accordingly, would there be any benefit to switching to "different" (but less nutritious/inferior) food occasionally? Of course not. Again, variety does not supersede quality.

Likewise, it is foolish to change from a highly efficient exercise (such as *decline dumbbell triceps extensions*) to a less efficient exercise (like *triceps kickbacks*), and expect to either load the muscle more, or achieve better development. The muscle will simply perceive that change as "inferior," and will benefit less from it—even if it results in more muscle soreness.

For a number of years, I went along with the belief that I needed to use a variety of exercises, changing exercises frequently. Eventually, however, I realized that this did not make sense. Once I understood what constitutes "superior biomechanics" of an exercise, and I identified the best one or two exercises for each muscle, I began using only that one (or two) exercises for each muscle, every time I worked those muscles.

The result was better development, less wasted energy, and less joint soreness (less joint strain). It has not resulted in my muscles changing their genetically determined shape, as some might expect. In fact, I have successfully trained for competition using those same exercises—without any sort of "variety"—and my results are better than when I did rotate my exercises.

There are other aspects of your workout that you can change, based on the timetable of your goal, including varying the intensity of an exercise (more weight/more repetitions/less rest between sets, etc.), as well as increasing the overall volume of work (i.e., more total sets)—both of which do benefit the muscle. There is no real benefit, however, to doing multiple exercises, per body part, per workout, nor in changing exercises every four to six weeks.

In fact, pectorals and trapezius are the only two muscles which can benefit from performing two exercises/two different angles (i.e., direction of movement and direction of resistance). All other muscles only require one exercise—a second exercise being redundant. This does not mean that doing two or three exercises per workout, per muscle, would be less productive—although it may be (depending on the exercises selected). Rather, it is meant to suggest that performing two or three exercises per muscle, per workout, is not necessary. It is not more advantageous than doing one good exercise, per muscle, per workout, and it would likely result in some wasted effort and/or a higher risk of injury. Of course, this analysis assumes the same total number of sets are used in both scenarios.

## Testing the Theory

The reason the following statement can be said with confidence—"*no one has ever tested the theory*"—is because relatively few people are willing to do only one exercise, for each physique muscle, for an extended period of time (six months or more), as an experiment. Even fewer would know how to conduct the test properly.

To be clear, the test would not be comparing the results of performing one random exercise for a six-month period of time, against the results of performing four other random exercises in rotation, for a six-month period of time. Rather, the test should be designed to compare the results of doing one single exercise that rates a "10" (in terms of efficiency) for a given muscle, against the results of doing four different exercises that rate less than 10, in rotation, for that same muscle. As such, a person would need to know what constitutes a "10," in terms of exercise efficiency.

The following scenario describes how such an experiment would be done wrong. A person uses one "random" triceps exercise, consistently, for the first six months—and that exercise that happens to rate a "5." For the following six months, four other triceps exercises are randomly selected, and they rate a "4," "6," "7," and "8."

The outcome of this process would be misleading. The results would be better (in terms of muscle growth) during the second half of the experiment, but not for the reason you would likely assume. The result would not be more successful, because the exercises were rotated. It would be more successful, because the four exercises used for the second half of the experiment had an average rating of 6.25, which is higher than the 5 rating of the exercise used for the first half of the experiment.

Conversely, if the triceps exercise selected for the first half of the experiment rates a "10," and the same other triceps exercises ("4," "6," "7," and "8") are used for the second half of the experiment, the result would be very different. The single triceps exercise that rates a "10" would produce a better result in the first six months, as compared with the four triceps exercises that average a "6.25" rating, over the course of the next six months.

Efficient exercises (those that rate a "10") load the muscle most, waste the least amount of energy, have the most productive resistance curve, do not strain the joints, and create the least risk of injury—even when they're used exclusively. In reality, it is NEVER more productive to switch from an exercise that rates a "10" to an exercise that rates a "5" or "6."

## Summary

Assessing an exercise from the perspective of biomechanical efficiency (maximum load on the target muscle, minimum wasted/unproductive effort, minimal injury risk) requires knowledge of three categories:

- "Ideal" anatomical motion for each physique muscle, based on:
  - Target muscle insertions moving directly toward target muscle origins
  - Movements occurring in ways that are most "natural" to the muscles and joints
  - Sufficient range of motion/dynamic muscle contraction
- "Ideal" direction of resistance, in order to provide:
  - Alignment
  - Opposite position loading
  - Early phase loading/optimal resistance curve
  - Relief from mechanical disadvantage, where necessary
  - Mostly "active" levers working for the target muscle, mostly "neutral" levers working for the non-target muscles
- Basic muscle physiology:
  - Selecting a resistance curve that matches the strength curve of the muscle
  - Utilizing dynamic exercise, instead of isometric exercise
  - Utilizing "independent"/unilateral exercise, whenever possible
  - Working "with" reciprocal innervation—avoiding it when necessary, and incorporating it when useful

An exercise that complies with all of the aforementioned prerequisites is more productive, more efficient, and more safe. The degree to which an exercise fails to comply with these prerequisites results in a commensurate loss of efficiency, compromised productivity, and/or a tendency to cause injury or strain. In other words, the more "imperfect" the exercise is (in terms of its biomechanical components), the less beneficial it is, as well as the more risky it is.

Accordingly, you can thus determine which exercises are "best" for each physique muscle, which exercises are compromised, and to what degree they are compromised. This evaluation allows you to establish which exercises are "bad," "good," "better," and "best."

A compound exercise can also be evaluated this way. The exercise could be deemed "good," if its individual components (its various moving parts) are each optimally productive and safe. Conversely, a compound exercise that combines two or more motions, of which one or more motions are contorted, out of alignment, not 100 percent natural, or have a compromised resistance curve, must be valued less, for that reason.

A muscle typically produces one primary "ideal" motion. In other words, it moves its muscle insertion directly toward its origin during the concentric phase, and directly away from its origin during the eccentric phase. This factor literally defines the pathway of the limb that is operated by that muscle. Further, an ideal motion does not contort the joint that that muscle operates.

When an ideal anatomical motion is combined with the ideal direction of resistance, it is not necessary to use more than one exercise for that muscle, per workout—or ever. That one exercise stimulates the muscle to the optimum degree. A second exercise would either be inferior or redundant.

In reality, there aren't "multiple ways" a muscle needs to be worked for the goal of physique development and general fitness. When a highly rated exercise is used, the entire muscle is stimulated. There aren't parts of the muscle that do not get simulated, simply because multiple exercises were not used. The only exceptions to this rule (and only to a degree) are the pectorals and the trapezius, which require two different directions of motion.

Furthermore, a muscle cannot change its genetically-determined shape, regardless of which exercises are used.

A muscle also does not get "accustomed" to an exercise, such that it no longer benefits from that exercise. If an exercise has excellent biomechanical components, a muscle will always benefit from that exercise, even if that exercise is used exclusively. Switching from an excellent exercise to an exercise that has inferior biomechanical components will benefit the muscle less.

A muscle "super-compensates" (adapts up/improves) to accommodate the stress it experienced from a recent exercise session. Super-compensation results in an increased level of muscle strength, muscle fiber thickness, muscle endurance, etc. This process only takes three to six days. After that, the muscle begins "deconditioning," if not exercised again. It returns to its baseline after approximately 14 days, which is why you need to work a muscle again every three to six days, if you want the hypertrophy to continue.

As such, there's no need to "shock" the muscle with a new exercise. A muscle is "shocked" every time it is exposed to the stress of an exercise, whether that exercise is different or not. The muscle is constantly adapting up and deconditioning down from its last exercise-induced stress. If you want to "shock" a given muscle more, simply allow it to rest for a week or two, and the same exercise will be perceived as "new" again. This technique is more productive than switching to an inferior exercise.

What benefits a muscle most (from the perspective of hypertrophy/development) is that the biomechanical components of an exercise be optimal, which include the following:

- An exercise that moves the target muscle's operating lever toward the origin of that muscle (during concentric contraction) is BETTER than one that does not.
- An exercise that provides full (or relatively full) range of motion is BETTER than one that only provides static muscle tension for that muscle or an insufficient range of motion.
- An exercise that provides alignment of the direction of movement; the direction of resistance; and the origin/insertion of the target muscle is BETTER than an exercise that does not provide that alignment.
- An exercise that allows simple and direct muscle contraction, without joint contortion, (twisting/straining), is BETTER than an exercise that overcomplicates the movement and contorts (twists/strains) the joint.
- An exercise that provides a direction of resistance that is directly opposite the target muscle's origin (i.e., "opposite position loading") is BETTER than an exercise that provides a direction of resistance that is not directly opposite the target muscle's origin.
- An exercise that provides "early phase loading" is usually BETTER than an exercise that does not. The exception would be exercises that coincide with an "unusual"* mechanical disadvantage.

**Note: "Unusual," because it only occurs with flexion muscles, and only during part of its range of motion. Muscles that always work with mechanical disadvantage—extension muscles—are not in this category.*

- An exercise that involves a mostly "active" (perpendicular) operating lever (limb) is BETTER (more efficient) than an exercise that utilizes a partially active lever, or a mostly neutral operating lever (i.e., a limb moved by the target muscle).
- An exercise that employs a longer lever (not diminished by the "doubling back of a secondary lever," like a forearm or lower leg), is usually BETTER than an exercise that provides a shorter lever length/less resistance magnification.

# CHAPTER 18

# PECTORALS AND THE SERRATUS ANTERIOR

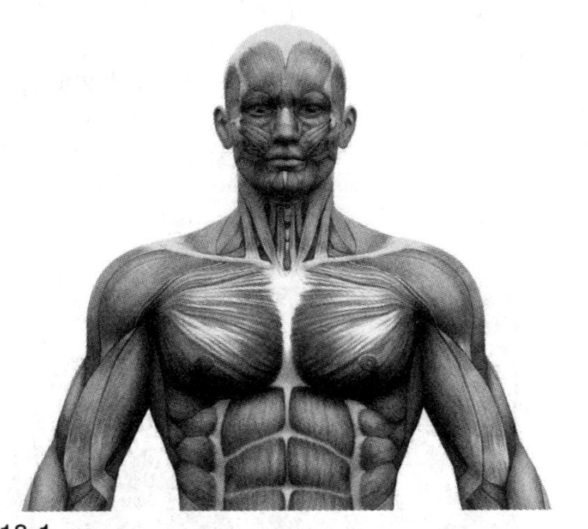


Figure 18-1

The "pectoralis major" is a fan-shaped muscle that covers the top third of the front of the torso. Technically, it is categorized into three parts—the "clavicular" fibers (Figure 18-2 "A"), the "sternal" fibers (Figure 18-2 "B"), and the "costal" fibers (Figure 18-2 "C"). These names identify the origin of each particular group of fibers. The largest percentage of pectoral fibers are those that originate on the sternum, while a smaller percentage originates on the clavicles and on the "costals" (the ribs). The insertion of ALL the pectoral fibers is on the upper part of the humerus (Figure 18-2 "D")—just below the humeral head.

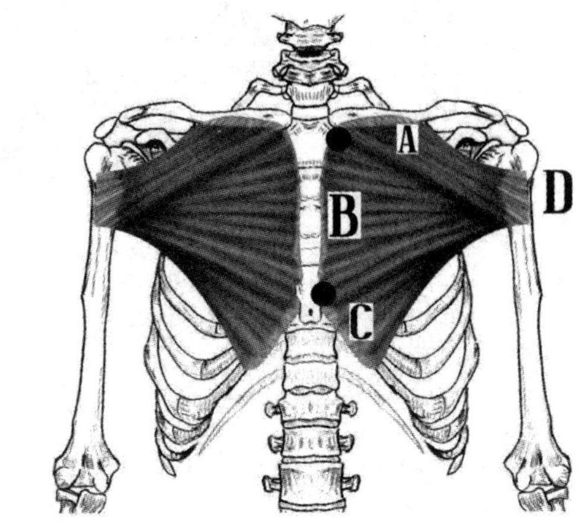


Figure 18-2

When the arms are outstretched, it's easy to see that all of the pectoral fibers are situated below the arm line (i.e., the line that extends from one shoulder joint to the other shoulder joint). The pecs are situated between the clavicles (which are parallel to the arms) and the lowest point of the anterior ribs. In fact, not one bit of the pectorals is situated above the clavicles.

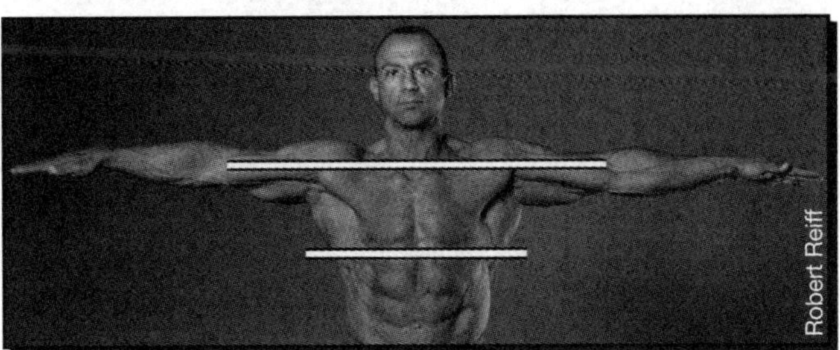


Figure 18-3

The conventional wisdom, regarding the best exercises for the pectorals, has been to use an incline angle for the "upper pecs," a flat bench for the center of the pecs, and a decline angle for the "lower pecs." This recommendation, however, is not entirely correct.

That recommendation would make sense, if half the pectorals were situated above the arm line, and the other half of the pectorals were situated below the arm line. As you can see, however, that is not the case. Figure 18-4, left image, illustrates a graphic that has been circulated, suggesting which part of the pectoral muscle the various angles benefit. When this graphic is placed alongside an actual human figure (Figure 18-4, right image), you can see how misguided this belief is.

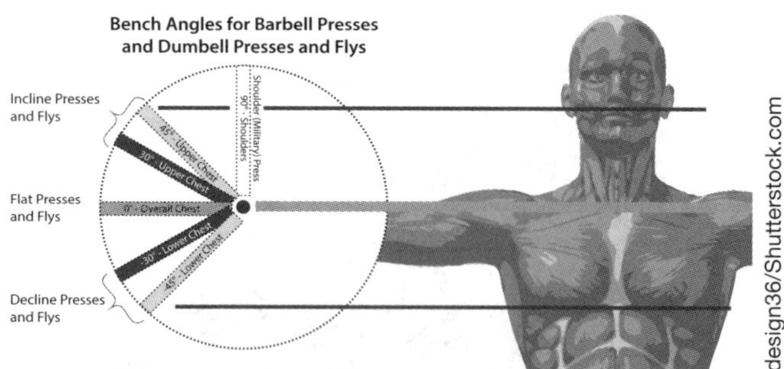


design36/Shutterstock.com

Figure 18-4

For a pectoral exercise to be productive, the humerus must move toward the pectoral origins. There would have to be pectoral origins above the arm line for an incline-angled movement to be productive, but there are no pectoral origins there. Therefore, an incline angled press is almost useless for pectoral stimulation. Only the flat and decline angles move the humerus toward pectoral muscle fiber origins.

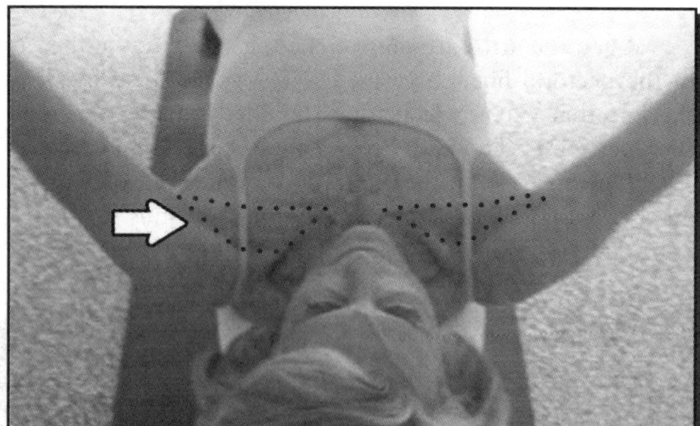

Figure 18-5

In Figure 18-5, the arrow is pointing to this woman's clavicular pectoral fibers, which are clearly visible (notice how they originate on her clavicle bone). These are the pectoral fibers that are highest on the chest. Yet, as you can plainly see in this photo, a *flat bench (supine) dumbbell press* engages them perfectly well, because those fibers are parallel with the direction of humeral movement (in conformance with the rule of alignment), and the humerus is moving toward the fiber origins of the clavicle.

Remember the analogy of the "Leaning Tower of Pisa," that was presented in Chapter 9. In the image in Figure 18-5, you could substitute her left arm for the "Tower." You would be standing on her left clavicle (on the opposite side of the tower's lean), pulling the rope (the clavicular pectoral fibers), preventing the tower from falling, or pulling it upward.

A *flat bench (supine) press* (with dumbbells) is the "highest" angle you should ever use, but a good argument could be made that an angle which is slightly more "decline" would actually be better. The "flat" angle moves the humerus toward the highest fibers on the chest—the upper half of the sternum, and also the clavicular fibers—but very little else. In other words, it loads too few pectoral fibers.

In Figure 18-6, you can see an individual doing a *flat dumbbell press*, from a side view. From this angle, you can see that his upper arms have moved toward the highest part of his sternum. You know this, because there are no pectoral fibers visible "higher" (to the left of his arm), yet there is quite a bit more pectoral muscle visible to the right of his arm—all the way to the line that's been placed there.

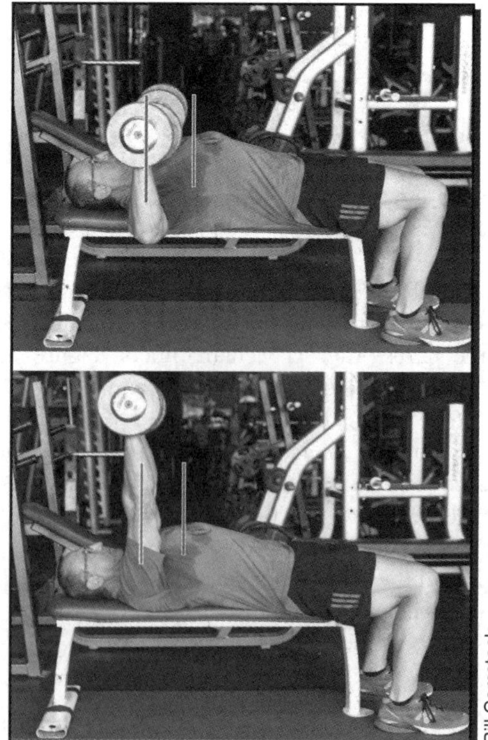

Bill Comstock

Figure 18-6

## The Best Anatomical Movement for Pectoral Exercise

In Figure 18-7, you can see the man performing a *decline dumbbell press*. Notice how his arms are moving toward the center of all of his pectoral origins (indicated by the arrow)—the area that is directly between the highest and lowest parts of his pectorals.

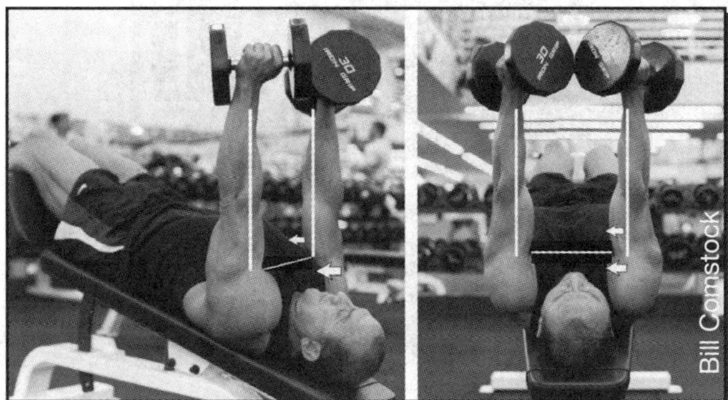

Figure 18-7

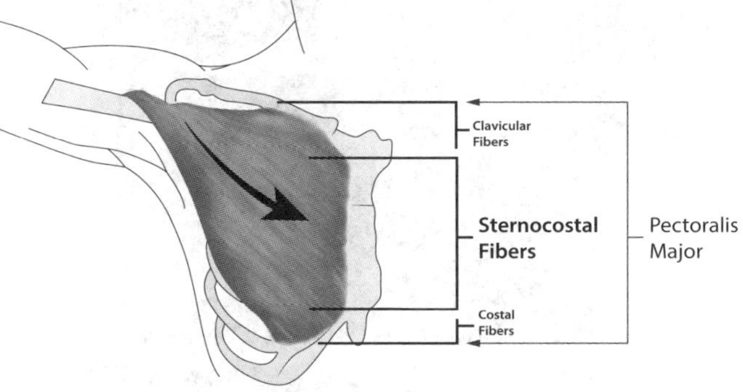

Figure 18-8

When you perform a *dumbbell press*, at a decline angle of approximately 30 degrees (Figure 18-7), you activate the largest number of pectoral fibers, because you are moving the humerus toward the area where the greatest number of pectoral origins are situated. All three "parts" of the pectorals—the clavicular, sternal, and costal fibers—contract when the arms are moved toward the area that is in the middle of the sternum. This angle is the single best direction of humeral motion for engaging the greatest number of pectoral fibers at one time. As such, if you only want to do one pectoral exercise and stimulate the greatest number of pectoral fibers, this exercise—a 30-degree *decline dumbbell press*—would be a very good choice.

If you think it's necessary to do two exercises for the pecs, I would recommend either a *flat bench dumbbell press* or an *extreme decline* angle, using *cables*. Later in this chapter, you'll see an exercise I recommend for anterior deltoids, which also targets the clavicular pecs.

## The Myth of Incline Movement for the Upper Pecs

Figure 18-9 shows a side view of an individual doing an *incline dumbbell press*. Hypothetically, imagine that you can see through his right arm. As such, you'd notice that his arm is aligned with his chin and his neck, which is the direction in which his humerus is moving. Are there pectoral fibers on his chin or on his neck? Of course not. While a small number of pectoral fibers may be assisting, it's impossible for them to play much of a role. Remember the example of the man in the previous chapter pulling the rope attached to the heavy box? There's simply no way for that man (i.e., the pectoral fiber origins) to pull that box (i.e., that humerus) in a direction (i.e., toward his chin) that is different from where he's standing (i.e., on the upper part of the sternum and the clavicles).

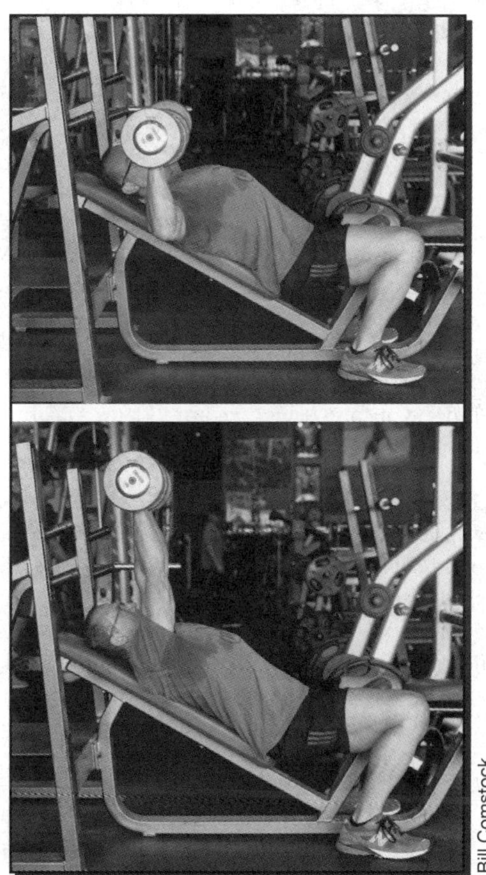

Figure 18-9

The next time you're working out with a friend, try this experiment. Place your hand on the highest pectoral fibers on your colleague's chest, when they're doing an *incline dumbbell press*. Then, do the same thing when they're performing a *flat dumbbell press*. You're bound to feel that there's more pectoral contraction occurring in the upper fibers, when your friend is doing a *flat dumbbell press*.

There is another little experiment you can try. If you're standing, flex one side of your "upper pecs," with whatever arm position best allows you to feel that area contracting. Chances are that you will not move your arm toward your chin or neck. You'd move your arm more straight across your torso, maybe even a little lower.

In fact, the next time you're watching bodybuilders doing incline work at the gym, watch how—after they finish a set and check their "pump"—they move their humerus across the middle of their chest, around the place it would be if they were doing flat bench or a slight decline press. Instinctively, you KNOW which direction arm movement best contracts your upper pecs, and it is not by putting your arm up near your neck or chin.

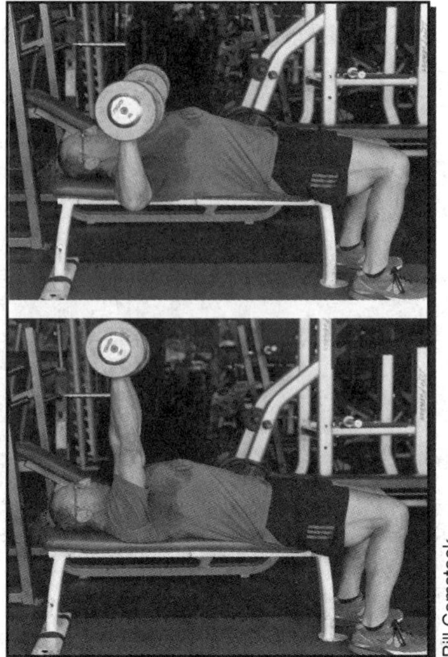
Bill Comstock

Figure 18-10

## Evaluating Other Angles for Pectoral Exercise

It is important to be clear about what "angles for pectoral exercise" actually references. In fact, the pectorals don't "know" whether you are lying on a flat bench or on a decline bench, or even if you're standing. They only "know" the direction in which they are moving the upper arm bones (the humerus), in relation to the torso. The rule of Alignment (which includes "opposite position loading"/"the line of force") requires that the direction of resistance be directly opposite the anatomical direction of movement. So, whichever angle you choose to move your arms, just ensure that the direction of resistance you are using accommodates "alignment" and "opposite position loading."

Accordingly, when you're doing a *supine (flat bench) dumbbell press* (Figure 18-10), the "angle" that you're using is "perpendicular to the torso" (i.e., straight forward), even if you are not using a flat bench and free weight. You could be pushing at a perpendicular angle (relative to your torso), but be sitting upright, using cable resistance that is opposite to your direction of movement. Both of these are utilizing the same "angle," even though they appear different.

Figure 18-11 shows how you can position your body any way you like (presumably a position that is most comfortable), and set the pulleys so that the cables pull directly opposite the direction of anatomical movement you've selected. As noted previously, your pectorals only "know" the direction they're pushing, relative to your torso. They don't know which way your torso is facing.

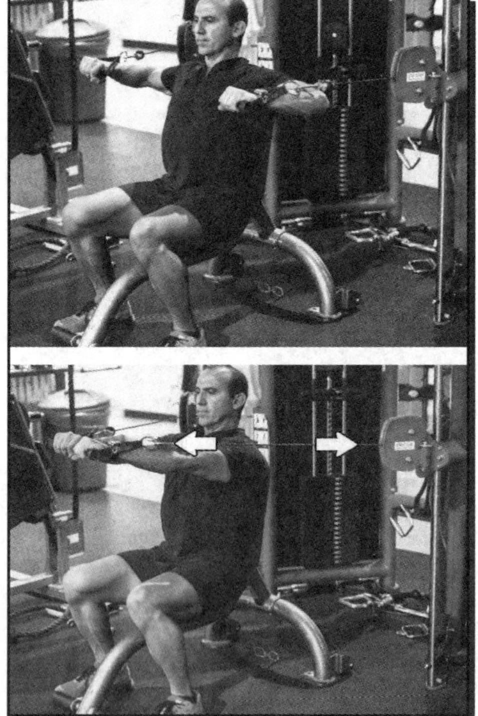
Bill Comstock

Figure 18-11

In both of the aforementioned examples, the arms are being moved straight forward by the pectorals. Relative to the torso, the direction of arm movement is the same in both exercises. Both of these would be called a "flat" direction of push—a description that references a "flat bench" as a direction of arm movement, but does not actually require a flat bench.

In Figure 18-12, I'm doing a *decline dumbbell press*. What matters, however, is NOT the bench I'm using. What matters is the direction in which I am moving my arms, relative to my torso. Since I'm using gravity as my resistance in this instance, and gravity is always vertical, I need to position myself on a decline bench so that I can push directly opposite gravity, and still toward the center of my sternum.

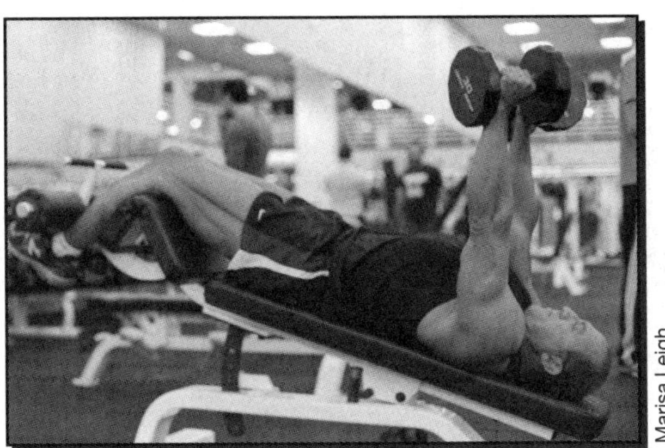
Marisa Leigh

Figure 18-12

Figure 18-13 also depicts a "decline angle press," although using cables instead of dumbbells. Despite having the torso in a completely different position, as compared to being on an actual decline bench, the angle of humeral movement—relative to the torso—is very similar to the angle used in the previous example. The cable is moving in a horizontal direction, but the angle of the bench is tilted back about 20 degrees from vertical (when viewed from this perspective). So this is the same angle of movement as occurs during a "decline angle press." If the bench were completely vertical, the movement would be considered "flat bench cable press."

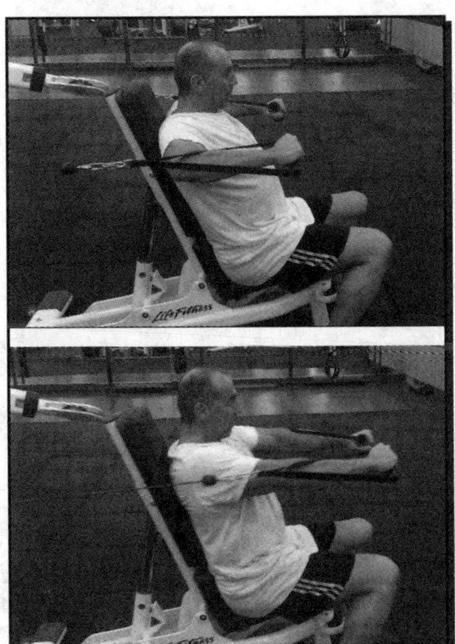
Figure 18-13

Accordingly, from this point forward in the book, when a reference is made to an "incline" angle, a "flat" angle, or a "decline" angle—in terms of pectoral training—the discussion is about the direction of humeral movement, relative to the torso. It is not necessarily specifying that a particular bench is being used.

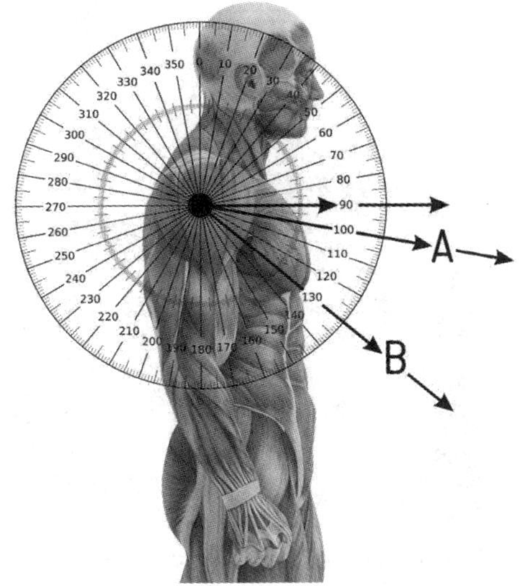

DM7/Shutterstock.com

Figure 18-14

Figure 18-14 includes three arrows, starting at the shoulder joint, indicating the best directions of humeral movement for training the pectorals. This is not to suggest that all three directions need to be used. It just means that any direction of "push" (humeral movement) that ranges between "flat" to "extreme decline" is acceptable for pectoral training. The directions of humeral movement depicted in Figure 18-14 all move the arms toward the origins of the pectoral fibers.

Note that an "incline" angle of push is NOT included in Figure 18-14. A "flat" direction of humeral movement already moves the humerus toward the highest pectorals fiber origins. Since there are no pectoral origins above the shoulders or clavicles, there's no need to move the arms in that direction.

Personally, I feel that even the "flat" movement isn't necessary. As shown in Figure 18-14, the second arrow ("A") and the lowest arrow ("B") are the angles that I believe are best. These two directions of humeral movement will work ALL of the pectoral fibers, including the clavicular fibers. Nevertheless, if you enjoy doing a "flat" angle press, it's acceptable.

Obviously, it would be very difficult to perform an "extreme decline" angle press (arrow "B" in Figure 18-14) on a bench set at such an extreme angle, with dumbbells. In fact, it would be difficult enough just getting ON a bench that is set at such a steep angle. Then, getting a pair of heavy dumbbells in position to begin the exercise, without getting injured in the process, would be even more challenging. Furthermore, having your body turned so "upside down" would also be very uncomfortable. Fortunately, you can easily recreate that same angle by using cables, as illustrated in Figures 18-15 and 18-16. Notice how I'm moving my arms in the "B" direction, as shown in Figure 18-14.

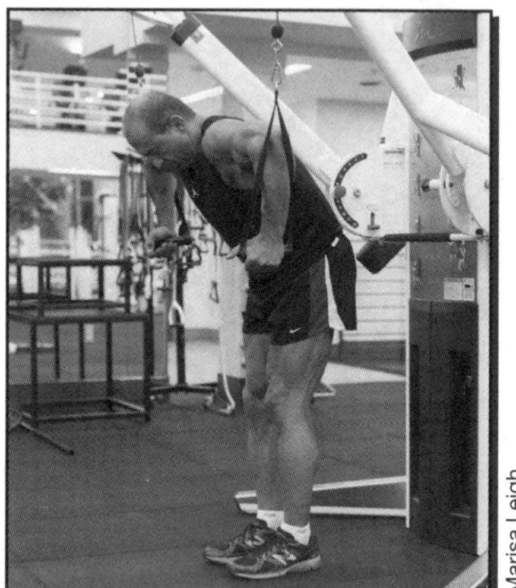
Marisa Leigh

Figure 18-15

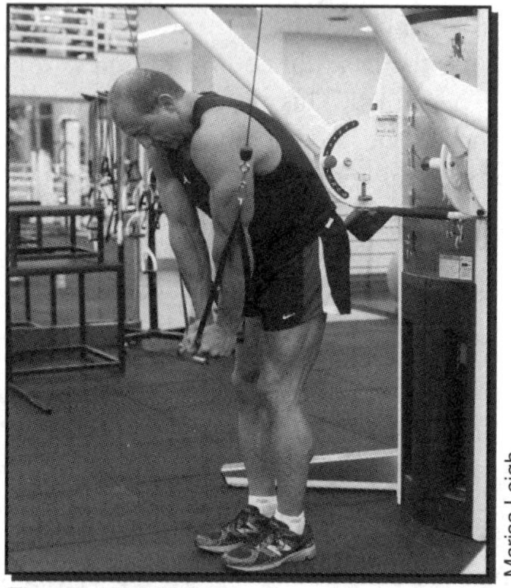
Marisa Leigh

Figure 18-16

This angle is somewhat similar to the direction of push used during *parallel bar dips*, but, in several ways, it's much better than actually doing *dips*. During *parallel bar dips*, it's impossible to maintain your torso at the angle shown in Figures 8-15 and 8-16. This is because the weight of the hanging legs pulls the torso into a more upright position. As much as you might try to hunch over like this, it's still not quite the same torso angle as shown in these figures.

Furthermore, when using cables like this, you can choose the exact amount of weight that is appropriate for the number of reps you want to do. I usually start very light, and perform 30 reps as part of the warm-up process. Then, I add a bit more weight and do 20 reps. I keep adding weight, and decreasing the reps, until I get to a weight that challenges me for six or four reps. In contrast, it's impossible to have resistance options that allow a rep range of 30 to four, when doing *parallel bar dips.*

Most importantly, I can bring my arms out—laterally—as I stretch my pecs, and then I can bring my arms inward ("medially"—toward the midline of my body), as I contract my pecs (Figure 18-17). This technique is impossible when doing *parallel bar dips*, because the bars don't move. Some people "think" that keeping the elbows wide when doing dips does the same thing. It does not. The hands, along with the forearms (not just the elbows), need to move laterally (out to the sides), and then inwardly, until the hands are together at the midline of the body.

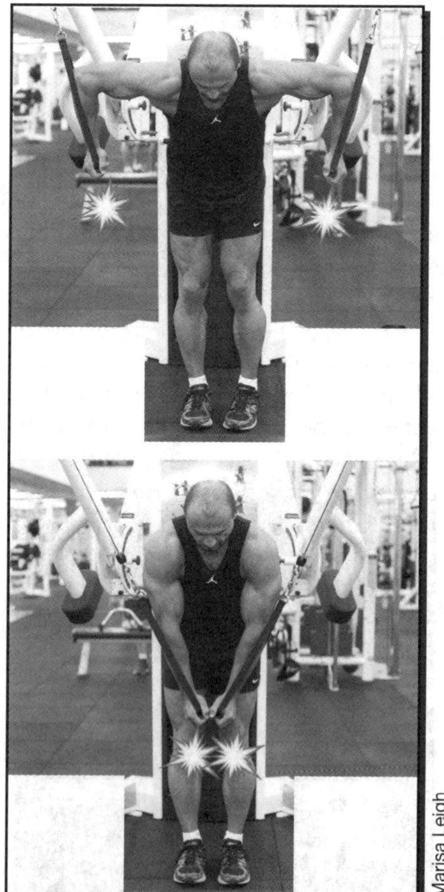
Marisa Leigh

Figure 18-17

In addition, the direction of resistance, when doing *dips*, is vertical, which is not quite ideal. When doing a *decline cable press*, the direction of resistance is upward, but with a distinct outward (lateral) angle. This technique provides more resistance (opposition), when the pectorals are contracted, as compared with a vertical resistance. By keeping the forearms parallel to the cables throughout the movement, you can maintain the forearms in the "neutral" position (as the secondary lever) and focus all your attention on loading the pecs.

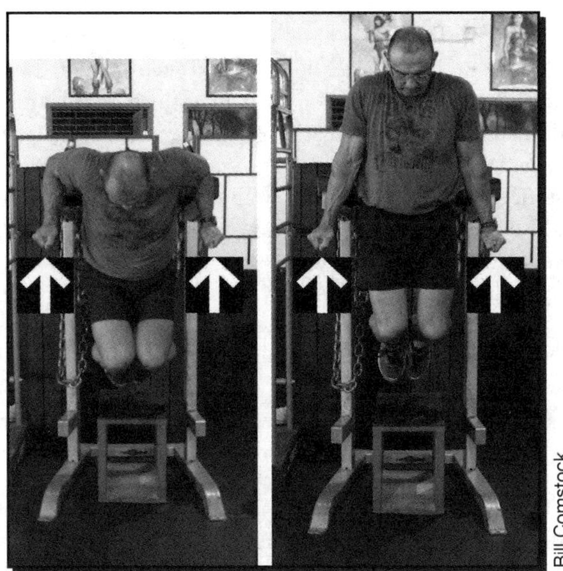

Figure 18-18

In Figure 18-18, you can see that the upper arms and elbows of the person doing *parallel bar dips* tend to go "back," when he descends, rather than "out" (laterally). This factor occurs because the dip bars don't move outward. The best way to work the pecs is by allowing the humerus to move outward (laterally)—away from the pectoral origins on the sternum—and then inward, toward the midline of the body—toward the pectoral origins.

The starbursts shown in Figure 18-17 (upper image) show the width between the hands and elbows, when in the stretch phase of a *decline cable press*. Compare that to the arrows in Figure 18-18 (left image), showing the width between the hands and elbows, when in the stretch phase of *parallel bar dips*. In Figure 18-17 (lower image), the starbursts show where the hands are upon completion of the movement, when doing a *decline cable press*. Compare that to the arrows in Figure 18-18 (right image), showing where the hands are upon completion of the movement during *parallel bar dips*. This comparison should make the advantage of a *decline cable press,* over *parallel bar dips,* abundantly clear.

When doing dips, it's impossible to make the humerus go out laterally, and still keep the hands and forearms under the elbows. In other words, the hands, forearms, elbows, and upper arms should ALL move outward, laterally—in order to follow the pathway of the pectoral fibers. On the other hand, because dipping bars are restrictive in this sense, the tendency is to move the humerus posteriorly (toward the rear), which loads the anterior deltoids, more than the pectorals. If you force the elbows out to the sides, when doing parallel bar dips, the forearms are no longer "neutral" (parallel with the direction of resistance), so a percentage of the load shifts away from the pectorals to the triceps. Still, you are not able to fully contract the pectorals, against a resistance that is pulling outwardly.

In Figure 18-19, I am demonstrating a *decline dumbbell press*. From this perspective, you can see that I am keeping my forearm neutral (vertical/parallel with gravity), throughout the entire range of motion, from beginning to end. You can also see the ideal range of motion. The point of maximum descent should not go lower than indicated in Figure 18-19, upper image, when using a very heavy weight. Stopping the eccentric movement at this point avoids excessive mechanical disadvantage, which reduces the risk of pectoral rupture and shoulder joint strain. Going lower than this would be acceptable when the weight is "light," and you are mostly warming up—but it would not be acceptable when the weight being used is "heavy."

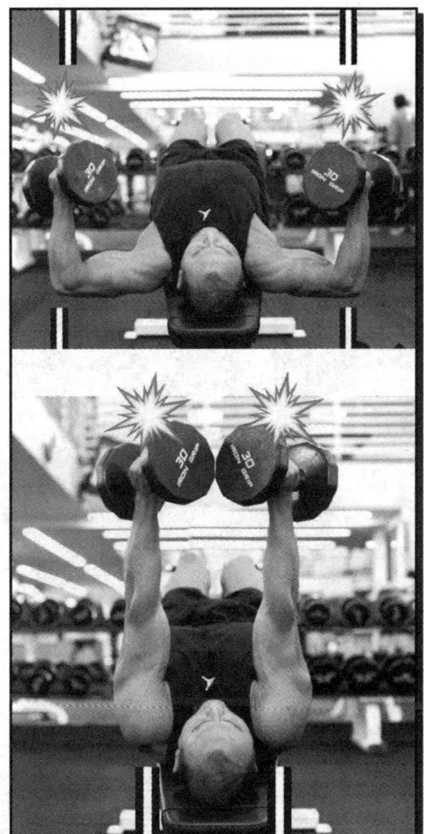

Figure 18-19

Although the angle of the average decline bench can be varied between 20 degrees and 35 degrees, I prefer an angle of approximately 20 degrees. This point corresponds to the aforementioned "A" angle. I refer to it as a "slight" decline.

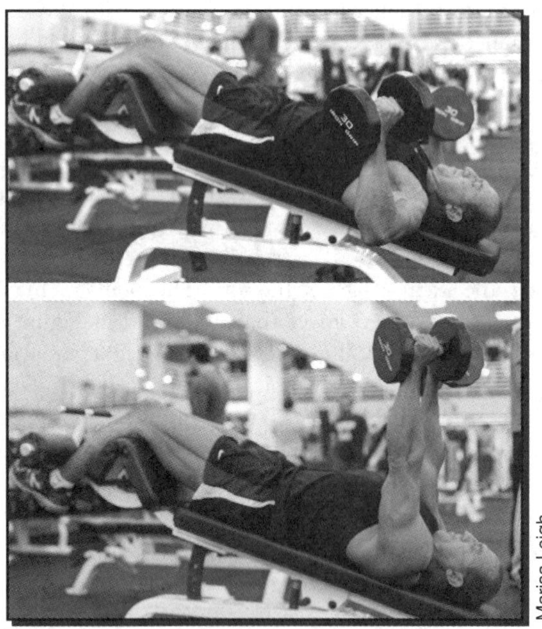
Marisa Leigh
Figure 18-20

An exercise we commonly see performed in the gym as part of a Pectoral workout is the "*cable crossover*," illustrated in Figure 18-21. This angle of humeral movement is fine; it's like the "extreme decline" angle ("B") shown in Figure 18-14.

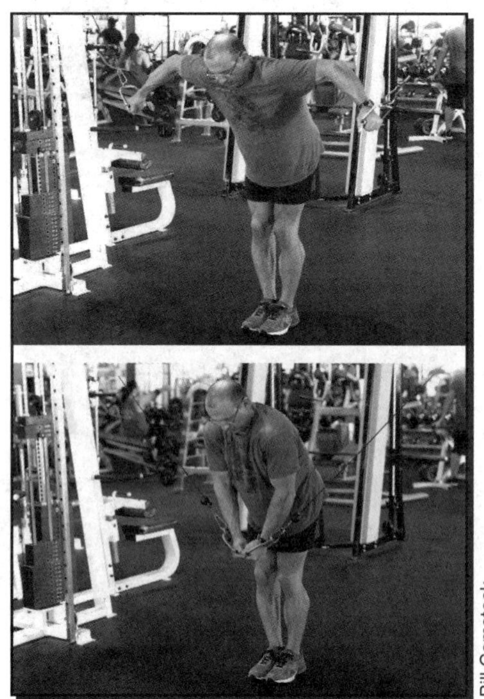
Bill Comstock
Figure 18-21

However, the direction of resistance is not especially good. The pulleys are too far apart, and too much to the side, rather than "behind" the user. This creates a resistance curve that provides too much resistance at the conclusion of the range of motion (at the point of contraction), and not enough resistance at the beginning of the range of motion (the point of elongation). This is out of sync with the muscle's natural strength curve.

The principle of "early phase loading" requires that the resistance be greater during the beginning of the range of motion—certainly during the first third of the range of motion. That is the phase where skeletal muscles usually have their greatest strength capacity. In order to create this type of resistance curve when using cables (for pecs), the resistance should come more from behind, rather than from the sides. As such, the pulleys would need to be closer together, than the standard "cable crossover machine" allows—and the user needs to stand father out in front of the pulleys. Notice the pulley machine I'm using in Figures 18-16 and 18-17 allows the pulleys to be about three feet apart, rather than the standard (and immovable) width of eight feet, which is standard for a cable crossover machine.

Furthermore, the forearm (as the "secondary lever"), should ideally be "neutral" (parallel with resistance/parallel with the cable) throughout the entire exercise (when working the pecs). During traditional *cable crossovers*, however, it's impossible to keep the forearm parallel with the cable, because the cable is coming more from the side, than from the rear. This factor causes the forearm to be more perpendicular with the cable, which makes it too "active" during most of the range of motion. As a result, the biceps are loaded as much as, or perhaps more than, the pecs. At best, this is distracting. At worst, it's the "weak link" in the chain.

Ultimately, the "backward" resistance curve provided by the *cable crossover* is its most glaring flaw. It insufficiently loads the pecs during the early phase of the range of motion (where the pecs are the strongest), and excessively loads the pecs during the latter part of the range of motion (where the pecs are weakest). In addition, the excessive, but mostly unproductive, biceps participation that occurs during this exercise further lowers its value.

Personally, I would rate the *cable crossover* a "5" (on a scale of 1 to 10) for pectoral training. While it's not a terrible exercise, it's certainly not one of the better exercises for the pectorals.

Changing directions a bit, pectoral exercises that involve the use of a barbell—instead of dumbbells or cables—are compromised for several reasons. Using a barbell for a pectoral exercise restricts full range of motion, eliminates the potential for "cross education" (i.e., cross-over benefits caused by independent limb use), and alters the mechanics in a way that adds "friction force" unproductively.

For example, when performing a "*bench press*" (i.e., using a barbell on a flat bench), the humeral movement stops far short of full pectoral contraction at the conclusion of the repetition (the "top" of the motion). This is because the hands are "stuck" on the bar, nearly 3 feet apart from each other. Since the hands cannot be brought together at the midline of the body—as would be the case when using dumbbells or cables—the humerus is unable to complete its final 20 degrees of the pectoral's full range of motion.

As a rule, an incomplete range of motion is generally considered "not productive"—compared to using a full range of motion. This factor cannot be ignored, when evaluating an exercise. If we "forgive" (overlook) the incomplete range of motion of a *bench press*, we would be obligated to also "forgive" an incomplete range of motion during every other resistance exercise. That would certainly not be a good strategy.

In Figure 18-22, you can see the difference in the ending positions, between using a barbell and using dumbbells. The dumbbells allow a much greater pectoral contraction (more complete range of motion), than does the *bench press*.

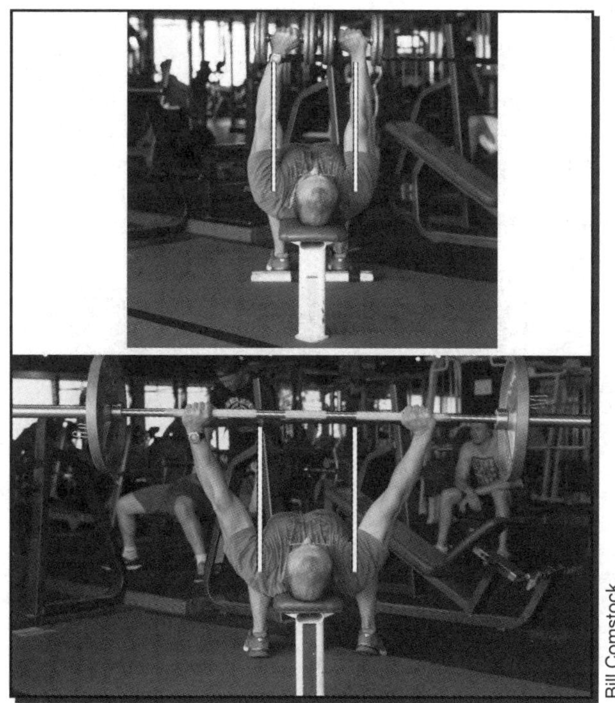


Figure 18-22

Furthermore, when using a barbell, individuals tend to focus on the bar touching their chest in the descended position, rather than on what feels comfortable and natural for the shoulder joint, and what causes "enough" or "too much" pectoral stretch. Conversely, when using dumbbells, since there is no barbell that can touch the chest, exercisers tend to focus on the stretch of the pectorals, as well as the comfort of the shoulder joint.

Generally speaking, the humerus should not be brought much "lower" than the level of the torso, during a pectoral exercise. Barbell *bench pressing* tends to cause too much stretch at the bottom of the range of motion, because of the perceived need to "touch the bar to the chest." It also provides an insufficient range of motion at the top of the movement, because the hands cannot be brought together. Using dumbbells allows the user to use the ideal range of motion, without concern for the perceived need of "touching the bar to the chest," and without being restricted from bringing the hands together at the top of the movement.

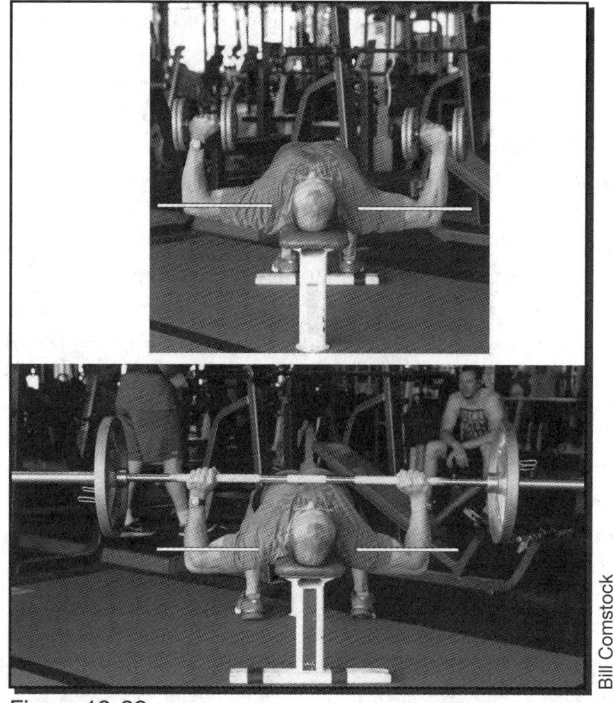


Figure 18-23

Another problem that occurs when using a barbell during an exercise that is intended for pectoral development, is the principle that was discussed in Chapter 6—"ground reaction force"/"friction force." When using a barbell, individuals are essentially obligated to push the hands upward and *outward*, because they are unable to pull the hands inward, toward the midline of the body, as the use of dumbbells allows. This outward angle of humeral push engages the triceps more and the pectorals less than would be the case when using dumbbells. As a result, the pectorals actually get a lesser percentage of the load, when using a barbell, as compared to using dumbbells. So, even though it may seem that you're working the pectorals harder, because you're able to use more weight than you could use with dumbbells that is not an accurate assessment.

In addition, there is also the lack of humeral "independence," when using a barbell for a pectoral exercise. When the two arms share a single instrument (as in the bench press), the muscles that operate that limb lose much of the crossover benefit that could be gained from having the arms working independently of each other, as would be the case when using dumbbells.

The *butterfly machine* (shown in Figure 18-24) is another exercise which is often included in a pectoral workout, among those individuals who are seeking to improve their physique. While it's not a "bad" exercise, it is not especially good either. There are several versions of this machine. The version that allows the arms to move toward a slight "decline" direction is a bit better than those that move the arms straight forward.

One of the main "problems" with this exercise (regardless of whichever version you're using) is that there is a tendency to allow the elbows to "drop," i.e., to be held lower than the hands and the shoulders. This factor creates misalignment, and causes an external rotational force to be applied to the humerus/shoulder joint. This strains the shoulder, unnecessarily. This factor is influenced, to some degree, by the position of your hands on the handles of the machine. If the handles are held so that the palms of your hands are facing forward, it will automatically tend to rotate your elbows downward—which will then cause the resistance from the machine to force an external rotation of your upper arm bone (thereby straining the shoulder joint). Conversely, if you grip the handles so that the palms of your hands are facing downward, it will automatically tend to rotate your elbows upward. That will allow your elbows to be better aligned with your hands, and your shoulders, and the trajectory of your movement, and the direction of the resistance. It's important to keep the elbows up. Also, the height of the seat should be set so that your hands and your shoulders are at the same height.

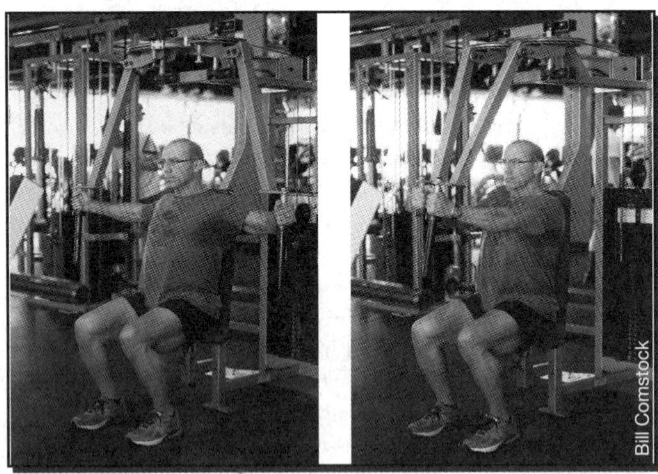

Figure 18-24

Most butterfly machines have a "cam," which provides more resistance at the beginning of the range of motion and a gradual diminishment of the resistance, as the range of motion nears its completion. This feature is good, because it would comply with "early phase loading," provided it diminished

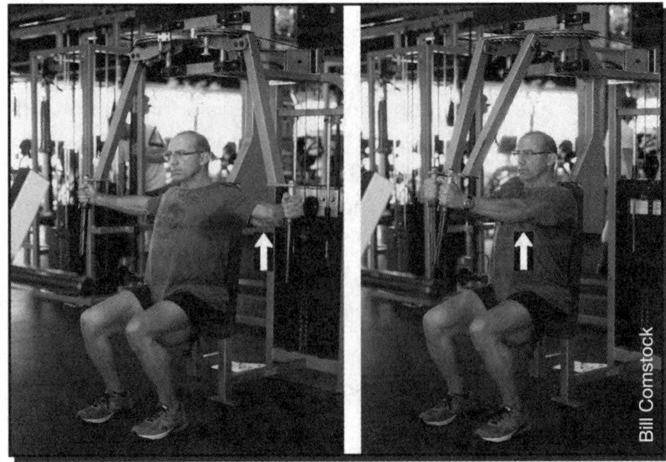

Figure 18-25

the resistance enough. Generally speaking, however, I have never encountered a *butterfly machine* that provides enough diminishment of the resistance, toward the end of the range of motion. The result of this is that by selecting a resistance level that allows you to complete the range of motion (including the weaker end phase), it will likely be insufficient resistance for the early part of the range of motion, where the pectorals are stronger.

The exercise shown in Figure 18-26—the *seated cable front press*—is primarily an anterior deltoids exercise. During this exercise, the humerus moves from a low position (alongside the torso), straight forward and upward—TOWARD the clavicles—but not higher than the clavicles. Since the origin

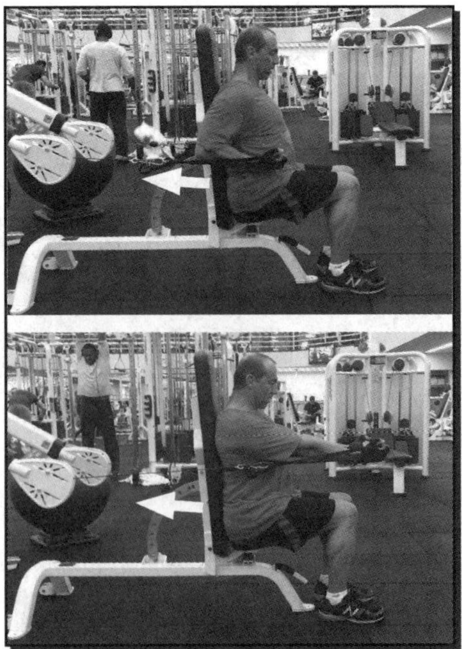
Figure 18-26

of the anterior deltoids, as well as that of the clavicular pecs, is on the clavicles, both of these muscles will be engaged. So, even though this exercise does not look like a typical "upper pectoral" exercise, it does engage the clavicular pectorals very well. It does not, however, engage the upper sternal pectoral fibers very much, because the humerus is not moving inward (medially)—toward the sternum.

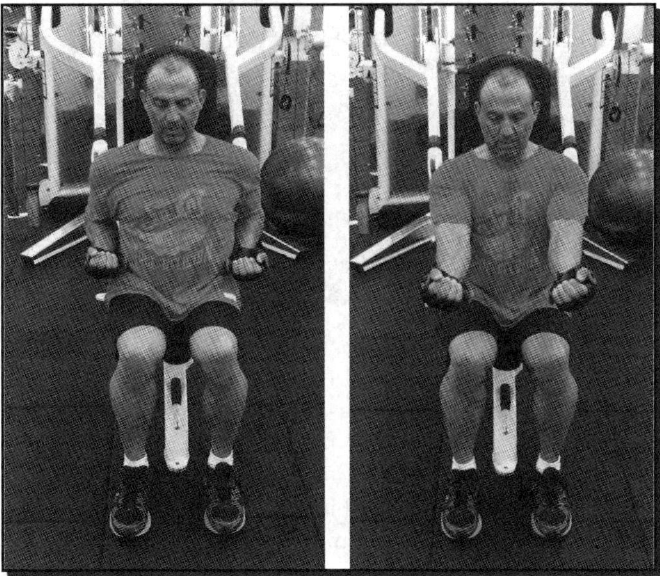

Figure 18-27

The anterior deltoid's origins are on the lateral aspect (outer half) of the clavicles, while the clavicular pectoral origins are on the medial aspect (inner half) of the clavicles. For this reason, the anterior deltoids and the clavicular pectoral fibers participate together in certain movements.

## Anatomy and Function of the Pectoralis Minor

The pectoralis minor is not commonly discussed in bodybuilding circles—with good reason. It is not a primary physique muscle. In fact, it is arguably not even a "voluntary" muscle. You cannot deliberately control it, because it does not cross a joint you can intentionally move. It is a small muscle that lies beneath the pectoralis major, and cannot be seen, because it is not near the surface of the skin.

Its origins are on the third, fourth, and fifth ribs (Figures 18-28 and 18-29), and its insertion is on the coracoid process of the scapula. Because it does not tie into the humerus at all, it has no effect on the humerus (the upper arm), the way the pectoralis major does. Rather, it stabilizes the shoulder blade, pulling it forward against the thoracic wall. Its contraction is involuntary, and it generally works synergistically with other muscles. Furthermore, it has essentially no capacity for growth. As such, it's not a muscle with which you need to concern yourself.

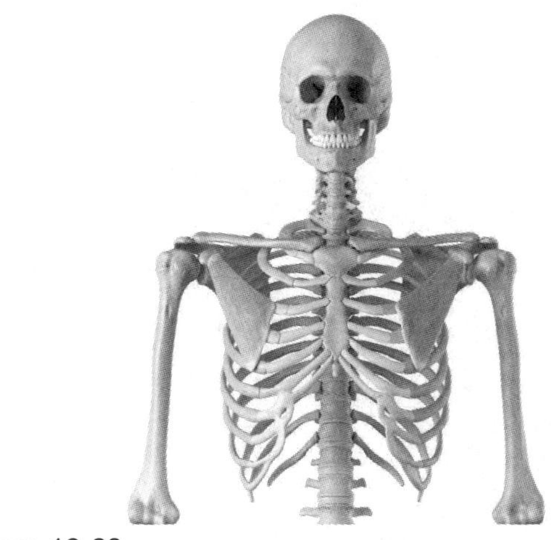

Figure 18-28



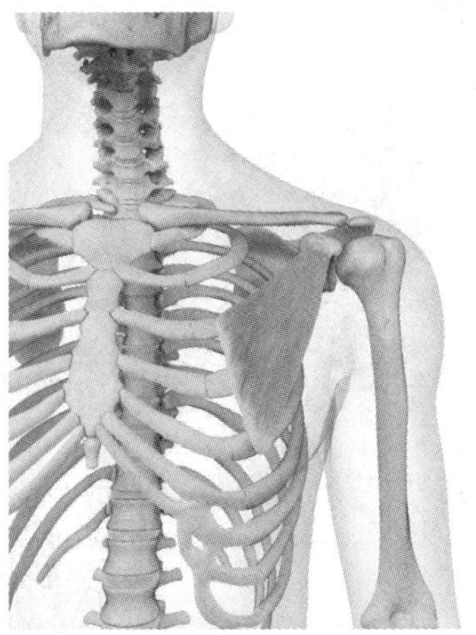

Figure 18-29



## Anatomy and Function of the Coracobrachialis

The coracobrachialis is a very small muscle, which crosses the shoulder joint. Accordingly, it participates (mildly assists) in humeral flexion and adduction. These are movements during which the pectorals and anterior deltoids do the primary work, which is why I chose to include it in the "pectoral" section—even though it's hardly worth mentioning from the standpoint of pectoral development. It appears as if it's part of the biceps, except that it plays no role in elbow flexion, because it does not cross the elbow joint.

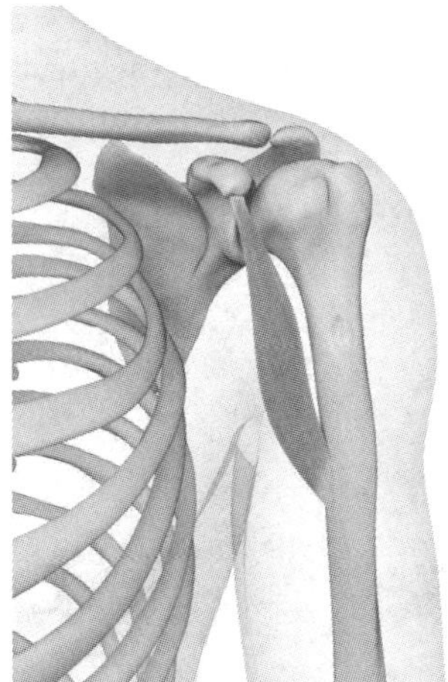


Figure 18-30

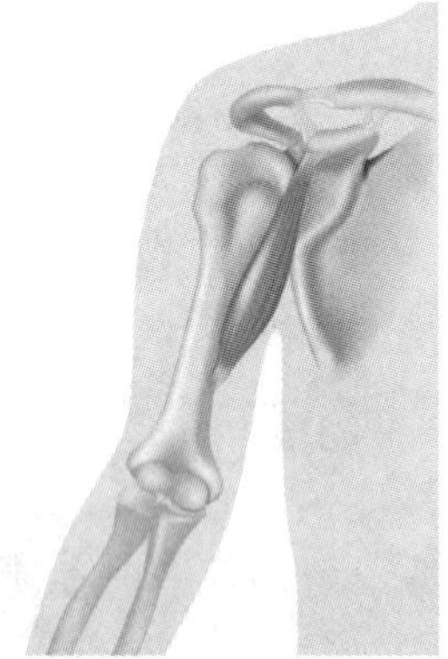


Figure 18-31

This muscle helps pull the humerus forward, upward and slightly inward, and it stabilizes the humeral head in the glenoid socket. Its origin is on the coracoid process, and it inserts onto the humerus. It is not a muscle that can be isolated. It only works in conjunction with other muscles, and only as a minor assistant. In Figure 18-32 (yes, it's my arm), you can see that it looks like a short rope, at the upper end of the biceps, right before it tucks under the outer edge of the pectorals.

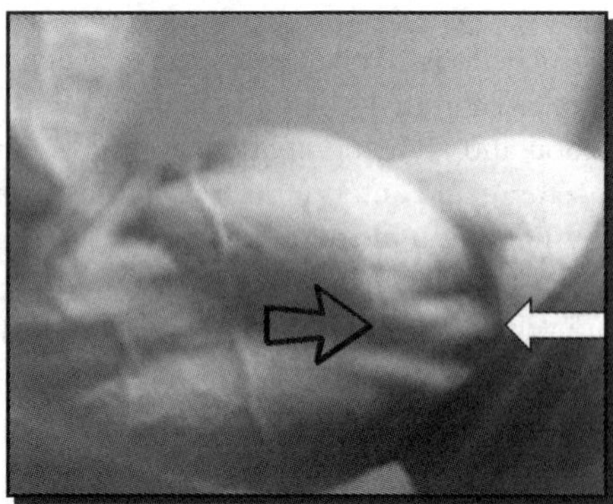

Figure 18-32

## Anatomy and Function of the Serratus Anterior

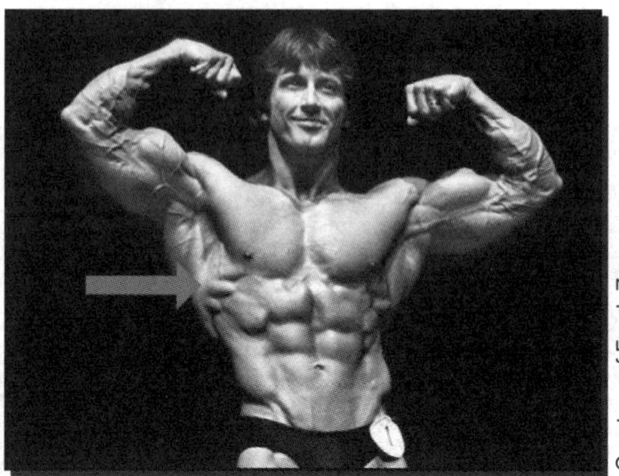


Figure 18-33

The serratus anterior is a muscle that originates on the upper eight ribs, stretches back posteriorly, and attaches to the medial (the inside) edge of the scapula. The attachment on the ribs is its "origin," while the attachment on the scapula is its "insertion." The reason for this distinction is that an "origin" always refers to that which is more stable, while an "insertion" refers to that which is more mobile.

The serratus anterior does not move the ribs back toward the scapula. Rather, it pulls the scapula forward, toward the ribs. It stabilizes the scapula, and pulls is against the back of the ribcage—against the posterior side of the "thoracic wall."

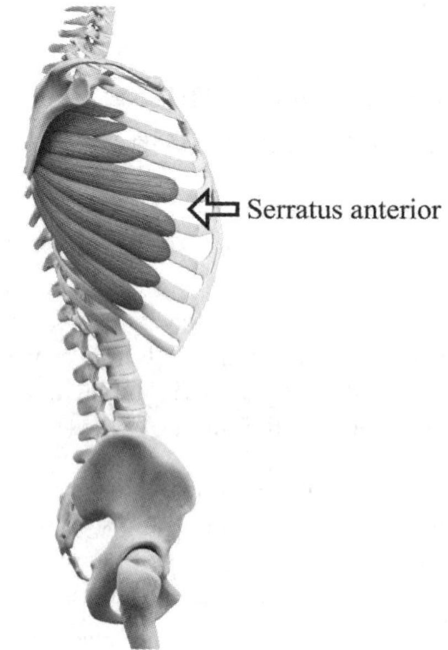


Figure 18-34

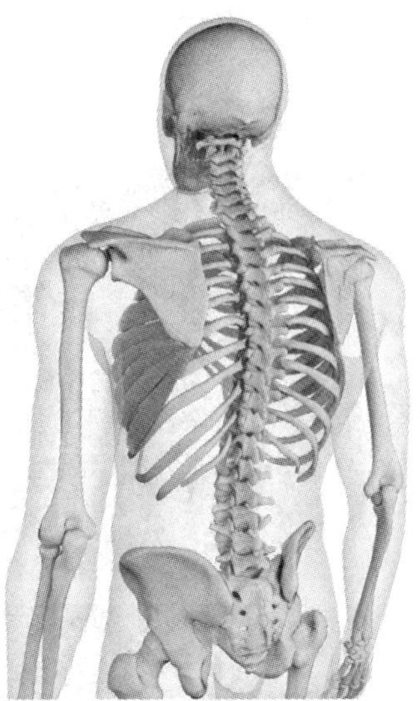
SciePro/Shutterstock.com

Figure 18-35

This muscle is sometimes called "the boxer's muscle," because boxers tend to have well developed serratus muscles. Note the serratus anterior, which is clearly visible on professional boxer Manny Pacquiao, shown in Figure 18-34. Also notice that despite this muscle being so vast, only the smallest part of it is visible through the skin. In fact, most of the serratus anterior is covered by layers of other muscles.

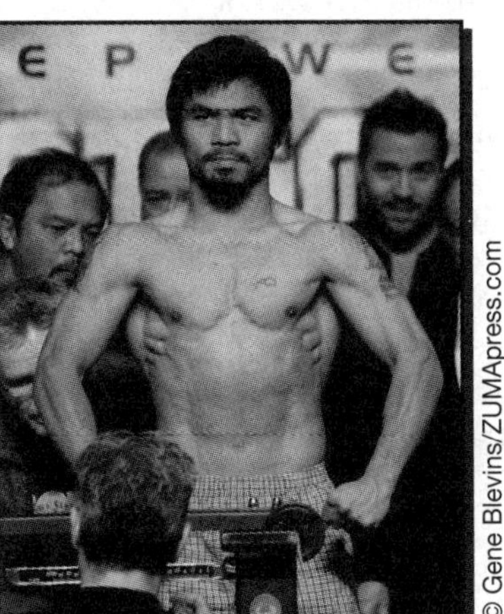
© Gene Blevins/ZUMApress.com

Figure 18-36

It's extremely difficult to isolate the action of the serratus anterior, because it performs mostly a stabilizing function, rather than a deliberate movement. Unlike the biceps or the triceps, where the movement produced by that muscle is easily identified and executed, the serratus primarily acts as a stabilizer, while other muscles perform their primary task. The closest thing to a "movement" that can be associated with the serratus anterior is a thrusting forward of the shoulder carriage, as would occur when "punching." Even this action, however, is not solely executed by the serratus anterior.

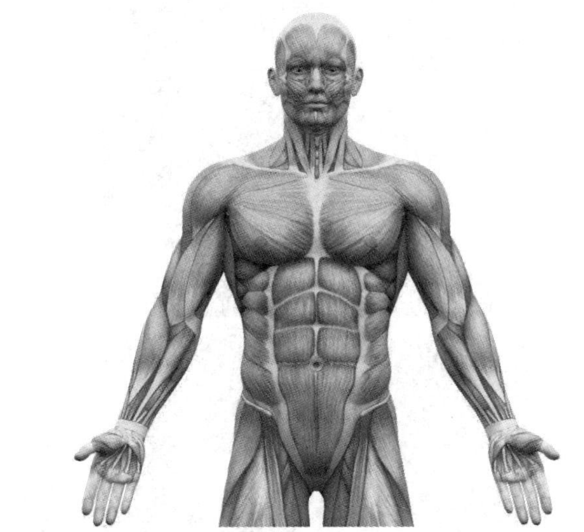
decade3d - anatomy online/Shutterstock.com

Figure 18-37

The exercise shown in Figures 18-38 and 18-39—a forward thrust of the shoulder carriage, while lying on a flat bench—is sometimes recommended for development of the serratus anterior. This action "protracts" the scapula, which means that it rotates the scapula forward. While this movement may be useful to a boxer, for the purpose of improving the effectiveness of his punches, it's doubtful that it would cause a significant improvement in the visible development of the serratus anterior for the bodybuilder.

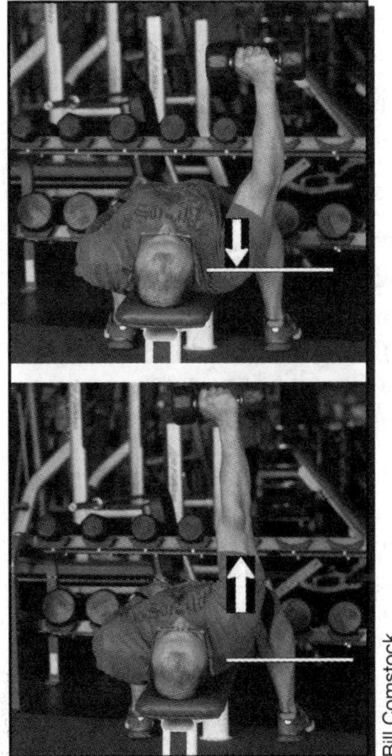
Bill Comstock

Figure 18-38

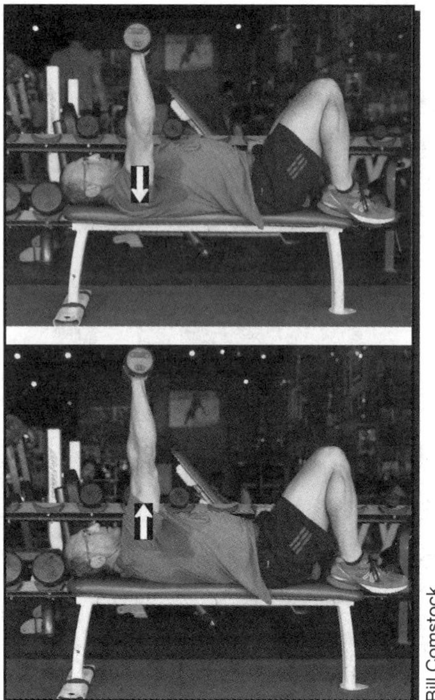

Figure 18-39

It's safe to assume that Frank Zane, the legendary bodybuilder shown in Figure 18-33, never did this movement—yet his serratus anterior was among the most notable in the sport. In fact, Zane and the other bodybuilders of the era all performed the same basic exercises, but Zane was the only bodybuilder whose serratus anterior were so pronounced. This situation suggests that it was mostly a genetic advantage, which allowed Zane's serratus to be so impressive.

The serratus anterior engages during several traditional "weight training" exercises. For example, the movement illustrated in Figures 18-38 and 18-39 could be considered the final part of a *flat bench (supine) dumbbell press*. After the humerus is fully extended upward, the shoulder carriage can then be pushed forward as well (… as opposed to leaving the scapula flat on the bench). Still, it's highly doubtful that Frank Zane intentionally added this extra movement to the end of his standard *flat bench dumbbell press*.

The serratus anterior engages any time the scapula needs stabilizing, which includes most pectoral exercises. This is the reason this muscle is included in this chapter. This muscle also engages during some anterior deltoid exercises.

Some people (mostly "old school" lifters) believe that a good exercise for the serratus anterior is *pullovers* (shown in Figure 18-40). Because the scapula requires stabilizing during *pullovers*, the serratus may participate here as well. Given that the *pullover* movement, however, is not a natural movement for the shoulder joint, it may result in shoulder joint strain. The questionable value of a pullover, in terms of helping develop the serratus anterior, makes assuming the risk of shoulder joint strain all the less worthwhile.

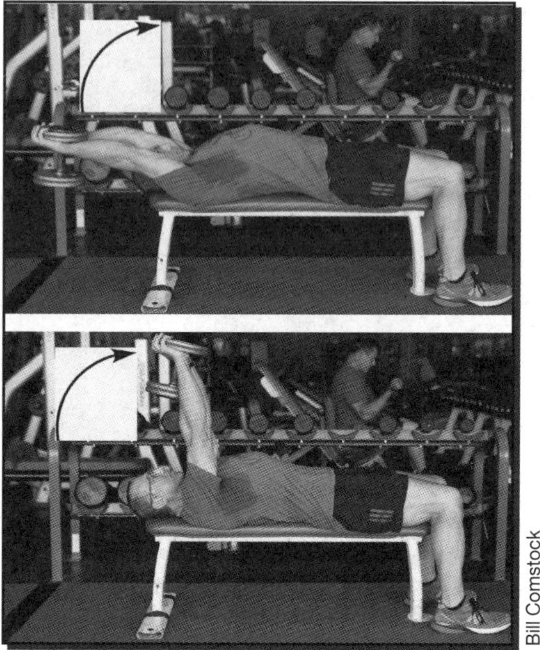

Figure 18-40

In my 40-plus years of competing in competitive bodybuilding, my observation has been that some people naturally develop their serratus anterior by doing exercises for their other major muscle groups, while other people are unable to achieve "outstanding" serratus anterior development, regardless of their best, most targeted efforts.

Therefore, I recommend that you not focus much (if any) direct effort on developing the serratus anterior, unless you are participating in a physical therapy program to correct a "winged scapula" (a shoulder blade that protrudes posteriorly, when simply standing), or addressing some other skeletal dysfunction. The serratus will become activated, to the degree that your genetics allows, simply by performing exercises for the other major muscle groups of your body.

## Summary

The ideal anatomical motion for the pectorals, for the purpose of optimally loading the greatest number of fibers, is a slight decline angle "press" (anterior humeral adduction), which allows the hands to come all the way together (for optimal pectoral contraction), ending with the humerus at the mid-sternum level. This could be achieved with dumbbells (on a slight decline bench), or with cables, using a bench/pulley arrangement that achieves the same angle.

The ideal direction of resistance, which should then be applied to the ideal direction of anatomical motion, is directly opposite the slight decline motion of the humerus—and slightly outward, by about 20 degrees. In other words, instead of having the resistance come from a "straight back" direction—as would be the case when using dumbbells—the angle of the resistance would be such that the left arm is using resistance that comes slightly more from the left, and the right arm is using resistance that is coming slightly more from the right. This creates a resistance curve that provides a little bit less resistance at the early phase (when mechanical disadvantage is occurring), and a little bit more at the late phase/point of contraction. This angle of resistance can only be achieved by using cables that are appropriately set.

The decline dumbbell press (set at a 20-degree angle decline) could be considered a close "second alternative," but not quite the very best pectoral exercise. This factor is because the direction of resistance, when using "free weight/gravity," is straight down (vertical), which provides a slightly less than optimal resistance curve for the pectorals—a little too much at the beginning of the range of motion, and not enough (essentially zero) at the conclusion of the range of motion.

Of course, it's easier to find a gym that has a decline bench and dumbbells, than it is to find a double-adjustable pulley, which allows just the right setting to create the perfect angle of resistance, as well as the perfect resistance curve for the pectorals. To reiterate, the decline dumbbell press is a very close "second alternative"—perhaps a "9" on the scale of "1 - 10." Don't fret, if this is the only option available to you.

On the other hand, if a double-adjustable pulley is available to you, it is an ideal option for training the pectorals. In addition to providing the optimal resistance curve, it is also more comfortable to sit upright on a bench, as compared to being semi-inverted, with your hips higher than your head. Furthermore, it's much easier to get in and out of an upright bench, as well as picking up the cable handles, as compared to climbing in and out of a decline bench, and picking up a pair of heavy dumbbells (or bringing them down with you). Although using cables is not as "impressive" to watch, as it is to see a person bench pressing a slightly bending bar, holding six or eight rattling 45-pound plates, you can load the pecs just as much or more, using cables. You can use as much weight as you want, even to the point where four reps is challenging (or even one repetition, although that would not necessarily be productive).

If you want to use a second (additional) exercise, a good option is the *extreme decline cable press*. This exercise would target the lowest clavicular fibers a little bit more than the *slight decline cable press* (or the *slight decline dumbbell press*), although not significantly more.

Given that the *slight decline cable press* (or the *slight decline dumbbell press*) moves the humerus toward the middle of the sternum (the mid-point between the highest pectoral fibers and the lowest pectoral fibers), it engages all the pectoral fibers. Accordingly, it should, therefore, be considered the "primary" exercise for the pecs. As such, the most number of sets should be devoted to that exercise/angle (i.e., 5 to 10 sets, depending on one's current level and ambition). The *extreme decline cable press*, therefore, would only require four or five sets. It should not be treated as the "primary" exercise.

All other angles of humeral movement, and all other directions of resistance (including that provided by a cam/machine) would be compromised, in comparison to the two aforementioned exercises. They may be "worth doing," but with the understanding that either the direction of humeral movement is less than optimal, or the direction of resistance (i.e., the resistance curve/alignment, mechanical disadvantage, etc.) is less than optimal—or both.

# CHAPTER 19

# LATISSIMUS DORSI AND "UPPER BACK" MUSCLES

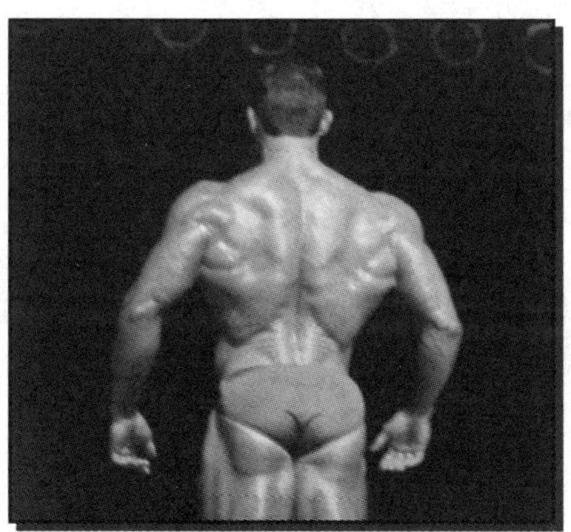

Figure 19-1

In bodybuilding "jargon," people usually classify the lats and other muscles of the upper back, collectively, as the "back." For example, if someone asks a gym buddy which muscles they're working today, the answer would likely be something like "chest and back," or "back and biceps." What's important, of course, is to know the individual muscles of the "back," and to understand their distinct functions, so that you can determine which exercises are BEST for each of those muscles.

Most people are familiar with the latissimus dorsi—the "lats." Beyond that, however, most bodybuilders, and even most trainers, do not know the names nor the exact functions of the other muscles of the upper back. How do I know this? Because virtually no one exercises their BACK muscles "correctly"—a fact that will be obvious in relatively short order.

## Anatomy of the "Lats"

The origins of the latissimus dorsi are located on the lower two-thirds of the spine (thoracic 7 through lumbar 5), and on the lower third and fourth ribs, as well as on the bottom tip of the scapula and on the upper-posterior part of pelvis (the iliac crest). All of these fibers then insert onto the upper-inner part of the humerus, just below the humeral head.

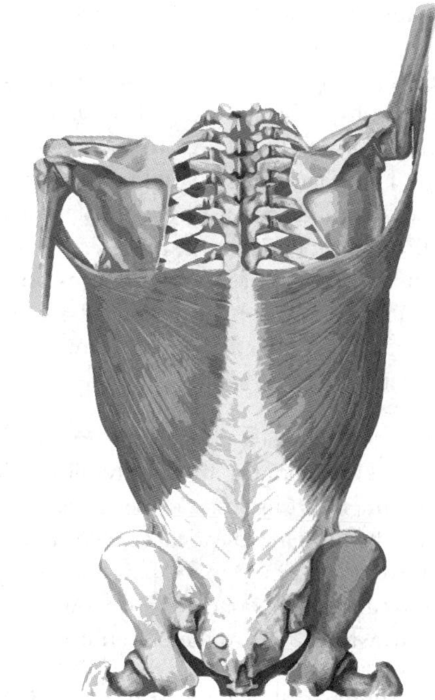

Figure 19-2

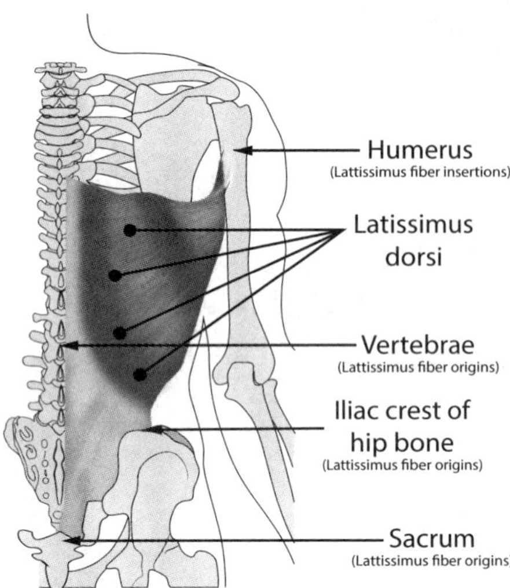


Figure 19-3

Common exercises for the lats include *chin-ups* and various types of *pulldowns* (wide grip with a straight bar, narrow grip, with an A-bar handle, etc.), as well as various *rowing* movements (*one-arm dumbbell row, seated cable row,* etc.). As such, our mission, in this instance, is to determine if these are actually good exercises for the lats, or if there are better exercises.

## Determining the Ideal Anatomical Motion for Exercising the Lats

The three "clues" outlined in Chapter 17 can be used to determine what the ideal motion for the lats would be. These clues are: the origin and insertion of the muscle; the direction of the muscle fibers; and the apparent design of the shoulder joint. In that regard, the most immediately obvious indication is the direction of the lat fibers. As you can see, they are mostly diagonal. That factor alone would suggest a diagonal movement, as well as a diagonal direction of resistance. In fact, none of the aforementioned exercises are "diagonal" movements with a diagonal resistance. For example, *chin-ups* and *pulldowns* are vertical movements with a vertical resistance. While they're better than rowing movements (for the lats), they are still not quite ideal.

The second most obvious clue is the origins and the insertion of the lats. The origins are mostly all on the spine and on the upper-inner part of posterior pelvis. Since "muscles always pull toward their origin," the ideal concentric anatomical motion of the lats would be a movement that causes its operating lever (the humerus/upper arm bone) to move inwardly, toward the spine, and downward—toward the posterior pelvis.

The next question that should be asked is: "FROM which direction should that motion come?" Naturally, it should come from a direction that is directly opposite the concentric motion. Since the concentric motion is headed toward the spine (in a diagonally downward angle), it should originate from a position that is directly away from the spine—away from the fiber origins that are on the spine. That placement would point to a starting "location" that is diagonal, upward from the torso at an angle of approximately 30 or 40 degrees. Furthermore, it should come from an angle that is slightly in front of the torso—approximately 45 degrees to the front—in order to prevent excessive external humeral rotation, when the arm in the descended position and the elbow is bent.

Finally, it would be helpful to consider the shoulder joint for a minute, and ascertain what its design tells us about the ideal motion of the lats. As such, in Figure 19-4, focus your attention on the right humerus (upper arm bone), which is pointing almost straight up. Then, look at the attachment of the latissimus, on the humerus, when the humerus is at that angle. Do you see the mechanical disadvantage there? The arm must rotate outwardly (refer to the curved arrow) around the shoulder pivot, but the lats cannot pull in that direction. The lats can only pull toward their origins.

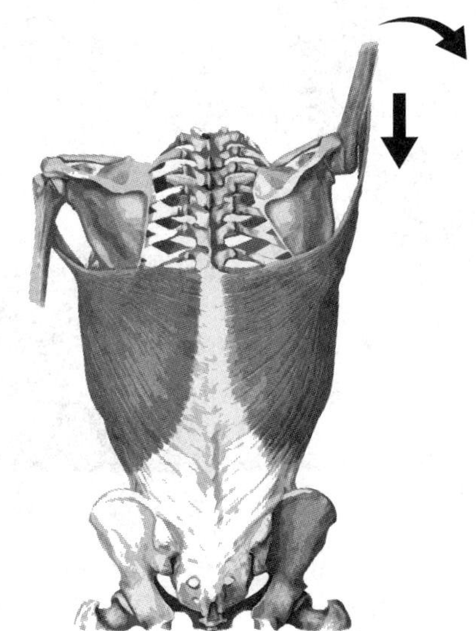

Figure 19-4

When the humerus is elevated that high, the latissimus is forced to pull on the humerus from a mostly parallel angle, which is the most extreme angle of mechanical disadvantage. The force requirement, when this situation occurs, is approximately six to seven times greater than what it would be if the muscle were able to pull on its corresponding bone perpendicularly. For this reason, starting a *chin-up* or a heavy *lat pulldown*, with a humerus that is angled that high (70 to 80 degrees), has a fairly high risk of injury.

Figure 19-5 shows you what this scenario looks like during an actual *chin-up*. From this starting position, the first 40 degrees of the humerus' trajectory experiences a significant mechanical disadvantage. On the other hand, when the upper arm is about 30 degrees up from horizontal (refer to the dotted marker on the protractor, Figure 19-6), the lats are able to pull on the humerus more perpendicularly. That is the point at which the lats can pull on the humerus from a better mechanical advantage, and can more effectively pull the upper arm toward the spine, toward the latissimus origins. This factor makes it more productive, as well as more safe.

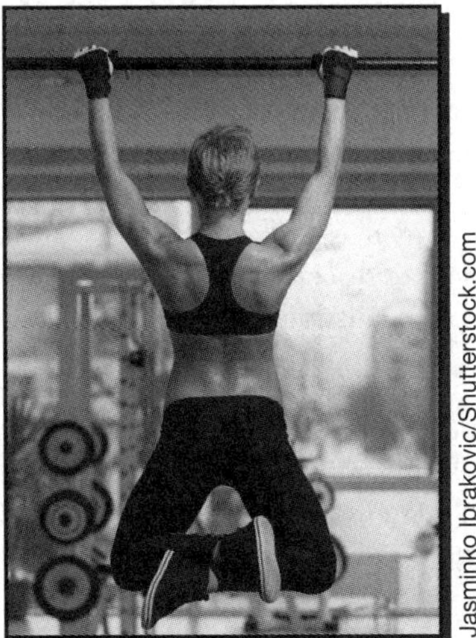

Jasminko Ibrakovic/Shutterstock.com

Figure 19-5

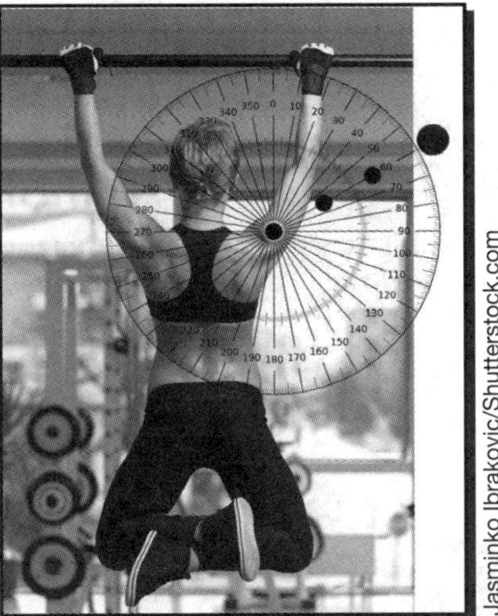

Jasminko Ibrakovic/Shutterstock.com

Figure 19-6

As noted previously, *chin-ups* and *pulldowns* engage the lats better than do any of the *rowing* movements, but *chin-ups* and *pulldowns* both have mechanical shortcomings. They both use a vertical resistance (rather than a diagonal resistance); they both begin their range of motion, with the humerus too high; and then they complete their trajectory too soon, before the humerus has completed its full inward/downward trajectory, and the lats are able to fully contract.

If you use a wide grip, when performing either *chin-ups* or *pulldowns*, you reduce the mechanical disadvantage, when the arms are fully extended upward. On the other hand, you also limit your ability to bring the humerus all the way down and inward, which prevents complete contraction of the latissimus. If you use a narrow grip, you'd be able to bring your humerus farther inward (alongside your torso), which provides a better latissimus contraction. The narrow grip, however, results in a more severe mechanical disadvantage when the arms are up.

In both cases, using a wide grip or a narrow grip, it's impossible to keep the forearm (as the secondary lever) in the neutral position (i.e., parallel with the direction of resistance). This factor is because the lats each have a separate direction of movement (the left lat pulls downward and inward to the right, and the right lat pulls downward and inward to the left). In addition, each requires a different direction of resistance (ideally speaking), which is impossible unless two separate resistance sources are used.

The *chin-up* is further problematic because it forces you to use your entire bodyweight. As such, you don't have the variety of resistance options you should have. Ideally, you should be able to warm up with a resistance that is light enough to do 20 or 30 repetitions, without too much effort. Then, you would gradually increase the resistance, until you're only able to perform six to eight challenging repetitions, with good form.

*Note: A chin-up machine, which provides "assistance," would be helpful in this regard. However, there are still two additional problems with chin-ups that must also be considered.*

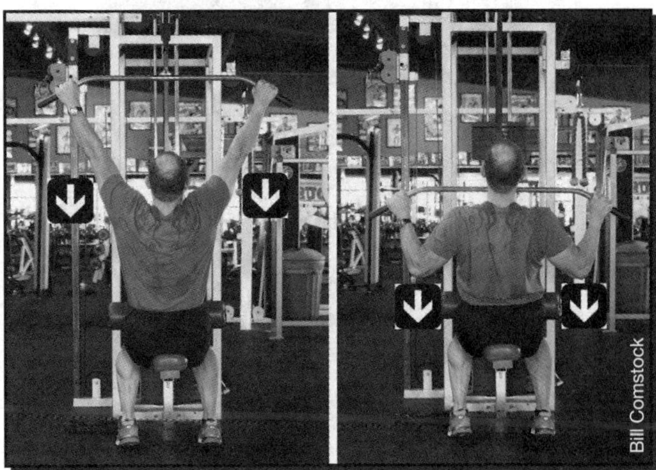

Bill Comstock

Figure 19-7

Another "problem" with *chin-ups* is that it forces your body to hang vertically, which then causes the humerus to pull from a less-than-ideal angle. Ideally, the humerus should pull from a slightly forward angle. This factor can be achieved, when doing *lat pulldowns*, simply by leaning back about 20 degrees. It is impossible, however, to angle your torso 20 degrees from vertical, when doing *chin-ups*. Adding additional resistance, when doing *chin-ups* (by way of a belt or chain around your waist), further exacerbates this problem.

Because *lat pulldowns* allow "more resistance options" and a "better direction of humeral movement relative to the torso," it is a better exercise than *chin-ups* for working the lats. *Lat pulldowns*, however, still have an imperfect direction of resistance, as well as a couple of other disadvantages associated with using the "single instrument" (the lat pulldown bar), as opposed to each arm working independently.

Again, the ideal anatomical motion for the lats would be a movement that has the humerus (upper arm) starting at about 30 degrees above the shoulder, and angling toward the front about 45 degrees (halfway between "straight to the side" and "straight to the front"). This positioning allows the movement to start from a point where the latissimus is optimally elongated, yet avoids mechanical disadvantage, and also avoids any possible shoulder impingement.

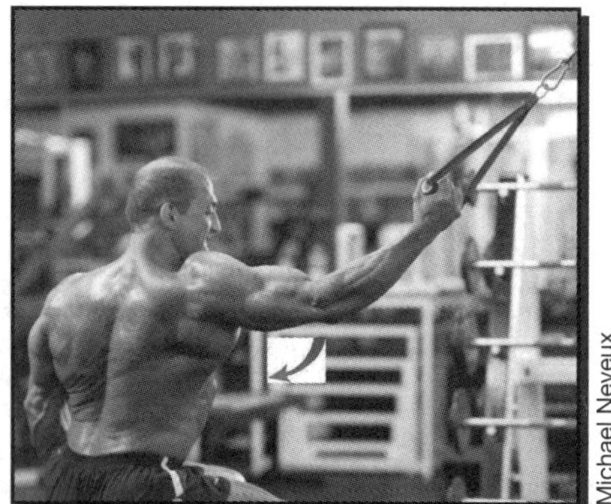

Figure 19-8

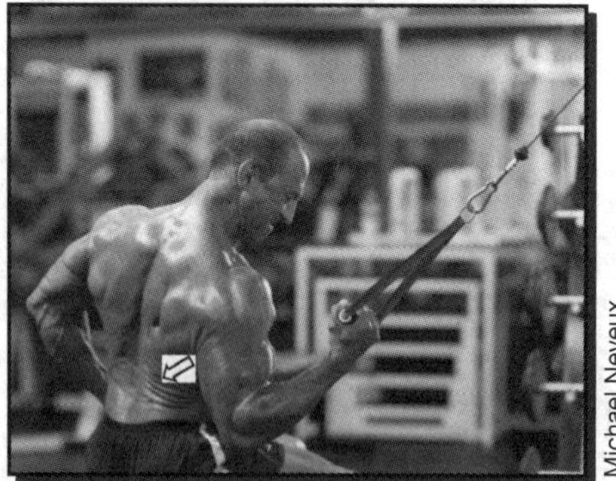

Figure 19-9

The concentric movement would then bring the humerus downward and inward, toward the exerciser's side (Figure 19-9), which allows the humerus to move toward the latissimus origins on the spine, as well as on the upper-posterior part of the pelvis. The movement ends with the elbow almost touching the hip bone, for full latissimus contraction. This scenario represents the most pure, most natural latissimus function, without shoulder joint strain. That ideal direction of movement, combined with the ideal direction of resistance, is best achieved with a *one-arm cable lat pull-in*, shown in Figures 19-8 and 19-9.

In contrast, the direction of movement that is performed when you do any kind of *rowing* exercise is straight back—posteriorly. The lats, however, do not directly produce a "straight back" direction of "pull." As such, the typical *rowing* motion fails to move the operating lever of the lats (i.e., the humerus/upper arms) toward the latissimus origins on the spine. Furthermore, the "straight forward" direction of resistance, which is typically present during most *rowing* exercises, is neither directly opposite the latissimus origins, nor is it parallel to the latissimus fibers.

Instead of working mostly the lats, *rowing* motions work mostly the posterior deltoids. While the lats participate to a degree, they are not able to do the majority of the work, because neither the motion, nor the direction of resistance, are correct enough to qualify as "good" for the lats.

## Determining the Ideal Direction of Resistance for the Lats

As you know, the direction of resistance determines the "resistance curve" of an exercise. It also plays a role in alleviating (or exacerbating) a mechanical disadvantage, depending on the direction of resistance you select.

The latissimus attachment on the humerus is similar to that of the biceps brachii on the radius (forearm bone). When either of these muscles are fully elongated, they are forced

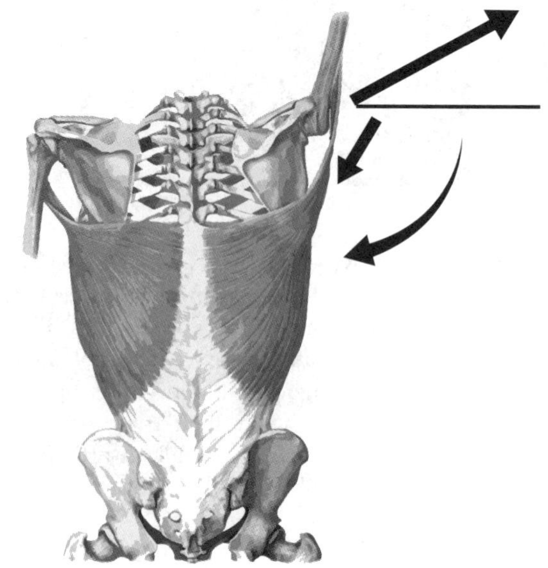
Figure 19-10

to pull on their operating levers from a more parallel angle. This factor increases the force requirement to a degree that could be dangerous. As a result, in both instances—when you're working the biceps or the lats—it is better to provide a direction of resistance that is mostly parallel to the operating lever, at the beginning of the range of motion, where the risk is the highest.

In Figure 19-10, an arrow has been placed pointing from the shoulder joint, upward at a 30-degree angle. If you were to begin the movement with your humerus at that angle, with the direction of resistance that is also at that angle, they would be parallel. Technically, this positioning would make the humerus a "neutral lever." On the other hand, since the lats would be pulling on the humerus from a mostly parallel angle (more parallel than perpendicular), at that starting point, the increased force requirement from this would compensate for the mostly "neutral" angle of the humerus, relative to the direction of resistance.

This situation is very much like starting a *standing dumbbell curl* with a neutral forearm. When you start the motion, even the slightest "perpendicular-ness" to that forearm magnifies the load tremendously, because of the mechanical disadvantage. In other words, the fact that the operating lever is "less active" (mostly parallel to gravity) is offset by the fact that the force requirement is increased by the mechanical disadvantage.

As the operating lever (the humerus) moves downward and inward, during *one-arm cable lat pull-ins*, it becomes progressively more "active" (more perpendicular with the cable). It reaches the most perpendicular angle about halfway into the range of motion. This factor allows the latissimus to pull on its operating lever from a better mechanical advantage, which balances out the resistance curve nicely. As you get "stronger" (i.e., as you gain mechanical advantage), the humerus becomes more "active" (i.e., more perpendicular with resistance), which makes the resistance "heavier" (i.e., increases its percentage of load on the lats).

Another benefit of this particular exercise (*one-arm lat pull-ins*)—using only one arm at a time, with a resistance that comes from the recommended angle—is that you can pull your upper arm "down-and-inward" farther than you would be able to during standard *lat pulldowns*. This exercise allows a more ideal range of motion—less ROM at the top, where it's risky, as well as more ROM at the bottom, for a better contraction.

At this point, you should understand what constitutes the ideal anatomical movement for optimally engaging the lats, as well as what constitutes the ideal direction of resistance which should accompany that anatomical movement. Accordingly, you should be able to clearly see why rowing movements are not very good for optimally engaging the lats. In that regard, it can be helpful to examine the biomechanical shortcomings of one particular rowing exercise that is very commonly used during latissimus workouts—the *one-arm dumbbell row*.

Keep in mind that the goal—during any resistance exercise—is to have the operating lever of your target muscle (i.e., in this case, it's the humerus) move toward the target muscle's origins (i.e., in this case, the latissimus origins on the lower two-thirds of the spine), during the concentric phase of the movement. Then, during the eccentric phase of the movement, the goal is to have the operating lever move directly away from the latissimus origins on the spine. Furthermore, the direction of resistance should originate from an angle that is directly opposite the latissimus origins on the spine, and on the same plane as the target muscle's origin and insertion, in accordance with the principle of alignment and of "opposite position loading" (i.e., the line of force).

The first problem with this exercise is that the typical angle of the torso, during *one-arm rowing*, is about 30 degrees from horizontal, with the top of the spine higher than the lower part of the spine. This situation means that resistance (gravity) is pulling more from below the shoulder, rather than from above the shoulder. As a result, instead of pulling concentrically downward, toward the lower vertebrae and posterior part of the pelvis, the concentric pulling is moving toward the upper back and shoulders.

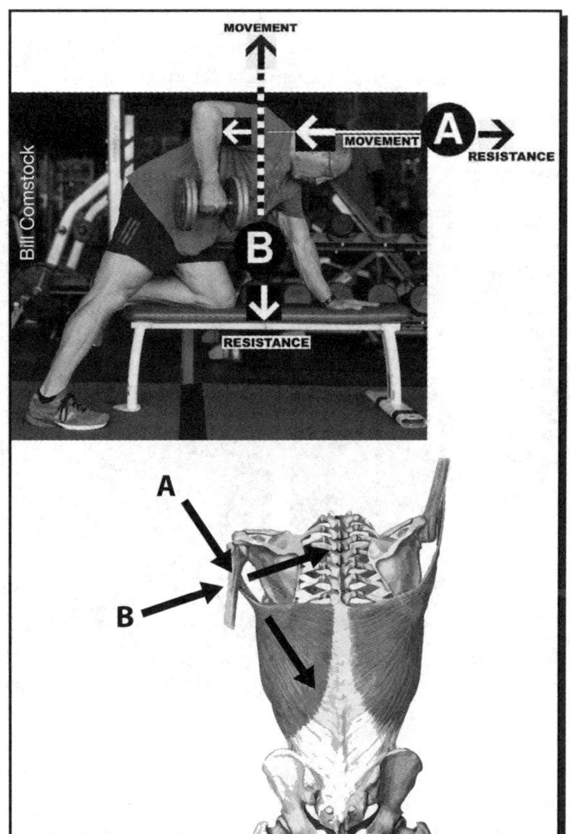


Figure 19-11

In Figure 19-11, the "A" arrow indicates the direction of "pull" that would optimally engage the latissimus, because that would move the humerus more toward the latissimus origins. On the other hand, having the torso at this angle causes the humerus to move more upward (the "B" arrow), toward an area where there are no latissimus fibers. This factor is not the only problem with the *one-arm dumbbell row*, however. In order to optimally engage the lats, the humeral movement needs to be toward the spine, but that is not the direction of the humeral movement that occurs during *one-arm dumbbell row*.

When performing a *one-arm dumbbell row* (Figure 19-12), people usually rotate their torso in a direction that holds the shoulder of the working side higher (farther from the ground) than the shoulder of the side that being used for support (i.e., the straight arm that is braced against the bench). This factor results in a direction of humeral movement that is not toward the spine.

As you can see, the direction of the exerciser's arm movement is toward 12:00, but the origin of his lats are on his spine, where a dot has been placed. It's obvious that he's not moving his arm toward that dot (toward the spine, and the latissimus origins). By the time he finishes the repetition (the conclusion of the concentric motion), he has further rotated his torso, such that his spine is even farther away from the trajectory of his arm. When he begins the motion (Figure 19-12, left image), the dot is in the 2:00 position. By the time he finishes the repetition (Figure 19-12, right image), the dot is in the 4:00 position—farther away from the 12:00 trajectory of the humerus, than it was when it was in the 2:00 position.

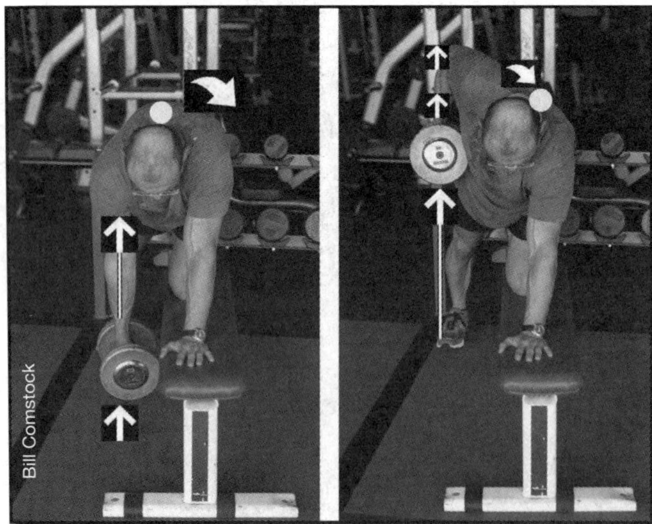

Figure 19-12

As a result of this misalignment, during *one-arm dumbbell rowing*, the latissimus is not participating nearly as much as it's assumed. Rather than having the humeral movement heading toward the origin of the latissimus, it is heading toward the posterior deltoid and the teres major.

While you might be thinking, at this point, that the solution would be to not rotate the torso, it would be impossible to hold the torso in the "correct" position, given the direction of the resistance/gravity (straight down, vertical). The torso would need to be held in such a way as to have the hips higher than the shoulders and the shoulder of the working arm lower than the shoulder of the non-working arm, in order to produce a humeral movement that is directly opposite gravity, and moves toward the lower two-thirds of the spine.

For maximum benefit, "opposite position loading" requires that the direction of resistance come from a "place" that is directly opposite the origins of the target muscle. When targeting the lats, the resistance should come more from the side (lateral to the torso), and from higher than the shoulder, while the humerus moves in a direction that is downward and inward, toward the origins of the latissimus.

Almost all standard rowing exercises (e.g., *T-bar rowing, seated cable rowing, one-arm dumbbell rowing*, etc.) involve a straight forward-pulling direction of resistance, which is very inadequate for optimal loading of the latissimus. As was discussed in Chapter 8 ("Opposite Position Loading"), whatever muscle origin is directly opposite resistance will be the most loaded, whether that is the exerciser's intention or not. As such, if a muscle origin is NOT directly opposite resistance, it will NOT be the most loaded by that resistance.

For this reason, most rowing exercises would rate a "4" or a "5," in terms of efficiency for latissimus training. An "unsupported" rowing exercise (e.g., *low pulley rowing*, or *bent-over barbell rowing*) would rate even lower, because of the additional strain on the lower back.

## The Muscles of the "Upper Back": Middle Trapezius, Teres Major, Infraspinatus, and Teres Minor

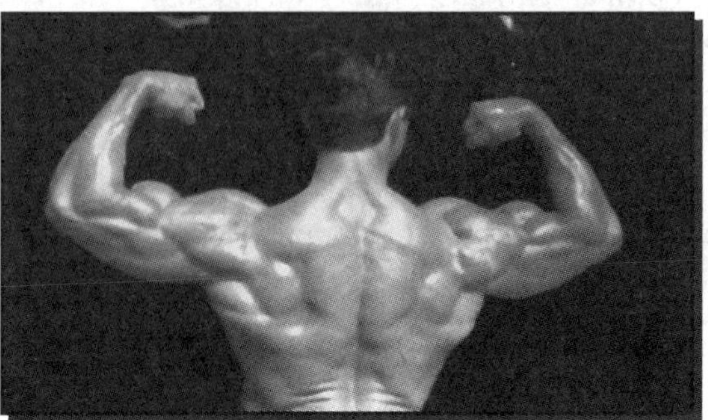
Figure 19-13

As was noted at the beginning of this chapter, most people are typically not able to identify the muscles of the "back," beyond the lats. Even among those individuals who can identify the muscles of the upper back, they typically don't understand the action those muscles produce. This group includes, by the way, most competitive bodybuilders and most personal trainers, even though they devote vast amounts of time and effort doing "back" exercises, or teaching "back" exercises to other people.

In fact, most of the exercises that have been traditionally used to work the "upper back" are NOT as productive as we've all been led to believe, which you'll soon see for yourself.

In Figure 19-14, you can see that the middle trapezius is the second most prominent muscle of the back—second only to the lats. It covers nearly a third of the entire back—from the base of the neck, down to the mid-spine, and from the outer edge of one scapula to the outer edge of the other scapula. As such, in Figure 19-15, you can see how significant the trapezius are in this *"back double biceps"* pose.

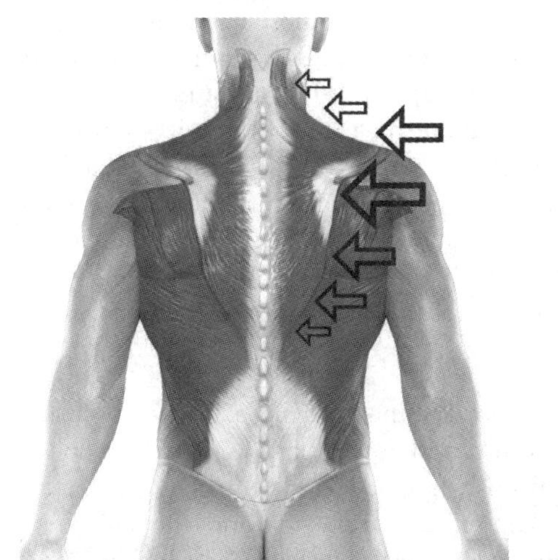
CLIPAREA I Custom media/Shutterstock.com

Figure 19-14

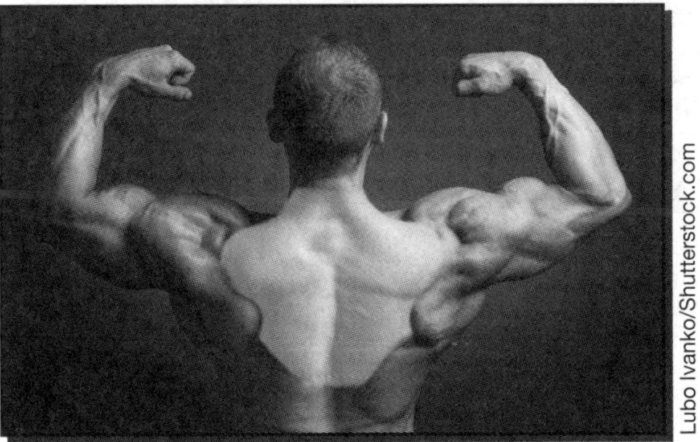
Lubo Ivanko/Shutterstock.com

Figure 19-15

The second and third most prominent muscles of the upper back—the teres major (Figure 19-16) and the infraspinatus (Figure 19-17)—are significantly smaller than the middle trapezius. The teres major is a triangular section, just above the outer part of the lats. The infraspinatus is in the middle, between the trapezius, the posterior deltoid, the teres major, and the latissimus. The only remaining muscle of the upper back is the teres minor, which is very small and cannot be seen in these figures. Nonetheless, it will be reviewed in a moment, as will the rhomboids.

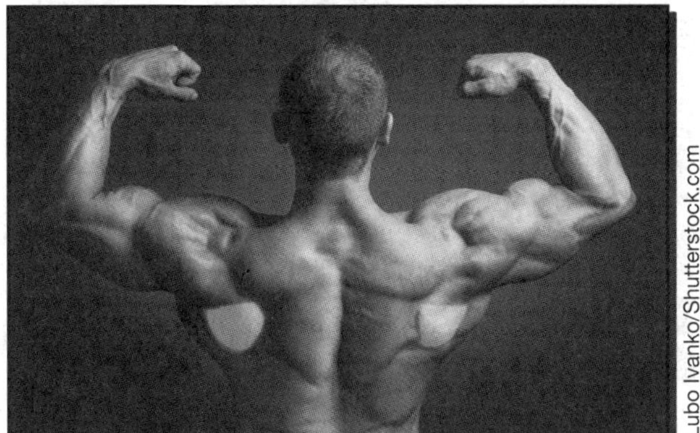
Lubo Ivanko/Shutterstock.com

Figure 19-16

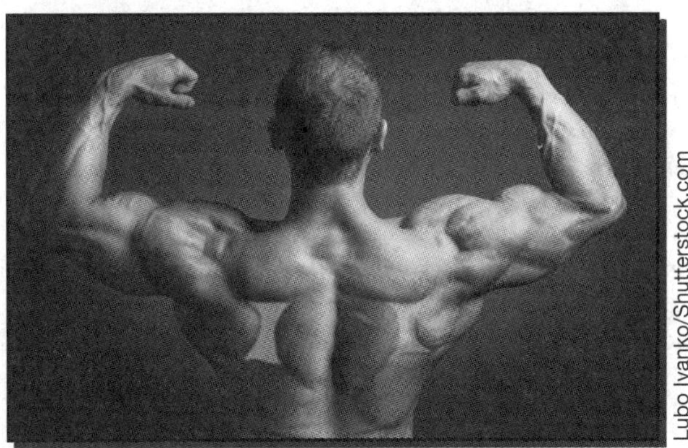
Lubo Ivanko/Shutterstock.com

Figure 19-17

Given that you are now aware of the names and locations of the primary "upper back" muscles, the next step is to identify the anatomical movement that each of these muscles produce. Then, you'll need to ask yourself the key question: "Are you doing the right exercises for these muscles, given their primary functions?"

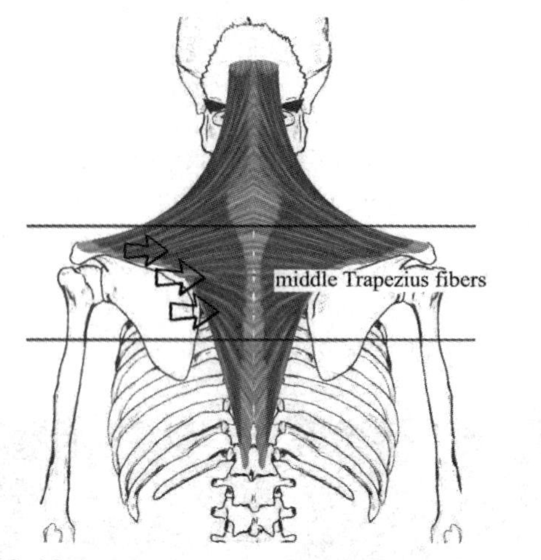


Clint Smith/E2 Systems, Inc.

Figure 19-18

The origins of the trapezius are situated on the upper two-thirds of the spine, beginning at the base of the skull (the occipital bone), down to the lower thoracic vertebrae (T6 through T12). Its fibers then extend laterally, converge and attach onto the outer portion of scapula (the shoulder blade), as well as the outer portion of the clavicle (collar bone). None of the trapezius muscle fibers attach onto the humerus (the upper arm bone). This factor is important, as you'll soon see.

The direction of the trapezius fibers are indicative of the muscle's actions. The upper trapezius fibers pull the scapula and the outer end of the clavicle upward. The middle fibers pull the scapula backward and inward, toward the spine. The lower fibers pull the scapula downward and inward.

The trapezius is assisted by the rhomboid major and minor. The levator scapulae also assists the trapezius in pulling the scapula upward. The rhomboids and the levator scapulae, shown in Figure 19-19, are beneath the trapezius. As a result, they cannot be seen, even if that person is very lean.

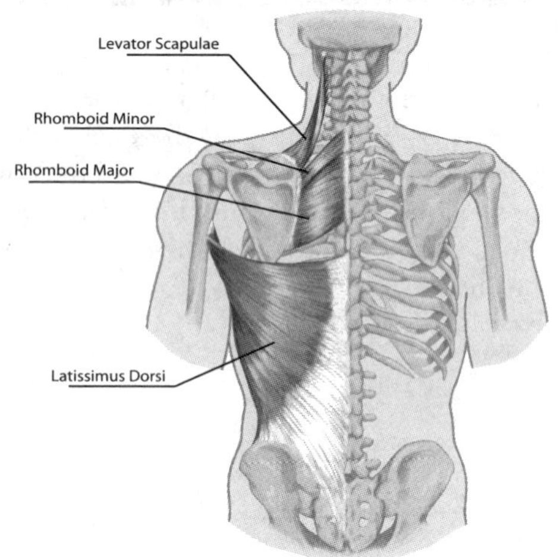


stihii/Shutterstock.com

Figure 19-19

Both of these muscles—the rhomboids and the levator scapulae—are significantly smaller than the trapezius, and have very little capacity for growth. You should note that they attach to the inner edge of the scapula, whereas the trapezius attaches to the outer edge of the scapula. Therefore, they cannot play as strong a role in elevating the scapula, as compared with the trapezius. All in all, they are not muscles with which you need to concern yourself, because they participate anytime you engage the trapezius, whether you are aware of it or not.

In regard to the development (visible growth) of the middle trapezius, you should ask yourself the following question: "*How much of a role does the middle trapezius play—during a rowing exercise—given that the middle trapezius does NOT connect to the arms?*" Since *rowing* exercises mostly involve arm movement, the answer to that question is "a very small role."

Next time you're at the gym, watch people as they perform any of the following exercises: "*seated cable rowing,*" "*one-arm dumbbell rowing,*" "*T-bar rowing,*" or any other type of rowing exercise, including those done on rowing machines. What you'll see is that a rowing movement is about 90-percent arm motion. The trapezius (the largest muscle of the "upper" back) cannot pull on the arms, because it is not connected to the arms. As such, the traps play NO role whatsoever in the arm-part of a rowing motion. The middle trapezius is only involved in stabilizing the scapula (preventing the scapula from collapsing forward), during any standard rowing exercise. It is not the middle trapezius that pulls the arms backward—nor is it primarily the lats.

Despite the fact that *rowing* exercises are considered a standard part of a traditional "back workout" for bodybuilding, they are obviously not "ideal" for either the lats or the middle trapezius. The middle trapezius and the lats are the two largest, most prominent muscles of the "back," yet neither of those muscles gets fully activated or fully loaded during standard *rowing* exercises.

As was discussed in Chapter 8, the rowing motion is produced mostly by the posterior deltoids. In addition, because the posterior deltoids (and the teres major) are positioned directly opposite the forward-pulling resistance of most *rowing* exercises, they are also the muscles that are most loaded.

Of course, some people try to "squeeze" their shoulder blades together when they perform *rowing* exercises, in an effort to flex (contract) the middle trapezius. That's a noble intention, but it ends up being an incidental part of a *rowing* exercise, despite a person's best efforts. When the resistance is pulling the arms straight forward, the automatic thing to do is to pull in the opposite direction of that forward pull, which must be a "straight back" direction of movement.

Squeezing the scapula together requires a different direction of movement—one that is more "inward"—NOT "straight back." It is physically and psychologically difficult to add that secondary motion, in a slightly different direction, when a heavy resistance is pulling you straight forward. Even if you're able to do it, it would not entirely solve the problem, because the target muscle origins are not positioned directly opposite the direction of resistance. As a result, the middle trapezius would not be loaded by a large percentage of the resistance being used.

You'll recall that in Chapter 8, an example was discussed demonstrating that when a rope is thrown over a tree branch, and then someone pulls that rope straight downward (in a 6:00 direction), that force will mostly load the 12:00 area of the branch. As such, if you want to "load" (apply force) to the 2:00 part of the tree branch, you must pull the rope from an 8:00 direction.

The origins of the trapezius fibers are all on the spine, which is located at the 3:00 and 9:00 position, relative to each of the arms. The line of force, from a forward-pulling resistance, is opposite the back of the shoulders—the posterior deltoids and the teres major. Those are not the intended target muscles of a rowing exercise, however. The muscle origins of the trapezius and of the latissimus (the intended target muscles of a rowing exercise) are on the spine, and therefore not positioned directly opposite the line of force of a forward-pulling resistance.

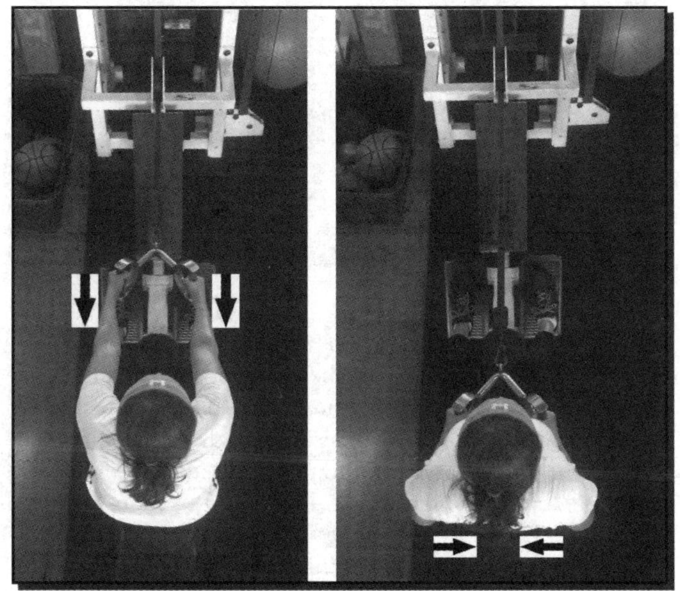
Figure 19-20

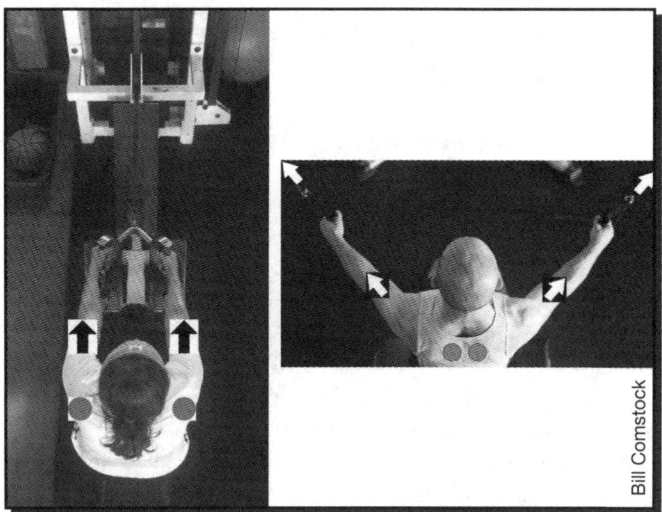

Figure 19-21

In Figure 19-21 (left image), the arrows are pointing in the direction of the resistance, which is opposite the backward-pulling direction of the arms. In contrast, in Figure 19-21 (right image), the two arrows are indicating the direction the resistance SHOULD occur, for the middle trapezius to be optimally loaded and challenged for its designated function—pulling the scapula inward, toward the spine. It is very difficult to move the arms "backward," and the scapula "inward" simultaneously—two different directions of movement—while fighting against a forward-pulling.

Next, focus your attention on the two dots on Figure 19-21, left image, which show where the load of the forward-pulling resistance goes—onto the posterior deltoids and teres major. In turn, the dots on Figure 19-21, right image, indicate where the load of a diagonal direction of resistance goes—onto the middle trapezius—because those origins are now directly opposite resistance.

"Opposite position loading" requires (for maximum efficiency) that the resistance come from a direction that is mostly opposite the origins of the middle trapezius fibers. Since those origins are on the spine (the center of the torso), the resistance should come from a more lateral (side) angle. The anatomical motion would then be mostly scapular, because that is the only motion the middle trapezius produces. As such, the emphasis should be on squeezing the shoulder blades together, with a much lesser emphasis on pulling with the arms.

*Note: The minimal arm movement that would occur during this exercise would engage the highest fibers of the latissimus (and only to a fairly small degree), assisted by the teres major. The posterior deltoids would play a much smaller role, and would be much less loaded, as compared to a standard rowing exercise.*

## The Best Exercise for the "Upper Back"

The *scapular retraction* exercise (shown in Figures 19-22 to 19-24, from three angles) is the best exercise for targeting the middle trapezius of the upper back. It provides a direction of resistance that comes from an outward angle—level with the exerciser's shoulders. Then, the anatomical motion of the scapula is backward and inward, toward the spine. This movement would be directly opposite the direction of resistance. The objective would be to feel the middle trapezius contracting (as if trying to squeeze a pencil between the shoulder blades), during the concentric phase, and then to move the scapula forward and outward (laterally), during the eccentric phase. Using the arms (bending the elbows) a little bit helps the scapula move better, in addition to engaging some of the uppermost latissimus fibers. The elbows should NOT be pulled past the sides of the torso, however.

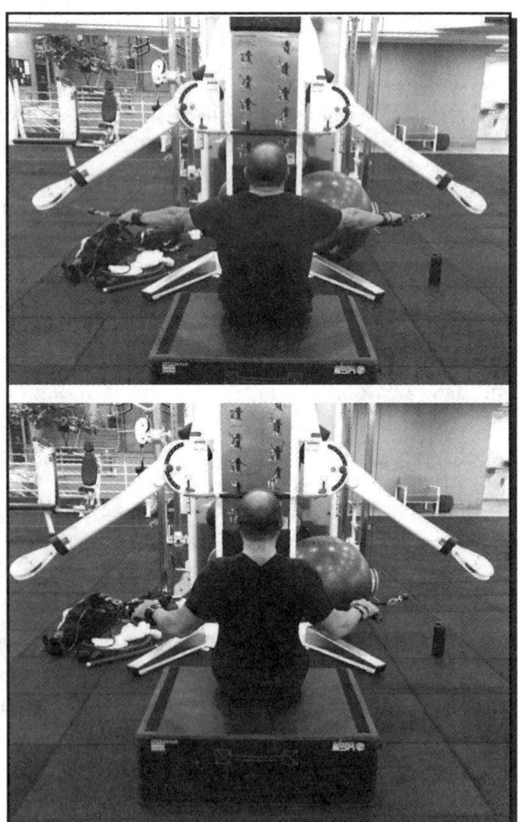
Figure 19-22

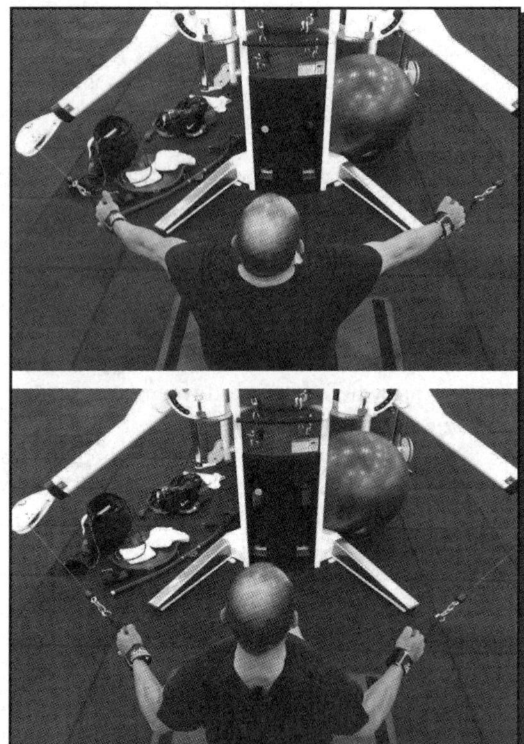
Figure 19-23

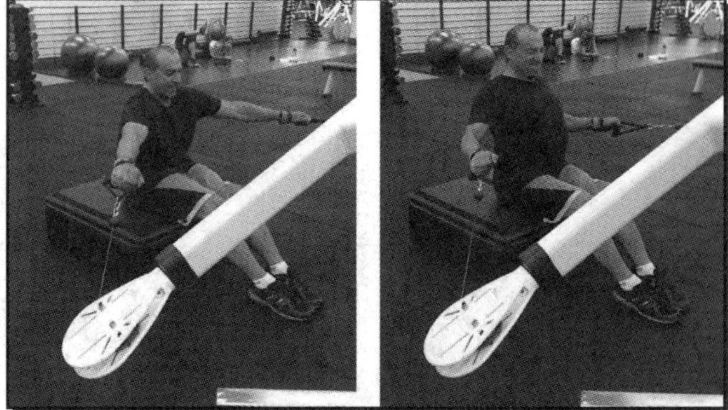
Figure 19-24

Of course, many people do not have access to this type of pulley system, which allows the height and the width of the two pulleys to be adjusted. If that's the case, it's unfortunate. What's even more unfortunate, in this instance, is that gym equipment manufacturers are not designing equipment properly. A machine that is designed like the set-up demonstrated in Figures 19-22 to 19-24 should be in every gym—ready to use. Unfortunately, this type of machine is not being made yet. If you want to perform this exercise, and don't have access to this type of pulley system, you can try to do it with a single pulley (one side at a time), but it will be difficult to prevent your torso from rotating, once you begin using substantial resistance.

*Note: Ironically, there are some "rowing" machines that start narrow and end wide. This type of design is the opposite of "ideal," because the motion is moving away from the spine, instead of toward it.*

The fact that "scapular retraction" machines don't exist yet, and that a person has to set up this type of arrangement in order to do it, does not negate the fact that this is the correct movement, as well as the correct direction of resistance, for best loading and contracting the largest muscle of the upper back—the middle trapezius. This type of exercise rates a "10" for development of the middle trapezius.

In contrast, a standard *low-pulley row* would rate a "5," at best. During a *low-pulley row*, the middle trapezius would only be loaded with about 40 percent of the resistance being used. In addition, the movement that naturally occurs during a *low-pulley row* is NOT one that moves the appropriate limb (i.e., the scapula) toward the spine. Rather, it causes the arms to move straight backward, which is toward the origins of the posterior deltoids.

In comparison, a *scapular retraction* (with a semi-lateral resistance) would load the middle trapezius with the greatest percentage of the load. It would load the posterior deltoids with about 80 percent less load than a *low-pulley row*. It would also load the lower back, with about half the load (less strain) than a *low-pulley row*. Thus, performing *scapular retractions* would result in you getting more of what you want—more load on your target muscle (the middle trapezius), and less of what you don't want—excessive load on your non-target muscles (the posterior deltoids and the lower back).

In fairness, a standard *rowing* machine, that is chest-supported, is adequate and safe enough for people who are "low-level" fitness participants. I'm not suggesting that equipment manufacturers discontinue making simple rowing machines, even though they are not "ideal." Standard "rowing" requires less coordination, is simpler to understand, and provides the user with a useful strength increase in that kind of motion (i.e., straight pulling). For those individuals who are motivated to pursue optimal muscular development, however, there should be a dedicated *scapular retraction* machine that makes it easy to perform this exercise, without having to set it up each time.

The teres major (highlighted in Figure 19-25, and shown on the anatomical illustration in Figure 19-26) is a relatively small muscle that originates on the lower/outer edge of the scapula, and attaches onto the humerus—just below the humeral head. It's like a "mini-latissimus," except that it originates on the outer edge of the scapula (close the shoulder joint), instead of on the spine. Therefore, it pulls in a direction that is more similar to the posterior deltoid, than to the latissimus. Therefore, it participates strongly in all movements which engage the posterior deltoids, but it also participates in all latissimus-related exercises like *pulldowns, chin-ups*, and *lat pull-ins*. This muscle does not need any focused attention, in terms of exercise. It gets plenty of work "peripherally."

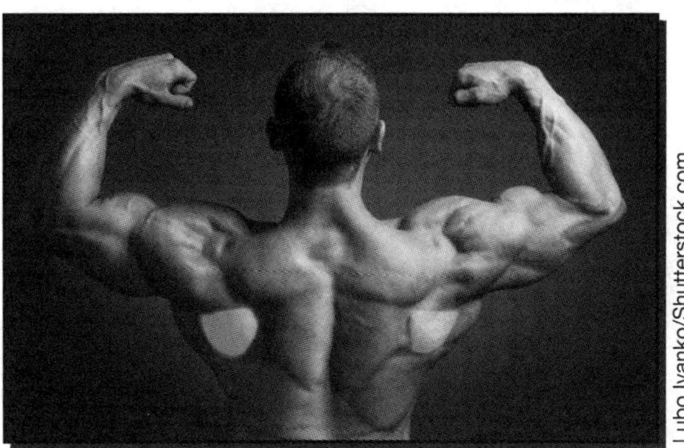

Lubo Ivanko/Shutterstock.com

Figure 19-25

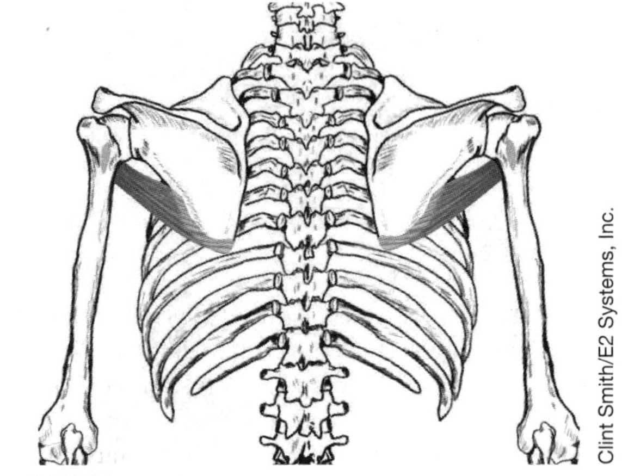

Clint Smith/E2 Systems, Inc.

Figure 19-26

The teres minor (Figures 19-27 and 19-28), which is an even smaller muscle, is generally not considered a "physique muscle." It lies between and beneath the teres major and the infraspinatus. It originates on the outer edge of the scapula, and attaches onto the posterior side of the humeral head. This factor is important to note, because since its attachment is so high on the humerus, it has essentially no leverage on it. In other words, this muscle cannot participate much in "pulling" movements of any kind—whether they're *pulldowns, chin-ups,* or *rowing*. Because the teres minor wraps around the posterior side of the humeral head, and it originates on the lateral aspect of the scapula, its primary function is to rotate the humerus externally. This muscle works in conjunction with the infraspinatus, which is the larger, stronger external rotator of the humerus.

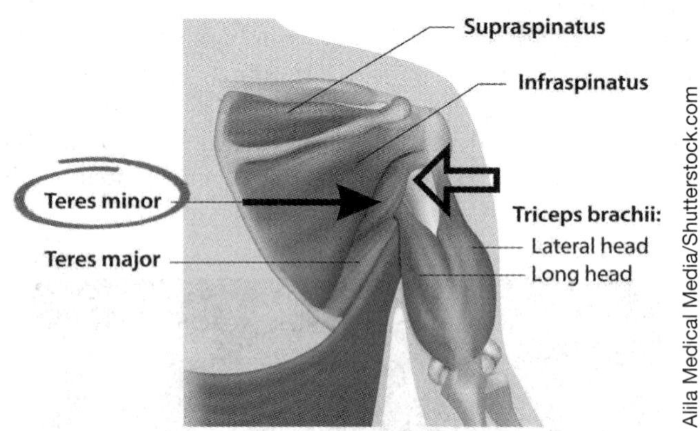


Figure 19-27

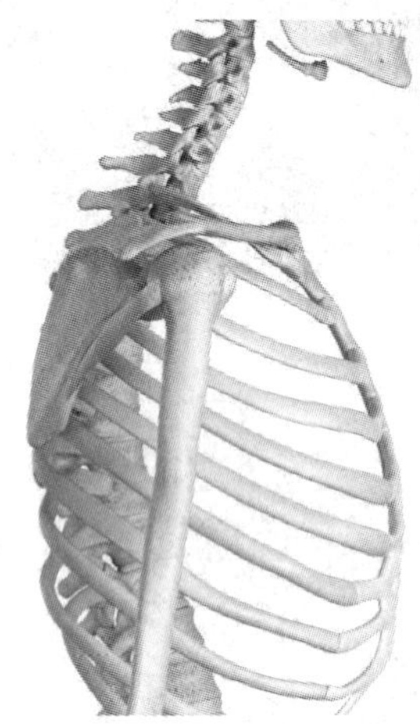


Figure 19-28

The infraspinatus (highlighted in Figure 19-29, and shown in the illustration in Figure 19-30) is the primary external rotator of the humerus. As you can see, it originates on the medial edge (closest to the midline of the body) of the posterior side of the scapula, and then attaches onto the humeral head, just above the attachment of the teres minor.

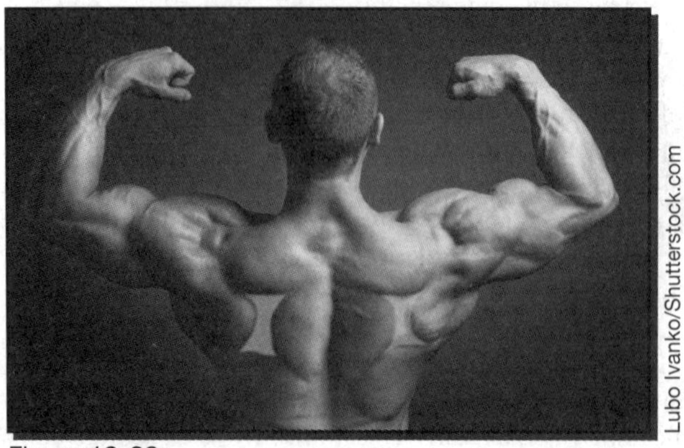


Figure 19-29

When it contracts, it rotates the humerus "externally." Like the teres minor, it has essentially no leverage on the humerus, because its attachment is so high on the humerus. Therefore, it cannot participate much in humeral adduction (pulling the arm downward, backward or inward), in movements like *pulldowns, chin-ups,* and *rowing.* Accordingly, although the infraspinatus looks as though it is one of the primary "back" muscles, it actually does not participate much in any of the exercises typically associated with "back exercises."

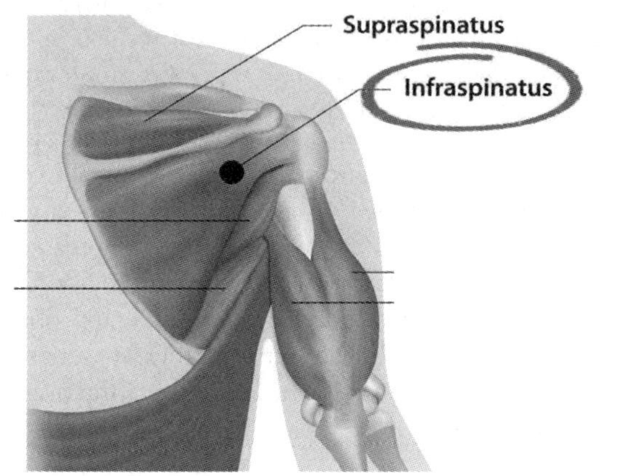


Figure 19-30

Ironically, the infraspinatus participates more during posterior deltoid exercises, especially when the alignment of that movement is not correct. In those instances, it works as an isometric "external rotation" exercise, preventing forward rotation, against resistance.

This muscle is definitely worth exercising, along with the teres minor (both external rotators), primarily for functional benefit. The external shoulder rotators are usually weaker than the internal rotators, because day-to-day activities typically require inward shoulder rotation, but rarely require external rotation. For this reason, the infraspinatus is more vulnerable to injury. This muscle, as well as the other "rotator cuff" muscles, will be further discussed in Chapter 25.

So, as you can see, *chin-ups, pulldowns, T-bar rowing, low pulley rowing,* and *one-arm dumbbell rows* are not optimally efficient exercises for either the latissimus or the middle trapezius. Despite this, however, many people are able to achieve a respectable level of latissimus and middle trapezius, using these exercises. It's not that traditional exercises do not work at all—it's that these exercises are not the most efficient, or the most productive, or the most safe. Exercises that are "half as efficient/half as productive" may require twice as much effort, but eventually can produce the same result as the better exercises. It's wiser to select exercises, however, that are mechanically better, because they'll produce the same result (or a better result) with less effort, less time, and less risk of injury.

## What About the Upper Trapezius?

The upper trapezius can be seen from the front as well as from the back, especially when that part of the trapezius is well developed. The upper trapezius fibers play an important role in the aesthetic of an individual's physique, because they fill in the space between the neck and the shoulders. You can see the aesthetic need for this in Figure 19-31, as well as in the photo of Frank Zane (Figure 19-32).

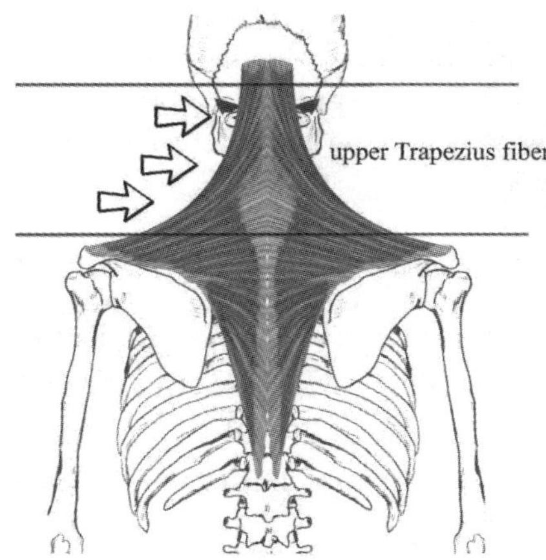


Clint Smith/E2 Systems, Inc.

Figure 19-31

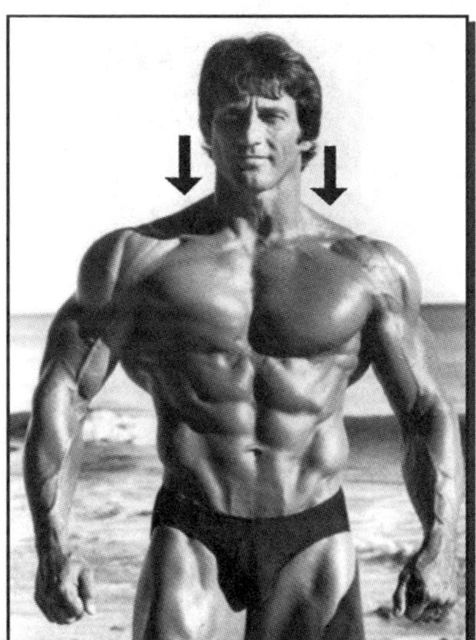

Figure 19-32

Depending on a person's genetics, these fibers can either grow quite a lot, or just modestly. The degree to which this muscle grows is not entirely within an individual's control. All anyone can do, in this regard, is to ensure that they are performing the correct movement, with the correct direction of resistance, with sufficient range of motion, and with sufficient intensity (volume/number of sets). The rest is determined by genetics.

In Figure 19-33, you can see a more massively developed upper trapezius, flexed in a typical "crab" pose, by Dexter Jackson. In Figure 19-34, I am hitting the same pose, but with upper trapezius that are much less massive. I have never been able to develop much "thickness" in this particular muscle, as compared with other more massive bodybuilders. I share a similar genetic structure to that of Frank Zane (seen in Figure 19-32), who also was known more for his symmetry than for his mass.

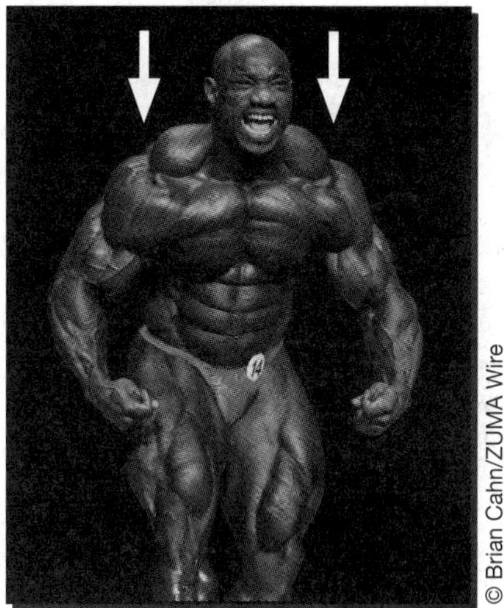

© Brian Cahn/ZUMA Wire

Figure 19-33

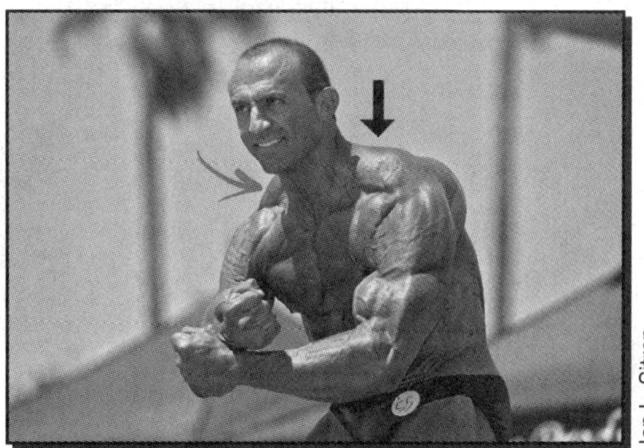

Ian L. Sitren

Figure 19-34

Some people "prefer" the aesthetics of a less massive upper trapezius, while others believe "the bigger, the better." Either way, the way each person's individual body develops—in terms of "thickness" and shape—is determined mostly by genetics, all other factors being equal.

Anatomically speaking, the upper trapezius fibers are relatively easy to work, because their ideal anatomical function is not complicated. They simply pull the shoulder carriage (i.e., scapula and clavicles) upward and slightly backward. As such, most traditional "shrugging" exercises will suffice for developing these fibers.

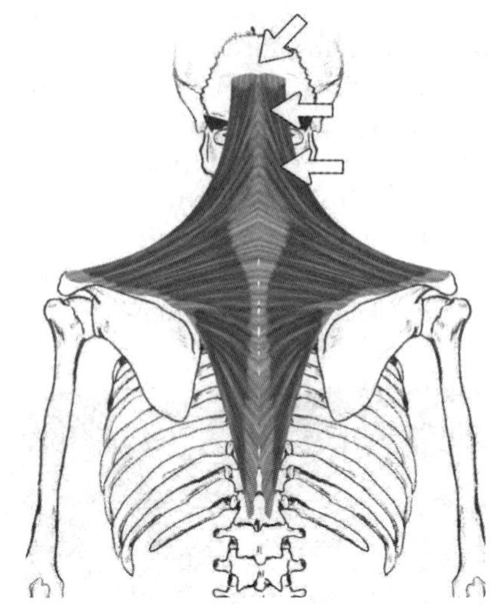

Clint Smith/E2 Systems, Inc.

Figure 19-35

In Figure 19-35, you can easily see that the origins of these fibers are all on the upper part of the spine (cervical). Some fibers even originate at the base of the skull, on the occipital bone.

All these upper fibers then attach to the upper ridge of the scapula ("A" in Figure 19-36), as well as the outer part of the clavicles ("B" in Figure 19-36). When these fibers contract, they pull the scapula and clavicle upward. Of course, this contraction pulls the humerus up as well, because the humerus is attached to the scapula and to the clavicles by way of tendons and ligaments.

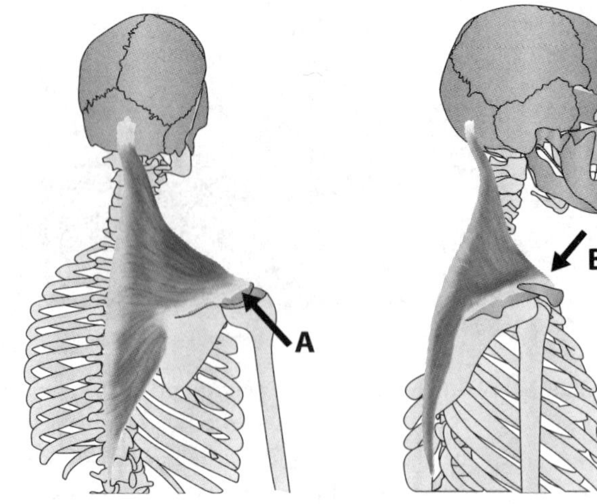


Figure 19-36

The trapezius muscle produces extremely divergent directions of movement. The upper trapezius fibers pull the scapula upward; the middle fibers pull the scapula backward; and the lower fibers pull the scapula in a downward-backward direction.

Although all the fibers of the trapezius are collectively considered "one muscle," it produces nearly 150 degrees of scapular/clavicular movement. No other muscle in the body produces such a wide range of directional movements. As such, the pectorals are a distant second place, in this regard. These are the only two muscles that produce a range of movements, because they are the only ones that are fan-shaped. Their insertion is at one specific point, their origins are spread out over a broader area, and the joint over which their fibers cross is multidirectional.

In terms of selecting a direction of movement for exercising the trapezius, you need only concern yourself primarily with TWO directions: straight "up" (upper trapezius/0-20 degrees) and straight "back" (middle trapezius/90-100 degrees).

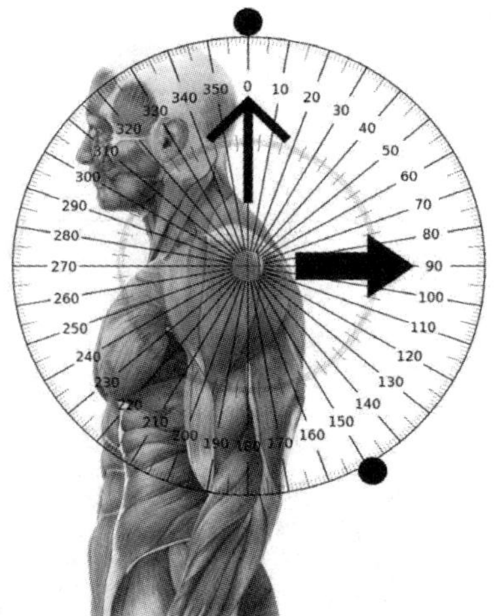

DM7/Shutterstock.com

Figure 19-37

The middle and lower fibers are best worked with an exercise that requires scapular retraction, which was demonstrated earlier in this chapter. The upper trapezius fibers are best worked with a simple upward-shrugging exercise. It is not necessary to pull in every single direction in which the trapezius fibers run. This is because a large percentage of muscle fibers participate, whenever either of the two directions of movement is performed.

The most common upper trapezius exercise is the *standing dumbbell shrug* (shown in Figure 19-38). This exercise is fine. In fact, it is preferable over *barbell shrugs*, because using dumbbells allows the weights to be held alongside the torso and hips, which helps keep the spine stable.

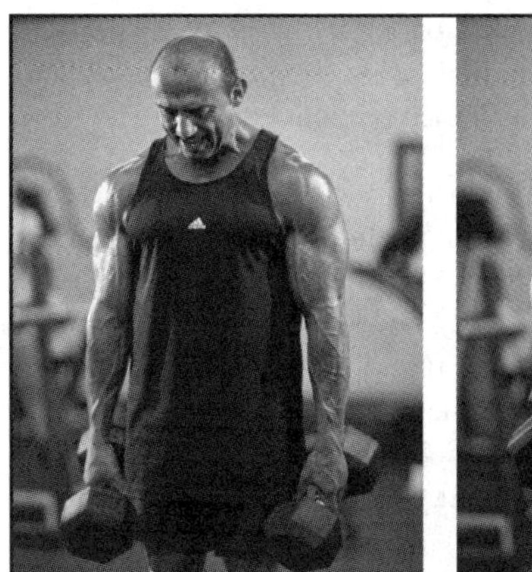
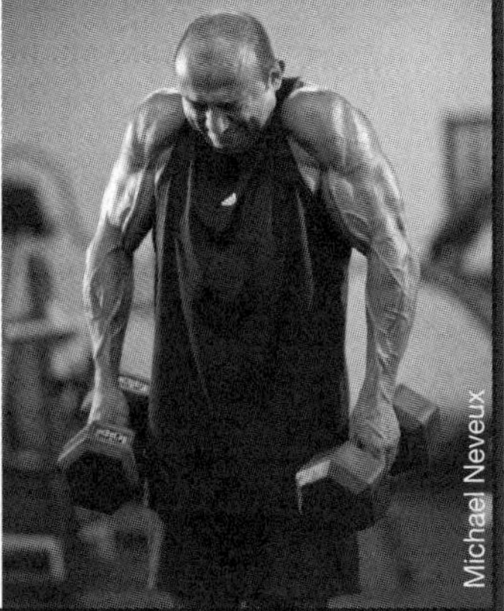


Figure 19-38

Figure 19-39 shows a person using a barbell for *shrugs*. As you can see, because the barbell is typically held IN FRONT of the torso and hips, it tends to pull the torso forward to some degree. This factor is not a problem for most people, especially if the weight being used is moderate. If the weight being used is "very heavy," however, it tends to pull the spine forward, into a slight forward flexion, which would put stress on the intervertebral discs. Since there is no biomechanical advantage in using a barbell for this exercise, taking this risk is unnecessary. Holding a barbell behind your back restricts freedom of movement, due to the gluteus blocking the upward movement of the barbell.

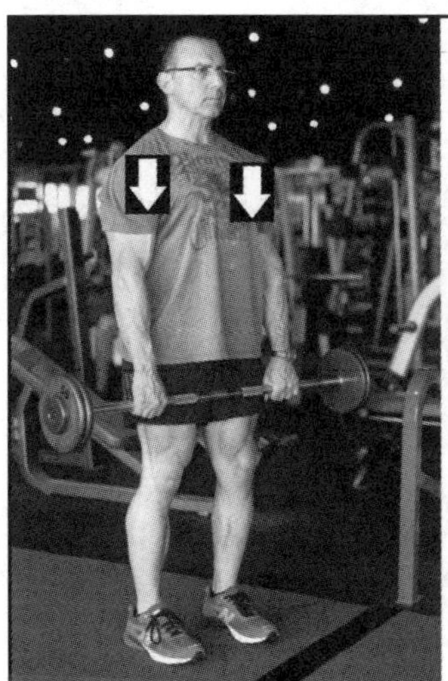
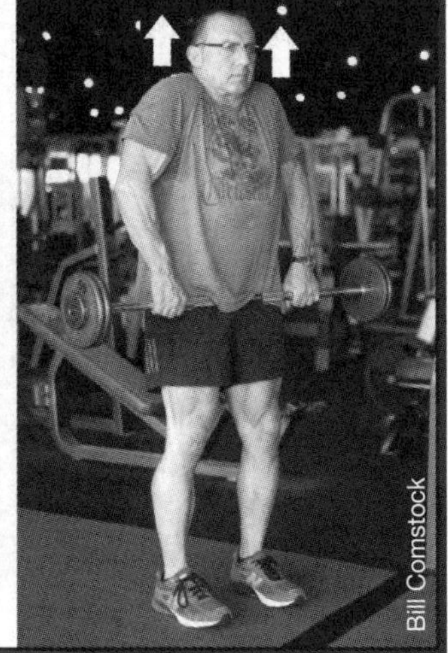


Figure 19-39

My personal preference, for the upper trapezius, is the *standing cable shrug* (Figure 19-40). This exercise allows you to keep the resistance alongside your hips—as if using dumbbells—so there is no strain on the lower back. In addition, because the pulleys can be set slightly wider than your shoulders, you don't have to deal with dragging the dumbbells (or your hands) against the sides of your legs, on the way up and down. Using cables also allows you to step slightly forward, or slightly backward (thereby slightly altering the direction of resistance), which allows you to adjust for spinal comfort. This factor also allows you to "aim" (shift) the resistance either straight upward, or slightly backward.

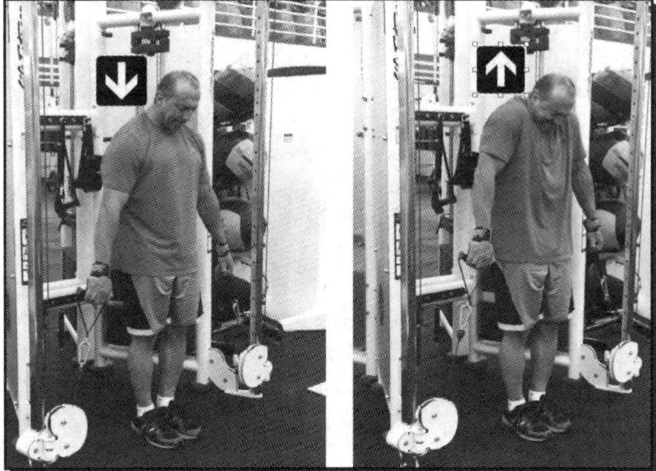

Figure 19-40

If you step back a bit (Figure 19-41)—so the pulleys are slightly more in front of you—it directs the resistance slightly more toward the trapezius fibers at 80 and 70 degrees, due to "opposite position loading." Notice that you can also lean back as you do this, which would not be possible, while using dumbbells (i.e., you'd fall backward). This positioning allows you to protect your lower back, by using your bodyweight as a "secondary resistance" to offset (reduce) any forward pull on your lower back.

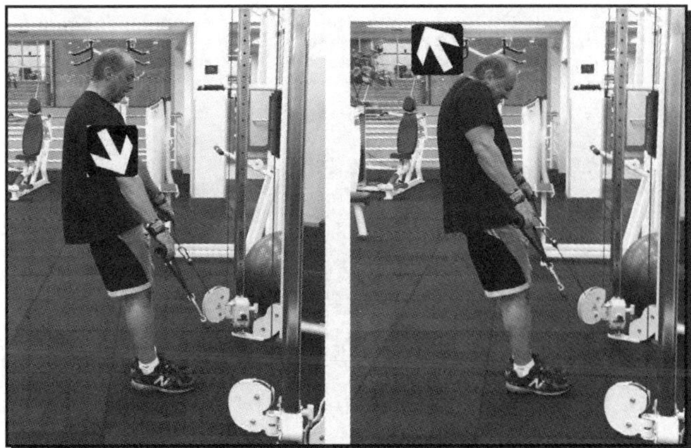

Figure 19-41

Leaning backward like this is not necessarily "better," in terms of directing the resistance more toward the posterior trapezius fibers. Those fibers will get a significant load, even when doing a straight vertical shrug, with a straight vertical resistance. It is fun, however, to play with this feature a bit. It can also help you find an angle that allows more lower back comfort.

Even though the trapezius is able to pull the scapula in various directions, it would be a mistake to pull the shoulders upward, and then ROLL the shoulders backward, during a shrugging exercise. Some people do this with the mistaken belief that it will engage some of the middle trapezius fibers. As noted previously, however, anatomical movement should always move directly opposite resistance. Since the resistance during a vertical shrug is straight downward, the direction of movement should be (exclusively) straight upward. Rolling the shoulders backward has almost no benefit, because the middle trapezius would not be loaded by a downward-pulling resistance. Only the muscle fibers that are positioned directly opposite the direction of resistance are loaded.

It is best to perform shrugs with both arms/scapula simultaneously, even when using dumbbells or cables. Since this movement typically allows a significant amount of weight to be used (often as much as 100 pounds per side, 200 pounds or more, in total), loading only one side at a time would cause a forceful asymmetrical pull on the spine, which would increase the risk of injury to the intervertebral discs. As such, shrugging both sides simultaneously provides better balance and stability, very much like engaging both arms simultaneously during a *supine dumbbell press*.

CHAPTER 20

# DELTOIDS—LATERAL, ANTERIOR, AND POSTERIOR

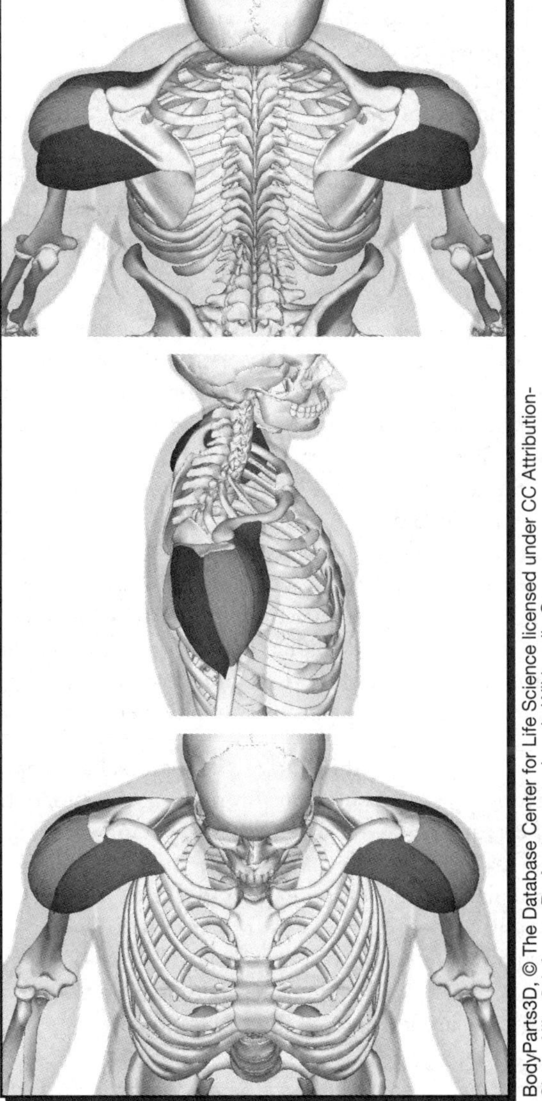



Figure 20-1

In gym jargon, the deltoids are often referred to simply as "shoulders," which includes the three deltoid "heads" (Figure 20-1). Each of these heads has a separate function (direction of movement), although some overlap exists. For example, a movement might involve the frontal part (anterior deltoid), as well as the side part (lateral deltoid). Another movement might involve the rear part (posterior deltoid) and the lateral deltoid. The posterior and anterior deltoids, however, produce movement in opposite directions, so they would not both engage simultaneously.

By identifying the origin and insertion of these three muscles, as well as the structure of the shoulder joint, we can determine the "ideal" anatomical movement of each of these three muscles. Then, you can see whether the exercises that are usually performed for these muscles are "ideal," or whether there are other, better exercises.

## Anatomy of the Lateral Deltoids

The lateral deltoid originates on the outer edge of the acromion process, on the scapula, and its insertion is on the deltoid tuberosity, on the humerus (Figures 20-2 and 20-3).

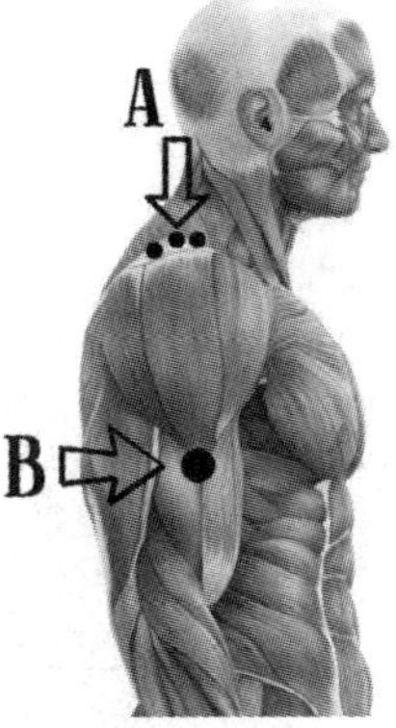




Figure 20-2

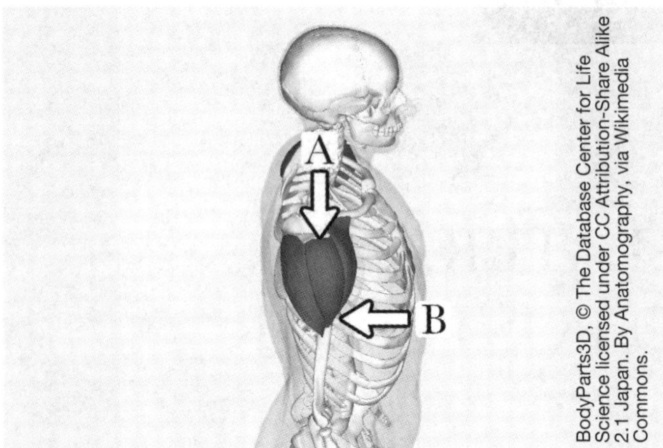


Figure 20-3

Note that the direction of the fibers of the lateral deltoids is parallel with the plane that runs through the origin and the insertion of the muscle. When the lateral deltoid contracts (shortens), it brings the muscle insertion upward, toward the origin, thereby creating the movement known as "lateral abduction of the humerus"—i.e., raising the arm sideways (Figure 20-4). That motion is the "ideal" anatomical motion of the lateral deltoid. It is the simplest, most natural function of the muscle, without requiring any twisting or rotation of the humerus, nor any distortion of the shoulder joint.

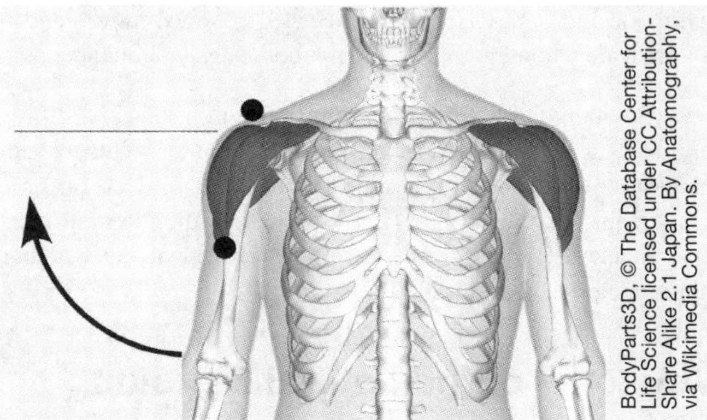


Figure 20-4

The ideal pathway and range of motion for the lateral deltoid, therefore, is moving the humerus laterally, from the side of the torso, up to a point where the humerus is almost perpendicular with the torso (Figure 20-5), and no higher. By that point, the lateral deltoid is fully contracted, assuming the scapula (the location of the muscle origin) has been held in place (i.e., that you have not raised your scapula/clavicle/shoulder carriage). The primary goal of any exercise should be to cause its muscle fibers to go from "fully extended" (i.e., fully lengthened) to "fully contracted" (i.e., fully shortened). This factor would cause the limb that is operated by that muscle to move toward the origins of that muscle—and then returning that limb to a position where the target muscle fibers are optimally elongated.

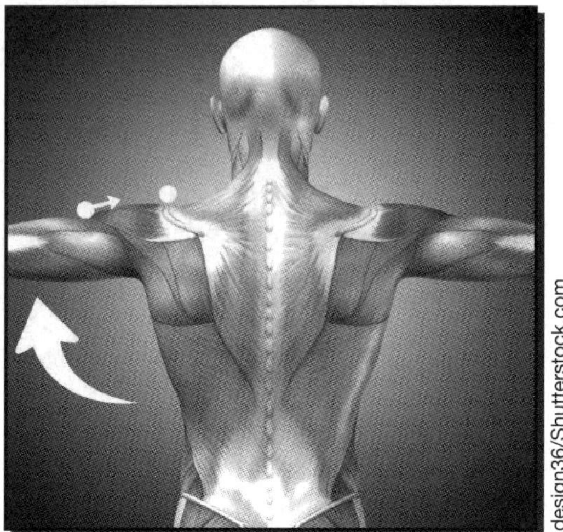


Figure 20-5

In fact, the lateral deltoid can be fully contracted before the humerus reaches a perpendicular angle with the torso, provided the scapula and clavicle are held down. If the scapula and clavicle are allowed to rise up during the movement (which is what most people do, by "shrugging" their scapula/clavicle upward), then the origin of lateral deltoid moves away from the approaching humerus. As a result, the muscle insertion has to "chase" the retreating muscle origin, making muscle contraction more elusive.

Some people mistakenly believe that raising the arm higher than the point where it is perpendicular with the torso makes the "range of motion" more complete. It does not. The range of motion of the lateral deltoid is complete when the muscle fibers are fully shortened (contracted), regardless of how far the arm travels. Optimal shortening/contraction of the lateral deltoid occurs when the humerus is raised laterally to an angle that is between 10 to 20 degrees "less" than perpendicular with the torso, provided the scapula and clavicle are not allowed to rise. If you allow your scapula/clavicle to rise up (shrugging the scapula and clavicle upward), however, optimal contraction of the lateral deltoid is delayed (until the arm reaches a higher point) or is avoided entirely.

You can test this factor for yourself. Simply have someone put their hand on top of your clavicle/outer edge of the scapula (on the side of the working arm), and hold it down firmly to prevent it from rising. Then perform a lateral abduction (side raise) with that arm. You will discover that you can only raise your arm up to a point that is approximately 80 degrees to the torso—maybe even a little less—which is where the lateral abduction motion should end, if you are keeping your scapula down.

That is the point where the lateral deltoid muscle fully contracts. Going beyond that point does not provide a better contraction of the lateral deltoids. Furthermore, moving the humerus beyond that point may result in shoulder impingement—the pinching of the supraspinatus tendon, as it gets squeezed between the humerus and the acromion process. The higher the humerus is raised—beyond the perpendicular position—the greater the risk of shoulder impingement.

The bottom end of the range of motion begins with the humerus right at your side. Although you could bring the humerus inward, crossing in front of the torso, doing so distorts the shoulder joint to a degree, and does not significantly increase the benefit to the lateral deltoids.

## "Lateral Abduction" Is the Ideal Direction of Anatomical Movement for the Lateral Deltoids

Raising the humerus laterally, with the aforementioned range of motion and the appropriate direction of resistance, is all that is necessary to engage the lateral deltoids perfectly. There is no better movement for this muscle.

Any movement other than lateral abduction, which you might consider doing, should prompt the following questions:

- Does that variation improve the mechanics of the lateral deltoids, beyond that which is provided by a simple *side raise* (lateral abduction) movement? For example:
    - Does it position the lateral deltoid better, with regard to "opposite position loading?"
    - Does it improve the alignment?
    - Is it a more safe/more natural joint movement?
    - Does it provide a better resistance curve?

If an alternate movement (exercise) does not provide any of these four mechanical components, then it is not a "better movement." In reality, it is not even "equally good," as a simple lateral abduction, for the lateral deltoids or the shoulder joint. In fact, it is a "less natural" movement.

Doing an exercise that allows you to move more weight is not a legitimate reason for selecting that exercise. How much weight you're able to move during any given exercise is not indicative of how much a particular muscle is loaded.

There are a number of mechanical factors that allow a heavier weight to be lifted, even when a particular muscle is less loaded. By way of comparison, a person can lift a heavier rock by using a pry bar (Figure 20-6), than they can by lifting a lighter rock with only their arms. Does that mean that they are "working harder" when they're using the pry bar because the rock is heavier? Of course not. The individual is simply using "mechanics" that minimizes the workload and maximize the output (amount of weight lifted). For example, *overhead presses* and *upright rows*—two common exercises performed for the lateral deltoids—allow a heavier weight to be used, but do not load the deltoids any more than do simple *side raises*.

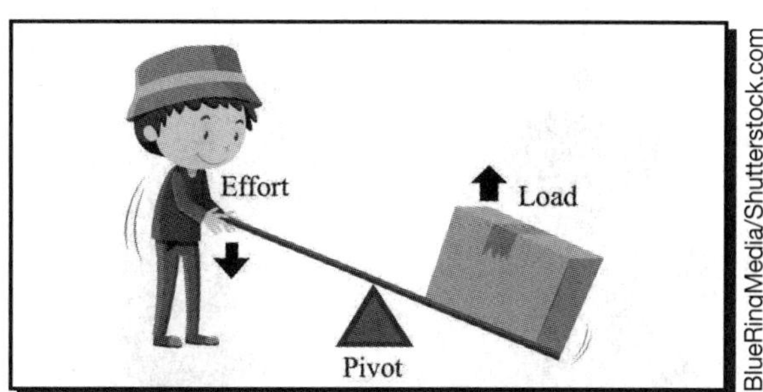

Figure 20-6

The *overhead press* (Figure 20-7) uses shorter levers (bent arms instead of straight arms), which reduces the magnification of the load to the deltoids. It also alters the alignment, such that the origin and insertion of the lateral deltoids are not on the same plane as the direction of resistance. Furthermore, it engages other muscles that assist (i.e., anterior deltoids and triceps) on the exercise, but are not as productive for those assisting muscles, as other (better) exercises, for those assisting muscles, would be. The *overhead press* not only causes a significant strain to the infraspinatus (explained more thoroughly in Chapter 17), it also increases the likelihood of developing impingement syndrome.

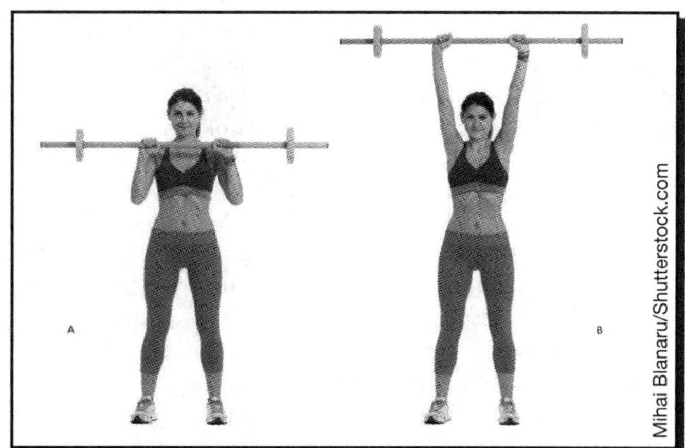

Figure 20-7

During *upright rows, either with a barbell or with dumbbells* (Figure 20-8), the forearms—acting as a secondary lever—double under the upper arms (which are the primary levers for the deltoids), which effectively reduces the length of the humerus (upper arm bone), which reduces the magnification to the lateral deltoids. As a result, the amount of load against which the deltoids must work is reduced, even as a heavier weight is used. *Upright rows* also strain the infraspinatus (because of the forward rotation of the humerus), the wrists (because they're forced to bend sideways), and the lower back (because more weight must be used to compensate for the reduced load magnification, and that additional weight pulls the torso forward, which could strain the lower back).

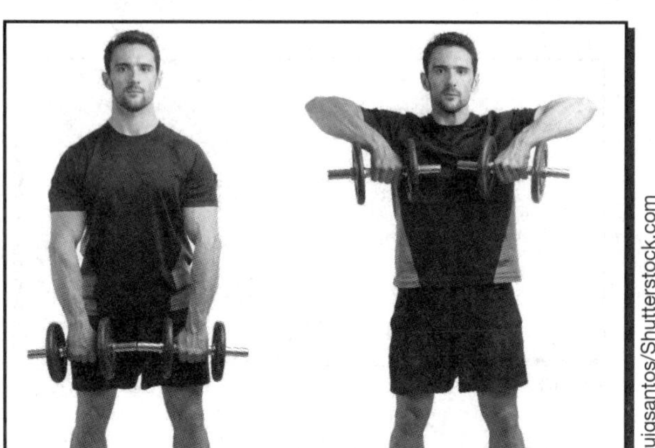
ruigsantos/Shutterstock.com

Figure 20-8

A person is able to lift more weight when doing an *overhead press* or *upright rows* (as compared with *side raises*) because shorter levers are being used, and other muscles are forced to assist ("peripheral recruitment"). The deltoids are not necessarily getting any more load than they would if you simply performed a lateral abduction. *Overhead presses* and *upright rows* utilize less efficient levers, which then requires the use of heavier weight. This increases the skeletal strain and the risk of injury.

Some people do multiple exercises for a given muscle, because they "want to do more sets." If that's the case, it would be better to do three times more sets of *lateral abduction*, than it would be to do three exercises—one of which is a good exercise (e.g., *side raises*) and another two which are not good exercises (e.g., *overhead presses* and *upright rows*).

Lateral abduction of the humerus ("*side raise*") is the purest, most natural anatomical motion produced by the lateral deltoid muscle and the shoulder joint. A "*side raise*" (lateral abduction) moves the muscle insertion directly toward the muscle origin, and utilizes perfect alignment. There is no need to perform a motion that is more complicated, nor would there be any advantage in doing so.

Now that the ideal direction of anatomical motion of the lateral deltoids has been determined, the next critical factor to determine is the ideal direction of resistance which will provide the "ideal" resistance curve, proper alignment, and optimal lever (limb) efficiency.

When someone talks about a "*side raise*," the first exercise that usually comes to mind is the *standing side dumbbell raise* (Figures 20-9 and 20-10). That exercise, however, is not the "best" option for the lateral deltoid. While the movement of the humerus is ideal, the direction of resistance is not ideal.

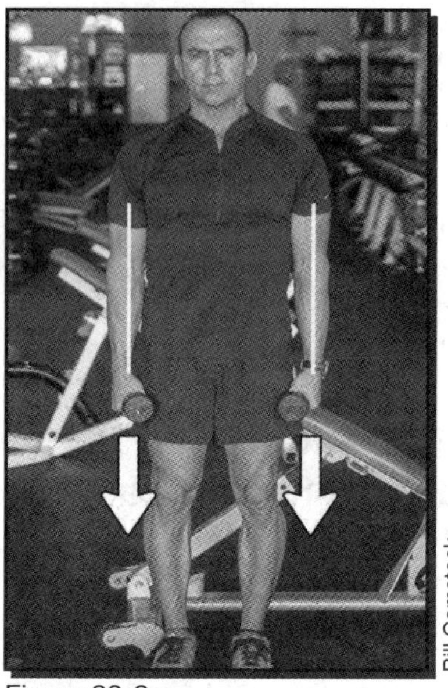
Bill Comstock

Figure 20-9

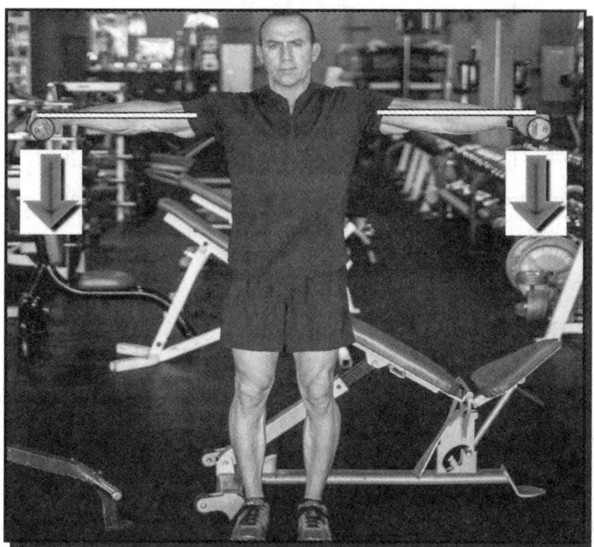
Bill Comstock

Figure 20-10

Since the individual is using "free weight gravity" (a straight downward direction of resistance), and because he is standing vertically, the resistance curve of THIS exercise is "late phase loaded." In other words, it is lightest at the beginning of the range of motion and heaviest at the end of the range of motion, because the exerciser's arms are parallel with resistance at the beginning, and perpendicular with resistance at the end of the range of motion. This resistance curve is the opposite of ideal.

## Identifying the Ideal Direction of Resistance for "Lateral Abduction"

Instead, what is needed is an exercise that provides "early phase loading"—i.e., an exercise that provides more resistance at the beginning of the range of motion, and less resistance at the end of the range of motion. The exercise shown in Figures 20-11 to 20-13—"*lying one-arm side dumbbell raise*"—is one viable option.

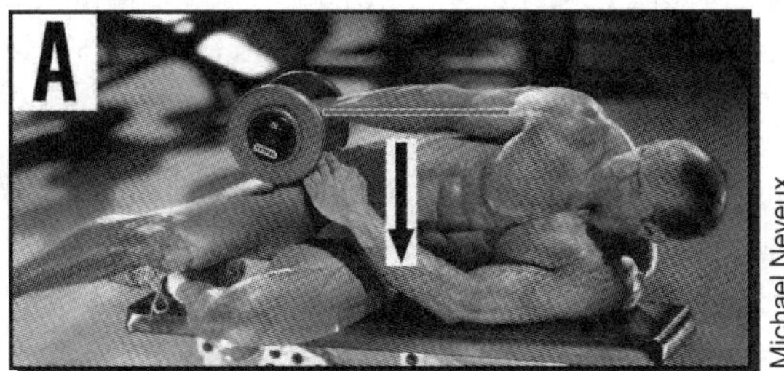

Figure 20-11

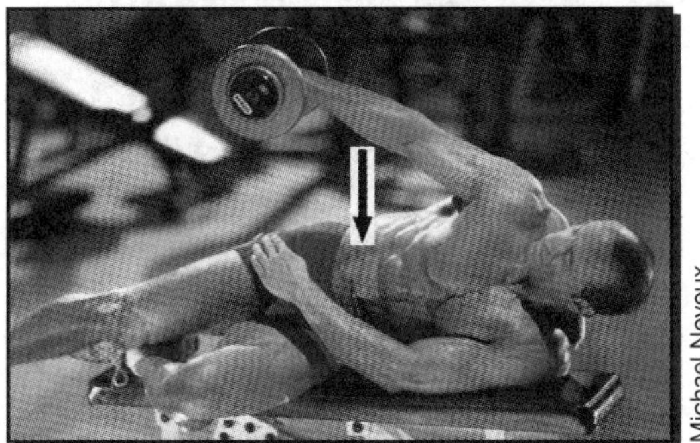

Figure 20-12

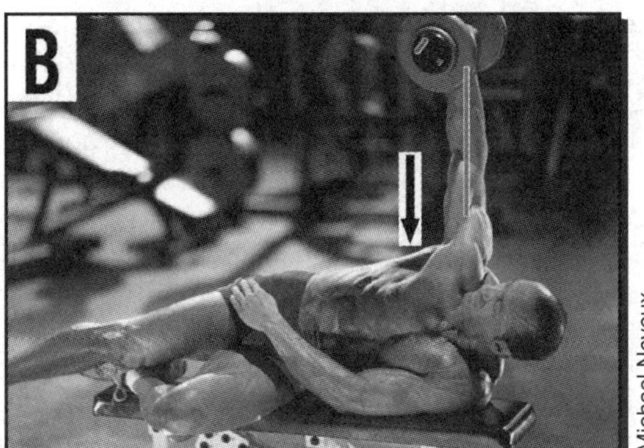

Figure 20-13

This exercise (Figures 20-11 to 20-13) provides a resistance curve that is the opposite of that which occurs during the *standing side dumbbell raise*. In this version of a *side raise*, the humerus is perpendicular with gravity at the beginning of the range of motion ("A"), and is parallel with gravity at the end of the range of motion ("B").

The "*standing one-arm side cable raise*" (Figures 20-14 and 20-15) is an even better option. In fact, this exercise is the best lateral deltoid exercise for several reasons. The standing position is more comfortable than lying on your side, where your other arm is pinned underneath you.

Furthermore, the resistance curve, in this instance, does not diminish all the way to zero at the conclusion of the range of motion. It diminishes (which is good), but still provides about 40 percent of the original resistance (depending on the height of pulley) at the conclusion of the concentric movement. The reason there is still "some" resistance, although less, at the top of the movement is because the cable (as the indicator of the direction of resistance) is not fully parallel with the upper arm, in that "late phase" of the repetition. The angle of the arm, relative to the cable, goes from perpendicular (maximum resistance) to about a 30-degree angle.

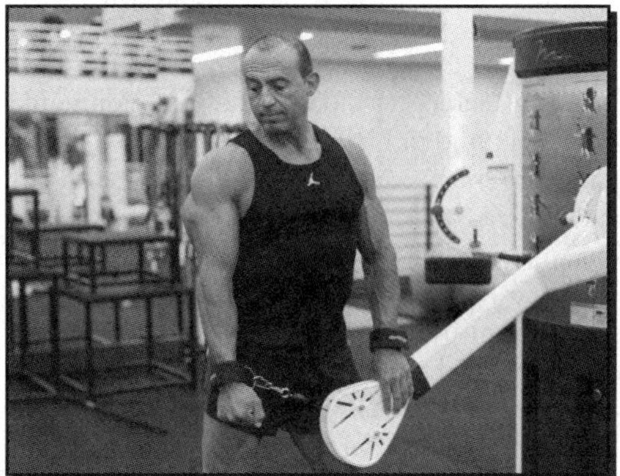

Figure 20-14

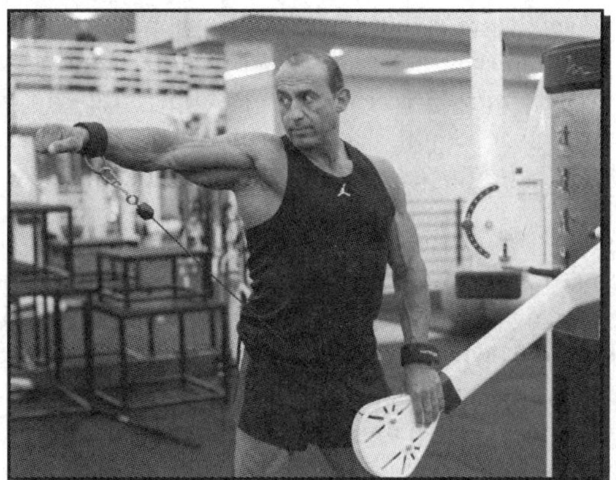

Fig ure 20-15

Perhaps, more importantly, using cables allows you to use wrist straps with the D-ring attachment, which you see in Figures 20-14 and 20-15. This factor allows you to bypass the weaker muscles of the forearms and fingers—the weaker link in the chain, so to speak. The lateral deltoids can handle much more resistance than the forearm extensors and fingers can accommodate. If you are using a significant amount of resistance on this exercise, the forearm and fingers will either fatigue first or become so achy during the exercise that it will distract from the deltoid work.

Typically, the use of wrist straps on this exercise can be compared to leg extensions, in which the resistance is applied at the ankle. Can you imagine trying to "hold" a weight with your feet or toes? In this instance, the resistance is applied at the wrist, which is a more solid way of applying resistance, than holding it with your fingers.

Ideally speaking, the height of the pulley should be about at the same height as the wrist (of the working arm) in the starting position, thus allowing the cable to be perpendicular with the forearm during the early phase of the movement. This angle would cause the resistance curve to be "heaviest" at the beginning of the range of motion (where the muscle is strongest), and "lightest" at the conclusion (where the muscle is weakest).

Obviously, some gyms do not have an adjustable pulley, like the one pictured in Figures 20-14 and 20-15. If that is the case, using the *lying side dumbbell raise* is a reasonably good substitute for the *cable side raise*. It can be done anywhere, even if it isn't quite as comfortable, nor quite as effective, as using cables. Unfortunately, using a dumbbell will likely prevent you from using as much weight as your deltoids can handle, because of the limited strength of the fingers and wrist extensors. On the other hand, it's still a much better exercise than the standing version of the *side dumbbell raise*.

An additional advantage of doing an early phase loaded *side raise exercise* (like a *standing cable raise* or *lying one-arm dumbbell side raise*), is that the upper trapezius muscle will then NOT be "opposite resistance" (as it would be during *standing side dumbbell raise*). As a result, the upper trapezius will be loaded much less. This factor further eliminates distraction, and allows better focus on the lateral deltoids.

When you perform a *standing* (or *seated*) *dumbbell side raise*, the trapezius muscle is positioned on the "opposite side" of the downward resistance the entire time. Ironically, the lateral deltoid, which is the target muscle of this exercise, is only positioned opposite resistance at the conclusion of the range of motion (when the arm is up, which is not even half the time). In essence, it could be argued that the trapezius works harder (although isometrically) during a *standing* (or *seated*) *dumbbell side raise*, than do the lateral deltoids. As such, the two early phase loaded exercises (Figures 20-11 through 20-15) reduce the trapezius load to almost zero, because the traps are not positioned "directly opposite" the direction of resistance.

What about *overhead presses and upright barbell rows* for working the "shoulders"? They are not very efficient (requiring that more weight be used than is actually necessary), and have a higher risk of injury, but they are perfectly acceptable for people who don't mind spending more energy than is necessary, don't mind incurring a higher risk of injury, and are more concerned with lifting heavy weights than they are with working their muscles most "efficiently." In other words, using them is not very wise.

If you are a person who prefers to keep your workouts more "fun," more casual, and more flexible, and don't want to be limited to doing only the one or two exercises (for each muscle/"body part") which rate a "9" or higher, that's fine. Go ahead and mix it up, including exercises that are less efficient, less productive, and have a higher risk of injury. What's most important, however, is to not delude yourself into thinking that all exercises are equally productive, equally efficient, and equally safe. They are not.

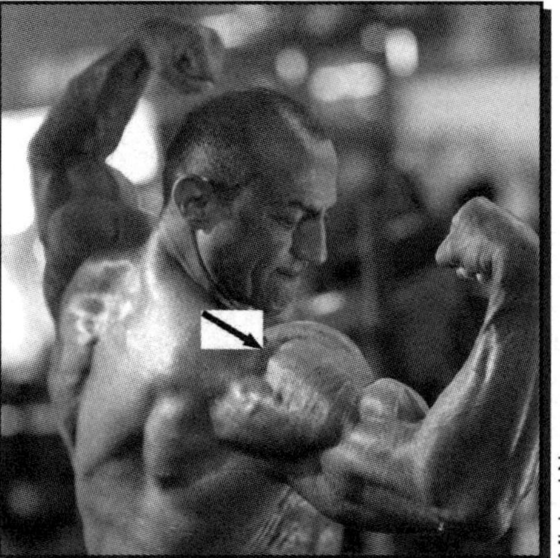
Michael Neveux

Figure 20-16

In Figure 20-16, you can see that my deltoid development is not lacking. Most people would automatically assume, upon seeing this photo, that my deltoid workouts included *overhead presses* and *upright rows*. However, I have not done either of those exercises since 1991, which is 23 years before this photo was taken. The lateral deltoid development you see in Figure 20-16 was achieved entirely with one single exercise—the *standing cable side raise*.

Typically, I do between 15 and 20 sets of this exercise, starting with the lightest possible weight (using higher reps and/or a lower level of effort), as part of the warm-up process. Subsequently, I gradually add weight and decrease the reps, and increase the percentage of maximum effort. I alternate between the right side and left side, ranging in reps from 30 reps (during the warm-up) down to as low as four reps (with the heaviest weight possible), often doing two sets with the same weight for the same number of reps. By the time I'm finished with this sequence, my deltoids are "fried" (totally exhausted... which is indicative of a successful workout), yet the shoulder joint has not been strained at all.

Of course, this type of routine is not the ONLY way to develop world-class deltoids. There have been many outstanding bodybuilding champions who have used the more conventional method of training their "shoulders," who have achieved excellent results. I am not claiming that conventional methods "do not develop the deltoids." What I am saying is that the conventional method is not the most efficient way of developing the deltoids.

What the math (physics) and logic clearly indicates—and the deltoids development I've achieved using this method proves—is that doing *overhead presses* and *upright rows* is not necessary, even though this has been the conventional wisdom for decades. "Efficiency" relates to the energy cost (weight used) and the injury risk, as compared to the actual muscle loading and the ultimate result (muscle development). The wisest approach is to achieve optimal development (optimal muscle loading), while not spending more energy (not lifting more weight) than is necessary, and reducing or eliminating the risk of injury.

Why work harder than you need to? Why not get the most benefit, with the least amount wasted effort? Why risk injury, unproductively? There are far more efficient exercises for developing the deltoids, than *overhead presses*. This concept makes perfect sense to most people, but many individuals refuse to believe it, and are not willing to even try it. Still others might believe it, but only after they've seen enough other people do it successfully.

Many people have already injured their shoulder joints so badly, from doing *overhead presses*, that they are simply unable to do *overhead presses* anymore. Not surprisingly, these people tend to be more receptive to a more sensible way of training their deltoids.

Unfortunately, training your deltoids properly (efficiently, productively, and safely), AFTER your shoulder joint has been severely damaged, will not make your shoulder joints "good as new" again. On the other hand, it will allow you to train your deltoids without as much pain, and without creating further joint damage.

## Exercise Options for the Lateral Deltoids

In my opinion, the best exercises for the lateral deltoids, in descending order, are as follows:

- *Standing one-arm side cable raise*, with the pulley set at hip height, and using a wrist strap with a D-ring (Figures 20-14 and 20-15)
- *Lying (horizontal) one-arm side dumbbell raise*, on a floor mat (Figures 20-11 to 20-13)
- *Standing one-arm cable side raise*, with the pulley at ankle height (when an adjustable pulley is not available, while a low pulley is—Figure 20-17)
- *Incline one-arm side dumbbell raise* (the lower the incline angle, the better—Figure 20-18)

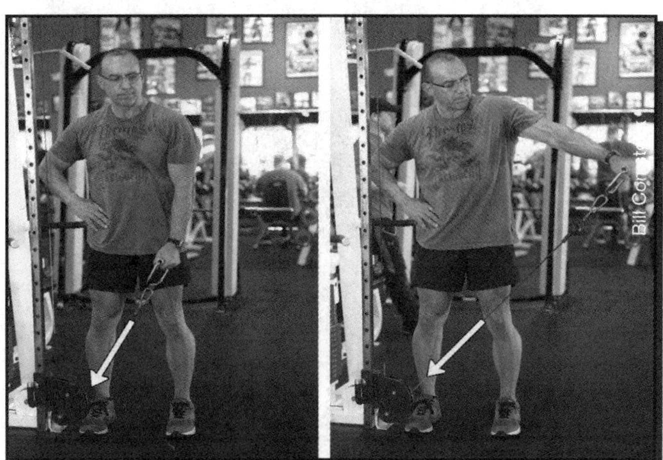


Figure 20-17

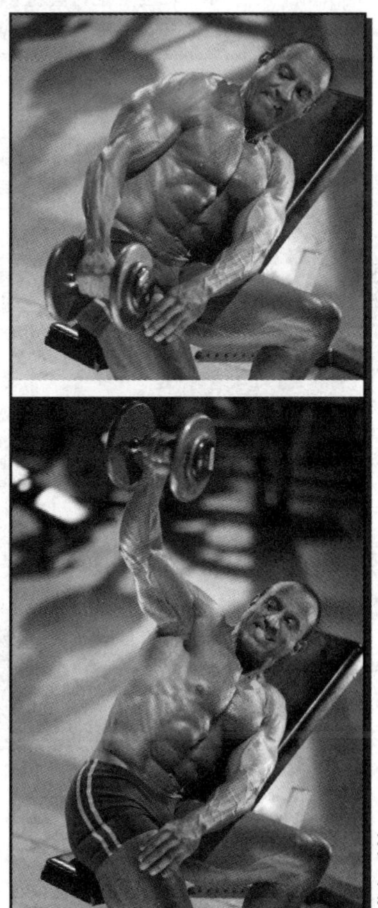


Figure 20-18

- *Side deltoid raise* on a machine (assuming it's a well-designed machine, that you position the seat correctly, and that you push laterally only with your humerus—Figures 20-19 and 20-20)

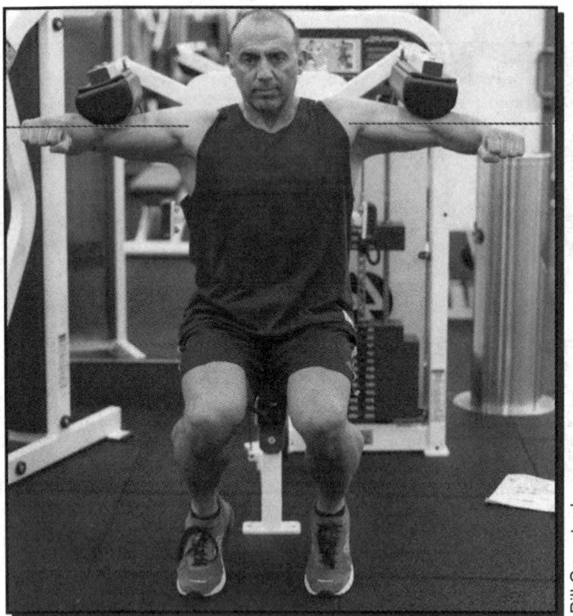
Bill Comstock

Figure 20-19

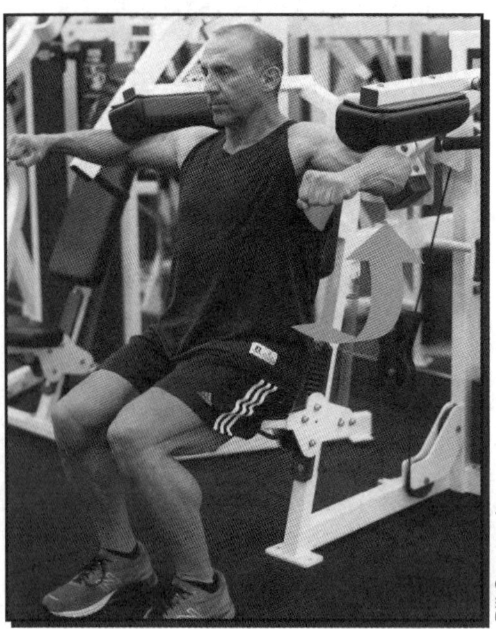
Bill Comstock

Figure 20-20

A well-designed lateral raise machine will have a cam that allows the resistance to diminish toward the end of the range of motion. Furthermore, it will have its pivot points set correctly to match a person's shoulder width, which is difficult because people's shoulder width differs. In other words, the machine's pivot points and the person's shoulder joints should line up ... allowing the machine's lever arm and the person's humerus to travel the same arc. As such, the seat height should also be set so that a person's shoulder joints are neither below, nor above, the machine's pivot points.

Most of these machines also have a handle, which should, however, not be used for anything more than to keep the humerus from rotating during the movement. The lateral force should be applied only by the humerus against the arm pads of the machine's levers. Furthermore, the humerus should not be raised higher than perpendicular with the torso.

When performing any kind of *side raise* exercise, if possible, you should always try to end the range of motion at the point where you actually "feel" the deltoid contract. Although the technical guideline is to move the arm up to the point where it's approximately 80 degrees from the torso, the ultimate determinant of where the range of motion ends is the sense that the muscle has reached its point of optimum contraction. This is no different than when you perform biceps curls, triceps pushdowns, or leg extensions. Since these are hinge joints, however, it's easier to know exactly where the range of motion ends. It's not quite so obvious with the deltoids, since the shoulder joint has much more mobility.

As such, you should not abandon your sensory/kinesthetic connection to the exercise, and rely only on "external" cues, with regard to where a range of motion should end. In reality, using both "internal" (sensory) and "external" (anatomical knowledge) cues is best.

One of the great advantages of doing an "early phase loaded" *side raise*, is that, since the resistance diminishes toward the end of the range of motion, the muscle contraction can actually be felt, as well as be held. On the other hand, this factor is not true when doing an exercise that is "late phase loaded," such as *standing side dumbbell raises*. Since that particular version of a lateral deltoid exercise is "too heavy" at the end of the range of motion, it's impossible to feel and hold the contracted position at the conclusion of the range of motion.

## Anatomy of the Anterior Deltoids

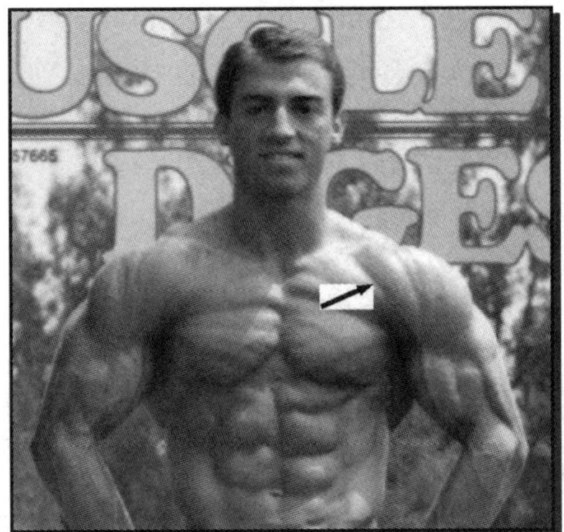

Figure 20-21

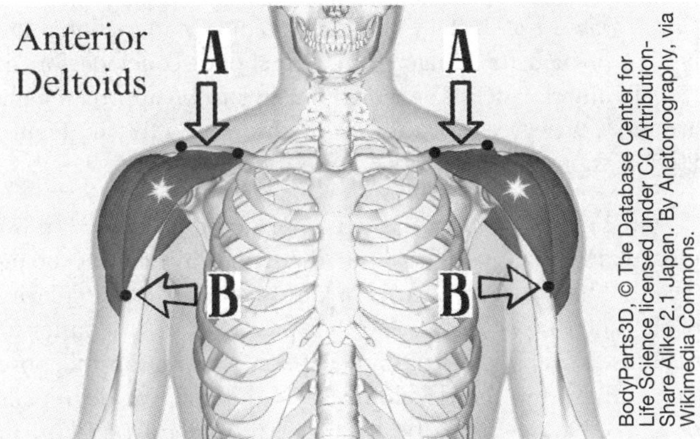


Figure 20-22

The anterior deltoid is also known as the "front deltoid." As you can see in Figure 20-22, it originates on the outer half of the clavicle ("A"). Its insertion is on the deltoid tuberosity on the humerus ("B"), right next to (slightly in front of) the insertion of the lateral deltoid.

## Identifying the Ideal Anatomical Motion for the Anterior Deltoids

The anterior deltoid participates in any movement in which the humerus is pulled forward and/or upward, toward the clavicle—where the muscle originates. These movements include all chest exercises, as well as *parallel bar dips* and *overhead presses* (both of which involve the anterior deltoid quite a lot, but not in the safest/most productive way). Even a few biceps exercises engage the anterior deltoids, if the humerus is brought forward during the curling movement—or to hold the humerus steady (preventing it from moving backward), as the biceps performs its dynamic work.

The important question is, "What is the IDEAL movement, for the anterior deltoid?" In other words, which anatomical motion—in the form of an exercise—engages this muscle better (more efficiently and safely) than any other?

In that regard, the most basic guideline detailed in this book—that "muscles always pull toward their origin"—should be the first factor you should consider in order to identify the most natural way of engaging the anterior deltoid. As such, imagine the insertion of the muscle being pulled directly toward the muscle origin, in as simple and straightforward a manner as possible. That action would produce a movement that takes the humerus from a starting point, somewhere alongside the torso (actually, slightly posterior to the sides of the torso)—forward and slightly upward (more forward than upward)—moving the humerus toward the muscle origin on the clavicle.

This description might make you think of the exercise known as the *standing front barbell raise* (Figure 20-23). Most people think that this is a "good" exercise for the anterior deltoids, but there are actually several problems with this exercise, including the following:

- It's not the ideal range of motion (insufficient early phase range of motion, and the movement typically concludes beyond the point of contraction).
- It's not opposite position loaded (the muscle is not positioned opposite resistance, because the humerus is not rotated properly).
- It's not early phase loaded (it's late phase loaded).
- It's loading a non-target muscle more than the target muscle (i.e., lateral deltoids).

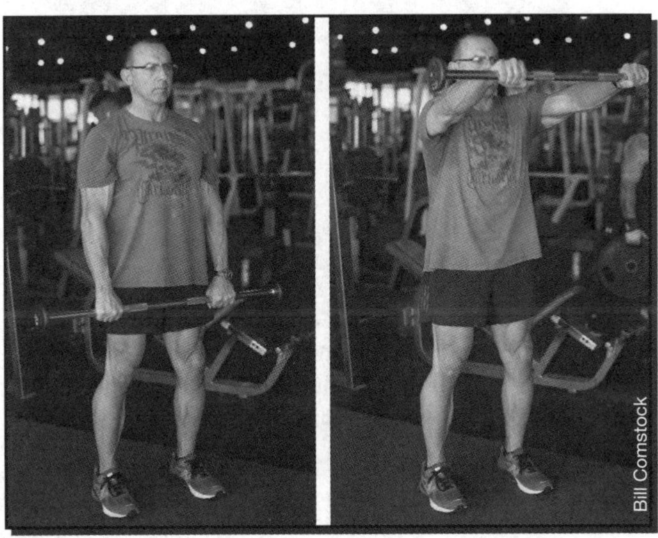


Figure 20-23

The ideal range of motion would take the anterior deltoid (or any other muscle) from a stretch position—or least "sufficient elongation"—to the point of contraction. The stretch position for the anterior deltoids requires the humerus to angle back (posteriorly), approximately 30 degrees from the torso. In Figure 20-24, you can see how the front deltoid stretches, when the arm is allowed to angle posteriorly.

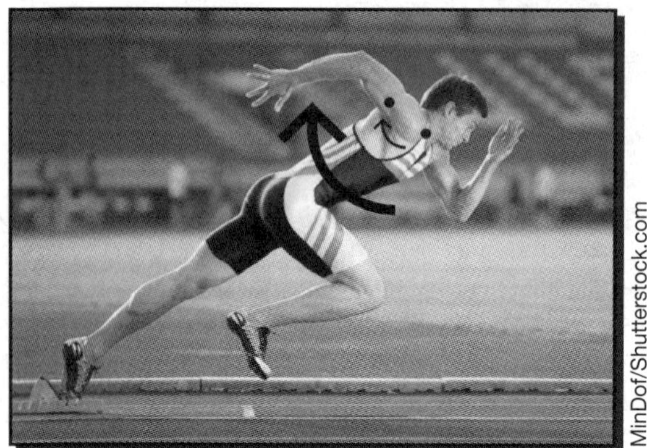

MinDof/Shutterstock.com

Figure 20-24

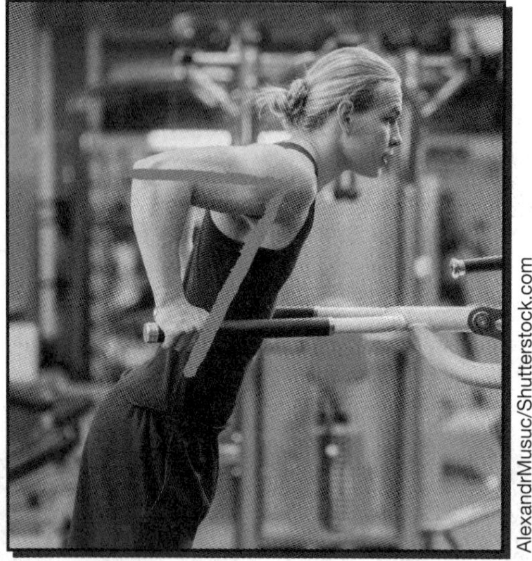

AlexandrMusuc/Shutterstock.com

Figure 20-25

Previously, the fact that *parallel bar dips* "over-stretch" the anterior deltoids was discussed. In that regard, you can see in Figure 20-25 that, during parallel bar dips, the upper arm angles posteriorly as much as 80 degrees to the torso. That is much too far for a "reasonable" anterior deltoid stretch. In reality, the maximum amount of posterior angling of the humerus, for a reasonable amount of anterior deltoid stretch, is about 40 degrees back from the torso ("A" in Figure 20-26).

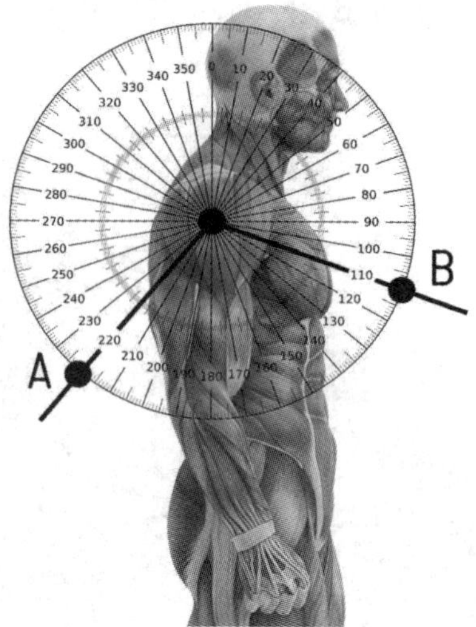


DM7/Shutterstock.com

Figure 20-26

The point of contraction for the anterior deltoids is farther forward/upward than occurs when performing *parallel bar dips,* but NOT as far as typically occurs during the *standing barbell front raise*. In fact, the ideal point of contraction—the point at which the range of motion should conclude for an "ideal" anterior deltoid exercise—seems to be approximately around 70 degrees forward from the torso ("B" in Figure 20-26)—not quite perpendicular to the torso.

In Figure 20-27, in which I am doing a "crab"/"most muscular" pose, you can see the anterior deltoids being flexed. This pose, in part, is meant to show the muscularity of the anterior deltoids. No other pose "flexes" the anterior deltoids as well as this particular pose. The reason this pose so clearly shows the development of the anterior deltoids is because that seems to be the precise humeral position, in which the anterior deltoid best achieves its full contraction—about 70 degrees in front of the torso (i.e., slightly below perpendicular with the torso).

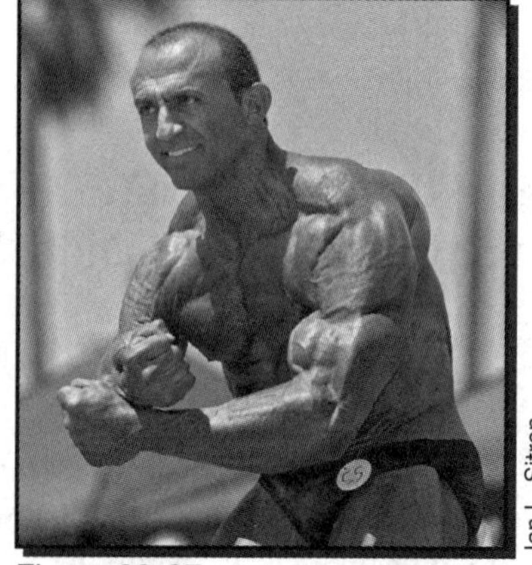

Ian L. Sitren

Figure 20-27

As such, when doing an anterior deltoid exercise, the arms should not be raised much higher than they would be during a "crab" pose. It would also be wise to try to feel the anterior deltoid contraction, at the conclusion of each repetition of an anterior deltoid exercise.

The exercise shown in Figures 20-28 and 20-29—the *seated anterior deltoid cable press*—is the best exercise (in my view) for achieving the ideal range of motion, both in the stretch position and the contracted position. It also provides "early phase loading" (the humerus is perpendicular to the cable, "early" in the range of motion). In addition, it ensures "opposite position loading" (the anterior deltoid is positioned directly opposite the direction of resistance), as well as perfect alignment (the direction of resistance, the direction of anatomical movement, the origin and insertion of the target muscle, are all on the same plane).

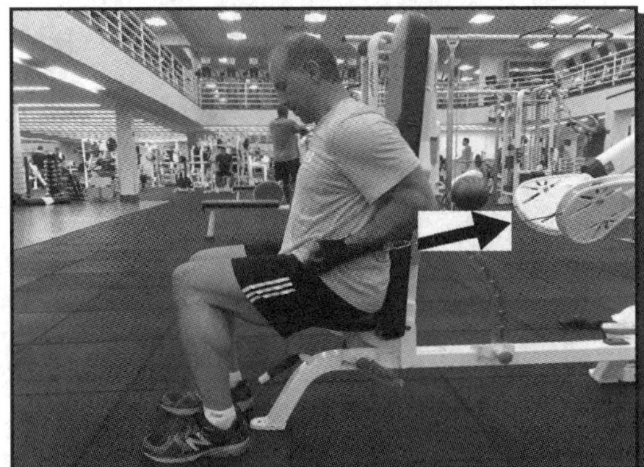
Figure 20-28

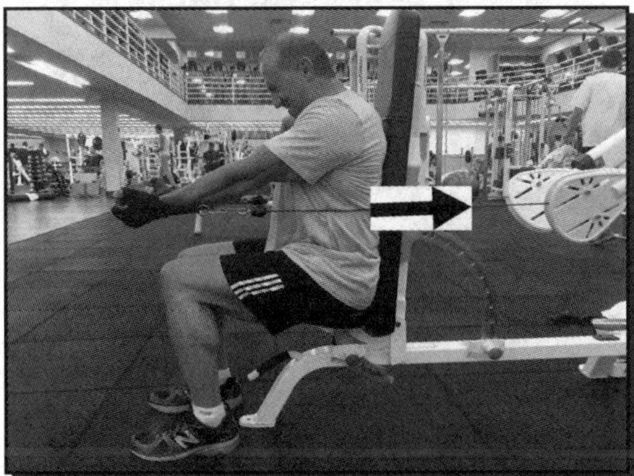
Figure 20-29

You should note that the elbows should be kept close to the sides of the torso. This is the "ideal" humeral pathway of the anterior deltoid muscle, because it causes the muscle insertion (i.e., on the deltoid tuberosity on the humerus) to move directly toward the muscle origin (i.e., on the lateral aspect of the clavicle), from a stretch position, in the simplest possible way.

This "elbows-in" pathway of the arms also minimizes the participation of the pectorals, which would otherwise dominate the recruitment, if the elbows were brought out laterally. The "elbows-wide" pathway is the primary track of the pectorals, because that motion would be parallel to the pectoral fibers, and because it would cause the humerus to move toward the sternum, where the pectoral origins are situated.

You should also take note of the "palms-up" grip, which allows the humerus to be rotated externally, thereby allowing the anterior deltoids to be positioned opposite the resistance. Conversely, the *standing barbell front raise* exercise is typically done with a palms down grip, which rotates the humerus internally. That internal humeral rotation causes the lateral deltoid to be positioned more opposite resistance than the anterior deltoid. In order to ensure "opposite position loading," the anterior deltoid must be positioned directly opposite the direction of resistance. This occurs best with a "palms up" grip—with the humerus externally rotated.

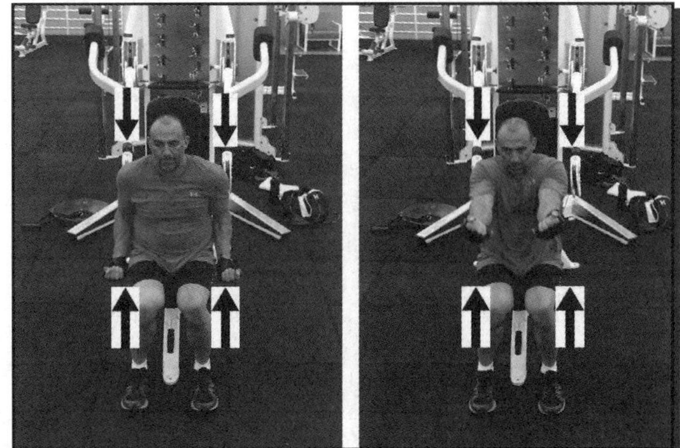
Figure 20-30

The starting position of the *seated anterior deltoid cable press* (Figure 20-30, left) begins with a mostly "active" lever (humerus), indicated by the mostly perpendicular angle of the cable relative to the humerus. This positioning allows the anterior deltoid to be loaded more at the beginning of the range of motion, where the muscle has more strength potential. Subsequently, the resistance diminishes as the humerus moves forward and becomes more parallel with the cable. This is good because as the anterior deltoid contracts, its strength potential diminishes.

Conversely, the *standing barbell front raise* begins with a mostly "inactive" lever—the humerus is parallel with gravity. As a result, no part of the deltoids experience any load during this early phase, even though this early phase is where skeletal muscles have their greatest strength potential. Subsequently, as the arms are moved forward (during *barbell front raise*), the humerus begins encountering "perpendicularly-ness" with gravity, thereby progressively increasing the resistance. Simultaneously, however, the deltoids become progressively weaker (i.e., lose strength potential), because the muscle is approaching the "late phase" of its range of motion. Therefore, this particular resistance curve (i.e., lighter at the beginning and heavier at the end) is the opposite of ideal. This flawed resistance curve, combined with the inappropriate alignment of the anterior deltoids relative to gravity, essentially disqualifies the *standing barbell front raise* as a "good" exercise for the anterior deltoids.

Another advantage of the *seated cable front press* is that it's done in the vertical position, with the resistance coming from behind (perpendicular to the torso, instead of from below or parallel to the torso). Consequently, there is NO load on the lower back, as there would be with the *standing barbell front raise.*

When setting up the pulleys for the *seated cable front press*, it is important that the pulleys be set at the right height, as well as the right width apart. Notice in Figure 20-30 (indicated by the arrows), that they are set at exactly shoulder width. This positioning allows perfect alignment between the direction of resistance, the direction of arm movement, and the origin and insertion of the anterior deltoids.

The exercise shown in Figure 20-31—a *supine (flat bench) dumbbell front press*" is a good second alternative to the "*seated anterior deltoid cable press.*" It allows you to use the same range of motion, with a good resistance curve (i.e., "early phase loading"). Note that the palms of the hands are facing "upward" (toward the head, rather than toward the feet), which makes it possible to keep the elbows in close "in," as they move along the sides of the torso.

Compare this exercise, shown in Figure 20-31, with the *standing front barbell raise*, Figure 20-32. In both instances, the upper arm (humerus) is moving forward, but that is the only similarity. Most of the other mechanical factors, however, are distinctly different:

> *Note: The fact that the elbows are bent during a "supine dumbbell front press"—in the stretch position—is irrelevant, because the anterior deltoid only pulls on the humerus. It does not "know" whether the elbows are bent or straight.*

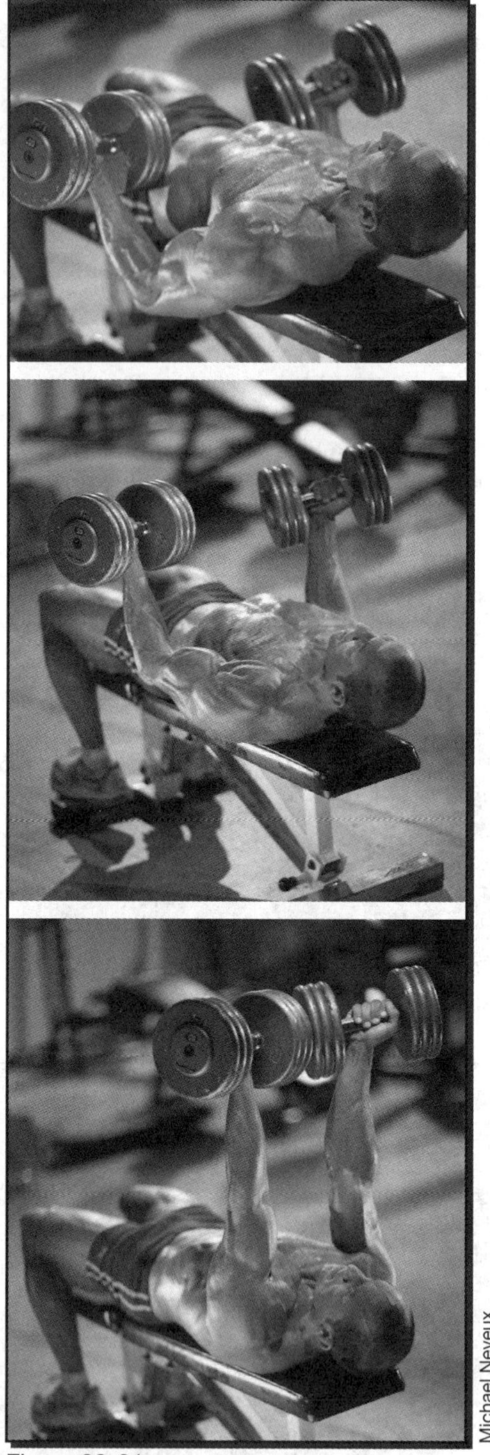

Michael Neveux

Figure 20-31

- The *supine dumbbell front press* is early phase loaded; the *standing front barbell raise* is late phase loaded.
- The *supine dumbbell front press* has a better range of motion (better stretch/better contraction), than the *standing front barbell raise.*
- The *supine dumbbell front press* has the anterior deltoid in a position that is opposite gravity (because the palms of the hands are facing upward, the elbows are tucked into the sides, and the humerus is therefore rotated into the correct position); the *standing front barbell raise* has

the lateral deltoid more in a position that is opposing resistance—instead of the anterior deltoid, which is the intended target muscle.

- The *supine dumbbell front press* is benefitting from unilateral resistance (independent arms); the *standing front barbell raise* uses a single instrument, and therefore is compromised due to the non-independence.
- The *supine dumbbell front press* keeps the lower back stable; the *standing front barbell raise* loads the lower back when the arms are raised (as such, it loads a non-target muscle more than the target muscle).

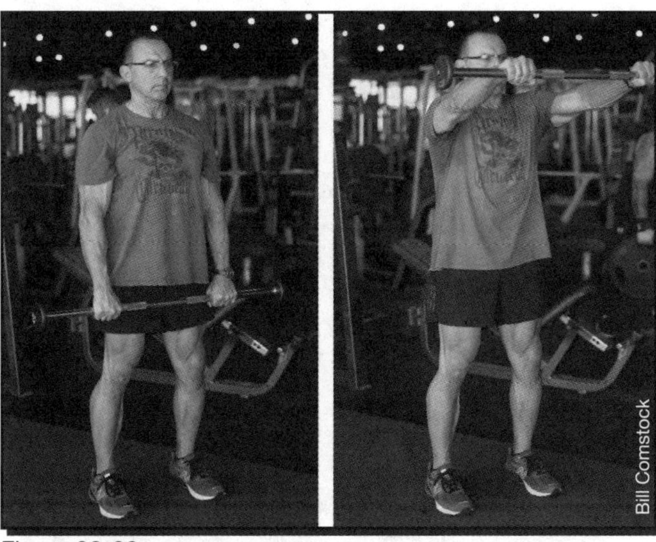
Bill Comstock
Figure 20-32

Yet another version of an *anterior deltoid front press*, which is performed using cables, is shown in Figures 20-33 and 20-34 (please ignore the bench that is there—it is not a required part of the exercise). The same criteria for evaluating the exercise are employed:

- The pulleys are set at shoulder-width (thereby providing "alignment").
- The resistance is mostly perpendicular with the humerus at the beginning of the range of motion ("early phase loaded").
- The anatomical motion of the arms is such that the humerus travels alongside the torso (moving the operating lever toward the target muscle origin).
- The anterior deltoids are "opposite position loaded" because the humerus is externally rotated (elbows in/ palms up).

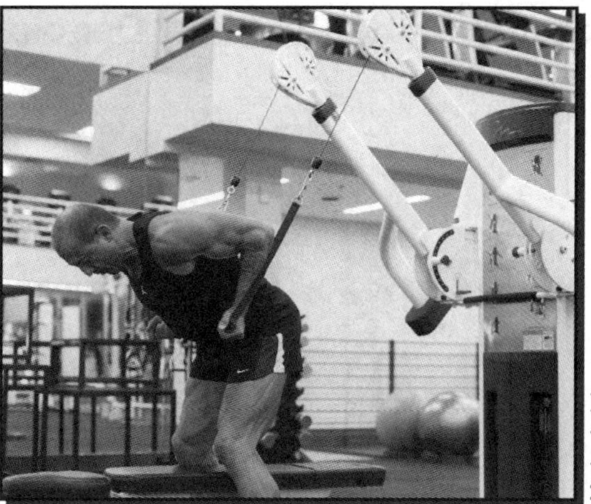
Marisa Leigh
Figure 20-33

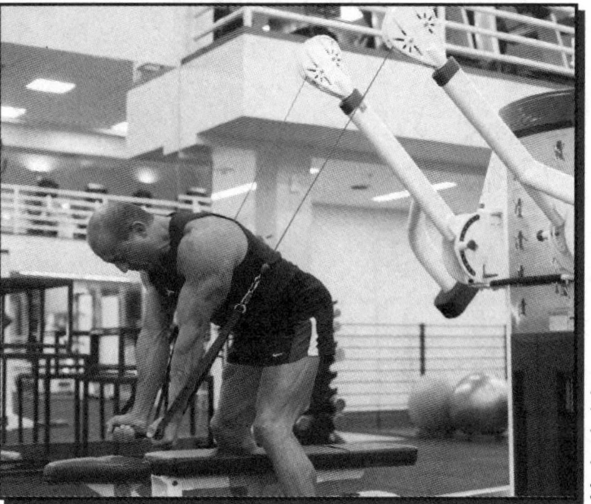
Marisa Leigh
Figure 20-34

## Exercise Options for the Anterior Deltoids

Therefore, the best anterior deltoid exercises, in descending order, are as follows:

- *Seated cable front press* (assuming you have access to this type of pulley system, and you don't mind taking the trouble to set it up)
- *Standing (bent-over) cable front press*
- *Supine (flat bench) dumbbell front press*
- *Slight decline bench/dumbbell front press* (head slightly lower than hips)
- *Slight incline bench/dumbbell front press* (head slightly higher than hips)

## Anatomy of the Posterior Deltoids

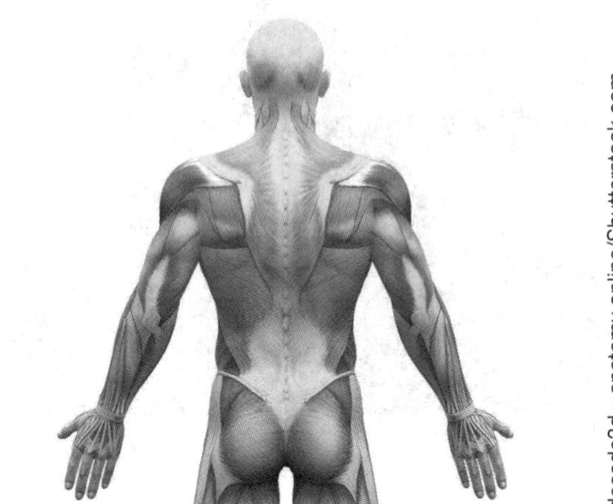



Figure 20-35

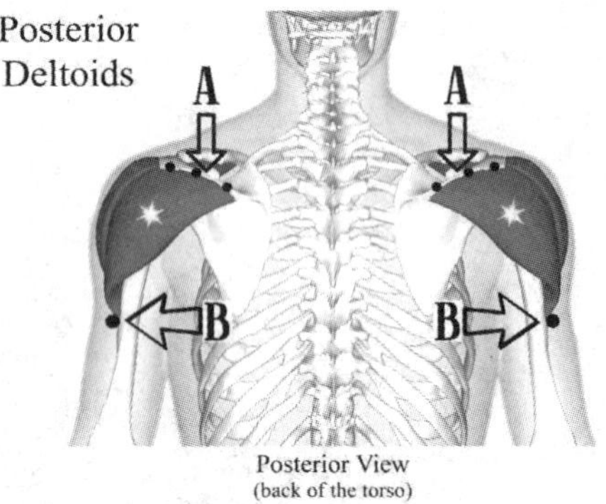




Figure 20-36

The posterior deltoids are commonly referred to as the "rear deltoids" or simply as the "rear delts." As you can see in Figure 20-36, they originate on the upper ridge of the scapula ("A"), and they insert onto the deltoid tuberosity of the humerus ("B")—right next to, and posterior to, the insertion of the lateral detloids. Its primary function is to pull the humerus back (posteriorly)—toward its origin. It also helps to externally rotate the humerus, although this is a much lesser function. It's worth noting, as you look at Figures 20-35 and 20-36, that when the arm is down at the individual's side (as it is in these illustrations) the posterior deltoid fibers run diagonally, from origin to insertion.

## Identifying the Ideal Anatomical Motion for the Posterior Deltoids

At this point, the goal is to identify the "ideal" direction of humeral movement that is produced by the posterior deltoids, without bias—neither for nor against—traditional exercises. As before, the first step, in this regard, is to use the guideline of imagining the muscle insertion moving directly toward the muscle origin, in the simplest and most natural manner, in order to see what kind of movement that produces.

In Figure 20-37, a line has been drawn straight through the origin and the insertion of both (the left and the right) posterior deltoids. As discussed in Chapter 8 ("Alignment"), there should be alignment between the direction of resistance, the direction of movement, and the origin/insertion of the target muscle.

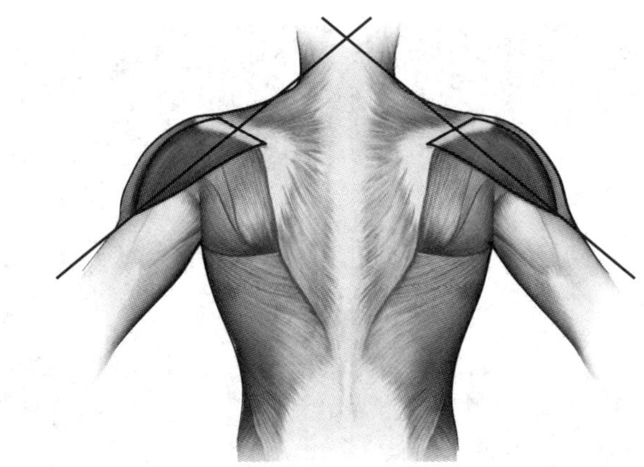

Figure 20-37

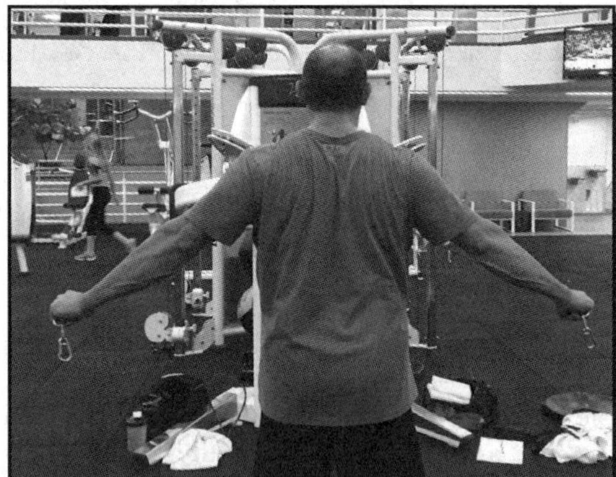

Figure 20-38

These lines represent PLANES, through which the resistance should travel, and through which your direction of anatomical motion should travel. Therefore, a movement that causes your humerus (i.e., the operating lever of the posterior deltoids) to travel diagonally—downward/backward—through that plane, would provide perfect alignment with the origin and insertion of the posterior deltoids. The image in Figure 20-38 demonstrates a perfectly good "ending position"—the point of contraction—for the concentric phase of the posterior deltoids' range of motion. The eccentric phase of the repetition would then move the arms in a forward/

upward/inward diagonal direction. In other words, there is NO need (no advantage whatsoever) in bringing the arms up so that they are perpendicular with the torso, as has been traditionally the norm for "rear deltoid" exercises.

The concentric motion should begin with both hands together—about the height of the xiphoid process (the lowest point of the sternum). Then, you would pull your arms backward, with a significant downward angle, ending with your hands around the level of your waist. This is all that is necessary to fully engage the posterior deltoids, through its full and correct range of motion.

The conventional wisdom has been to perform posterior deltoid exercises with the arms up, so that they are perpendicular with their torso. This, however, is entirely unnecessary, as you can see. That does NOT improve the mechanics of the posterior deltoid function. In fact, it clearly compromises it, because that motion is not nearly as "natural" a motion as is bringing the arms downward and backward, with a diagonal sweep.

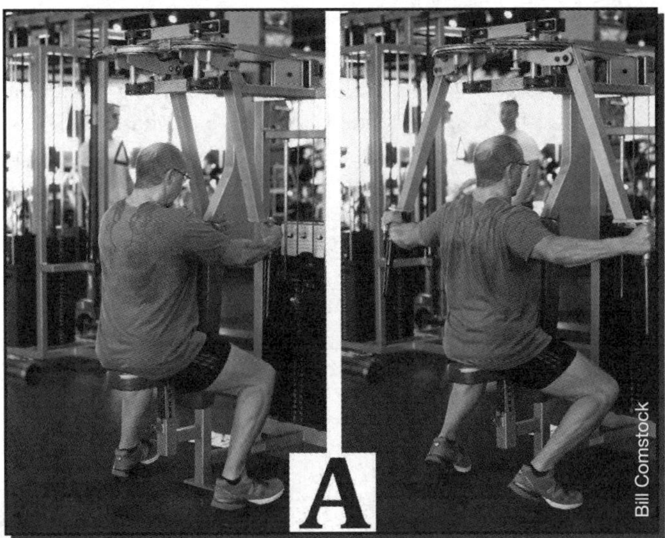


Figure 20-39

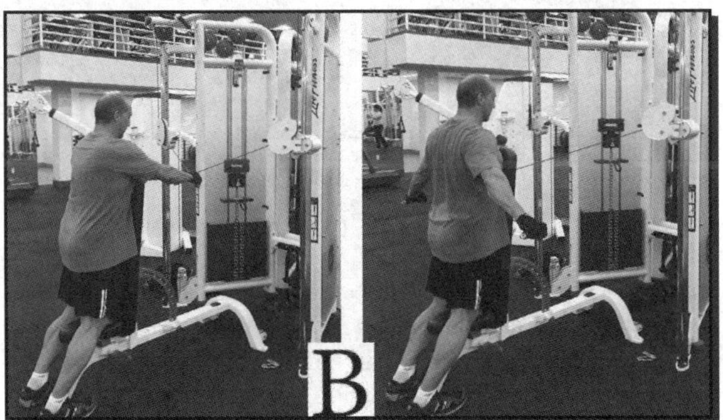


Figure 20-40

Figures 20-39 and 20-40 illustrate
comparison of the two movements. Clearly, movem
more "natural" than movement "A." As such, if you were to "flex" your posterior deltoid, to check how it feels, you would likely flex it with your arm low—the way it's demonstrated in Figure 20-40. That's the humeral position that allows the rear deltoid to contract most naturally.

From an evolutionary perspective, you could ask yourself the following question: "For what evolutionary purpose did the posterior deltoids evolve?" For what anatomical need did they adapt? Certainly, there were no "reverse butterfly" machines available, for our homo erectus ancestors to use in the wild. In fact, in all likelihood, it seems that the posterior deltoids evolved to allow our early ancestors to pull objects (branches, vegetation, fruit, climbing, etc.) downward and backward.

People participating in fitness and bodybuilding have obviously unnecessarily overcomplicated this movement for years. There simply is no logical reason to perform posterior deltoid exercises with the arms UP, so that they're perpendicular with your torso. There is no mechanical advantage, nor benefit, in doing so—and it is much less comfortable a movement.

Muscle elongation (stretch) occurs when a muscle insertion (on the operating lever/limb) moves away from its muscle origin. In the case of the posterior deltoids, that would require a diagonally forward/upward/inward movement of the humerus—parallel with the fibers of the muscle. This action moves the muscle insertion away from the upper ridge of the scapula, with a perfectly natural shoulder movement.

Figure 20-41 shows how this movement would look from the front. As you can see, this movement—which could be described as an upside down "V"—starts with the hands together (about chest high), and then moves the arms downward/laterally/posteriorly, ending with the hands about the level of the waist/midsection.

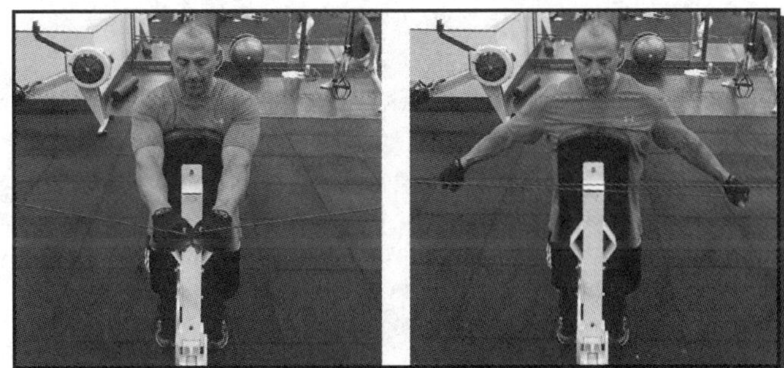

Figure 20-41

You should note that in Figure 20-41, although I am using the backrest of a bench as a brace, there is very little forward pull because the cables are not pulling straight forward. The resistance is pulling slightly forward, slightly across, and slightly upward. Using the backrest of a bench would help keep your torso still, but it is not actually necessary. It works perfectly well just standing, without the bench, although you would likely need to place one foot slightly forward, and the other foot slightly back, if a heavy weight is being used.

Having identified the ideal direction of motion produced by the posterior deltoids, you next need to establish the ideal direction of resistance. More specifically, you need to determine where to position the pulleys, assuming that you'll be using pulleys. Your objective is to create 1) "opposite position loading," 2) proper alignment and 3) "early phase loading."

Setting the pulleys at a height that is approximately the height of your head (slightly higher than your shoulders) provides an early upward resistance, against which the rear deltoids can pull downward. This helps provide "early phase loading." In terms of the width between the pulleys, they should be set at about a 45-degree angle from either side of the torso. This positioning provides an inward resistance, against which the rear deltoids can pull outward (laterally). As a result, this combination of the height and width of the pulleys provides the upward/inward resistance, against which your posterior deltoids can then pull the humerus downward/outward, with an excellent resistance curve.

Of course, it would be nice if this set-up (two pulleys, set at the correct height and width) existed as a pre-designed machine. This would allow you to simply put your body in place (either standing or seated), grab the handles, and perform the exercise. On the other hand, since a machine like this does not already exist, you must understand the concepts, so that you can adjust the pulleys yourself, assuming you have access to pulleys like these.

## Exercise Options for the Posterior Deltoids

The posterior deltoid exercises shown in Figures 20-42 to 20-47 are less "ideal" versions of the exercise described previously. They still "work" the posterior deltoids, but in varying degrees of being compromised. These are either less-efficient, less-safe, less-comfortable, less-precise (with regard to anatomical motion), not "early phase loaded," or it loads a non-target muscle (e.g., the lower back) more than the target muscle—the posterior deltoids.

The exercise shown in Figure 20-42—the *lying supine cable crossover*—is a relatively good option. The direction of humeral movement is not quite "ideal," because it's too perpendicular to the torso. It would be better if the movement were more "downward/backward," rather than straight back (like on a reverse butterfly machine). On the other hand, this "downward/backward" angle of movement can be easily arranged, simply by positioning the bench farther toward the exerciser's feet (which would be the same as moving the pulleys more "upward"). Then, when performing the exercise, move your arms in a "downward/backward/diagonally outward direction, opposite the direction of the cables' pull.

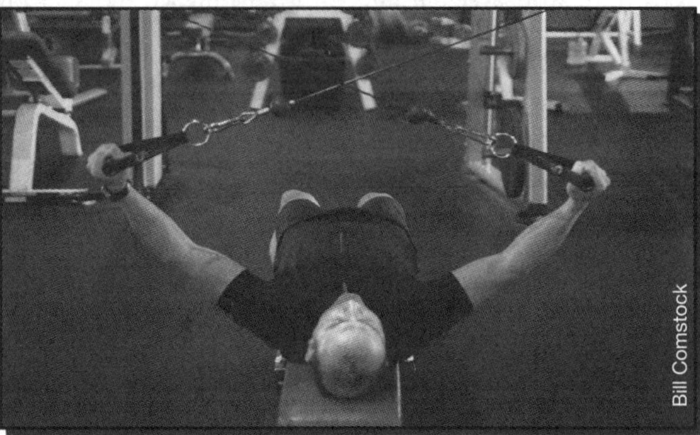

Figure 20-42

The crossing of the cable allows the resistance to come from a good angle (from the opposing side), which allows the early phase to be more loaded, and the late phase to be less loaded. This version also eliminates any possible strain on the lower back.

The exercise shown in Figure 20-43—the "*bent-over one-arm cable rear deltoid raise*"—is similar to the previous version, except that the lower back is much less supported. Using the non-working hand as a support against the knee is helpful, but not nearly as effective at relieving the stress on the lower back as the previous two versions. Nevertheless, the resistance curve on this exercise is good.

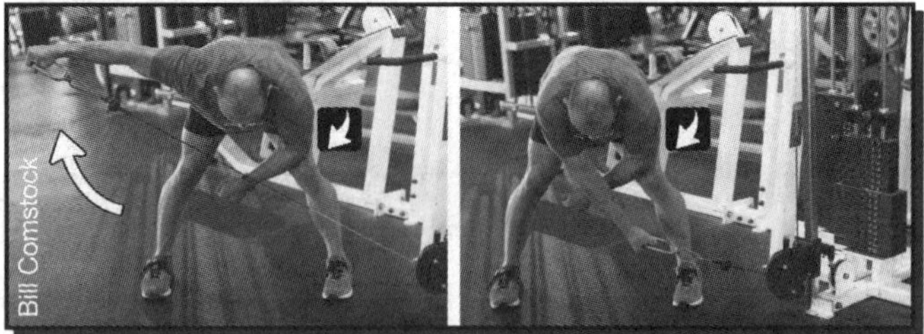

Figure 20-43

While the *reverse butterfly machine* exercise, shown in Figure 20-44, does not have an "ideal" direction of anatomical movement, it does have some advantages. For example, it does not load the lower back. In addition, it has a better resistance curve than the *bent-over dumbbell raises* (although still not as good cables provide), and it's convenient. You only need to adjust the seat height and lever arms, and you can begin the exercise.

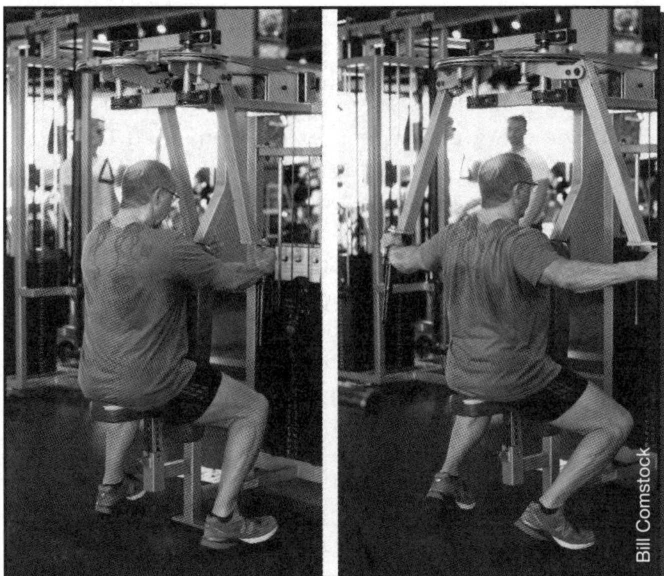


Figure 20-44

The exercise shown in Figure 20-45—"*incline supine rear dumbbell raises*"—has an anatomical motion that is worse (less natural) than the *reverse butterfly machine* or *bent-over rear dumbbell raises*. This motion starts low and ends high. Ideally, the motion should start high and end low, because that's the pathway that moves through the plane of the muscle origin insertion, and that motion more effectively moves the humerus toward the muscle origin. This motion is not nearly as natural for the shoulder joint, as is a motion that starts at chest level, and moves "downward" from there.

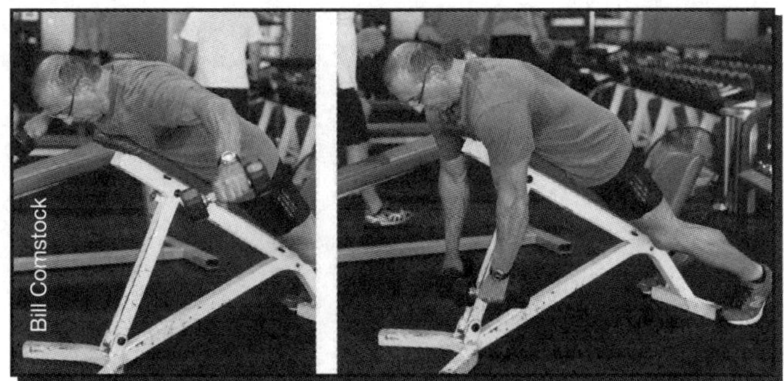


Figure 20-45

Furthermore, the position of the posterior deltoid—relative to the downward direction of resistance—prevents the posterior deltoid from being "opposite position loaded." As you can see, the muscle that is positioned at "12:00"—opposite the "6:00" direction of resistance (gravity)—is more the lateral deltoid, than the posterior deltoid. But, in fact, neither muscle is well positioned for optimum benefit. This mechanical flaw could be slightly remedied, by changing the trajectory of the arms, such that the humerus moves in a more downward/backward direction, angling the arms toward the feet, rather than straight upward. The biggest problem with this exercise, however, is that it's late phase loaded, rather than early phase loaded. In fact, it provides zero resistance where the target muscle is strongest, and completely misses the first 10 percent of the early range of motion. In reality, the only good thing about this exercise is that it doesn't load the lower back, although most of the other factors are compromised.

The standard "*bent-over rear deltoid dumbbell raise*" (shown in Figure 20-46) places more load on the lower back, than on the rear deltoids. This is becauses the lower back (erector spinae) is loaded with both the primary and the secondary resistance sources (the dumbbells PLUS the weight of the torso). To make matters worse, these two loads are applied to the torso perpendicularly, which means that the load on the lower back is maximally magnified.

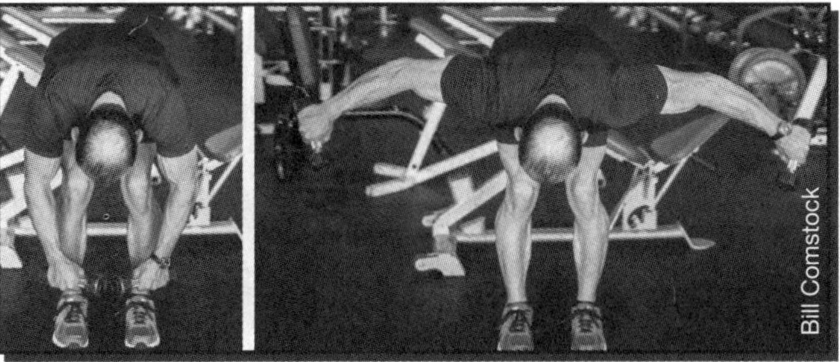


Figure 20-46

In addition, this version is also "late phase loaded"—like the exercise shown in 20-45, which greatly compromises the benefit to the posterior deltoids. It provides little or no resistance during the early part of the range of motion, which is where the target muscle is strongest, and where it most needs, and would most benefit from, "early phase loading".

Of course, it's very convenient to pick up a pair of dumbbells and perform this exercise, as compared with setting up a pair of pulleys, assuming you even have access to pulleys. On the other hand, that convenience does not negate the fact that the exercise is less-efficient, less-comfortable, and less productive as a rear deltoid builder, than the *cross cable rear deltoid* exercise shown previously.

The exercise shown in Figure 20-47—the *lying one-arm dumbbell rear deltoid raise*—is a relatively good alternative, if you do not have access to pulleys or a butterfly machine. It's an "acceptable" exercise (although not "great"), especially for someone who is not attempting to achieve maximum muscular development. It is "early phase loaded" (which is good), and it does not load the lower back. The angle of the body, however (relative to the direction of gravity), disallows a perfectly natural anatomical motion.

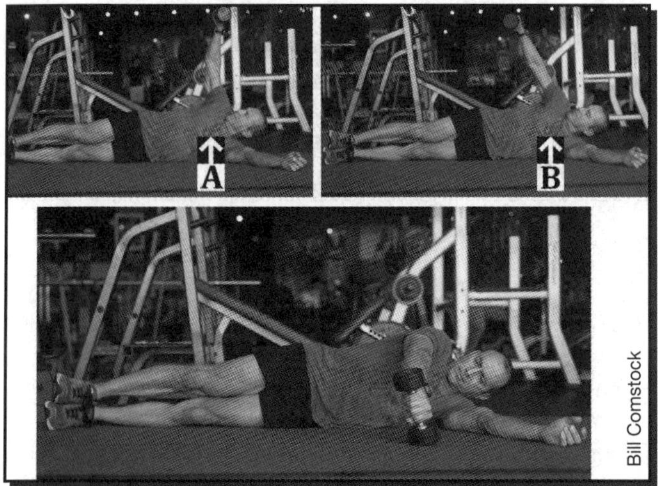


Figure 20-47

Notice that, in the "A" version, the arm is traveling straight up—vertically. In the "B" version, the arm is traveling at a slight diagonal. The "B" direction of arm travel is more anatomically natural (comfortable), but it's not aligned with the vertical downward pull of gravity. The "A" version is properly aligned with gravity, but that direction of anatomical movement is less comfortable—impossible, in fact, for some people (depending on their degree of shoulder mobility).

This creates the dilemma of forcing you to either move your arm straight upward (opposite resistance, which is good), but producing a less "natural" humeral pathway (which is not good)—or move your arm in the more natural direction, but be out of alignment with gravity.

If you are a trainer, you may have noticed that many individuals simply cannot move their arm straight upward, during this exercise. They tend to move their arm in the direction of the aforementioned semi-diagonal line, despite you telling them to move it straight upward. This scenario demonstrates that moving the arm straight up (when the torso is horizontal) is not a natural movement for the shoulder joint. The better humeral trajectory/shoulder joint movement, when working the posterior deltoids, is moving the humerus posteriorly, but in a downward direction—ending with the hand more alongside the navel (waist) rather than perpendicular to the torso.

If you decide to perform this exercise, it would be best to allow your arm to move in the direction of that semi-diagonal line, if that is more comfortable for your shoulder than moving it straight upward. As a result, the load will be shared by the posterior deltoid and the lateral deltoid, rather than loading mainly the posterior deltoid. This isn't "terrible," but it's not ideal. For novice individuals, whose goal is general fitness, it will suffice. On the other hand, if your goal is maximum muscular development, it's better to select an exercise that allows you to ensure both proper alignment and an ideal anatomical motion.

# CHAPTER 21

# Biceps, Triceps, and Forearms

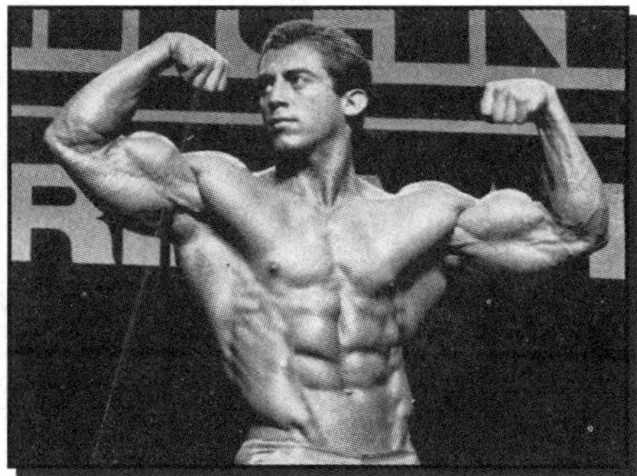

Figure 21-1

The biceps brachii is generally regarded as the muscle that most symbolizes "strength," even though it is neither the largest, nor the most powerful muscle of the body. Perhaps, this mindset is because of its curious "ball" shape, when the muscle is well-developed. In fact, many men prioritize "big arms," often to the neglect of other more functionally important muscles. Nevertheless, a complete physique requires well-developed biceps.

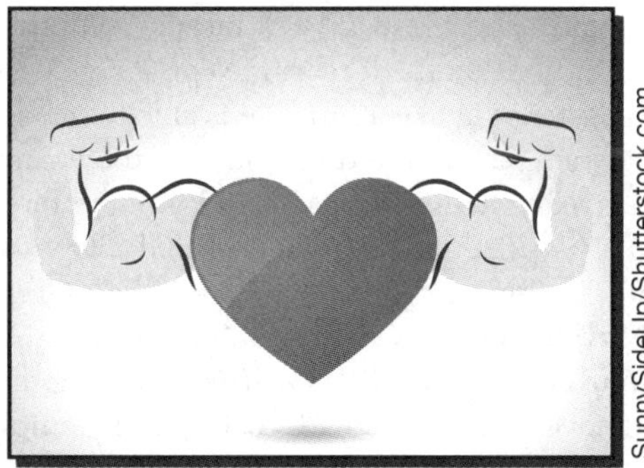

SunnySideUp/Shutterstock.com

Figure 21-2

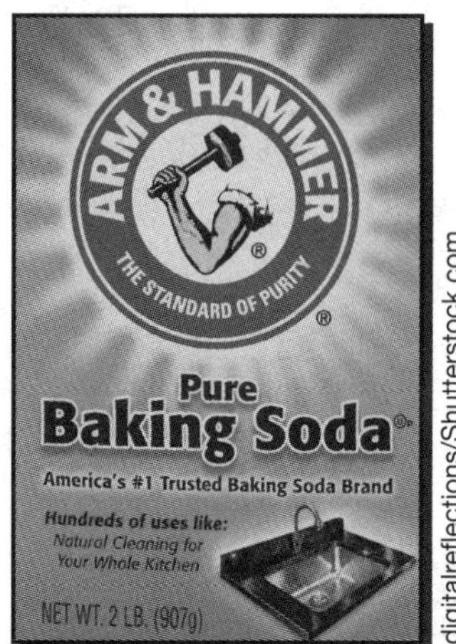


digitalreflections/Shutterstock.com

Figure 21-3

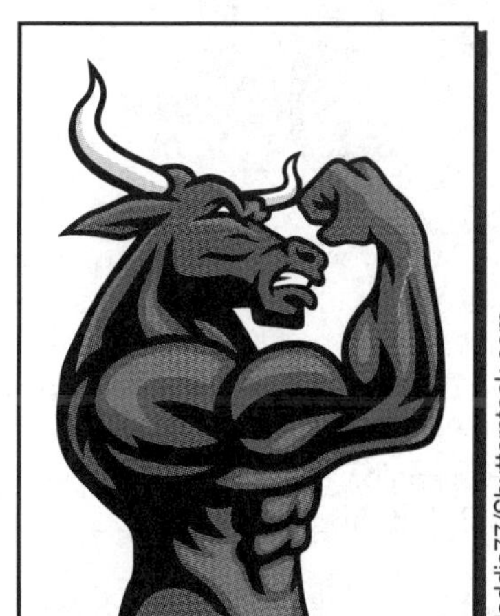

doddis77/Shutterstock.com

Figure 21-4

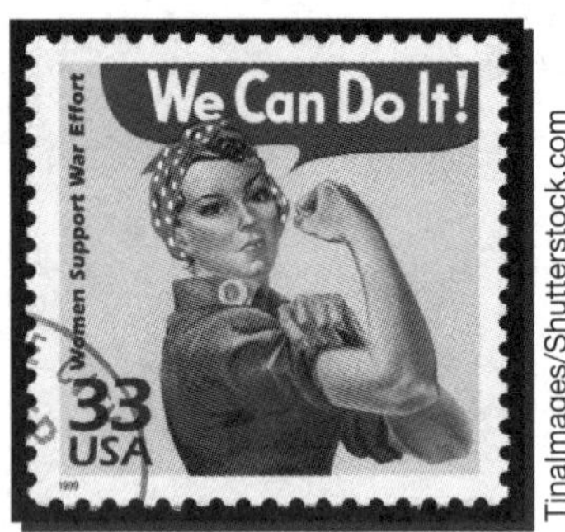

Figure 21-5

## Anatomy and Function of the Biceps Brachii

The primary function of the biceps is "elbow flexion"—bending the elbow. While two other smaller muscles assist in that action, the brachioradialis and the brachialis, neither plays as significant a role in elbow flexion, as does the biceps. The biceps also assists in shoulder flexion (raising the arm forward), although that is a very minor role for the biceps. The primary shoulder flexor is the anterior deltoid. It would be foolish, in fact, to perform "shoulder flexion" for the purpose of developing the biceps brachii—it's that minor a function.

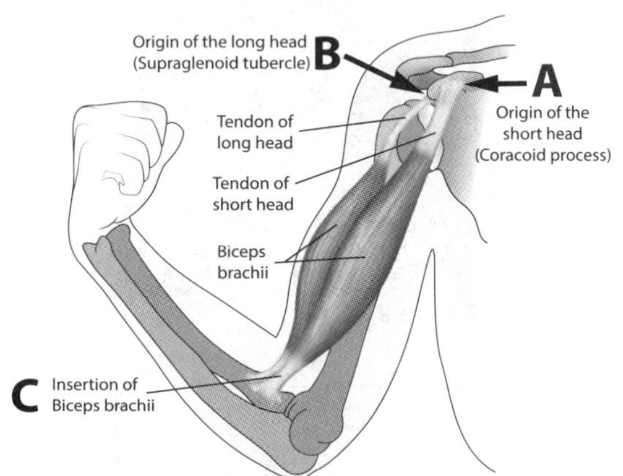

Figure 21-6

In Figure 21-6, you can clearly see that the biceps is comprised of two "heads"—two parts, so to speak. More specifically, it is a muscle with two origins. One of the heads is called "the short head" ("A"), while the other is called "the long head" ("B"). The short head originates on the coracoid process of the scapula, and the long head originates on the "glenoid tubercle" of the scapula.

As you can see in Figure 21-6, the originating tendon of the long head of the biceps wraps over the top of the humerus, and sits in a crevice called the "intertubercular groove." What is most important to note, however, is that both bicep heads CONVERGE near the elbow into one, single tendon, before crossing the elbow joint. This single biceps tendon then crosses the elbow, and connects to the radius of the forearm ("C").

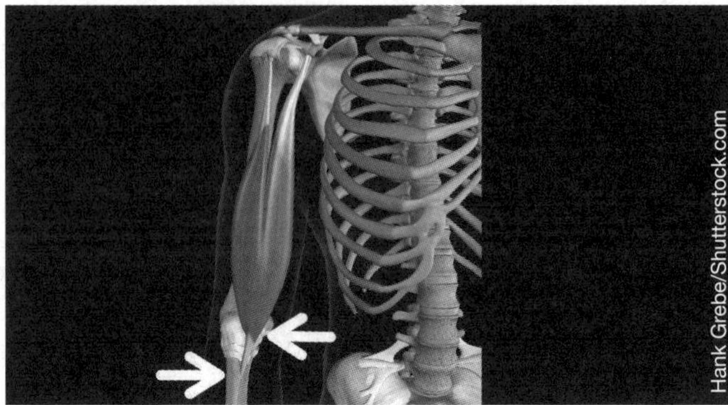

Figure 21-7

The reason this factor is important is because when the biceps bends the elbow, it entails the combined effort of both biceps heads. The elbow joint can only bend in one direction, just like a hinge. Therefore, it is impossible to isolate the "long head" (also referred to as the "outer biceps") or the "short head" (also referred to as the "inner biceps") of the biceps, because the same elbow action would occur in either case. There would be no functional purpose in one biceps head contacting more forcefully than the other biceps head, given that both biceps heads pull on the one single biceps tendon, and only in one direction.

It's common to hear people suggesting that a particular exercise will "emphasize" the outer head or the inner head of the biceps. This belief—that individuals can change the shape of their biceps by doing different biceps exercises—is pure fantasy. It is not supported by the mechanical facts. If it were possible to emphasize the "inner biceps" or the "outer biceps," there would have to be a mechanically different action that occurs at the elbow. It would require that the elbow be able to bend in more than one direction, as well as two separate tendons crossing the elbow, and two separate insertions on the forearm.

For example, in Figure 21-8 (left), I've modified the actual anatomy, imagining that—instead of there being only one biceps tendon—there are TWO biceps tendons, with two separate insertions on the forearm. Next, imagine that instead of the elbow bending like a hinge, it is able to bend like a ball-and-socket joint (i.e., multi- directional). If these circumstances were REAL, the "outer biceps" could pull the forearm more toward the outside, and the elbow would allow that kind of movement. In turn, the "inner biceps" could pull the forearm more toward the inside, with the elbow allowing that different angle of movement as well. As such, by choosing the direction of elbow-movement, you could, theoretically, emphasize one side of the biceps or the other. The real scenario, however, is depicted in Figure 21-8 (right): one biceps tendon, one insertion on the forearm, and one direction of elbow flexion.

*Note: Rotating the humerus at the shoulder—"curling to the inside" versus "curling to the outside"—does not constitute bending the elbow in a different direction.*

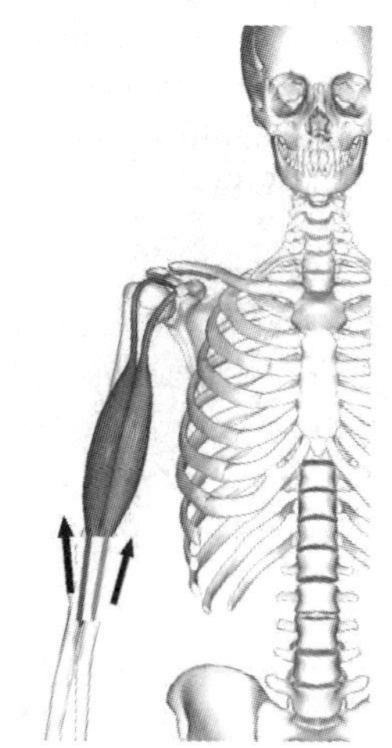

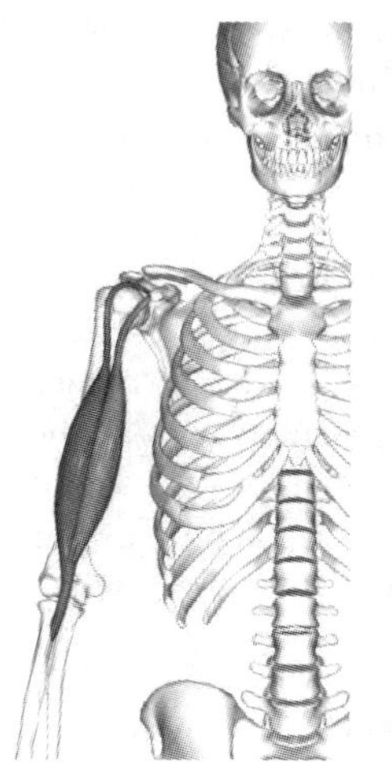



Figure 21-8

The reality is that both biceps heads act as one, when the elbow bends. They both pull simultaneously on the one single biceps tendon, which produces the one single action of elbow flexion, which only occurs in one single direction.

In other words, regardless of whether you use a barbell or dumbbells, whether you perform a *preacher curl* or a "*concentration curl*," whether you employ a hammer grip or a palms-up grip, or whether you do curls on an incline bench, the biceps works the same in all circumstances, in terms of its "parts" (long head/short head). As such, you cannot change the shape of your biceps by performing different exercises, aside from simply making your biceps larger (or allowing them to atrophy, i.e., to get smaller).

Of course, biceps exercises are not all "equal," in terms of effectiveness. Some exercises are "better" (more efficient/ more productive) than others, so they are not all the same in that regard. They are the same, however, in the sense that doing multiple exercises during a given workout for the biceps is redundant. The same action occurs in the biceps, from one exercise to the next, but to different degrees of efficiency, productivity, and risk.

If the two biceps origins have any separate functional purpose at all, it would more likely be related to minute, subtle participation during humeral movement of the shoulder, rather than the notion that different kinds of biceps curls (elbow flexion) can preferentially engage one head of the biceps more than the other.

## The Ideal Anatomical Motion of the Biceps

Since we've already established that the elbow performs only one action (elbow flexion), the question at this point is not so much "what action is the ideal elbow flexion?" as it is "what would constitute the ideal humeral/shoulder position, while the elbow is flexing," for the purpose of biceps development?

Our first clue is that "muscles always pull toward their origins," but that only tells us that the elbow must bend, in order to have the biceps insertion move toward the biceps origin. So, we'll consider the second clue—that the simplest (least contorted) action is usually the most natural. That would be the action for which a muscle has most likely evolved to perform, over the course of our evolutionary history. As such, the purest version of biceps contraction is simple elbow flexion, with the humerus at your side, as illustrated in Figure 21-9.

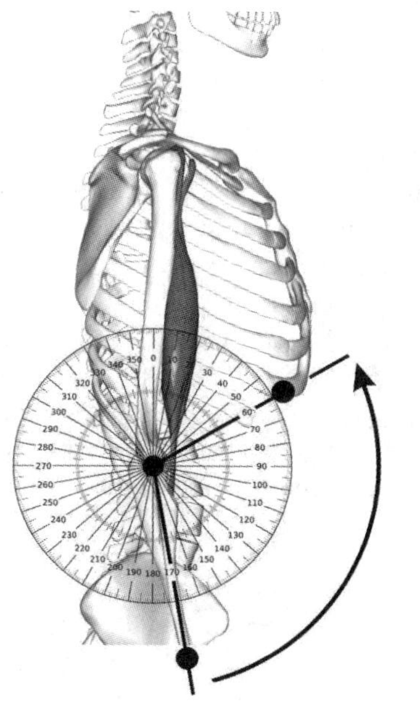



Figure 21-9

This motion—elbow flexion, with the humerus alongside the torso (or close to it)—would therefore be the most "natural" movement for a biceps exercise. That is the motion and humeral position that is the least contorted, and arguably the movement to which humans have most adapted, over millennia. Elbow flexion performed with any other humeral position could be characterized as representing varying degrees of "less natural"—some of which are acceptable, but none of which are "better"—with regard to being more productive or more safe.

Not surprisingly, the resistance curve that is produced when a free weight is curled, while a person is in the upright position, and their humerus is alongside their torso, synchronizes perfectly with the strength curve of the biceps. The mechanical disadvantage (i.e., increased force requirement) that occurs at the beginning of the movement coincides with the less "active" (less perpendicular) angle of the forearm. Then, the mechanical advantage that is gained halfway through the range of motion (i.e., the decreased force requirement) coincides with the more "active" (more perpendicular) angle of the forearm, which increases the resistance because of the greater moment arm.

When a *curl* is performed in the upright position, with "free weight" (i.e., dumbbell or barbell), the forearm begins in a neutral position (hanging straight down, parallel with gravity), precisely at the time when the mechanical disadvantage is the "worst" (i.e., biceps pulling parallel to the forearm). As the forearm begins its forward/upward trajectory, it enters into progressively more "active" (perpendicular) angles to gravity, which increases the load. This occurs simultaneous to the biceps entering into progressively "better" mechanical advantage with the forearm, which allows the increased resistance to be better managed by the biceps.

As has been previously discussed, the strength potential of a skeletal muscle generally diminishes as it shortens (contracts), and increases as it lengthens. This factor is true of the biceps as well. On the other hand, any mechanical disadvantage that may occur during an exercise also factors into the equation of "how much load" is placed on a muscle, as well as when it occurs (during the range of motion). For example, the increased force requirement of a biceps, when the elbow is straight (mechanical disadvantage), could be as much as six times (600 percent) greater than an equal amount of weight pulled from a mechanical advantage. Accordingly, even using a light resistance when performing a biceps exercise would be tremendously magnified, when the elbow is nearly straight.

Experimentation with different angle of *curls* can easily demonstrate that a standard, upright curling motion with dumbbells provides a very efficient resistance curve for the biceps, while a preacher-type of curl is typically "too difficult" at the beginning, and "too easy" at the conclusion. Performing curls with an upright (vertical) humerus, combined with "free weight gravity," provides enough resistance at the beginning of the range of motion, and a bit more of a challenge, when the biceps/elbow has entered into more of a safe zone, mechanically speaking. This ensures optimal safety, as well as an appropriate level of diminishing resistance toward the end of the range of motion.

Curiously, it seems that the strength curve of the biceps is not exactly like that of other flexion muscles—like the pectorals, for example. This factor can be easily proven. If you attempted to perform a heavy dumbbell *biceps curl* with your arm flat on a tabletop (with a horizontal humerus), you would quickly discover that the biceps do not have nearly as much strength at that angle, as do the pectorals—even though both situations represent the same degree of mechanical disadvantage when the muscle is elongated. This factor must be taken into consideration when selecting an "ideal" exercise for the biceps.

There is also an enormous risk factor, when the elbow is straight and the biceps is heavily loaded. As discussed in Chapter 3, the biceps and its tendon seem to be very susceptible to rupture when the elbow is straight or nearly straight, and the weight being used is considerable.

It seems that the mechanical disadvantage that occurs when the elbow is straight (i.e., the increased force requirement that it causes), more than off-sets the decreased level of "activeness" (perpendicular-ness) of the forearm, at the beginning of an upright, free-weight *biceps curl*. Even a very slight angle (from vertical) on the humerus and forearm, at the starting position, greatly increases the difficulty factor.

There are numerous biceps exercises that are commonly performed in a gym. Some begin with the humerus pulled back, like the *incline dumbbell curl* (Figure 21-11), while others are performed with the humerus in front of the torso, or out to the sides (Figure 21-10). You'll notice, however, that, regardless of the position of the humerus, the elbow still does the exact same thing in every exercise. Since bending the elbow is the primary function of the biceps, every biceps exercise must include elbow flexion. Therefore, the only other variables are the position of the humerus (relative to the torso), and the direction of resistance (relative to the humerus). In both of these cases, there are "good" (more productive/less injury risk) and "bad" (less productive/more injury risk) options—for humeral position and direction of resistance.

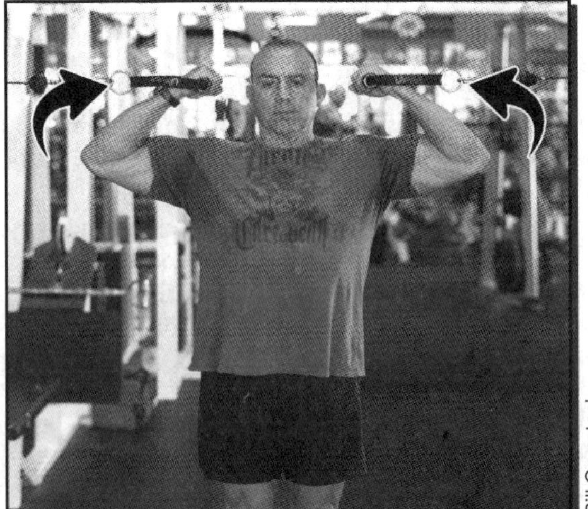
Bill Comstock

Figure 21-10

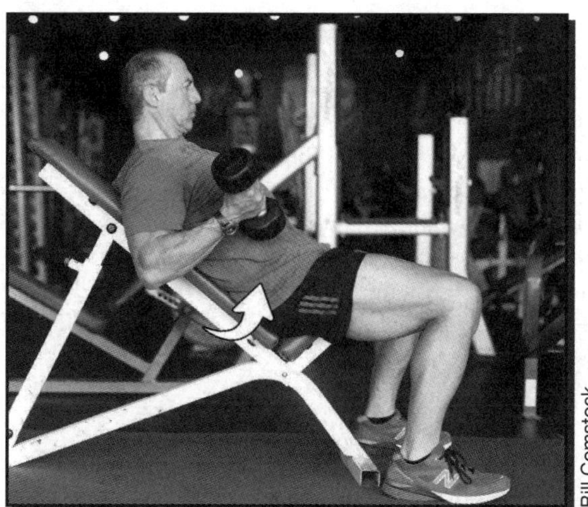

Figure 21-11

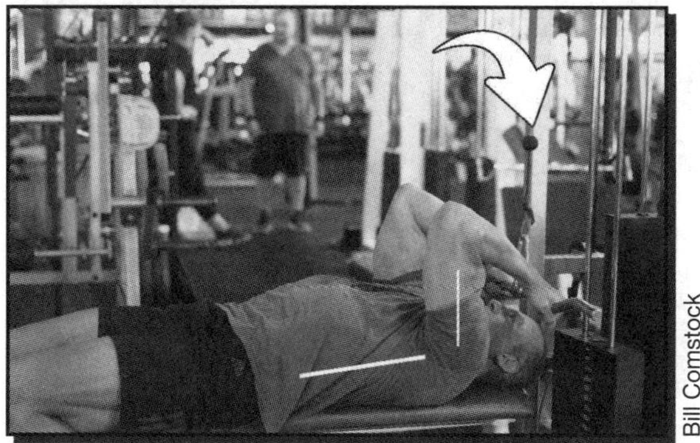

Figure 21-12

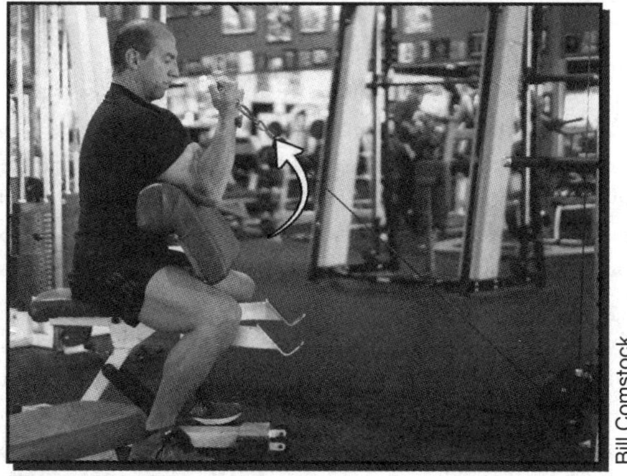

Figure 21-13

A good question to ask, therefore, is this: "Exactly what do these various humeral positions change, with regard to biceps activation, and are those changes good, bad, or insignificant?" Since the elbow bends the same, regardless of the humeral position, the only possible change is the amount of lengthening or shortening the bicep experiences, because changing the humeral position effectively moves the biceps insertion farther away from the shoulder (the place of biceps origin), or closer toward the biceps origin. This occurs because the biceps crosses the shoulder joint, as well as the elbow joint. If the humerus is pulled back, it increases the distance between the biceps origin and its insertion. If the humerus is pulled forward, it shortens the distance the biceps origin and its insertion—often excessively, to the point of "active insufficiency" (weakness), as was discussed in Chapter 4.

Despite the conventional wisdom, these changes in humeral position are not more productive. They do not change the shape of the biceps, nor do they cause any advantage whatsoever (mechanical, physiological, or neurological), above and beyond the benefit that is obtained with an *upright dumbbell curl*, during which the humerus is maintained alongside the torso. In fact, any humeral position other than "alongside the torso," compromises (to varying degrees) biceps function. This is because the optimum strength capability for the biceps occurs when it is neither excessively lengthened, nor excessively shortened. The biceps is strongest when the biceps "length" (the distance between the origin and the insertion) is at the length which occurs when the humerus is at the lifter's side—alongside the torso. We have apparently evolved to use our biceps most, and with the most amount of force, with this humeral position.

Biceps exercises that require the elbows to be significantly elevated, produce a stretch in the triceps, while the biceps is contracting, which may result in "passive insuffiency." This factor was discussed in Chapter 11. Stretching the triceps (while working the biceps) could interfere with contraction of the biceps, by limiting the elbow's ability to bend. In addition, stretching the triceps while the biceps is activated could signal to the central nervous system that "triceps over-stretching is occurring," which could cause a "relaxation synapse" to be sent to the biceps, in order to protect the triceps. Furthermore, there is also some shoulder discomfort, when doing biceps exercises, with the humerus significantly elevated.

While it may not be "bad" (risky or counterproductive) to perform biceps exercises with "other" humeral positions, there is no advantage in doing so, in terms of muscle development. At best, some alternative humeral positions are "equally productive." More often than not, however, they are less productive and more risky, than biceps exercises in which the humerus is simply held alongside the torso.

As such, if you enjoy doing biceps exercises with a variety of humeral positions, you should do them for the sake of enjoyment. You should not, however, perform them with the mistaken belief that they will provide a "different type" of benefit, or, any development advantage beyond that which is achieved with the humerus at your side.

## The Ideal Direction of Resistance for the Biceps

A variety of factors are influenced by the direction of resistance, during a given exercise, including the following:

- How "active" (degree of perpendicular-ness) is the operating lever (of your target muscle), during the range of motion
- Whether the resistance curve is productive, which means "early phase loading"
- Whether there is proper alignment, which implicates two important factors—"opposite position loading" (essential for efficiency), and also reduced injury risk (joint distortion/strain) which would be caused if alignment is not correct.
- Whether there is sufficient loaded range of motion (i.e., the movement does not encounter a "base" or an "apex" before the muscle is fully elongated or contracted), and ensuring there is relief from any mechanical disadvantage, if it occurs during a given exercise.

There are very specific ways of ensuring that you have the ideal direction of resistance (complying with the aforementioned requirements), for any target muscle. For the biceps, these include the following:

- Make sure that the forearm (as the operating lever of the biceps) crosses the direction of resistance perpendicularly, somewhere in the range of motion—but not in the beginning, due to the mechanical disadvantage that occurs, when the elbow is straight.
- Make sure that the direction of resistance is on the same plane as the trajectory of the forearm, as well as the origin and insertion of the biceps.
- Make sure that the biceps is loaded through most of the range of motion—that no "base" or "apex" occurs in between—and that the biceps is performing sufficient range of motion (at least 80 percent).

Since you are targeting the biceps—a flexion muscle—you are dealing with a muscle/joint that experiences a significant mechanical disadvantage, when the elbow is nearly straight. Therefore, you must factor this into the resistance curve, as part of the "early phase loading." In other words, you allow the forearm to be less active (more parallel with resistance), when the elbow is nearly straight, to compensate for the mechanical disadvantage that occurs at that point.

As such, when using free weight, starting the curling motion with a vertical forearm (torso upright and humerus vertical) loads the biceps enough, and also prevents the biceps overloading that would occur if the mechanical disadvantage (elbow nearly straight) occurred with a more horizontal forearm. Then, halfway through the motion, the forearm becomes more "active" (more perpendicular with gravity), as mechanical advantage (biceps pulling more perpendicularly on the forearm) is gained. In other words, the mechanical disadvantage that occurs when the elbow is nearly straight is used as part of the "early phase loading," although with a less "active" forearm, for the sake of safety. Then, when the mechanical disadvantage diminishes (becomes an advantage)—when the elbow is more bent—we allow the load to increase by having the forearm be more perpendicular to gravity.

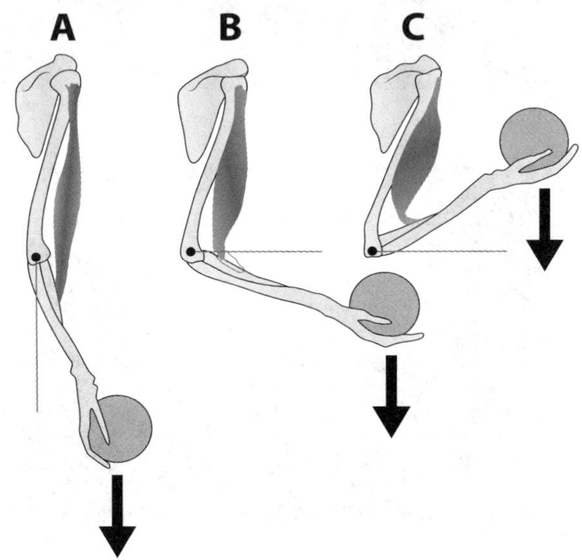


Figure 21-14

In Figure 21-14, you can see the elbow bending and the biceps contracting in three different positions. Note that the degree of mechanical advantage and disadvantage fluctuates as the elbow progressively bends. Simultaneously, as mechanical disadvantages/advantage fluctuates, the degree to which the forearm interacts with gravity (represented by the arrow), also changes:

- The forearm lever moves through various angles with gravity—from a mostly neutral (parallel) angle ("A"), to a mostly "active" (perpendicular) angle ("B"), and then slightly beyond perpendicular ("C").
- The biceps moves through various angles of mechanical disadvantage and advantage. Initially, it pulls on the forearm from a mostly parallel angle (the most extreme mechanical disadvantage—"A"). Then it changes to a mostly perpendicular angle (best mechanical advantage—"B"), and then it transitions toward a slight disadvantage again ("C").

In the initial stage ("A"), the resistance is less magnified by the forearm's interaction with gravity, but more magnified by the mechanical disadvantage. In the middle stage ("B"), the resistance is most magnified by the forearm's angle with gravity, but the biceps is at its strongest mechanical advantage with the forearm. In the final stage ("C"), the forearm's angle (relative to gravity) has started to reduce its load on the biceps (approaching a more vertical angle/more "neutral"), and the mechanical advantage has reverted back to a slight disadvantage.

While the math could be calculated on this scenario, it isn't necessary. You simply need to KNOW that there is an exchange occurring—one mechanical component is reducing the resistance to the biceps, while the other mechanical component is increasing it. Then, it reverses. As the first component increases the resistance to the biceps, the other decreases it. This is the reason why—although in most other circumstances (i.e., when working most other muscles), it is wise to begin a range of motion with the operating lever of the target muscle mostly perpendicular with the direction of resistance—doing so with the biceps would be very unwise.

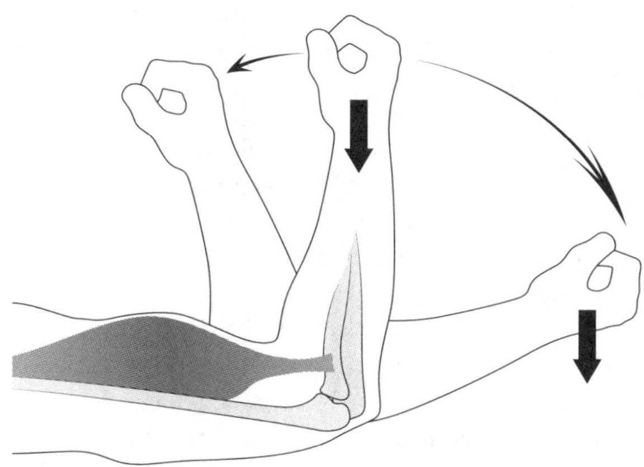

Figure 21-15

Figure 21-15 depicts a situation in which a horizontal forearm at the beginning of the range of motion (when the elbow is mostly straight) coincides with a maximum mechanical disadvantage (the biceps pulling on the forearm from a mostly parallel angle). This set of circumstances results in TWO resistance magnifiers occurring simultaneously—both at the beginning of the range of motion. Not only would this situation create a serious potential injury risk at the early part of the range of motion, it would also cause the forearm to reach the apex (neutral position) in the middle of the range of motion, precisely where the biceps is at its best mechanical advantage (strongest), and well before it has completed its range of motion. Going beyond that point (bending the elbow beyond the 90-degree angle) would result in the forearm "free-falling down the other side of the hill," toward the shoulder (without any opposing resistance)—if "free weight" is being used.

Although a *preacher barbell curl* (Figure 21-16) is less severe than the situation depicted in Figure 21-15, it also creates a flawed resistance curve. It is arguably too heavy (dangerously so) at the beginning of the range of motion (because of the mechanical disadvantage that occurs at that point)—and then fails to provide sufficient resistance at the top of the range of motion (when the elbow is fully bent), because the forearm is mostly neutral. Note the arrow that is placed under the weight, showing how, at the point where the mechanical disadvantage is the worst (when the elbow is straight), the forearm is at about a 50-degree angle, relative to gravity. Having the forearm this "active" would create too much load for the biceps, due to the mechanical disadvantage that is happening at the same time.

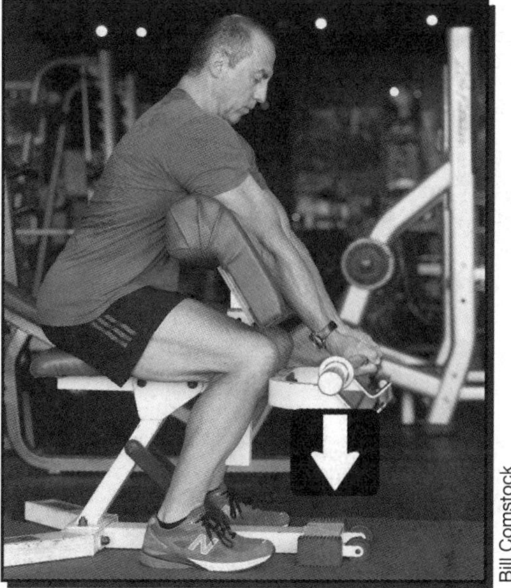


Figure 21-16

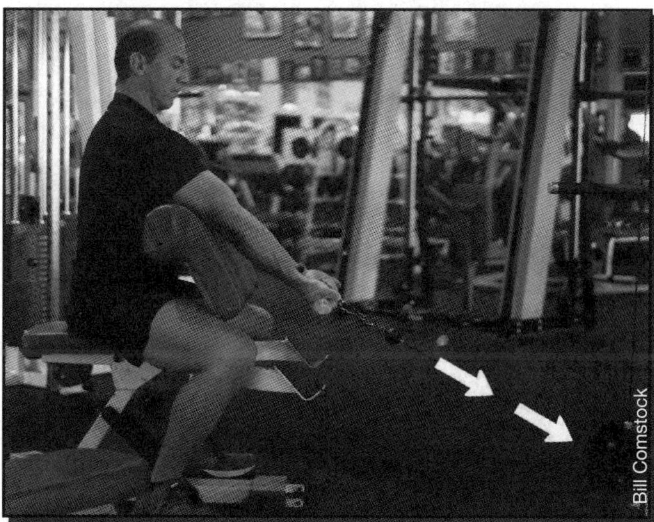


Figure 21-17

In Figure 21-17, a CABLE version of a *preacher curl* is depicted. In this version of the exercise, the direction of resistance is no longer "straight down." Rather, the direction of resistance is indicated by the cable, which is pulling toward the pulley. In this scenario, when the elbows are straight, the forearms would be almost parallel with the direction of resistance (i.e., the cable), indicated by the arrows. This alternate direction of resistance is much better, because it allows the biceps to experience a LESS "active" lever (forearm angle), when the mechanical disadvantage is at its worst (when the elbow is straight; the biceps pulling on the forearm from a mostly parallel angle). When the forearm has moved into a position that allows it to be more "active" (more perpendicular with the cable, about halfway into the range of motion), the increased resistance from the cable coincides with the improved mechanical advantage occurring at the elbow/biceps insertion.

Accordingly, when selecting the "ideal" direction of resistance for the biceps, it is best to select one that provides a direction of resistance that is mostly parallel to the forearm at the beginning of the range of motion, or at an angle that does not exceed 20 degrees from the neutral position. A 50-degree angle (Figure 21-16) arguably provides too much resistance, at the early stage of a *biceps curl*. That angle of resistance (relative to the forearm) is significantly less safe, and it is not more productive.

In Figure 21-18, I'm doing a "slight" *incline curl*, using an elbow support. This feature prevents the arm from reaching the fully vertical (neutral) position. As you can see in image A, my forearm is about 10 percent from the vertical position, which makes it a bit more "active" at the beginning of the range of motion, than would occur if the forearm were perfectly vertical. This angle of forearm (at the early stage of the range of motion), combined with the mechanical disadvantage that occurs at the elbow/biceps insertion, results in a bit more load on the biceps at the early stage, but still prudently safe.

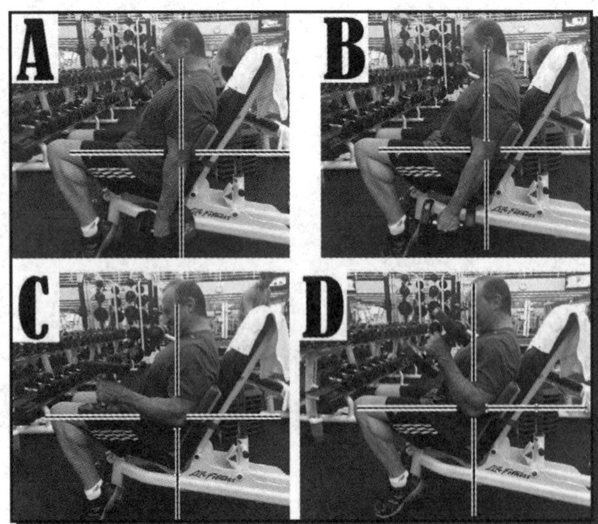

Figure 21-18

In Figure 21-18, image B, I've barely begun to bend my elbow, and already my forearm is about 20 percent active, which provides more than enough resistance at this "early stage" of this *curl*, because of the simultaneously occurring mechanical disadvantage. In image C, my elbow is bent at a 90-degree angle, which allows the biceps to be at its best mechanical advantage, but with the forearm slightly beyond the point at which it is 100 percent "active" (indicated by the horizontal line). In image D, my elbow is fully bent, my biceps is fully contracted, and the angle of my forearm is providing about 30 percent of the available resistance (to the biceps) at this point. As such, this exercise ("*slightly incline dumbbell curls with elbow support*") provides an excellent resistance curve for the biceps.

In addition to ensuring an ideal resistance curve, using an elbow brace like this also prevents an exerciser from using any momentum at all. It's nearly impossible to "cheat," i.e., to swing the weight up. Furthermore, it relieves the anterior deltoid from having to hold the humerus in the proper position, while the elbow is flexing. Using a starting angle (of the forearm) that is much more "active" (less vertical/more horizontal) than this, would greatly increase the risk of injury to the biceps tendon, and would not yield a greater benefit.

In Figure 21-19, I am using a pair of cables, which originate from pulleys that are directly alongside my ankles. In the starting position, my forearm and the cable are parallel, which allows me to start with zero resistance. As soon as my forearm angles slightly forward (still in the "early phase"), however, the load on the biceps significantly increases. This increase is due to the forearm becoming more perpendicular with the cable, combined with the mechanical disadvantage. Since the cable is pulling toward the pulley (not straight down, as "free weight gravity" would), the resistance increases sooner, and diminishes sooner, which are acceptable variations.

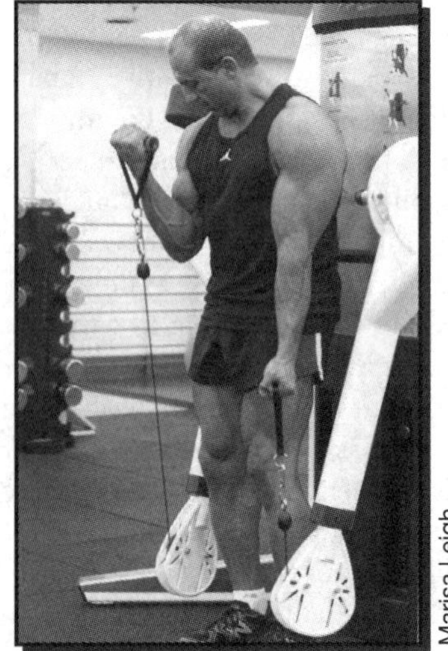
Marisa Leigh
Figure 21-19

In Figure 21-20, you can see a man standing slightly IN FRONT OF the pulleys. An arrow indicates the direction in which gravity would be pulling, IF he were holding free weight (a dumbbell). The slightly posterior direction of resistance of the cable (indicated by the larger arrow), however, provides a bit more resistance at the beginning of the range of motion, as compared with a straight-down direction of resistance. Rather than starting with zero resistance (a fully "neutral lever"), the movement begins with about 15 percent of the resistance—not accounting for the mechanical disadvantage. This direction of resistance results in the forearm reaching the "fully active" position (perpendicular with resistance) a bit sooner, and ending the range of motion with a bit less resistance, which is also an acceptable option.

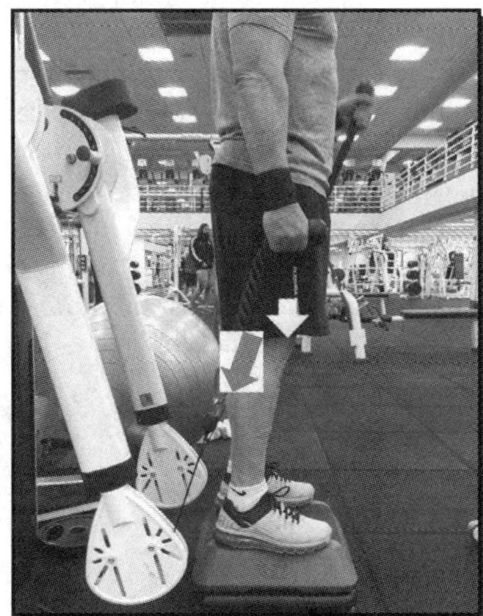

Figure 21-20

## Vulnerability of the Biceps/ Mechanical Disadvantage

When training the biceps, selecting a direction of resistance in which the forearm is more than 20 degrees from the neutral (parallel) angle—at the beginning of the range of motion (when the elbow is straight)—is not necessary, because the mechanical disadvantage that occurs at that position already magnifies whatever weight you're using. The "early phase" does not need much, if any, additional loading, by way of a more "active" lever (a forearm that is more perpendicular with resistance). Starting the range of motion with a forearm angle that is more than 20 degrees only increases the risk of injury.

As was discussed in Chapter 3, the vast majority of biceps ruptures occur when the elbow is straight, or nearly straight, and the biceps is loaded with a significant level of resistance. A ruptured biceps tendon is a serious injury, which usually requires surgical reattachment. If the biceps tendon tears off the bone, and is not surgically reattached, there will likely be some degree of permanent deformation, as well as varying degrees of function loss. Obviously, it would be wise to avoid tearing a biceps, in the first place.

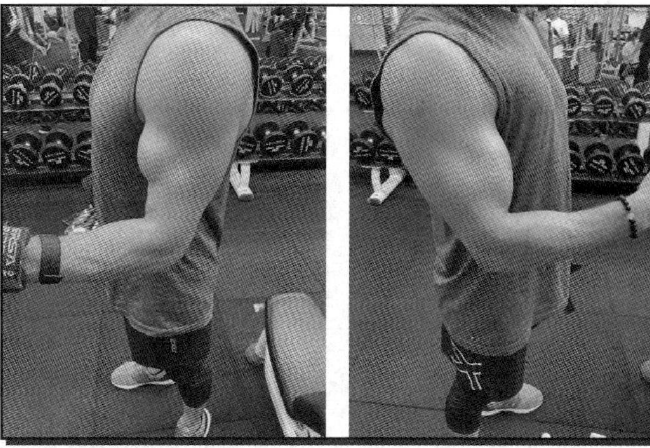

Figure 21-21

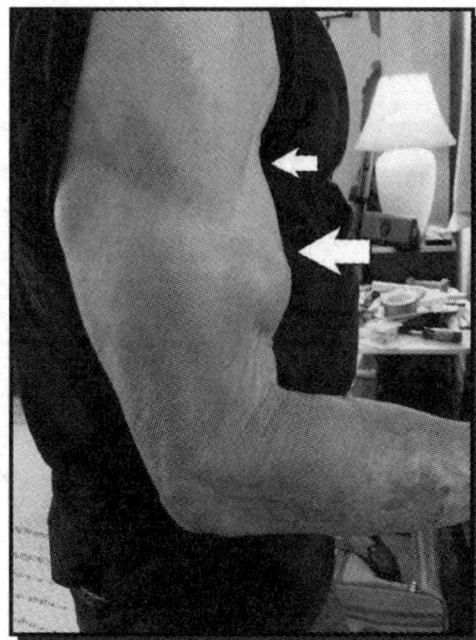

Figure 21-22

Figure 21-21 (left image) shows a biceps that ruptured on the lower end (i.e., the insertion, near the elbow). The image on the right shows this person's other biceps, intact. This type of tear causes the lower end of the biceps to slide upward, and "find a new home," i.e., to reattach itself wherever it can, by way of scar tissue. In contrast, Figure 21-22 illustrates a biceps that ruptured on the upper end (i.e., the origin, near the shoulder). This type of tear causes the upper end of the biceps to slide downward, and "find a new home," via the same method. In both instances, the appearance and function of the biceps are thus permanently compromised.

Knowing the circumstances that increase the odds of a biceps rupture is the first step in preventing this type of injury. You can exercise your biceps as intensely as you want, getting full benefits with minimal risk of injury, provided you understand the principle of mechanical disadvantage—when it occurs and how to compensate for it.

In descending order, the best biceps exercises are as follows:

- *Alternating standing cable curls* (Figure 21-23)
- *Alternating seated or standing dumbbell curls* (Figure 21-24)
- *Slight incline alternating dumbbell curls* (with elbow support) (Figure 21-18)
- *Preacher cable curls* (Figure 21-25)

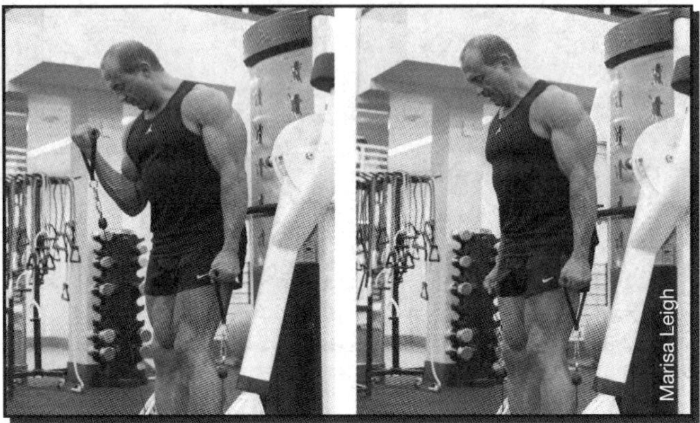


Figure 21-23

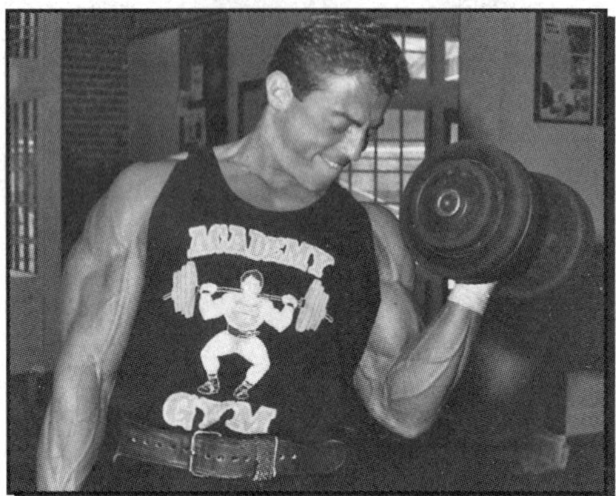


Figure 21-24

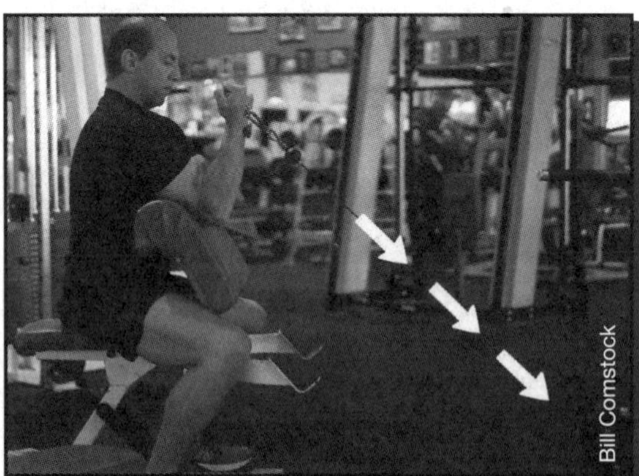


Figure 21-25

## The Effect of Hand/Wrist Position During Biceps Exercises

Some people believe that changing their hand position (when working their biceps), using either a "palms up" grip or a "hammer grip," will somehow work a different part of the biceps. It will not. The position of the hand (while doing a biceps exercise) has no bearing, whatsoever, on the shape that the biceps develops. On the other hand, the hand position does play a role in the percentage of force that is contributed by either the biceps brachii or the brachioradialis.

In Figure 21-26, you can see that the brachioradialis appears to be more of a forearm muscle, than an upper arm/ biceps muscle. Although it is situated more on the forearm, its primary job is to assist the biceps in elbow flexion. This factor is evidenced by the fact that it crosses only the elbow joint; it does not cross the wrist. The brachioradialis participates most when the elbow is flexed, while using a "hammer grip" hand position. When you do *curls* with a hammer grip, the biceps contributes a bit less force, and the Brachioradialis contributes a bit more force. When you utilize a "palms-up" grip (aka "supinated"), the biceps contributes a bit more force, and the brachioradialis contributes a bit less force.

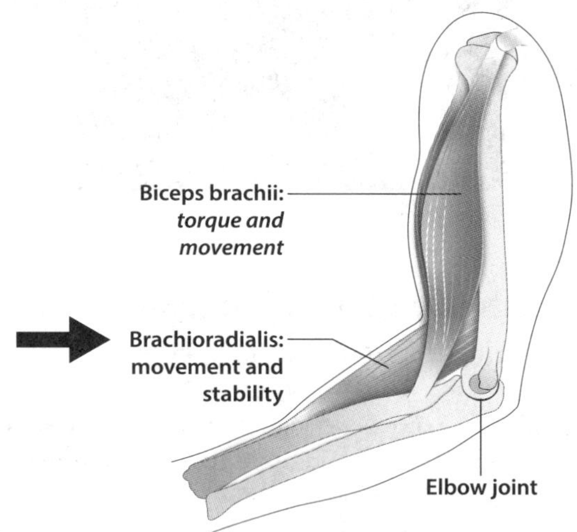


Figure 21-26

In my estimation, it seems that when using a hammer grip, the biceps does about 70 percent of the work, and the brachioradialis does about 30 percent of the work. In contrast, when you use a palms-up grip, the biceps seems to do about 90 percent of the work, and the brachioradialis does about 10 percent of the work. This estimation is based on my experience and "feel," not by way of an EMG analysis.

When the hand is supinated (rotated externally) to positions that are BETWEEN a "hammer grip" and a "palms-up" grip, it seems to result in a distribution of force (biceps brachii/brachioradialis) that is in between the aforementioned percentages, commensurate with the degree of hand supination. Regardless, however, the brachioradialis always contributes to elbow flexion, at least to a small degree. It's impossible to eliminate its participation in elbow flexion.

You might think that if you pronated (internally rotated) your hand all the way, so that your palm is facing downward—like you would use during a "*reverse barbell curl*"—that it would activate the brachioradialis the most. In fact, studies have shown otherwise. In reality, the brachioradialis is most active when the hand is in the neutral position (hammer grip), and less when the palms of the hands are facing downward.

Furthermore, it's very uncomfortable (unnatural) to fully rotate the palms of the hand downward ("pronation"), and then perform "elbow flexion" (a curling motion). It's virtually impossible to hold a straight barbell, with the palms facing downward, while keeping your elbows at your side. The wrists generally do not allow that degree of pronation, without rotating the entire arm, which then moves the elbows outward. Using an EZ Curl bar (Figure 21-27) eases the strain on the wrist to some degree, but there's still very little benefit in doing a "*reverse barbell curl.*" Given that it also greatly compromises the strength of the biceps, it doesn't make sense to do the exercise at all.

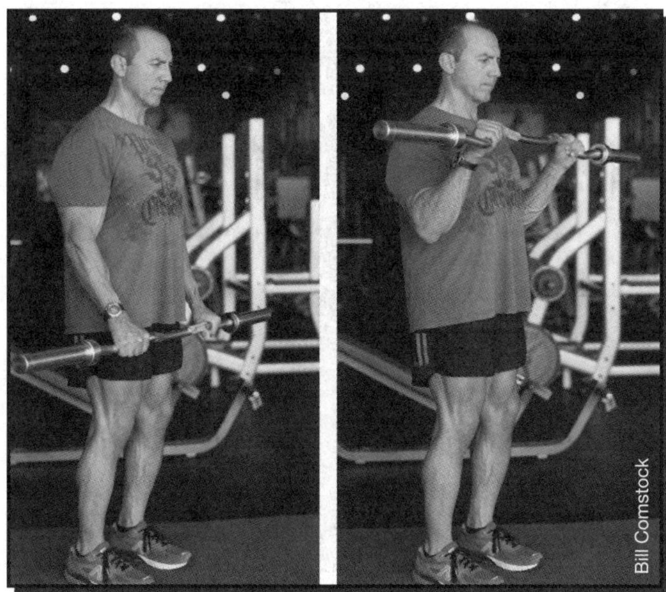


Figure 21-27

If you want to emphasize development of the brachioradialis, you should use a "hammer grip" on most or all of your biceps sets, whenever possible. As discussed in Chapter 3, the tendon of the biceps ruptures far more often when the palms of the hands are turned fully upward (supinated). It seems that when the biceps is heavily loaded without the full assistance of the brachioradialis, the biceps

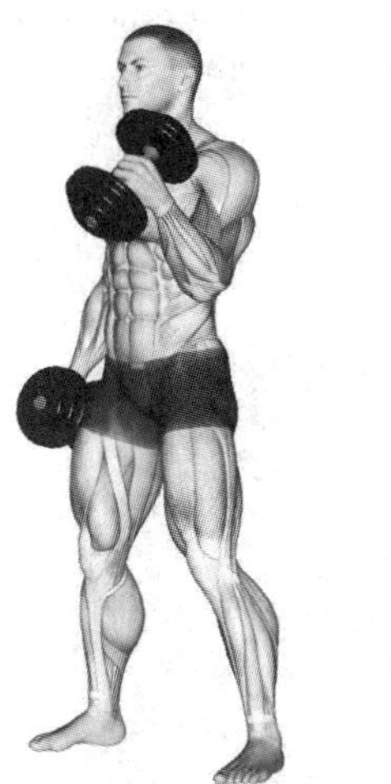
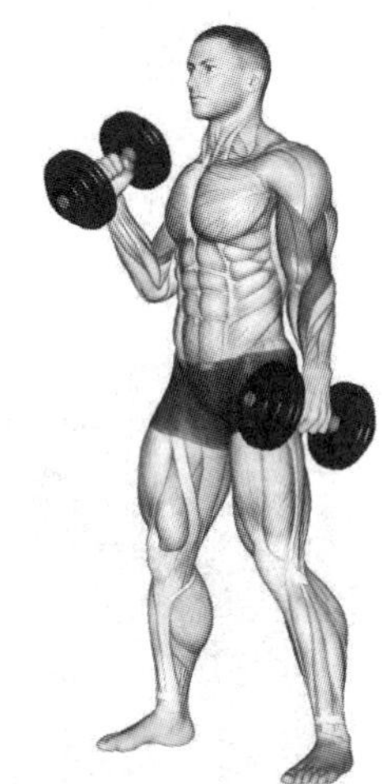

Makatserchyk/Shutterstock.com

Figure 21-28

is more vulnerable to injury, especially at the beginning of the range of motion. This factor might suggest that "nature" intended for individuals to load their biceps WITH the full assistance of the brachioradialis (employing a hammer grip), when exerting maximum effort.

The biceps is also assisted by another muscle during elbow flexion (in addition to the brachioradialis)—the brachialis (Figure 21-29), which lies beneath the biceps brachii. It is important to note, however, this "assistant" is not influenced by the position of the hand. Furthermore, since it does not cross the shoulder joint, it also plays no role in shoulder function, as does the biceps brachii (minor, though that may be). The brachialis' degree of participation during elbow flexion is constant, regardless of the grip an individual chooses to use, and regardless of the angle of the humerus, relative to the torso.

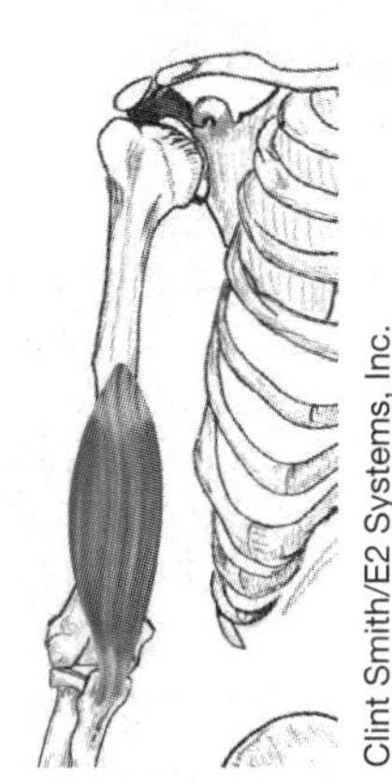

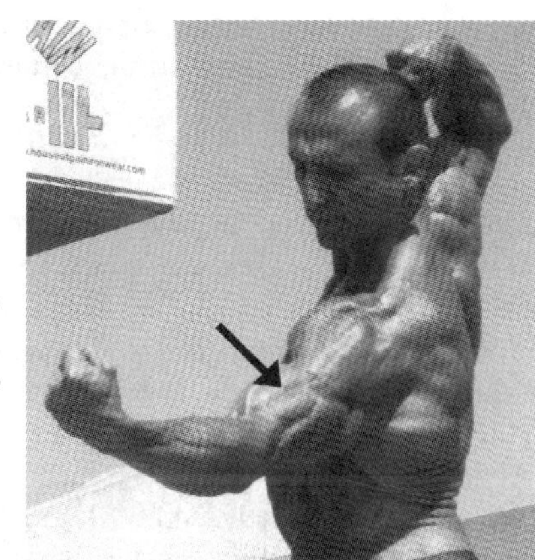

Figure 21-29

The brachialis originates midway on the humerus, just below the deltoid tuberosity. It crosses the elbow joint, and attaches onto the forearm, on the "coronoid process" of the ulna. It participates every time the biceps is activated, whether it is intended or not. It cannot be isolated or emphasized, nor can it be excluded from participating in elbow flexion.

## Anatomy of the Triceps

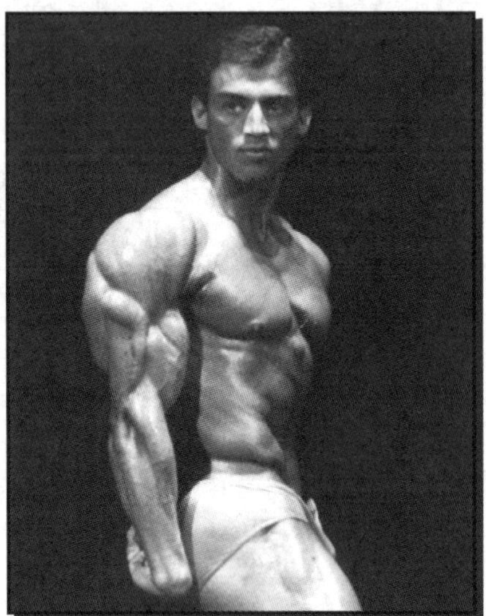

Figure 21-30

The triceps is the "antagonist" to the biceps. It is the muscle that operates (moves) the elbow in the opposite direction to that of the biceps. Its primary function is to extend the elbow. In other words, it "increases the angle" of the elbow joint, moving the elbow from the bent position to the straight arm position.

It is a single muscle, with one single insertion, but with three "heads." Each of these heads has a separate origin. For this reason, some people believe it is possible to preferentially emphasize one part of the triceps, more than another part of it. Logically speaking, and in the context of mechanics, that belief is not sensible.

Since the elbow is essentially a "hinge" joint (it only extends in one direction), and since there is only one tendon that causes that action, the entire triceps (all three heads) have to participate equally in that action. Similarly to the aforementioned analysis of the biceps, there would have to be three separate triceps insertions, each able to pull in a slightly different direction, and a joint that moves in multiple directions (like a ball-and-socket, rather than a hinge), for the heads to work separately. Although some triceps exercises (i.e., namely, those with the arms overhead) cause the long head of the triceps to stretch more when the elbows are bent, that would not necessarily cause the long head to grow any more than the other two heads.

In Figure 21-31, you can see the three triceps heads, as well as their origins. This image is a posterior view (seen from the back) of a right arm. The "lateral head" (aka the "outer head") and the "medial head" (aka "inner head") originate on the back of the humerus. The long head ("longus"), however, originates on the scapula, just below the shoulder socket. Because the long head is attached to the shoulder blade, it can participate (to a very small degree) in pulling the upper arm downward. The other two heads (the medius and the lateral) only participate in elbow extension.

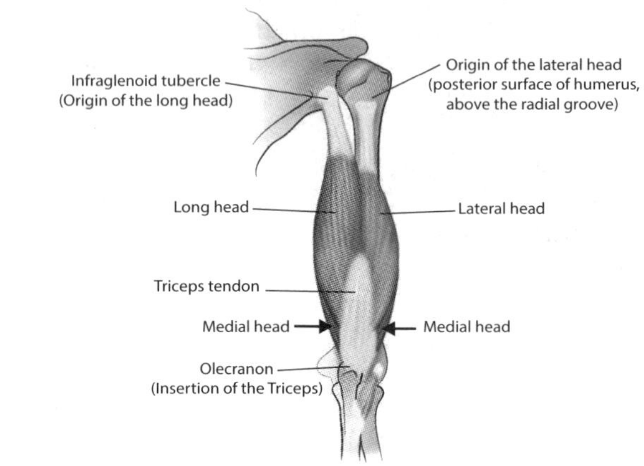


Figure 21-31

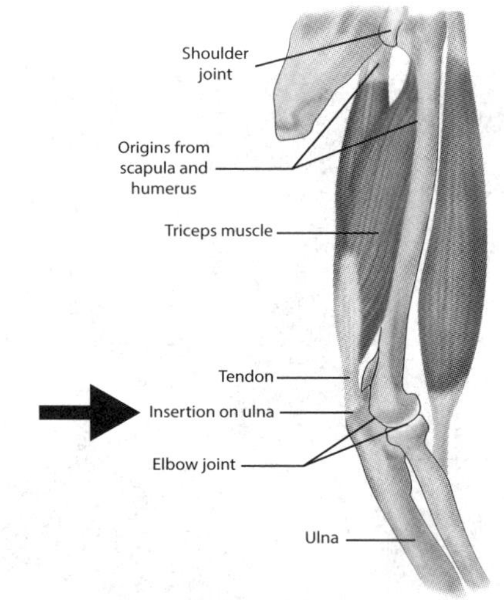


Figure 21-32

Figure 21-32 shows a side view of the triceps of the right arm. In this illustration, you can clearly see the insertion of the triceps tendon on the olecranon process of the ulna (the larger of the two forearm bones). Similar to the biceps tendon, the triceps tendon is singular. On that tendon, all three triceps heads converge and become one, before crossing the elbow joint.

Figure 21-33 shows a closer, more simplified view of the triceps/elbow mechanism. An arrow has been placed on the triceps, pointing from the olecranon process (the insertion point of the triceps), toward the origin of the triceps. This image shows the simplicity of how the triceps tendon pulls upward on the olecranon process, thereby extending the elbow.

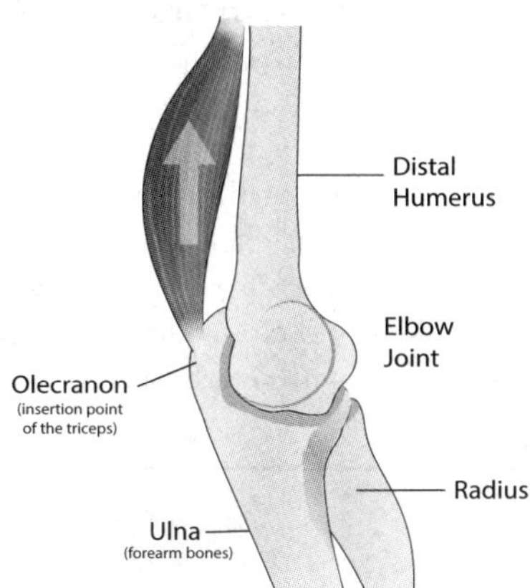


Figure 21-33

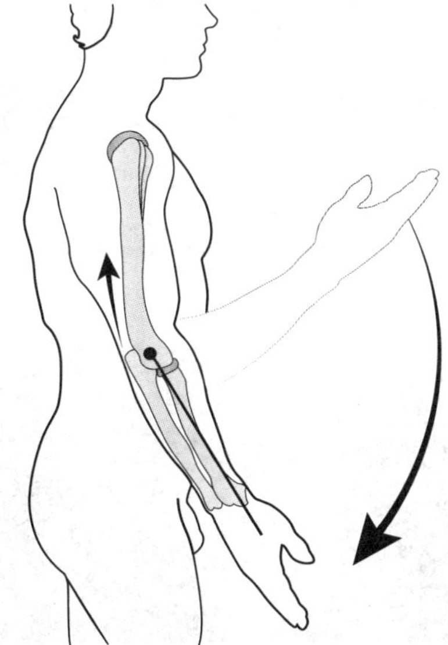

Figure 21-34

Figure 21-34 shows the extension of the elbow that is caused by the triceps pulling upward on the olecranon process.

Figures 21-33 and 21-34 show that, regardless of the triceps exercise you choose to do, this same mechanism occurs in every single exercise. There would have to be a significant, functionally different anatomical movement—other than unidirectional elbow extension, and also a dramatically different anatomical mechanism at the triceps/elbow joint—for any one of the triceps heads to preferentially contract with more force. All three heads must collaborate during elbow extension, given the single tendon triceps insertion and the unidirectional movement of the elbow.

Some people believe that using different hand positions will somehow emphasize one part of the triceps or another. Again, this does not make logical nor functional sense. When the triceps pulls "upward" on the olecranon process, it has no way of "knowing" the position of the hand. Changing the hand position does not alter the triceps tendon/olecranon/elbow mechanism. The same elbow extension action occurs, regardless of the hand position.

Believing that the triceps will develop differently, as a result of using a different hand position, is as baseless as believing that the triceps will develop one way if you face north, and a different way if you face south. Either way, the mechanism at the elbow is the same.

People are often seen in the gym, first doing a "*triceps pushdown with palms up*," then doing a "*triceps pushdown with palms down*," subsequently performing an "*overhead dumbbell triceps extension*," and finally doing a "*dumbbell triceps kickback*"—believing that each of these exercises contributes a different kind of benefit to the triceps. In fact, these exercises all extend the elbow the same way, but with different degrees of efficiency, productivity, and risk.

Using the example from Chapter 17, if you were an individual with a rope, acting as the triceps muscle, you would have no way of knowing what exercise is being done. All you would know is that you are pulling on that olecranon process (the triceps insertion on the forearm), which causes the elbow to extend. You could not possibly know which way the palm of the hand is facing.

The factors that the triceps does "know" (senses)—from one exercise or another—is the resistance curve, the range of motion, the amount of effort required, and the amount of fatigue. None of these elements alter the shape of a muscle. Furthermore, each of these factors has a "good," "better," and "best" version. So, why not just do the exercise that utilizes the "best" (most productive and most efficient) version of these factors, and skip the other exercises that utilize inferior versions of these factors?

## The Ideal Anatomical Movement for the Triceps

It has already been established that "elbow extension"—straightening the elbow—is the primary (concentric) function of the triceps. That only leaves two remaining factors—the "ideal" humeral (shoulder joint) position, and the "ideal" hand position (given that hand position affects the angle of the forearm/humerus/shoulder joint).

The most normal, natural position for the shoulder joint is with the upper arm at, or close to, the torso's side. Since this is the position most accommodated by evolution (humans and our ancient ancestors spent/spend more time with the humerus alongside the torso, than in any other position), it's logical to assume that it is the strongest position, as well as the safest position, from which to work the triceps. It follows, therefore, that any triceps exercise that *can* be done with the upper arm alongside the torso, or close to the torso's side, is the more "ideal" humeral position for working the triceps.

Of course, the aforementioned does not mean to suggest that a person is not capable of performing triceps exercises with other humeral positions, or that those other positions would be entirely unproductive or unsafe. It does suggest, however, that those other positions are not necessary for optimal triceps development, and that they are not "better" in some way. Not only are they not more productive, they are often less comfortable, and, on occasion, less safe.

This conclusion may fly in the face of conventional wisdom, but it would be a mistake to rely entirely on traditional beliefs for insight about the "ideal" way to work the triceps. We must rely on an analysis that is more rigorous than that. There simply is no logical nor scientific basis for someone to believe that they can preferentially influence the shape of their triceps by way of exercise selection.

Since it's impossible to change the shape of the triceps by way of doing different triceps exercises, the most logical strategy would be to do the triceps exercise(s) that is (are) most "natural"—the ones that are least contorted, and are most comfortable on the shoulder joint. Triceps exercises that allow the humerus to be alongside (or close to the side of) the torso, allow the triceps to work optimally well, with the least risk of injury and the least skeletal (i.e., shoulder joint) discomfort. In fact, any humeral position, other than the "arms close to torso's side" position, does not change the "triceps/elbow extension" mechanics in any way that could be construed as "better."

Some individuals erroneously believe that the "long head" of the triceps can be emphasized by performing *overhead triceps* extensions (Figures 21-35 and 21-36). This belief relies on the theory that pre-stretching the long head of the triceps will develop that part of the triceps better than an exercise that does not "pre-stretch" the triceps. There is no absolute evidence of that, however. It has just been conjectured.

If pre-stretching a muscle during a resistance exercise is "more productive," we would insist that every exercise, for every voluntary muscle, involve pre-stretch. Yet, we do not insist on that. In reality, pre-stretching does not result in better muscle growth. Furthermore, excessively stretching a loaded muscle increases the risk of injury, especially when a very heavy weight is being used.

From the standpoint of personal testimony, I performed overhead triceps exercises between the years of 1975 and 2000, because I accepted the conventional wisdom (the traditional belief), that it was "necessary" for the complete development of the long head of the triceps. Then I realized, logically, that that wasn't correct. From 2000 forward, I've done only triceps exercises that allow my humerus (upper arm) to stay near the side of my torso—no higher than perpendicular to the torso. The result? The long head of my triceps has continued to develop equally well. Today, at the age of 60, 20 years after discontinuing overhead triceps exercises, the long head of my triceps is as well developed as it ever has been. As a bonus, I've avoided the shoulder and elbow discomfort, as well as the potential injury associated with overhead triceps extensions.

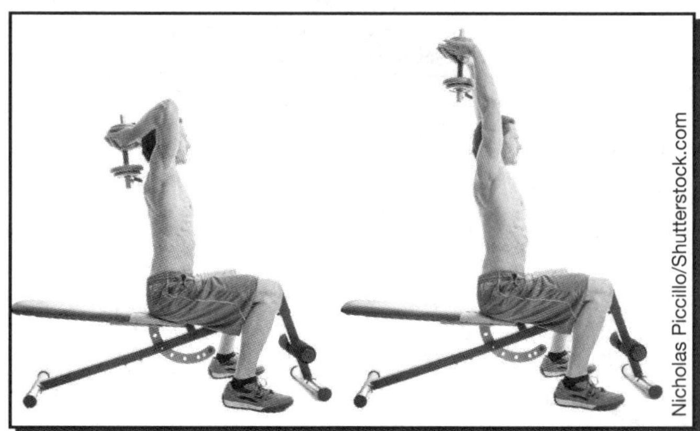

Figure 21-35

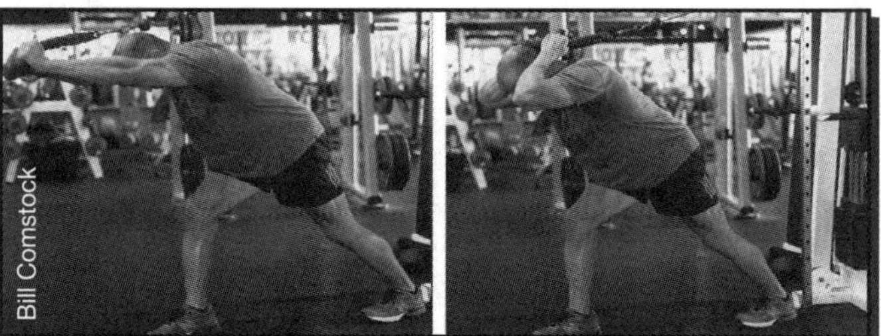

Figure 21-36

No one would ever claim that an *overhead triceps* exercise (two-arm or one-arm) is "more comfortable" than a *triceps pushdown*. Most individuals would agree that any triceps exercise performed with the elbows overhead is LESS comfortable than a triceps exercise with the arms down alongside the torso, or in front of the body. Yet, many people feel compelled to perform *overhead triceps* exercises, despite the discomfort. This is due entirely to the assumption that it provides a different type of benefit to the triceps, or that a variety of triceps exercises is "essential." Both of these assumptions, however, are false.

A number of years ago, I had been experiencing elbow discomfort when performing an *overhead triceps* exercise. Being the analytical person I tend to be, I started testing various humeral positions. I noticed that there was a progressive continuum of elbow discomfort, from the "humerus down" position (least discomfort) to the "humerus up"/overhead position (most discomfort), when doing various triceps exercises.

Essentially, I experienced NO elbow discomfort, when I extended my elbows while my upper arms were alongside my torso (e.g., *triceps pushdown* with cable). I experienced a bit more elbow discomfort when I extended my elbows with the humerus perpendicular to my torso (e.g., "*skull crushers*"/ *flat bench triceps extensions*, with barbell or dumbbells). I experienced the most elbow discomfort when I extended my elbows with my humerus angled upward, above my head—(e.g., *overhead triceps extensions* with a cable or a dumbbell).

Of course, this situation makes sense from an evolutionary standpoint. Early human ancestors (hominins) undoubtedly extended their elbows with their humerus in a variety of positions, but they probably extended their elbows least often with their arms overhead. It's likely they most often extended their elbows (engaged their triceps) in situations that required pushing downward, semi-downward, or straight forward. As noted previously, this factor suggests that activating a muscle from a skeletal position that is most "natural"—a position to which the body is most accustomed—would likely provide the most comfort, the least risk of injury, and the most strength potential.

Simply holding your upper arm (the humerus) alongside your head is not very comfortable for your shoulder joint, even without simultaneously extending your elbows with a heavy weight in your hands. If your triceps could talk, they might say something like, "why are you having me work from such an uncomfortable position, when I can do the same thing (extend your elbows) from a more comfortable position—like with your arms down alongside your torso?"

Getting back to the issue of elbow pain, it's worth pondering what might cause elbow pain, when the elbows are extended while the arms are overhead? One very likely answer is: the ulnar nerve. The ulnar nerve passes through a groove between the humerus and the ulna (Figures 21-37 and 21-38). It's obvious, however, that placing your arms overhead could cause the nerve to be more "taut" (stretched). When the arms are down, the ulnar nerve would be less taut.

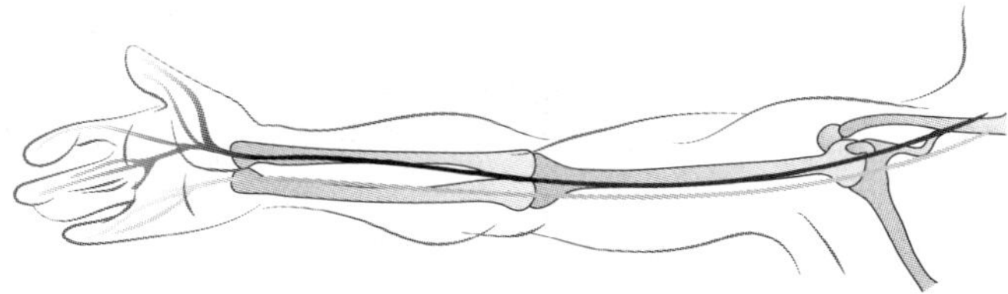

Figure 21-37

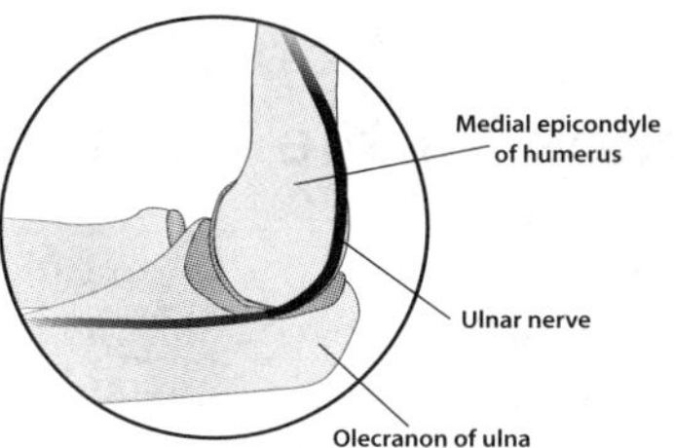


Figure 21-38

Regardless of what might cause elbow pain, performing an overhead triceps exercise is not a necessary part of developing the triceps muscle. Furthermore, since overhead triceps exercises might cause elbow pain, they are often uncomfortable on the shoulder joint, they do not change or "improve" the shape of the triceps, and they bestow no mechanical advantage whatsoever on the elbow/triceps mechanism, it's logical to avoid doing them.

Similar to the biceps, the long head of the biceps crosses two joints—the elbow and the shoulder. In other words, the position of the secondary joint (i.e., the humerus/shoulder) affects the length of the triceps. When the triceps is either excessively pre-shortened or excessively pre-stretched, the strength of the triceps is compromised. This is the reason why it's virtually impossible to "flex" the triceps muscle, such that you can feel the deliberate contraction, when the humerus is overhead: the triceps is excessively pre-stretched.

Consider the fact that when you intentionally flex your triceps (to savor a "pump" during a workout, or to check for soreness from a previous workout), you always flex your triceps with the humerus (your upper arm) down, alongside your torso, or close to it. You never flex your triceps with your humerus "up" alongside your head. The lower you hold your humerus, the better you are able to flex your triceps. As such, it's logical that the "humerus alongside the torso" position—or a humeral position not too far away from the side of the torso (certainly no higher than perpendicular with the torso)—is the "ideal" humeral angle for working the triceps.

It may be "fun" to do a variety of triceps exercises using other humeral positions. It may also be more practical, based on the availability of equipment. On the other hand, there is no logical reason to believe that performing triceps exercises with a variety of humeral angles, including those that require the humerus to be up, alongside the head, is "necessary" for optimal triceps development, nor more productive in any way, nor more safe.

## The Ideal Direction of Resistance for the Triceps

Having identified the best anatomical motion/humeral position for working the triceps, the next step is to identify the ideal direction with which to apply resistance, to the ideal motion/humeral position. The objective should be to select a direction of resistance that provides "early phase loading," proper alignment, and "opposite position loading."

Hypothetically, consider one particular triceps exercise that is commonly used, and see if it provides the "ideal" direction of resistance, or if it can be improved upon to some degree. In Figure 21-39, you can see the starting position of a standard *triceps cable pushdown*. Note that the cable (which indicates the direction of resistance) is almost completely parallel with the forearm. Remember that the forearm is the operating lever of the triceps. Since the forearm is nearly parallel with the cable at this stage, the forearm is mostly NEUTRAL in this starting position. Therefore, it is providing very little load to the triceps, at this point.

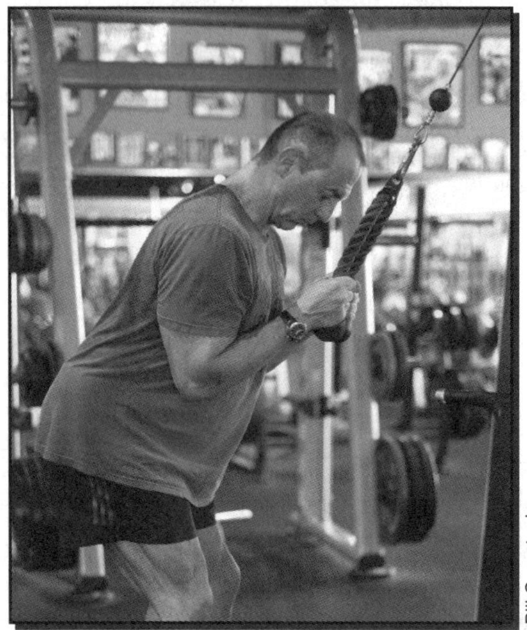
Bill Comstock

Figure 21-39

This "early phase" of the triceps' range of motion, however, is where the triceps is strongest. This point is where the triceps' lever (the forearm) should be most active (perpendicular), or mostly active (nearly perpendicular) with the cable. It's worth noting—ironically—that the humerus (the UPPER arm bone) is the limb that is mostly perpendicular with cable, in this starting position. The humerus, however, is controlled by the posterior deltoids and the lats. Accordingly, in the starting position of a standard "*triceps pushdown*," the rear deltoids and lats are more loaded than the triceps, and the triceps is loaded with only a small percentage of the resistance being used, precisely at the point in its range of motion when it is strongest and would most benefit from optimal loading.

In Figure 21-40, you can see the ending position of this exercise, and you can see that the forearm is closer to perpendicular than it was in the beginning. In this scenario, the forearm would reach the "most active" position about three quarters of the way through the range of motion. Thus, the standard *triceps pushdown* is more "late phase loaded," than "early phase loaded." In addition, the posterior deltoids are engaged the entire time, because the humerus is fairly perpendicular with the cable throughout the entire exercise.

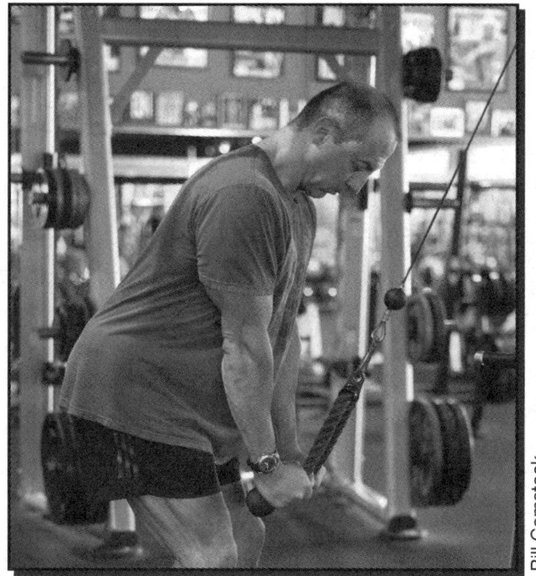
Bill Comstock

Figure 21-40

In other words, this anatomical movement is good (extending the elbows, while the upper arms are close to the torso), but this direction of resistance is not ideal. What's needed in this instance is a better direction of resistance—one that is MORE perpendicular with the forearm at the beginning of the range of motion, and LESS perpendicular with the forearm at the end of the range of motion. This "new" direction of resistance would therefore have to originate from slightly BEHIND this person, rather than in front of him.

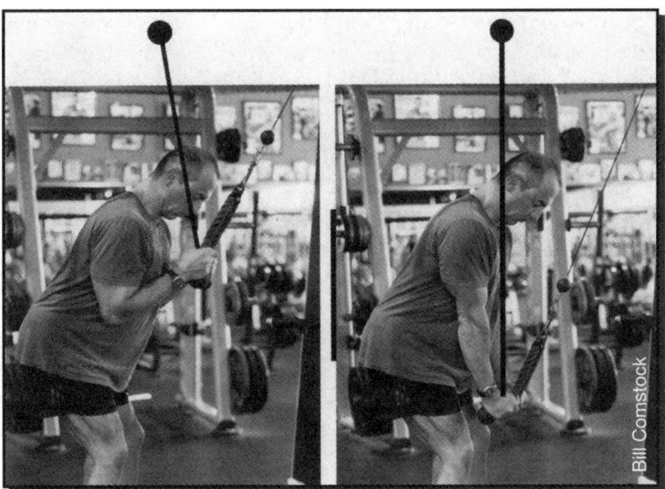


Figure 21-41

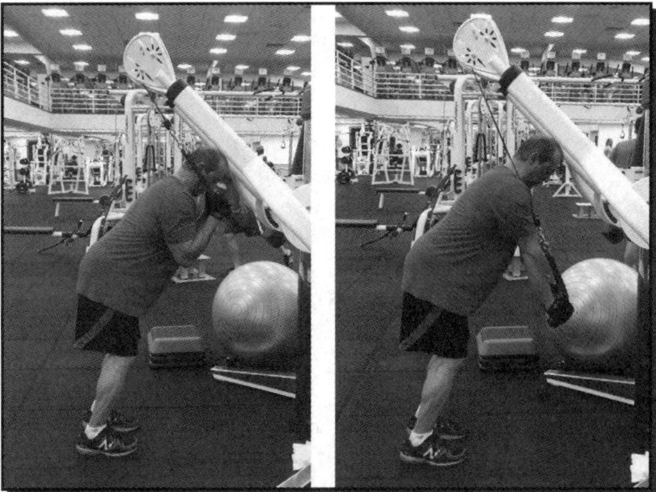

Figure 21-42

The line in Figure 21-41 indicates what that "better" direction of resistance would be. In addition to providing a better resistance curve for the triceps ("early phase loading" and a diminishing resistance in the "late phase"), this version also relieves the load on the posterior deltoids, because the angle between the cable and the humerus is now more parallel than it is perpendicular.

Of course, this angle of resistance would be difficult to set-up with a SINGLE cable/pulley, if you intend to do this as a two-arm exercise with both arms working simultaneously. The single cable would have to pass over the top of your head, or to either one side of your head or the other, which would make the exercise asymmetrical. In order to do a *two-arm cable triceps extension* (which could also be called a "*modified triceps pushdown*"), you'll have to use two, side-by-side pulleys—positioned shoulder-width apart, slightly behind you, and slightly higher than the top of your head.

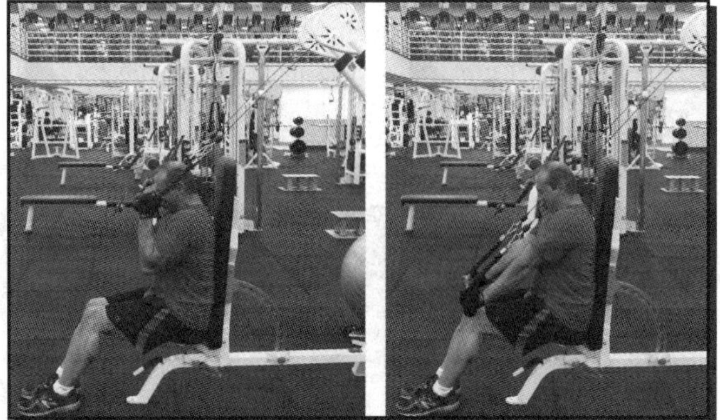

Figure 21-43

In Figure 21-42, you can see that the anatomical motion is similar to a standard *triceps pushdown,* with the humerus kept near the sides of the torso, but with a better resistance curve. With this version, the triceps encounters more resistance at the beginning, where it's stronger, and less resistance at the end, where it's weakest.

This exercise can also be performed while seated (Figure 21-43). It requires a bit more set-up (bringing a bench and setting it up), but it's also a bit more stable, and allows better focus on the triceps. This becomes more of a factor, when more weight is used. If this exercise is performed while standing, and a significant amount of weight is being used, it will pull you backward. You can offset this a bit by using a split stance (one foot in front and one behind, although that may feel a little asymmetrical). Using a bench—performing this exercise while seated—allows you to use a significant amount of weight, without having to struggle with balance.

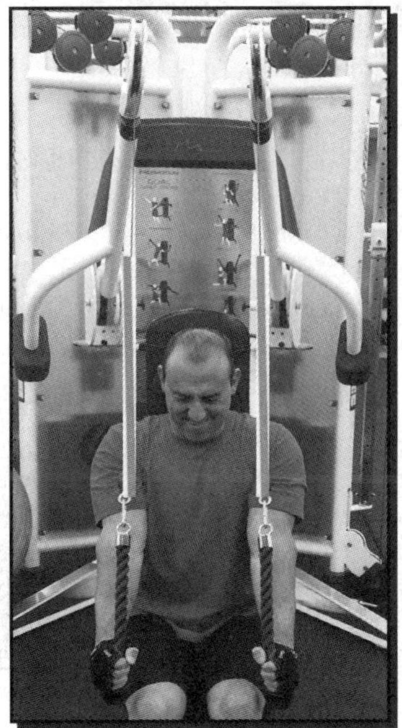

Figure 21-44

In Figure 21-44, you can see that lines have been drawn between the rope handles and the pulleys, along the cables. These lines are meant to show the alignment between the direction of resistance and the direction of movement, as well as the origin and insertion of the triceps. All are on the one plane, as they should be. To set up the pulleys for this exercise, you would set the pulleys so that they are directly behind your shoulders, and 20 to 30 inches higher than the level of your head. The angle of the cable should be about 45 degrees to your torso, when viewed from the side. Then, instead of pushing STRAIGHT down, the angle of push should be about 20 to 30 degrees forward (relative to the neutral/straight down angle).

Until the fitness equipment manufacturers figure out how to make this type of biomechanically correct *triceps pushdown* station, you'll have to set up this pulley arrangement yourself.

Another standard triceps exercise that's fairly good, but could be made significantly better, is the *lying dumbbell triceps extension*. While this exercise (Figure 21-45) has an excellent "early phase loaded" resistance curve, the humerus is a little farther away from the "natural" position than would be ideal.

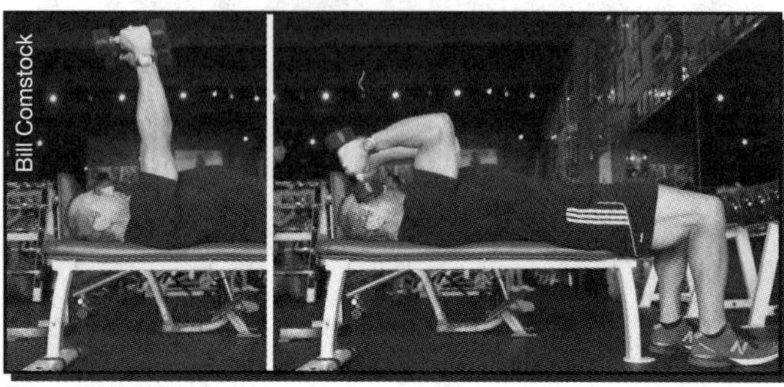


Figure 21-45

Many people notice that when they're performing this exercise, it's more difficult to "squeeze"/flex their triceps at the end of this range of motion, as compared with the *triceps pushdowns*. In fact, the farther an individual moves their humerus away from the "natural" position (along the side of the torso), the more elusive their ability to "squeeze"/flex their triceps becomes.

The solution in this instance is to use a decline bench that has a fairly steep decline angle (approximately 40 degrees), as shown in Figure 21-46. With your body at this angle, a vertically held humerus is closer to the more natural, "alongside the torso" position, similar to what you would use when performing *triceps pushdowns*. With the torso in this "decline" position (relative to gravity), the direction of resistance is similar to that of the modified cable triceps pushdowns shown in Figures 21-42 and 21-43 (45 degrees to the torso, coming from behind the torso). It allows the ideal direction of anatomical movement (with the humerus closer to the sides of the torso), as well as provides an ideal resistance curve ("early phase loaded").

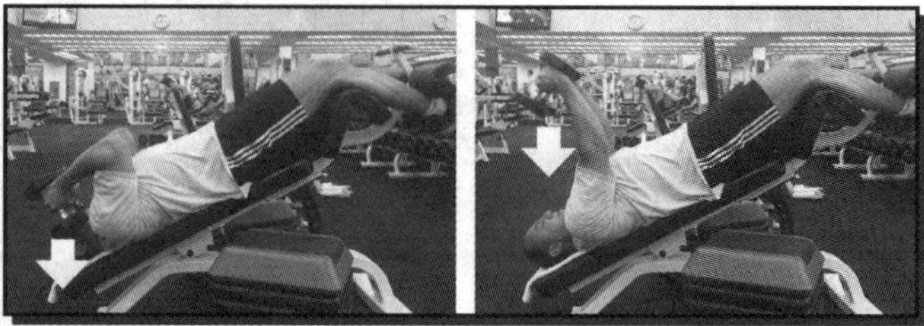

Figure 21-46

These are the two best triceps exercises—the "*decline dumbbell triceps extension*" and the *modified triceps pushdown*. They both provide a perfectly natural anatomical motion for the triceps/humeral position, and they both provide an ideal direction of resistance. *Supine dumbbell triceps extensions* would be considered "third best," and *standard triceps pushdowns* would be considered "fourth best."

While other triceps exercises contribute to triceps development, they are less efficient. They are less "ideal," in one way or another. They either strain the shoulder joint or the elbow joint; they may lack proper alignment; they may "late phase" load the triceps, instead of during the "early phase." As such, they may encounter a "base" or an "apex" (a neutral spot/no resistance) in the middle of the range of motion (as occurs with *triceps kickbacks*). Furthermore, they may fail to utilize a fully active forearm lever (as occurs with *parallel bar dips*, as well as with *bench dips*), which then requires that a heavier weight be used, without additional benefit.

You do not need to do both of the aforementioned "best" exercises in the same workout. Either one will serve the purpose, assuming enough sets are performed. Depending on your current level of condition and your future fitness-related goals, the right number of sets would range between 3 and 15 sets. Doing both of these exercises, in the same workout, would be redundant. Mechanically, they are very similar.

Many people are accustomed to doing three or four exercises for their triceps (per workout)—a habit that will probably be difficult for them to break. As a result, some individuals will cling to their ritual of doing multiple exercises for each muscle, during each workout. Others (those individuals who are driven more by logic, than by emotion or habit) will probably be delighted to know that they can perform "one great exercise" for their triceps, and be done with it.

The following are the top four triceps exercises (in descending order), combining the best anatomical motion and the best direction of resistance:

- *Modified cable triceps pushdowns*
- *Decline dumbbell triceps extensions*
- *Flat/supine dumbbell triceps extensions* (good resistance curve, but not quite "ideal" humeral position)
- *Standard cable pushdowns* (good anatomical motion, but not quite "ideal" resistance curve)

At this point, it can be helpful to look at some of the more compromised triceps exercises, so that you can fully understand the criteria that determines "good" and "bad," with regard to biomechanics:

❑ Bench Dips

A bench dip requires a very unnatural humeral movement, i.e., taking the upper arm to an excessively posterior position, which over-stretches and overloads the anterior deltoids. In fact, during this exercise, the anterior deltoids work much harder than do the triceps. This situation is due to the fact that the humerus (the upper arm bone) is the lever that is more perpendicular with gravity (much more so than the forearm), and the humerus is operated by the front deltoids, along this pathway.

This exercise is also very inefficient as a triceps exercise, from an effort and energy standpoint. This is due to the fact that the forearm, which is the operating lever of the triceps, is almost completely "neutral" (parallel or close to parallel, with gravity) throughout the entire range of motion during this exercise. As a result, the triceps only gets about 20 percent of the resistance being used (i.e., body weight).

There is a slight "ground reaction force/friction force" that occurs in this instance, which is caused by the arc through which the body passes, as it pivots around the heels of the feet. Note the slightly angled arrows in Figure 21-47, indicating the direction of "push," which is influenced by the direction of the body's trajectory.

❑ Parallel Bar Dips

This exercise has a similar problem as the bench dip. The direction of resistance is mostly vertical, and the operating lever of the triceps (i.e., the forearm) is also close to vertical, which makes it mostly neutral, as a triceps lever. In Chapter 2, it was established that the forearm is only about 11 percent active, as a triceps lever, during *parallel bar dips*. This factor results in the triceps being loaded with half as much resistance, as would occur during *supine dumbbell triceps extensions*, even while using four times more effort (body weight) than is required on the *supine dumbbell triceps extension*. In addition, like the *bench dips* in Figure 21-47, *parallel bar dips* also severely over-stretch and overload the anterior deltoids.

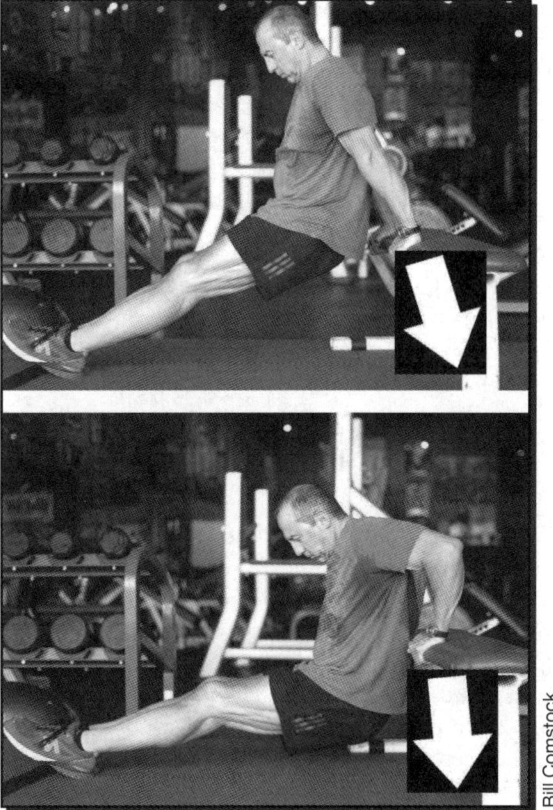


Figure 21-47

❑ Dumbbell Triceps Kickbacks

There are three major problems with the *dumbbell triceps kickback* exercise. For starters, it only utilizes half the range of motion of which the triceps is capable. It fails to load the first half of the triceps range of motion, which is the most important part of the range of motion for any muscle. It also is "late phase loaded," which means that it provides too much resistance in the latter part of the range of motion, and not enough in the early part. Finally, it loads the posterior deltoid more than the triceps. When the elbow is extended, and the arm is straight, the posterior deltoid receives the magnification of the weight in hand, multiplied by the entire length of the arm (the humerus PLUS the forearm). Meanwhile, the triceps only receives the magnification of the forearm's length, and only when the elbow is fully extended.

❑ Any Triceps Exercise That Is Performed Overhead

In reality, most overhead triceps exercises have a relatively good resistance curve. On the other hand, having the humerus positioned up, alongside the head, causes unnecessary shoulder and elbow strain. Furthermore, it is impossible to fully contract the triceps with the humerus in that position.

In addition, despite the increased stretch to the long head of the triceps (assuming you allow your elbow to fully bend, when it's in the descended position), there is no advantage to performing such an exercise. Overhead triceps exercises are more "efficient" than either *parallel bar dips,* or *bench dips,* or *dumbbell triceps kickbacks*, but they are also much less comfortable and have a higher risk of injury, without providing any additional benefit.

Finally, when doing any triceps exercise, it's always best to use a "hammer" grip, which is the most natural comfortable hand position, relative to the forearm/humerus. It allows the humerus to stay internally rotated, such that the elbows can stay "in"—aligned with the hands, forearms, and the origin and insertion of the triceps, and also with the direction of resistance.

A "palms-down" grip (palms facing away from you) externally rotates the humerus (to a degree), which forces the elbows to flare outward (laterally), which compromises alignment. A "hammer grip," or a grip that is slightly "palms-up" (palms facing slightly toward you, at about 45 degrees) is always better than a "palms-down" grip (for any triceps exercise), because it's easier to prevent the elbows from flaring outward. Keep in mind that using this "hammer grip" (or "palms facing slightly toward you" grip) does not alter the shape of the triceps, nor does it bestow any bonus benefit to the triceps. It simply allows triceps extension to be performed in the most natural manner, with the best possible alignment. For this reason, it's best to use dumbbells (held with a hammer grip), or a double rope, or single ropes, rather than utilizing a barbell or a standard cable handle.

## Anatomy and Function of the Forearms

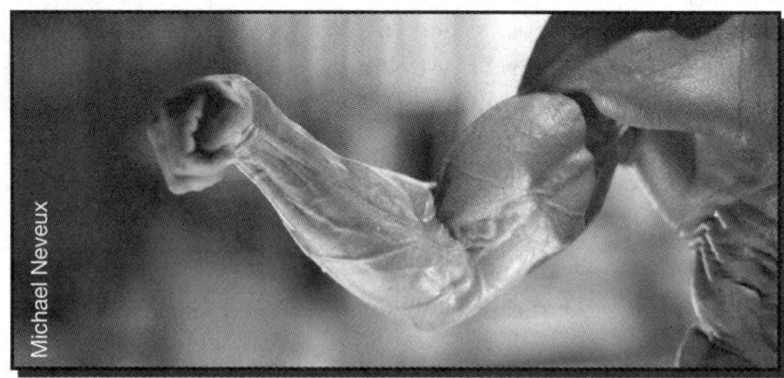


Figure 21-48

With the exception of the brachioradialis (which was discussed in the biceps section), the muscles of the forearms can be divided into four parts: the "flexors" (which flex the wrist), the "extensors" (which extend the wrist), the "rotators" (which rotate the hand in both directions), and the "extrinsic" muscles (which move the fingers, but are located on the forearms).

❑ Wrist Flexion and Extension

The "flexors" are the muscles on the side of the palm of the hand (Figure 21-49, image A). The "extensors" are the muscles that are the same side as the "back of your hand" (Figure 21-49, image B).

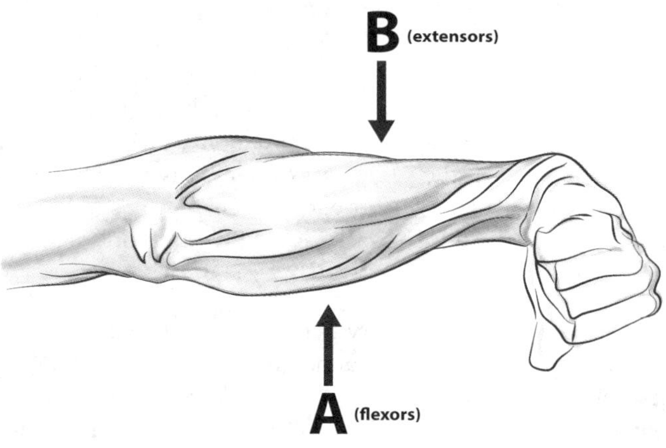


Figure 21-49

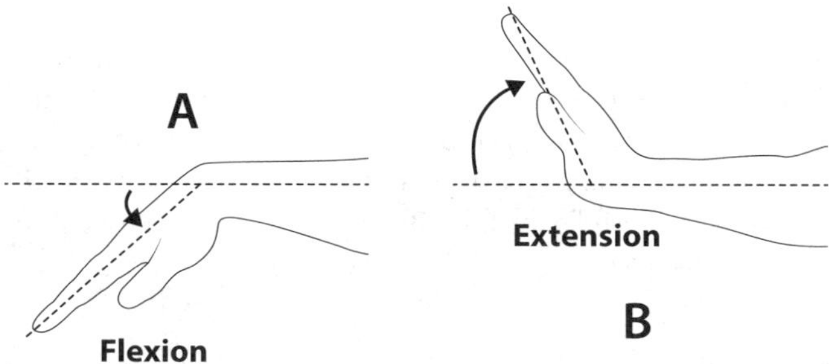


Figure 21-50

❑ Forearm Rotation

The forearm "rotators" supinate the hand (rotate it externally), as well as pronate the hand (rotate it internally)—shown in Figures 21-51 and 21-52.

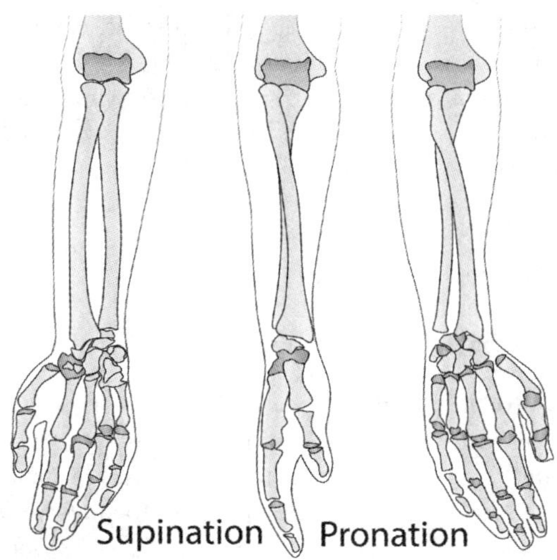


Figure 21-51

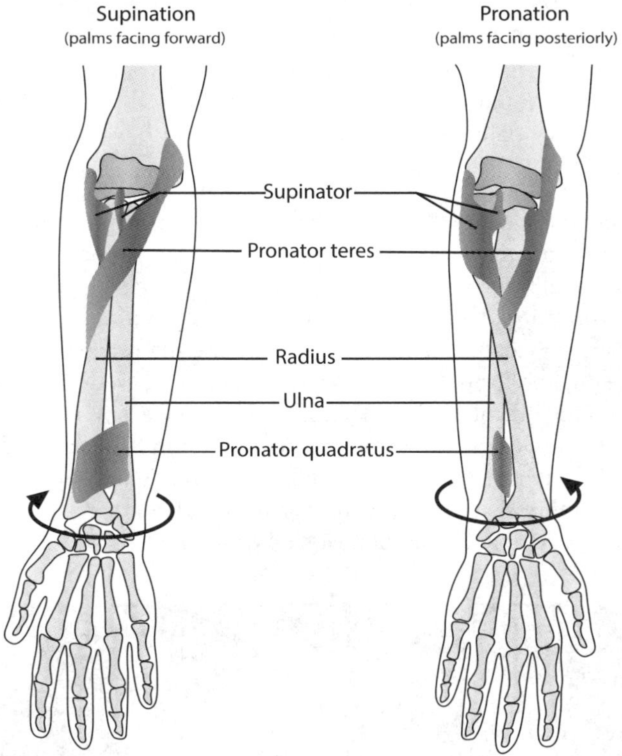


Figure 21-52

❑ Finger Movement

The fingers of the hand are moved by tiny muscles, divided into "extrinsic" (originating on the forearm) and "intrinsic" (originating on the hand itself)—Figure 21-53.

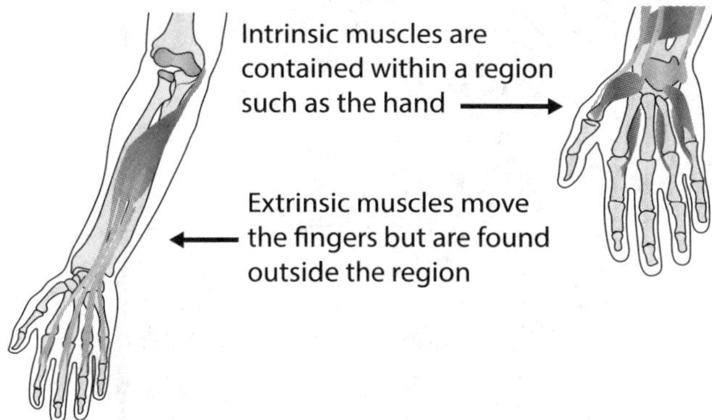


Figure 21-53

The anatomy of the forearm muscles is very complicated, with layers of tiny to moderately sized muscles crossing in many directions. The mechanics of the wrist, however, is very straightforward. Although the wrist is not quite like a hinge, it primarily bends forward and backward—"flexing" (Figure 21-50 "A") and "extending" (Figure 21-50 "B"). It is also capable of circular motion and side-to-side motion, but these functions are generally not very powerful. In fact, the primary musculature of the forearm simply flexes and extends the wrist.

The most common forearm exercises, for the purpose of physique development, are standard "*wrist curls*" and "*reverse wrist curls*." The exercise shown in Figure 21-54 is the standard "*barbell wrist curl*," which works the "flexor" muscles of the forearm, on the same side as the palm of the hand.

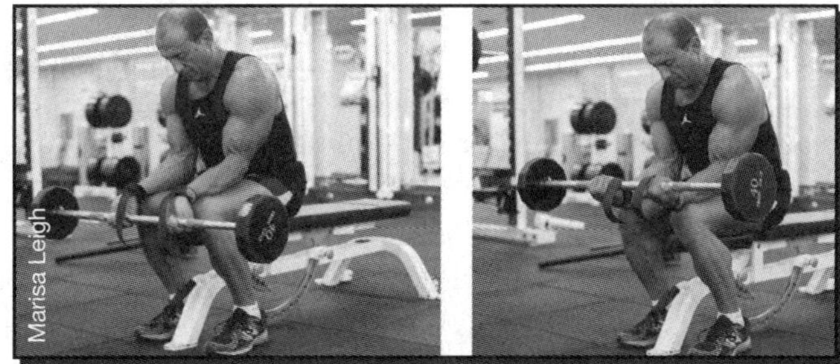


Figure 21-54

The exercise shown in Figure 21-55 is the standard "*reverse barbell wrist curl*" (using an EZ curl bar in this instance), which works the "extensor" muscles on the side of the back of the hand. While both of these exercises are generally good, each has some degree of mechanical difficulty.

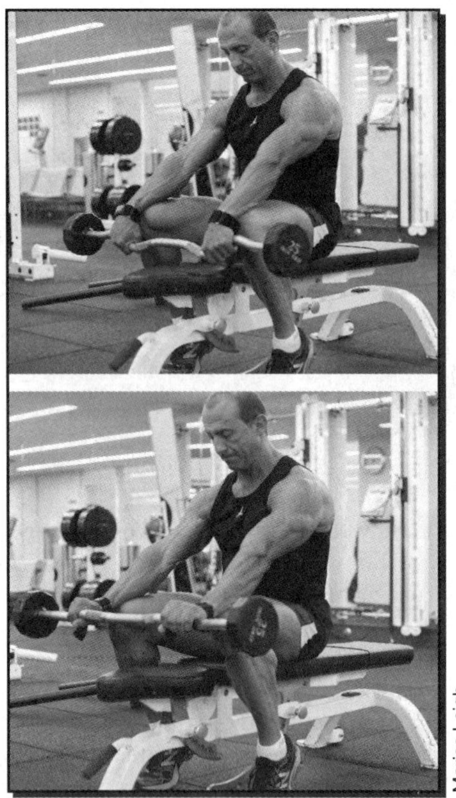

Figure 21-55

## Exercise Options for the Forearm Flexors and Extensors

As you can see in Figure 21-54 (*barbell wrist curls*), the two forearms must be kept parallel to each other, otherwise the two wrists will not bend on the same axis. For this reason, it may be easier (more comfortable) to do this movement with dumbbells (one-at-a-time or both simultaneously). This way, each wrist can bend on its own axis, which allows each wrist to move freely, without being forced (by the barbell) to bend on the same axis as the other wrist.

In Figure 21-55 (*reverse barbell wrist curls*), you can see that I'm using an EZ curl bar. If you experiment with this movement, you'll quickly notice that, as the hands "extend" upward, the knuckle of the pointer finger stays higher than the knuckle of the "pinkie" (the little finger). This factor makes utilizing a straight bar very difficult. Using an EZ curl bar (with the hands positioned properly on the bar) allows your hands to assume that natural position—leading with the pointer knuckle and trailing with the "pinkie" knuckle, which reduces wrist strain.

This movement can also be done using dumbbells (both simultaneously or one-at-a-time), and would likely be better for the same reason as the first exercise—it allows independent wrist movement, eliminating the wrist discomfort caused by using a barbell.

As you can see, I'm wearing wrist straps in Figure 21-55, so that my fingers do not fatigue (and fail) before the target muscles (the forearm/wrist extensors) do. Likewise, wrist straps would also be helpful when performing *reverse wrist curls* with dumbbells. When performing STANDARD *wrist curls* (wrist flexion), the weight sits in the palm of the hand, and finger strength is not critical. When performing *reverse wrist curls*, however, holding the weight relies mostly on finger strength (assisted by the thumb), but finger strength is inherently weaker than the wrist extension muscles.

It's worth noting that the muscles that extend the wrist (the muscles that are on the same side as the "knuckles" of the hand) have very little capacity for visible growth, in fact, almost none. Also, it is not possible to make dramatic strength increases by working these muscles, nor would it be necessary, for any type of day-to-day activity. Therefore, from the perspective of muscle growth, it is arguably not worth investing time and energy into working these muscles (by doing *REVERSE wrist curls*), unless it is for physical therapy or for the slight improvement of a sport that might rely on this set of muscles—like tennis (specifically, the "backhand"). On the other hand, the forearm flexors (the muscles on the same side as the palm of the hand), are indeed worth working.

Focus your attention on the "knuckle" side of the forearm shown in Figure 21-56. Notice that the brachioradialis is extraordinarily well-developed. This muscle, however, is not part of the "forearm extensors." The dramatic development of the brachioradialis you see here did not happen as a result of having done "*reverse wrist curls*," because the brachioradialis does not perform that function. In fact, you can see that—aside from the brachioradialis development—there is not much else that is noticeably developed on that side (the "knuckle" side) of the forearms. Accordingly, although you might assume that that impressive development was achieved by doing reverse wrist curls, that assumption would be incorrect.

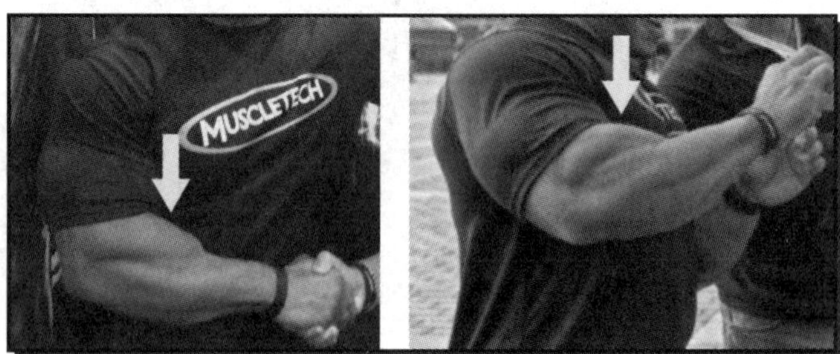

Figure 21-56

In Figure 21-57, top image, you can see that the brachioradialis extends all the way into the upper arm. Next, look at the lower two illustrations in Figure 21-57. You can clearly see that this muscle originates on the humerus (upper arm bone), crosses the elbow joint, and then attaches onto the "distal" end (the low end) of the radius (a forearm bone). It does NOT cross the wrist joint. Therefore, it does not operate the wrist. It plays no role whatsoever in "wrist extension." Its primary function is to assist the biceps in elbow flexion. (It also assists in rotating the forearm.) As was mentioned in the previously addressed biceps section, the most productive exercise you can do to develop the brachioradialis, which is the only muscle that really can be significantly developed on the "knuckle" side of the forearm, is *hammer curls* (i.e., *biceps curls* with a hammer grip).

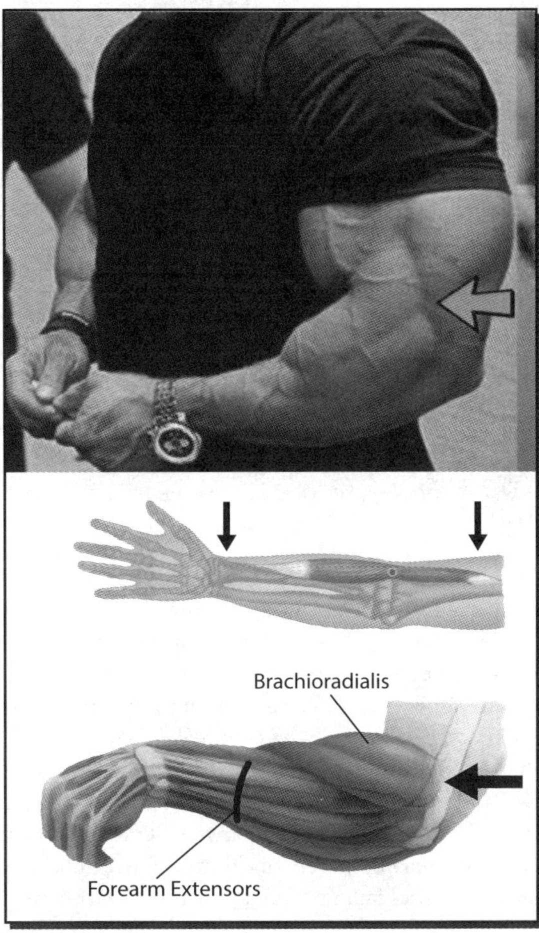

Figure 21-57

This situation is analogous to the fact that there is not much benefit in working the tibialis anterior (the muscle on the front of the "shins"/lower legs), even though there's a great benefit in working the calves (the muscle that is on the back side of the lower legs). The tibialis anterior causes the ankle to bend in the opposite direction as the calves, just as the forearm extensors cause the wrist to bend the wrist the opposite direction of the forearm flexors. Accordingly, it's worth working the forearm flexors, but not the forearm extensors, the same way it's worth working the calves, but not the tibialis anterior, when the objective is physique development and general fitness.

Other Forearm Exercises:

There's a variety of exercises that people do, in an effort to develop their forearm muscles. Very few forearm exercises, however, have "high value"—are optimally efficient, productive, and safe. Many forearm exercises have low value, because they are mechanically flawed, in one or more ways. Among the forearm exercises that fall short of being optimally beneficial for forearm development are the following:

- "Behind the Back Barbell Wrist Curls"

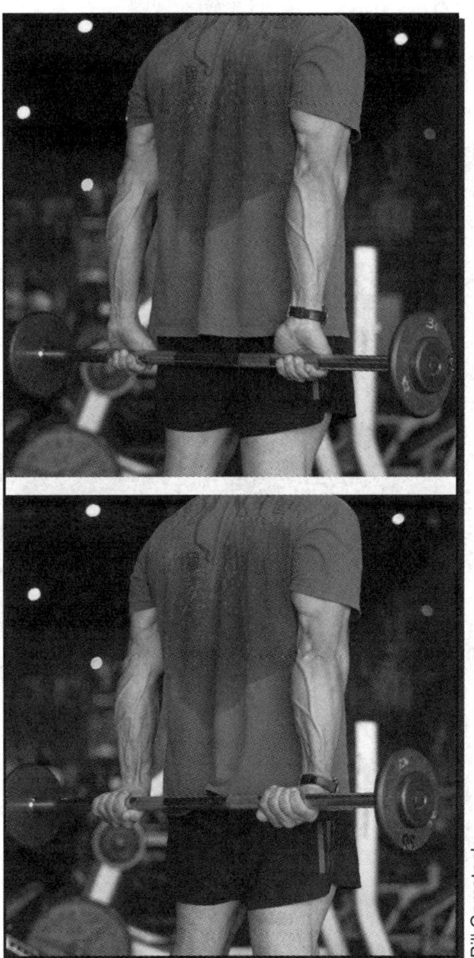

Figure 21-58

There are two significant problems with this exercise. The first is that it only works (loads) the second HALF of the range of motion. In Chapter 6 ("The Apex and the Base"), it was pointed out why it's wise to avoid exercises that have a base or apex (a neutral point) in the middle of the range of motion. This exercise is a perfect example of that.

*Behind the back barbell wrist curls* provide no load and no stretch during the "early phase" (the first half) of the forearm flexors' range of motion, which is arguably the most important part of the range of motion. The second problem is that this movement increases the resistance as the muscle contracts, and reduces it as the muscle elongates. This is the opposite of an ideal resistance curve. It's "late phase loaded," instead of being "early phase loaded."

❑ Radial Deviation

The anatomical movement shown in Figure 21-59 is called "radial deviation" (sideways wrist bending, pulling toward the thumb). This movement might have merit in specific physical therapy applications or it might be helpful for a particular job or sport. From a practical perspective, however, most people never experience a situation that causes them to think that they are "weak" in this particular motion.

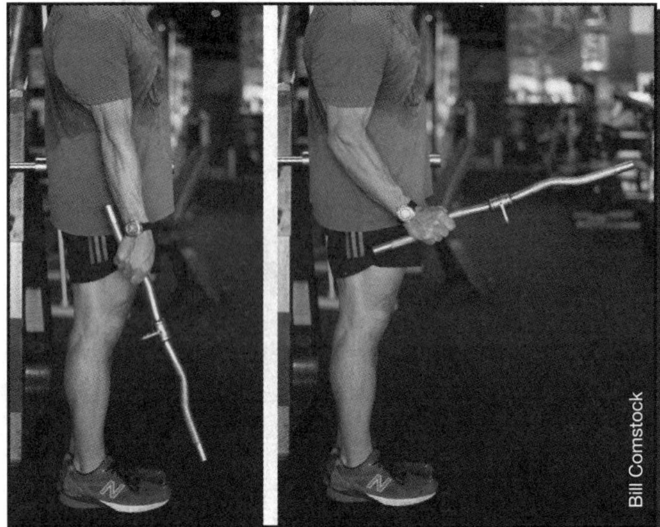

Figure 21-59

Furthermore, there is very little to be gained, in terms of visible muscle growth, from performing this type of motion. The muscles that produce this movement (the "extensor carpi radialis longus" and the "extensor carpi radialis brevis") are very small, and have almost no capacity for growth. In addition, the wrist mobility in this direction is very limited, so performing this motion, with resistance, could result in wrist pain or discomfort.

> *Note: Wrist motion in the opposite direction is called* "ulnar deviation"*—bending the wrist sideways toward the small/pinkie finger. Exerting this motion would have to be undertaken with the weight on the posterior side, rather than on the anterior side. This movement is produced by the "flexor carpi ulnaris" muscle, which is also a very small muscle, without much capacity for growth.*

❑ Wrist Rollers

The "*wrist roller*" is an old classic exercise, in which a weight is pulled up by winding a weighted rope onto the handle (Figure 21-60). The weight can be rolled in "both" directions. For example, the rope can be on the outside (in front) of the roller, which requires wrist extension (activation of the wrist extensor muscles) or on the inside (behind) the roller, which requires wrist flexion (activation of the wrist flexor muscles).

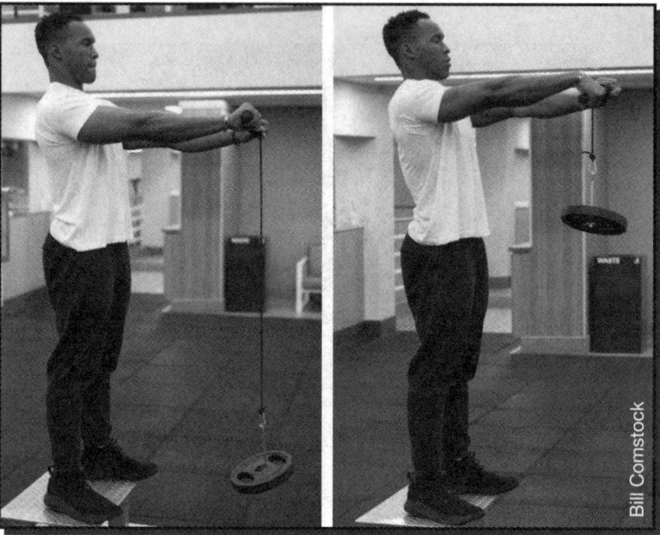

Figure 21-60

We have already established that performing wrist extension (working the wrist extensor muscles) is hardly worth doing. On the other hand, doing wrist flexions (working the wrist flexor muscles) is worth doing, but using this apparatus is not the best option. While it's better than nothing, it's not as good as performing *standard seated barbell (or dumbbell) wrist curls*. The lack of stability that exists with this exercise is the limiting factor. There's simply no way you could load the forearm flexors with this exercise, as much (with as much weight) as you could when doing standard seated barbell (or dumbbell) wrist curls, because the shoulders would fatigue (and fail) before the forearms.

In general, this exercise feels like it would be effective, because it produces quite a "burn" in the forearms. In reality, however, the amount of "burn" (localized fatigue) felt in a muscle, during a given exercise, is not directly correlated with the amount of visible development that is achieved. It may be a fun alternative to standard *barbell wrist curls* and *reverse wrist curls*, but it is much less productive, in terms of visible forearm muscle growth.

❑ Finger Exercises for Forearm Development

On occasion, people are seen doing exercises that involve finger movement with resistance, provided by springs or elastic bands—or by squeezing a rubber ball. These exercises might have application in some instances involving physical therapy/rehabilitation, or for sport-specific reasons, but they are not very useful for physique development. These exercises would certainly improve grip strength—to a degree. Rarely, however, is a lack of grip strength an issue with people who already perform resistance exercises.

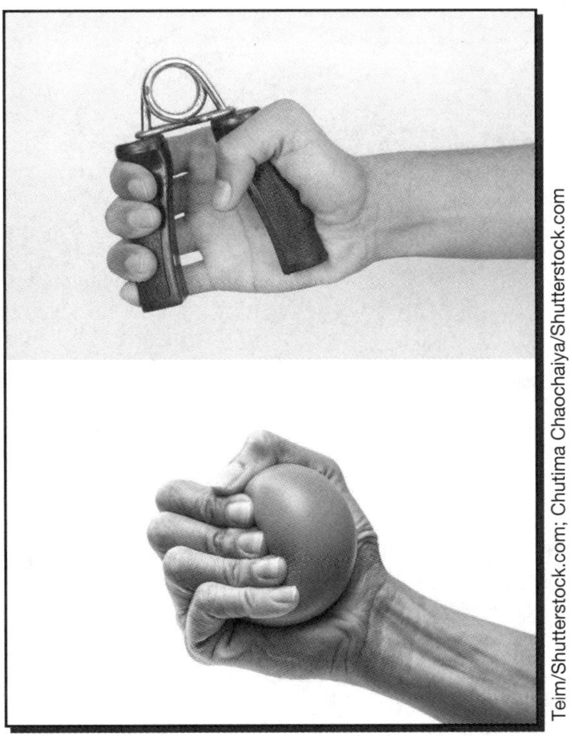

Teim/Shutterstock.com; Chutima Chaochaiya/Shutterstock.com

Figure 21-61

Some manufacturers of grip-exercise devices market their products by way of a photograph of a muscular arm and FOREARM, suggesting (subliminally) that using their product will result in visible muscular development of the forearm. Sometimes, their advertisements also claim that you'll achieve "super grip strength." While both of these claims may sound very appealing, they're very misleading.

In reality, gripping exercises do not produce any visible increase in the size of the forearm. Gripping involves the "extrinsic" muscles that operate the hand, but originate on the forearm. These muscles are very tiny (thin) and have very little capacity for significant growth. In terms of capacity for grip strength increase, there is a limit to how much it can improve. Expecting to achieve "super grip strength" (as in "super human" or far above "normal") would be very unrealistic. There is also very little need for "super grip strength" in day-to-day life, so investing much energy in that endeavor would not be very wise.

In recent years, thick rubber grips (like the ones shown in Figure 21-62) have appeared on the market, and are meant to be put on barbells and dumbbells. (Note: These are meant more for pulling exercises than for pushing exercises.) The underlying premise of this product is that a larger diameter (on a standard barbell or dumbbell) will challenge a person's ability to grip more, thus resulting in improved grip strength. Theoretically, this would give the user a "bonus" benefit, in addition to the benefit being provided to the target muscle of the exercise. In fact, both of these objectives would be compromised.

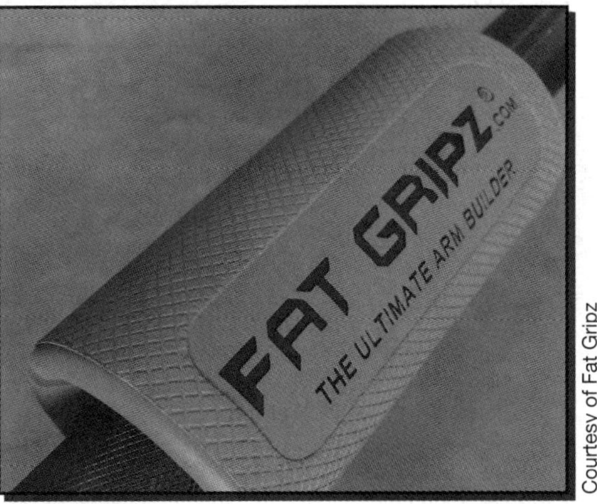


Courtesy of Fat Gripz

Figure 21-62

As noted previously, the gripping muscles are tiny, and do not have much capacity for visible growth, nor for a significant (or useful) increase of strength. Gripping strength is already sufficiently challenged and improved by the normal, day-to-day requirements of resistance exercise, e.g., holding heavy dumbbells, cables attached to heavy weight, moving benches and weights around in the gym, etc. More importantly, using a device that challenges the grip beyond what is normal would compromise your ability to do pulling exercises, because the grip would likely fail before the target muscle is fully challenged. If your goal is to maximally load and exhaust the larger physique muscles (for the purpose of growth), the more sensible approach is to AID the grip, rather than compromise it. Using wrist straps (Figure 21-63, top image), or even hooks (Figure 21-63, bottom image), would reduce the possibility of finger fatigue, allowing the target muscle to be adequately loaded and exhausted, without interference.

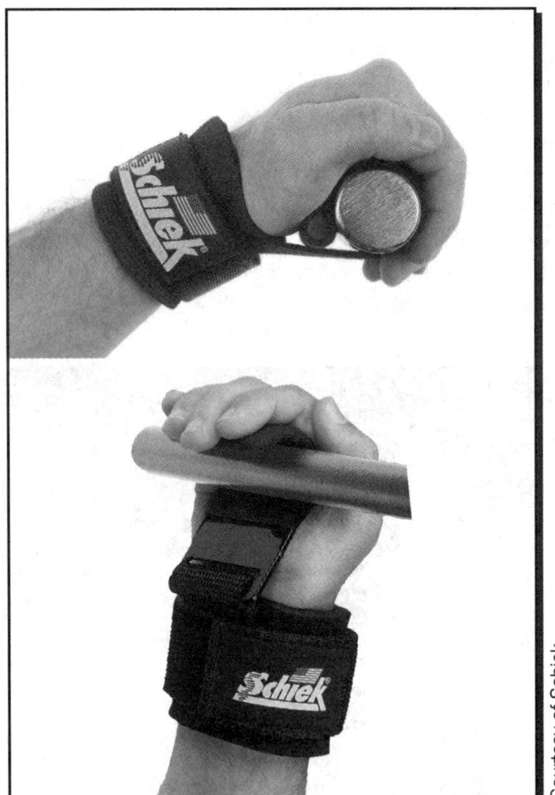


Courtesy of Schiek

Figure 21-63

# CHAPTER 22

# Quadriceps and Hamstrings

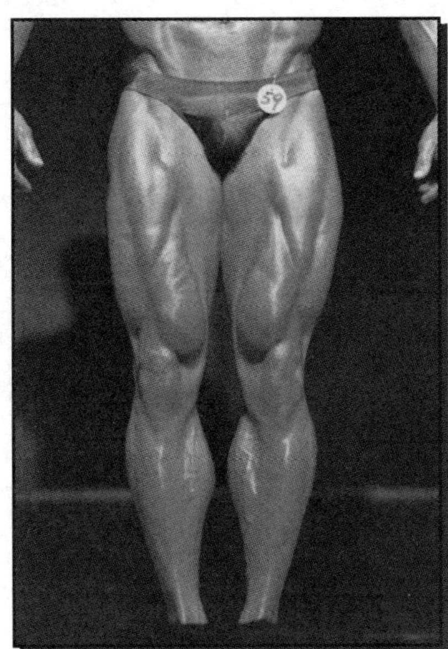

Figure 22-1

The legs are comprised of numerous individual muscles, but from the perspective of "physique development," the four primary muscle groups of the legs are the quadriceps, hamstrings, glutes, and calves. Less "primary" muscles of the legs, but still important, are the adductors and the hip flexors. This chapter addresses the "quads" and "hams."

The quadriceps muscle primarily extends the knee, similar to the way the triceps extends the elbow. Both of these are "extension muscles." Some individuals casually refer to the quadriceps as "one muscle," even though it is comprised of four parts, with a single insertion and four origins. One of the four parts of the quadriceps assists in a secondary function (in addition to its role in extending the knee)—it assists in flexing the hip.

This situation is similar to the triceps. It too is casually referred to as "one muscle," although it is comprised of three parts (with a single insertion and three origins). One of those three triceps "parts" assists in a secondary function (shoulder flexion), although its primary function is still elbow extension. For this reason, it's good to think of the quadriceps as the "triceps of the legs." This mindset will allow you to make reasonable comparisons, in terms of the "best strategy" for developing the quadriceps.

## Anatomy of the Quadriceps

In Figure 22-2, you can see the four heads of the quadriceps. Because the vastus intermedius lies beneath the other three muscles, it is not visible (on a person), even when the individual has very little body fat. The three visible "heads" are the vastus lateralis (the outer portion of the quadriceps), the rectus femoris (the middle muscle), and the vastus medialis (also referred to as the "teardrop" muscle, because of its shape).

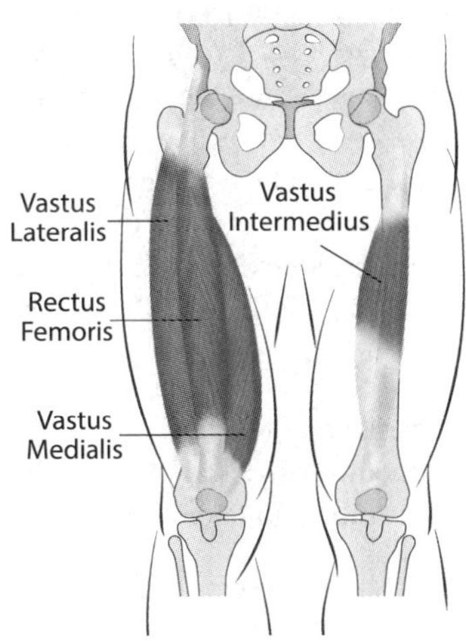


Figure 22-2

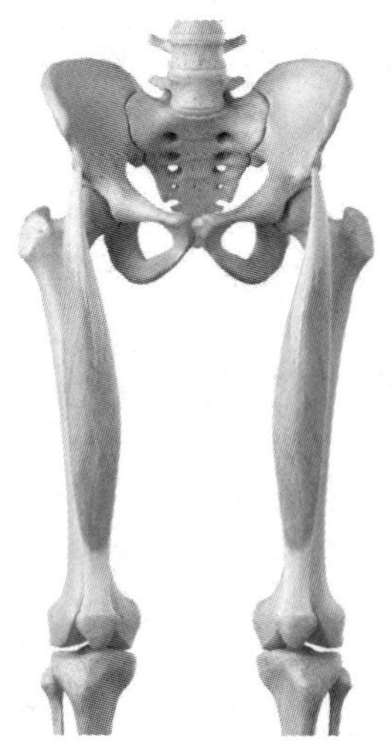


Figure 22-3

All four parts of the quadriceps converge at the singular quadriceps tendon, just above the knee. This juncture becomes the patella tendon below the knee, and then attaches onto the tibia of the lower leg, which is the "insertion" point of the quadriceps.

Three of the four quadriceps components originate directly on the upper end of the femur (the thigh bone). Only the rectus femoris does not; it originates on the pelvis, slightly above the hip joint. The fact that the rectus femoris crosses the hip joint is what allows the rectus femoris to also assist in flexing the hip joint. Thus, the three quadriceps heads that originate on the femur ONLY extend the knee. The one quadriceps head that also crosses the hip joint has the primary function of knee extension, as well as the secondary (less significant) function of hip flexion. This is very important, as you'll soon see.

Figure 22-3 provides a better view of the rectus femoris alone. In this instance, you can more clearly see its origin on the pelvis. It then extends down to the quadriceps tendon (just above the knee), where it converges with the other three parts. All four then join with the quadriceps tendon.

Most traditional "quadriceps workouts" involve mostly compound exercises, like *squats, leg presses, lunges*, etc. Often, but not always, leg extensions (on the *leg extension* machine) are also included. Lately, leg extensions have been maligned, for no good reason, which will soon be explained. The key question to ask is this: "Does a compound exercise that involves the quads, glutes, hamstrings, and adductors work the quadriceps 'better than,' 'not as good as,' or 'the same as' (but with a timesaving component) an isolated quadriceps exercise?"

In order to answer this question, we must establish whether the simultaneous activation of the "other" leg muscles (glutes, hamstrings, and adductors), when the quadriceps are working, "increases" or "interferes with" the optimal activation of the quadriceps, and explain the response either way (i.e., why it increases, or why it interferes with, optimal quadriceps activation).

Before we parse that analysis, let us first address the question of whether or not we can influence the shape of the quadriceps development, by selecting certain exercises, or by way of "modifying" certain exercises.

Whether "knee extension" occurs as an isolated incident or as part of a multi-joint activity, the action of the quadriceps is generally the same. All four parts of the quadriceps produce a unified effort, which pulls straight "upward" on the quadriceps tendon/patella tendon. This straight "upward" pull on the tibia results in extension (straightening) of the knee. Because the knee is a hinge-type joint, it only bends (extends/flexes) in one direction. Therefore, this single-action mechanism occurs the exact same way, regardless of the exercise that is being done. There is no way that one part of the quadriceps can be more activated than another part, while the knee only extends in one direction. It would have to result in a different action, but a different action is not possible.

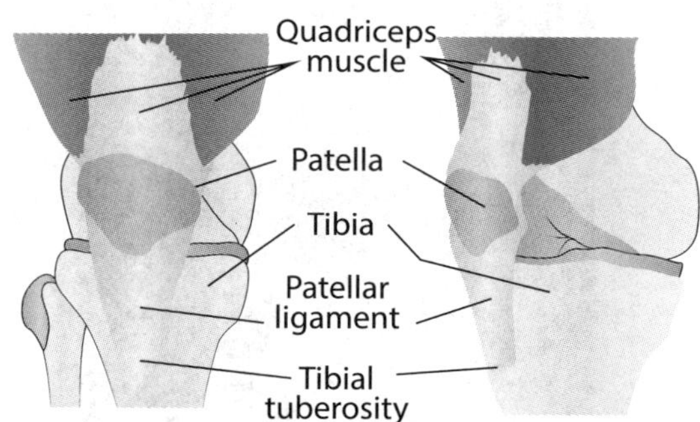


Figure 22-4

Figure 22-4 shows more clearly how the quadriceps tendon (above the knee) becomes the patellar ligament (also known as the patella tendon) below the knee, and attaches onto the tibial tuberosity on the front of the tibia. As such, whenever you extend your knee (straighten your leg), during any type of exercise that involves knee extension, all four parts of the quadriceps are activated. All four parts act as one, in terms of knee extension.

In other words, the quadriceps' role as a "knee extender" is as absolute as is the triceps' role as an "elbow extender." As such, when you work your triceps, would you consider doing anything other than "elbow extension?" Of course not.

You can see the similarity between the leg and the arm in Figure 22-5. Note that the quadriceps (Figure 22-5, left image) has the same configuration (origin/insertion) as does the triceps (Figure 22-5, right image). Both muscle groups have more than one origin and only one insertion. Furthermore, both muscle groups perform the same function, which is to extend a hinge-type of joint.

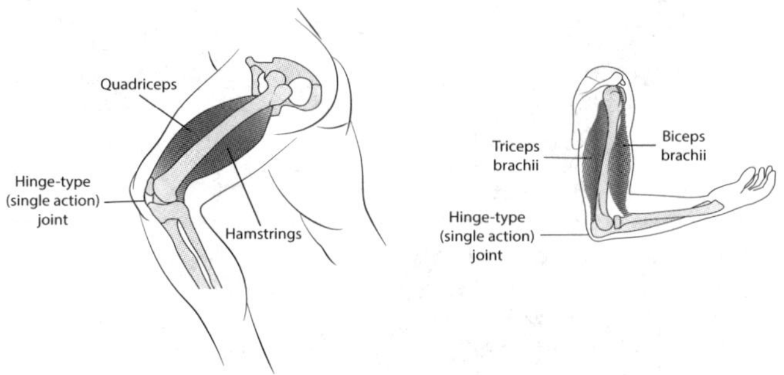


Figure 22-5

Any exercise that requires "knee extension" (straightening of the leg) activates the entire quadriceps muscle group. Therefore, doing multiple exercises for your quadriceps in a given workout—e.g., three or four exercises, all of which require the leg to straighten—involves quite a lot of redundancy, or worse. You'll soon see why.

Of course, quadriceps exercises all differ in terms of efficiency, productivity, and safety. They do not, however, stimulate the quadriceps "differently." It is foolish to believe that one exercise will develop "the outer sweep" of your quadriceps, while another exercise will develop "the quadriceps closer to the knee." The notion that some quadriceps exercises "build mass," while others simply "improve shape and definition" is also misguided. There is no science, nor any logic, that supports those beliefs.

Accordingly, when deciding which exercises (plural), or which single exercise you should do for your quadriceps, the factors to consider are as follows:

- "Efficiency" (cost/benefit—i.e., the load on the quadriceps versus the amount of weight necessary to provide that load, which is influenced by the lever (limb) length and the lever (limb) angle relative to the direction of resistance)
- "Full range of motion"
- "Early phase loading"/optimally productive resistance curve
- The reduction of unnecessary injury risk (i.e., excessive loading of non-target muscles, and/or excessive loading of the spine/joints)
- The avoidance of interference (i.e., avoiding reciprocal innervation)

Remember that all aspects of an exercise—mechanical and neurological—must be considered, when evaluating an exercise. We know that knee extension is the primary function of the quadriceps, just like elbow extension is the primary function of the triceps. Therefore, it would make sense to perform exercises that only extend the knee, just as we usually do triceps exercises that only extend the elbow.

If we combine knee extension with the movement of another joint/the engagement of another muscle(s)—a compound exercise—we must be able to justify it on a comparative basis. Is it better than, worse than, or "just as good as" an isolation exercise? The objective should be to find the "best" exercise, i.e., the optimal stimulation, for the quadriceps. Why bother doing exercises that produce inferior stimulation to the quads, or are inefficient (requiring much more weight to deliver the same load to the muscle), or are just redundant?

Consider this question: "Does the engagement of a secondary muscle group (i.e., the hip extensors, glutes, etc.), simultaneous to the engagement of the quadriceps, bestow any additional benefit to the quadriceps?" Aside from the misguided theory that it "saves time," there is NO additional benefit that the quadriceps will experience, as a result of simultaneously engaging the glutes and other hip extensors.

A better question, however, is: "Is it possible to compromise the activation of the quadriceps, by simultaneously engaging the glutes and the other hip extension muscles (the hamstrings and adductors)?" The answer to THAT question is, "absolutely!" During squats, leg presses, lunges, etc., exercises that load the glutes and the other hip extension muscles, the rectus femoris (the one quadriceps head that crosses the hip joint) is compromised. This situation is due to reciprocal innervation, which falls under the fifth criteria previously noted, the factors that determine the value of an exercise.

Hip extension is the opposite of hip flexion. These are antagonist movements. Reciprocal Innervation causes a muscle to "shut down" (partially or totally relax), when its antagonist is loaded and activated. Therefore, loading and activating the hip extensors (glutes, hamstrings and adductors), shuts off—at least partially—the hip flexors, which includes the rectus femoris (because it is one of the hip flexor muscles). The rectus femoris is one of the primary quadriceps muscles. As such, one quarter of the quadriceps is compromised in its knee extension efforts, during a compound leg exercise, by the simultaneous activation of the hip extensors. Obviously, this factor is counterproductive to a person's efforts to optimally stimulate their quads, during a quadriceps workout. Interference is the last thing you want, when you're pursuing optimal muscle stimulation.

Next, let's look at some of the most common exercises typically used for quadriceps development, and identify what's good about them and what's not so good about them:

## Analysis of Common Exercises for the Quadriceps

❑ Leg Extensions

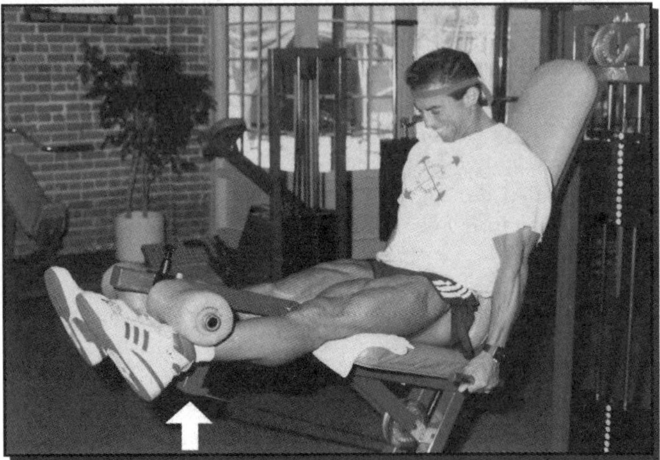

Figure 22-6

The "*leg extension*" (machine) is a standard exercise, included in most bodybuilding leg workouts. In fact, it's an excellent exercise, assuming the machine is designed correctly—with the machine's pivot correctly positioned and with a properly designed cam, providing a good resistance curve.

Unfortunately, many people don't appreciate how good this exercise is. They often consider it a "supplemental exercise," meant to compliment the more "foundational" *barbell squats* and *45-degree leg presses*. The reason that some individuals make this assumption is because they've been led to believe (misguided, in fact) that the quadriceps require a compound exercise for building mass. This assumption is entirely false.

By way of comparison, look at the two sets of images in Figure 22-7—*leg extensions* (image "A" for the quads) and *skull crushers/supine triceps extension* with dumbbells (image "B" for the triceps). Keep in mind that the quads (knee extension) and the triceps (elbow extension) are almost identical mechanisms. As you observe how similar these two movements are (when seen from this perspective), remember that "*skull crushers*" (aka *supine dumbbell triceps extension*) are considered one of the best exercises for the triceps. *Skull crushers* are not considered a "supplemental" exercise for the triceps. It is a "foundational" exercise for the triceps. The difference in the way these two exercises are regarded demonstrates bias, i.e., an irrational disregard of *leg extensions*, despite the same exact mechanics being highly regarded in the case of *supine dumbbell triceps extensions* ("*skull crushers*").

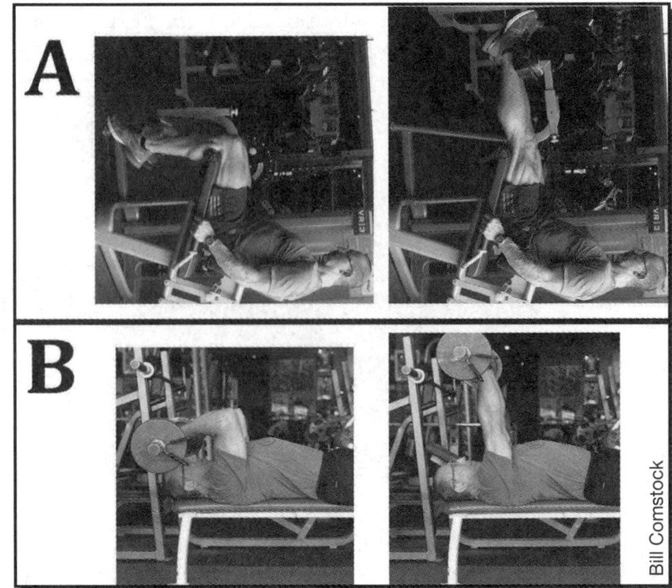


Figure 22-7

Since "*leg extensions*" (on the machine) is not a compound exercise, and it only works the quadriceps, it is often discredited. Consider the fact, however, that a *supine dumbbell triceps extension* (Figure 22-7, image B) is also not a compound exercise, yet this factor does not diminish its value as a triceps exercise. In fact, it is an excellent triceps exercise. Likewise, *leg extensions* is an excellent quadriceps exercise. It has the same mechanics as the *supine dumbbell triceps extensions*, and the triceps is the same type of extension muscle as is the quadriceps.

When the quadriceps are loaded and are contracting against resistance, they (the quadriceps) don't "know" whether the gluteus maximus and the adductors are also working. The quadriceps don't "know" if they are working alone, or as one of several muscles working in combination during a compound exercise. Either way, the quadriceps simply do their job—to extend the knee.

Since there is no added benefit to the quadriceps, in the simultaneous participation of the glutes (during a compound exercise), there is no diminishment of quadriceps benefit, when the glutes do not participate simultaneously.

In fact, the quality of the quadriceps stimulation is arguably better, when the gluteus (plus the hamstrings) are *not* working at the same time. This factor is due to the triggering of reciprocal innervation, i.e., the relaxation synapse (signal) that is automatically sent to a muscle (the quadriceps, in this case), when the antagonist muscle (the glutes and hamstrings, in this case) are simultaneously loaded and activated.

In terms of range of motion, when performing *leg extensions*, it is best to stay within the middle 80 percent of the range of motion. It is wise to forego the initial 10 percent and the final 10 percent, given that these are the areas of more potential knee strain, when using a heavy weight. Furthermore, there is no loss of benefit in omitting these parts of the range of motion.

The reason why there is potential knee strain in the final 10 percent of the range of motion is because the tibia (the lower leg bone) and the femur (the upper leg bone) have different shaped "condyles"—the tendinous linings that cover the ends of both bones. During the final part of the range of motion, a slight rotation of the tibia occurs. This action is sometimes referred to as "screw home rotation." As the knee concludes the final part of its extension, the tibia rotates, in order to accommodate the closing of the space between the upper and lower leg bones. The tibia and femur (the opposing condyles) will only "seat together," when this shift occurs.

This factor happens during leg extensions, but does not occur during squats or other types of leg press exercises, because of the "still opposing resistance" that is present during leg extensions. That "still opposing resistance" is beneficial for the quadriceps, and it's an absence of benefit that it does not occur during squats or leg presses. It does, however, encourage "screw home rotation," if the knee is fully locked out, i.e., fully straightened, when doing *leg extensions*. The simple solution is to just avoid the final 5 to 10 degrees of that range of motion.

If you repeatedly cause "screw home rotation," by fully extending the knees on heavy *leg extensions*—over the course of years—the condyles could eventually be eroded by the pressure and friction. It is not necessary, however, to fully straighten the knees. Omitting the final 5 to 10 degrees does not result in any loss of quadriceps benefit. As discussed previously, the early and middle parts of the range of motion are the most productive.

This fact is not to be misconstrued as an excuse to only perform 20 percent of the full range of motion during *leg extensions*. What is seen most often is people performing a range of motion that is ridiculous abbreviated, i.e., omitting the first 40 percent and the final 40 percent, and only doing the middle 20 percent. In reality, "full" range of motion requires at least 70 percent of the potential range, if not 80 percent.

Some people erroneously believe that fully flexing ("squeezing") the quadriceps, when performing *leg extensions*, improves the "definition" (i.e., clarity) of the muscles. The belief is that this will somehow "etch" greater striations into the muscle. This notion is false. Only a sufficient reduction of body fat improves muscle visibility. Muscles are comprised of individual fibers ("striations"). Whether these fibers are visible or not, depends on the person's body fat level. It does not depend on whether you "fully extend"/"fully flex" the quadriceps during *leg extensions*. Furthermore, body fat reduction cannot possibly happen "locally" (muscle group by muscle group, by an exercise that targets that muscle). It is a whole-body process, which occurs only by way of a caloric deficit, i.e., dietary caloric reduction and an increased caloric demand.

On a separate note, there are some individuals who believe that *leg extensions* are bad for the knees, because (as those people claim) it produces a "shearing effect." This factor refers to a displacement (or shifting) of the upper end of the tibia from the lower end of the femur. In reality, this belief is false, and is very easy to disprove. The "anchoring" effect produced by the upward-pulling quadriceps tendon (during loaded knee extension) is at least 20 times more forceful than the perpendicular resistance applied at the front of the ankle, by the machine's lever arm. For a full explanation of this factor, you should refer to the article I wrote on this topic, using the following link: *http://www.labrada.com/blog/workouts/is-the-open-chain-closed-chain-exercise-philosophy-shear-non-sense/* ("Is the Open Chain/Closed Chain Exercise Philosophy Shear Nonsense?")

If there is any real knee strain that occurs during *leg extensions*, it is due to the fact that *leg extension* machines are not designed correctly. They typically have one lever arm that provides the resistance to the ankles (by way of the padded roller against which both ankles are placed). This single lever arm rotates around a single pivot, which produces a straight forward trajectory—exclusively—of that lever arm. The knees, however, do not quite "match" the angle of motion produced by the machine's straight-forward trajectory.

In reality, the left knee angles slightly to the left (with a slight downward angle on the lateral aspect and a slight upward angle on the medial aspect), and the right knee angles slightly to the right (also with a slight downward angle on the lateral aspect and a slight upward angle on the medial aspect). This mismatch (between the machine's trajectory and a person's natural knee movement) produces a slight sideways torque on the knees. As a result, the knees are forced (by the machine's straightforward trajectory) to move in a direction that is not quite a natural direction of movement. What's needed, in actuality, is a machine that has two separate pivots and two lever arms, each producing a trajectory that matches each knee's natural "slightly outward/slightly diagonal" motion. Clearly, equipment manufacturers have failed to provide this type of *leg extension* machine design, up to this point.

❑ Barbell Squat

The *barbell squat* is considered by many people as the "primary" exercise for quadriceps development. In fact, the standard bodybuilding leg (quadriceps) workout typically combines various types of squats (*standard barbell squats*, *front squats*, *hack squats*), along with *leg presses* and *leg extensions*.

In Chapter 2 ("Active Levers and Neutral Levers"), it was pointed out that a lever (like the tibia/lower leg, in this instance) LEAST loads its operating muscle, when it is parallel with resistance, and it MOST loads its operating muscle when it's perpendicular with resistance. Since the tibia is the operating lever of the quadriceps, you should ask yourself the question, "How perpendicular with resistance is the tibia during *barbell squats*?" The answer to that question will determine how efficient the exercise is. For example, if the tibia is mostly parallel with resistance, the exercise is very inefficient. On the other hand, if the tibia is mostly perpendicular with resistance, the exercise is very efficient.

In Figure 22-8, you can see a side view of a *barbell squat*. Given the previous discussion, you should examine how "efficient" a person's levers (limbs) are, during this exercise. Remember that the direction of resistance is straight down in this instance (a 6:00 direction of resistance)—"free weight" gravity. Note also that a protractor has been placed at the bottom of the exerciser's tibia, showing the angle of tilt of his tibia.

A fully "neutral" tibia would be at a 90-degree angle (vertical), relative to the ground. That vertical angle could be called a "ZERO lever" (it delivers zero load to the target muscle—the quadriceps, in this case). The tibia is a fully "inactive" lever, when it is vertical. A fully "active" tibia would be horizontal. That particular position could be referred to as a 100 percent lever (it would deliver 100 percent of the available load to the target muscle—the quadriceps, in this case). A tibia that is halfway between vertical and horizontal (a 45 degree angle) could be considered a 50 percent lever (in a simplified, non-trigonometry estimation)—halfway between zero and 100 percent.

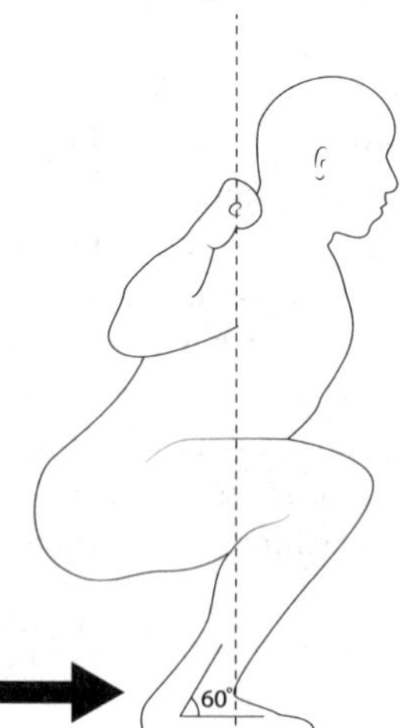


Figure 22-8

In Figure 22-8, you can see that this person's tibia, at this particular position in the movement, is angled at about 60 degrees. A 60-degree angle is 30 degrees from the "neutral" position. Each degree (between zero and 90) is 1.11 percent. Therefore, at this angle, the tibia is (approximately) 33 percent active, which is the MOST active angle that the tibia reaches during the range of motion of a typical squat movement. This is very inefficient, in the sense that 66 percent of the weight that is being used, i.e., 66 percent of the available resistance, is NOT loading the quadriceps, even though it is fully loading the skeleton (the spine and the joints).

> *Note: The math, in this instance, is not perfectly accurate, because, technically, a trigonometry formula would be used to calculate the exact percentage of load. On the other hand, the purpose of this book is not to teach trigonometry, nor is it meant to ascertain exact calculations. Rather, the purpose of this book is to gain an understanding of what delivers LESS resistance, as well as what delivers MORE resistance, with regard to lever/limb angles, during resistance exercise.*

In fact, the closer the tibia is to being parallel with gravity (i.e., vertical), the less resistance (as a percentage of the weight which is being used) that loads the quadriceps. In turn, the closer the tibia is to being perpendicular with gravity (i.e., horizontal), the greater the resistance (as a percentage of the weight being used) that loads the quadriceps. Of course, the exerciser does not have complete control of this factor, while squatting. This situation is because balance must be maintained, in order to not fall forward or backward. Still, the physics applies just the same.

In this example, you can see that the individual's quadriceps are only being loaded with about 33 percent of the "available resistance," due to the angle of the tibia, relative to gravity. In other words, a standard *barbell squat* loads the quadriceps with only about one-third of the "available resistance"—which is the weight of the barbell, plus the person's body weight.

Although this chapter is about the quadriceps, it's worth taking a quick look at the other levers (limbs) that are involved in *barbell squats* (their angles and the percentage of load that is placed upon their corresponding muscles), as long as we're on the subject of *barbell squats*. Then, we'll return to discussing the quadriceps.

Just as the tibia is the operating lever of the quadriceps, the femur is the operating lever of the gluteus. Hip extension—the downward pushing of the femur—engages the gluteus primarily, and also the hamstrings (by way of its assisting role in this action) and the adductors. The primary hip extension muscle, however, is the gluteus.

In Figure 22-9, a black line has been placed through this exerciser's FEMUR, with a protractor showing that it's at 10 degrees lower than the horizontal position. Having the femur 10 degrees below horizontal (i.e., the butt is lower than the knee) means that the individual has passed beyond the point where the femur is 100 percent efficient. Theoretically, this situation is good. It means that the muscle that is operating the femur (i.e., the gluteus, plus the adductors and hamstrings, to a lesser degree) is getting all or most of the "available resistance."

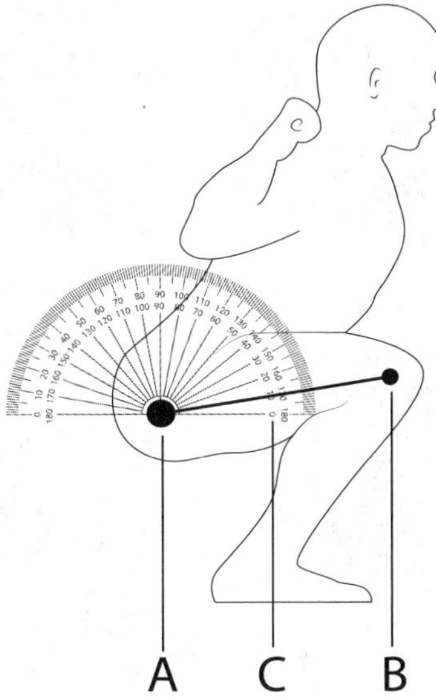


Figure 22-9

The angle of the limb, relative to the direction of resistance, is not the only variable, however. There is another important variable, which is the "effective" length of that lever (limb). As you know, a longer lever magnifies resistance more, while a shorter lever magnifies resistance less. When you do a standard *squat,* the lower leg (which is acting as the secondary lever to the femur) doubles under the femur, which reduces the femur's "effective" length. This factor was discussed in the first chapter of this book. Note that in Figure 22-9, the distance between line "A" and line "B" is the actual length of the femur. The distance between line "B" and line "C" indicates the degree of "doubling back" (length reduction) that the lower leg is causing.

Accordingly, the distance between line "B" line and line "C" is the amount by which the "effective length" of the femur is reduced. In turn, the distance between line "A" line and line "C" is the remaining effective length of the femur, as a result of this "femur length reduction." Technically, the distance (between A and C) is also called the "moment arm." As you can see, the effective femur length has been reduced by about 50 percent. As such, the magnification of the weight being used (which is loaded onto the gluteus) has, therefore, also been reduced by about 50 percent.

This factor means that although the femur does reach a maximally "active" angle with gravity (by reaching the perpendicular position to gravity), the effective length of the femur is only half as long as it could be. Thus, *squats* deliver less load to the glutes than an exercise that does not cause the femur's effective length to be reduced. This point will be discussed at greater length in the next chapter.

Let us now briefly examine the third lever ("limb") that plays a major role in *squats.* In Figure 22-10, you can see that the TORSO is angled at about 60 degrees (30 degrees from the vertical position), when a person is in this particular position, i.e., the fully descended position of a *barbell squat.* This angle results in the torso-lever being about 33 percent active, similar to the lower leg (in this particular scenario). Since the torso is longer than the lower leg, however, the magnification of the load that is produced by the torso lever is more than the resistance that is loading the quadriceps. Most of the load produced by the leaning forward of the torso loads the erector spinae, the muscles that run along the spine, with the greatest percentage of that falling on the lower back.

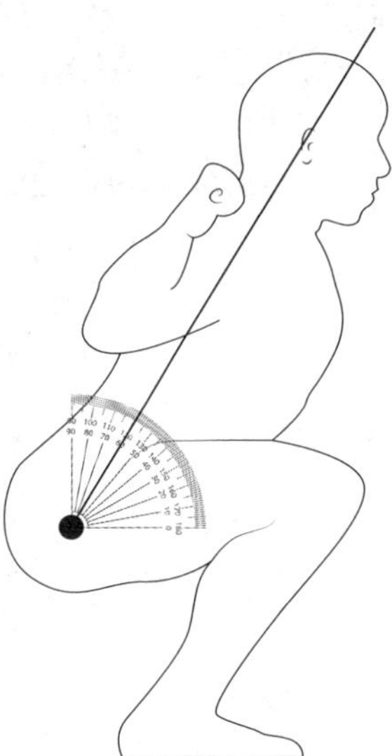

Figure 22-10

As a result of the respective mechanics of these three levers ("limbs"), during *barbell squats,* the quads and glutes are working, but not nearly as much as it might appear (as a percentage of the weight being used). In reality, the erector spinae (lower back) is working more than either the quads or the glutes. In addition, there is also a tremendous amount of spinal compression that occurs as a result of having a heavy barbell sitting at the top of the spinal column. This factor becomes especially problematic, when a heavy weight is being used. All of these issues must be considered, when deciding whether to do *barbell squats*—or not.

All factors considered, you'd have to conclude that the *barbell squat* is an extraordinarily inefficient exercise for the purpose of working the quadriceps and the glutes. The reduction of resistance (as a percentage of the weight being used) to the quads—caused by the mostly vertical tibia—and to the glutes—caused by the shortened femur length/"moment arm"—requires that more weight be used to compensate for the two reductions of efficiency. That increased load then compresses the spine and overloads the erector spinae. Yes, while you can "adequately" work/load the quads and the glutes with barbell squats, the "cost" is extremely high. In reality, there are far better (more efficient) ways of working the quadriceps and gluteus.

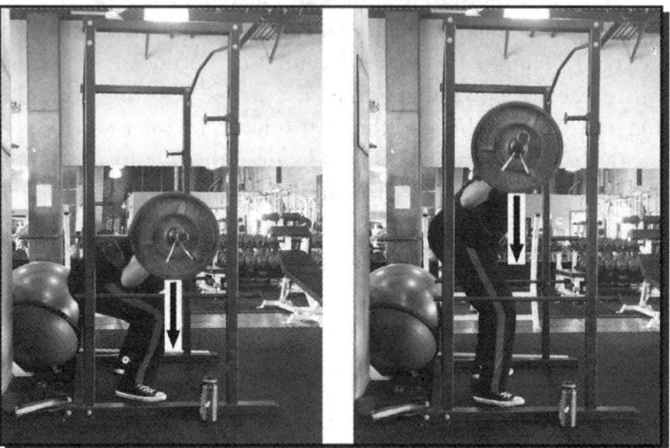

Figure 22-11

As you can see in Figure 22-11, this person's lower legs are almost entirely "neutral" (i.e., almost perfectly vertical/ parallel with gravity), even when he is in the most descended position. His tibia barely reaches an angle that is about 12 percent "active"—10 degrees from neutral. In other words, his quadriceps, which is presumably the muscles he most wants to target during this exercise, are only getting about 12 percent of the weight he's holding on his back.

Note in Figure 22-11, left image, that he is also ROUNDING his back, when he's in the descended (lowest) part of the movement. This factor (a forward-flexed spine that is loaded with weight) greatly increases the strain on the intervertebral discs. In essence, he's paying a huge price (exerting significantly more effort than is necessary, and being exposed to a potential spine injury) for a minuscule benefit to his quadriceps. This is absolutely foolish.

Again, you might think this kind of "bad form" is an amateur mistake. In fact, even experienced competitive bodybuilders often perform their *squats* like this, especially when they're using heavier weights.

The four sequential images in Figure 22-12 are of a veteran competitive bodybuilder with over 30 years experience. Yet, you can clearly see that he is rounding his back, and allowing his torso to tilt forward, much more than his tibia are tilted forward.

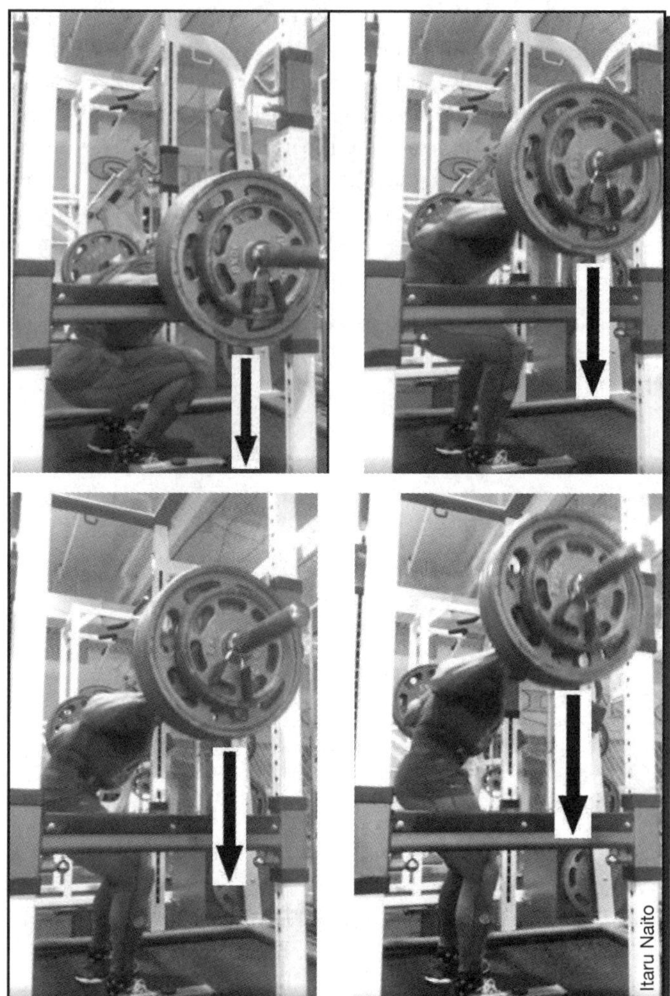


Figure 22-12

At this point, you may be thinking that performing "*front squats*" (Figure 22-13) would remedy this problem. It's true that *front squats* (holding the bar in front of the neck, instead of behind the neck) would allow a person to keep their torso more upright (i.e., more vertical), which would

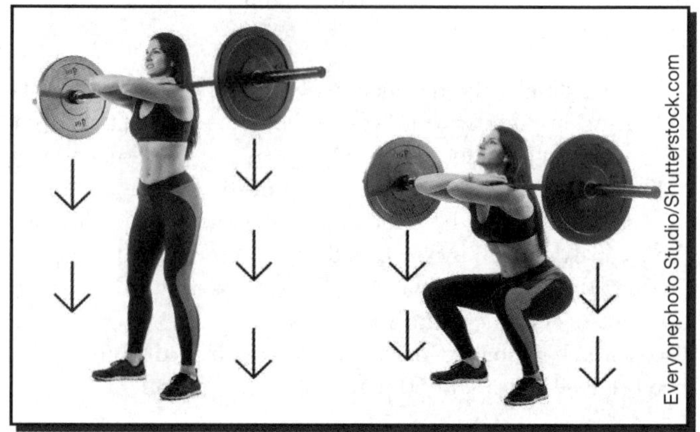


Figure 22-13

alleviate much of the strain in the lower back. It would not, however, eliminate the downward spinal pressure caused by holding a heavy weight at the top of the torso. Furthermore, it would not allow the tibia to be more "active," i.e., to be more perpendicular with gravity (to tilt forward more). In other words, *front squats* are still not "the solution" to the problem of inefficiently loading the tibia, for the purpose of providing optimal resistance to the quadriceps.

As you can see, the tibia is still not able to move beyond 30 degrees from the neutral (vertical) position. As a result, you would still be forced to use a heavier weight than necessary, in order to adequately load the quadriceps. The mostly neutral angle of the tibia (i.e., the fact that the tibia is more parallel with resistance, than it is perpendicular with it) minimizes the percentage of resistance being delivered to the quads. This mostly vertical tibia (lower leg lever) would thus cause you to feel that your quads are not being loaded enough, and you would then be compelled to use a heavier weight. Using a heavier weight would load the quadriceps more (compensating for the reduced inefficiency of the angle of the tibia), but the added weight would increase spinal compression.

Let's take a closer look at the spine, and see what happens when it is loaded with a heavy weight, bearing straight down on it. Figure 22-14 shows the natural curvature of a healthy spine. What do you suppose happens to these curves, when a heavy load pushes straight downward on the spine? Naturally, it would have an accordion-like effect, increasing the severity of those curves, thereby squeezing and distorting the intervertebral discs. Figure 22-15 shows the various problems that typically occur to the intervertebral discs of the spine, for a variety of reasons, even to people who do not perform heavy *barbell squats, deadlifts, front squats*, etc. You can be certain that loading 200 or 300 pounds of downward force onto the spine, every week, month after month, for years, would drastically increase the likelihood of these problems occurring.

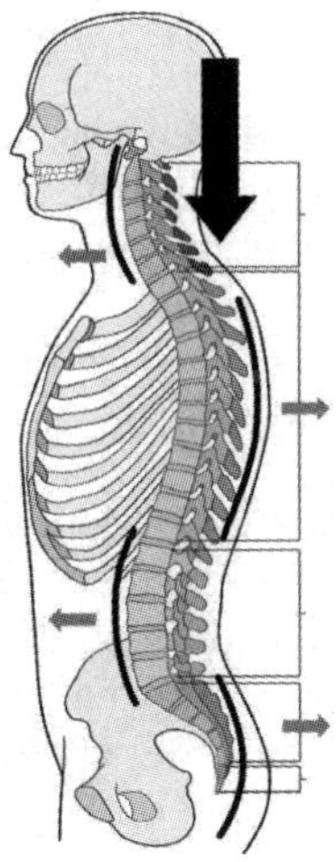

udaix/Shutterstock.com

Figure 22-14

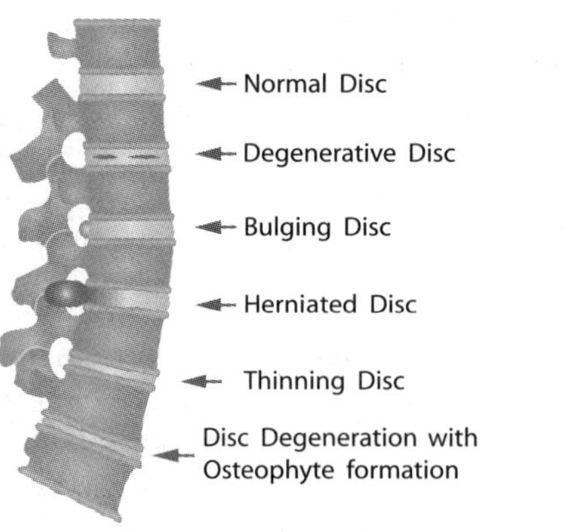


lotan/Shutterstock.com

Figure 22-15

Of course, the intervertebral discs can tolerate some degree of distortion, but there is a limit to how much they can be compressed and distorted. Eventually, loading a heavy weight onto the spine could (and often does) lead to spinal disc damage, which is not something that should be ignored. In fact, this is information that should not be withheld or omitted, when a trainer or a fitness publication "recommends" (to a client or fitness "student") an exercise that causes a forceful downward compression of the spine. Yet, people whose job is teaching physical fitness or bodybuilding to students rarely, if ever, mention it.

In a 2016 article for *Men's Fitness* magazine, author Jeremy Duvall, MS, CPT wrote: "*The* ***average Joe*** *should be able to squat 1.5 X his bodyweight. Two times bodyweight is golden.*"

This advice suggests that an average man who weighs 200 pounds—who is NOT exceptionally fit—"should" be able to *squat* 300 pounds. This suggestion is absolutely absurd.

If you are making efforts to *squat* as much weight as possible, because you are planning on competing in a powerlifting event (which includes the *squat*), or because you're doing it for ego satisfaction and bragging rights, and you are aware of the potential risk involved, and you accept that risk, it's fine. On the other hand, if you are pursuing muscular development or general fitness, performing heavy *barbell squats* (or any other type of *squats* that requires loading the spine), is not a wise choice. You can achieve better muscle loading of the quads, glutes, and adductors, without loading the spine and risking spinal injury (as well as potential hip and knee injury).

Believing that doing heavy *squats* is "necessary" for optimum fitness or for maximum muscular development of the quadriceps and gluteus, and that there is no risk of injury, or a low risk of injury, is simply naive. In fact, you do not need to do a compound exercise of any kind, in order to optimally develop the quadriceps, gluteus and adductors. Working these muscles with single-joint exercises is more productive and more safe.

As noted previously, the leg and the arm are similar mechanisms—each is comprised of two levers, connected by a hinge joint. Accordingly, an exercise that is good for the triceps would be very similar to an exercise that is good for the quadriceps. As such, knee extensions and elbow extensions involve nearly identical mechanical and muscular actions.

To prove this point, compare the two images in Figure 22-16. In the upper image, a person is doing a *barbell squat*, which is naively considered by many people as "the best exercises for the quads." The upward pointing arrow is the "ground reaction force," discussed in Chapter 6. The lower image shows the equivalent mechanics, performed with the arm. The forearm is the equivalent of the lower leg, and the upper arm is the equivalent of the femur. The angle of the forearm tilt is the same as the angle of the tibia tilt. No one would ever consider the lower image to represent "the best exercise for the triceps," because the forearm is not perpendicular enough to gravity to fully load the triceps. So, why should someone consider the same angle of the tibia, when doing *squats*, to be adequate enough for fully loading the quadriceps?

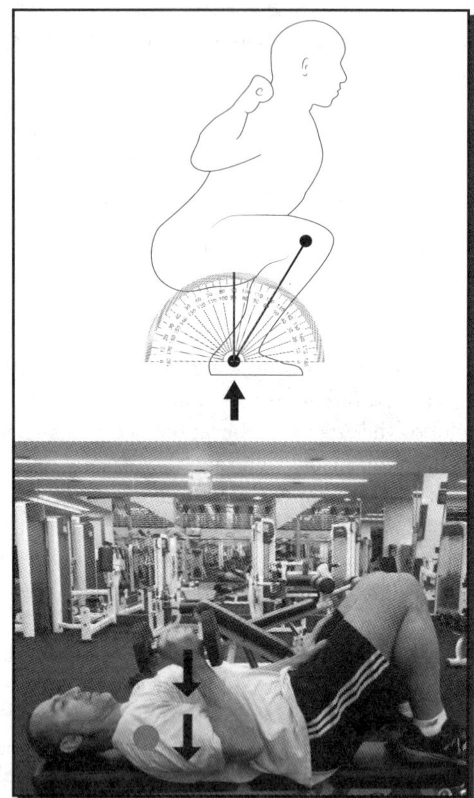

Figure 22-16

Figure 22-17 shows an image of what truly qualifies as "one of the best exercises for the triceps." What's the difference? The exercise represented in this image allows the forearm to enter into a completely perpendicular angle relative to gravity. Note that what allows this forearm angle is the fact that the upper arm bone (acting as the equivalent of the femur) is parallel with gravity. At this point, it's in the neutral position. In other words, improving the mechanics to the benefit of the triceps automatically reduces the involvement of the anterior deltoid (which is most responsible for operating the humerus, when it's alongside the torso, as in the previous image).

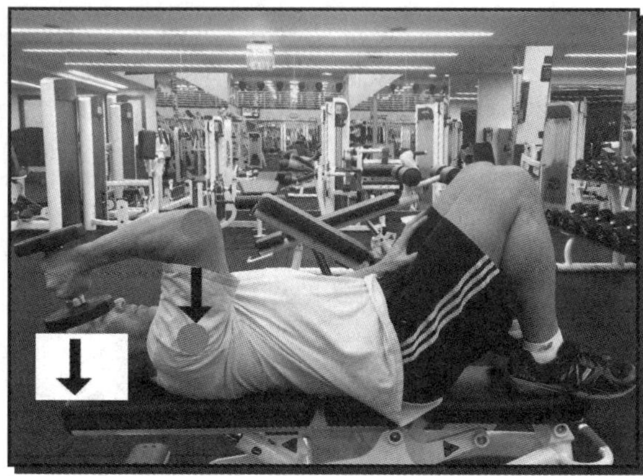

Figure 22-17

The same thing happens with the quadriceps/gluteus—by improving the angle of the tibia, to the benefit of the quadriceps, the angle of the femur changes in a way that eliminates the load on the gluteus. This is the paradox of compound exercises. Multiple muscles participating in a compound exercise usually do not derive as much benefit—individually—from that exercise, as they would from an isolation exercise.

This example demonstrates that, for muscle building purposes, isolation exercises are often better. While compound exercises might allow you to move more total weight at one time, they often compromise the stimulation to each participating muscle. As a rule, it's usually more productive for each muscle to work individually, without the compromise that is created by trying to simultaneously (and equally) benefit another muscle/other muscles.

There is one additional reason why it's better to work either the quadriceps OR the gluteus, during a given exercise, as compared to performing an exercise that involves both muscle groups at the same time. This issue relates to reciprocal innervation, which was discussed in Chapter 11, and will be addressed more fully toward the end of this chapter.

If you insist on using a compound exercise for the quads, the least you could do is select a better direction of resistance, so that the resistance loads your quadriceps more efficiently, and does not compress your spine. *Cable squats* (shown later in this chapter) is a wonderful alternative for regular (heavy) *barbell squats*.

The actual *squatting* movement—without the use of heavy weight—is fine, for the purpose of general fitness. This is especially true for cardiovascular benefit. *Squats* can be done safely with just bodyweight or with a moderate level of additional weight. "Moderate" would be in the realm of 20 percent to 50 percent of a person's bodyweight. Of course, this would typically be done for higher repetitions, e.g., 20 repetitions or more.

Doing bodyweight or light *squats*, with higher repetitions, is great for developing athleticism. "*Jumping squats*" (no added weight) can be exceptionally good for cardiovascular stimulation, as well as for sports that require vertical jumping.

*Squats* only become problematic, when you place a heavy barbell at the top of the spine, and try to maximally load the quadriceps by way of a tibia that is only 30 percent active. As such, the amount of total additional weight that you'd have to use in order to compensate for the inefficiency of the tibia angle dramatically changes the "cost/benefit" value of the exercise.

Accordingly, the main problem with a *barbell squat* (for the purpose of quadriceps development) is the angle of the tibia, relative to the direction of resistance, which is usually "straight down" gravity. This factor is what results in that 30 percent efficiency figure noted in the previous paragraph, rendering the tibia more "neutral" than "active," as the "loader" of the quadriceps. The secondary problem with a *barbell squat* is the spinal compression that it produces, which, when combined with the fact that more weight needs to be used in order to compensate for the inefficient tibia/gravity angle, results in a significant injury risk.

The third problem with a *barbell squat* (in descending order) is the fact that the angle of the tibia (as compromised as it already is for the benefit of the quadriceps) reduces the effective lever length of the femur, which results in a reduced load that the femur delivers to the gluteus. Paradoxically, if you could reduce the angle of the tibia (making it more vertical), it would benefit the glutes more, but it would further reduce (or eliminate) the load on the quadriceps.

The fourth problem with *barbell squats* is the fact that the exercise is often treated as a "test of strength," or as an effort to garner admiration, rather than as a method for the development of muscle. This mindset leads to using more weight than is reasonable or necessary, which subsequently leads to using very bad form (leaning the torso forward too far), which leads to an enormous amount of strain on the erector spinae.

The exercise shown in Figure 22-18 is called "*cable squats.*" Instead of using "free weight gravity," the added resistance is provided by cables coming from a low pulley, which are pulling in a diagonal direction. This direction of resistance crosses the tibia much more perpendicularly, than does "free weight gravity." In fact, nowhere in THIS range of motion is the tibia parallel with resistance (neutral). Even at the conclusion of the range of motion, the angle of the cable, relative to the tibia, is providing some degree of load to the quadriceps.

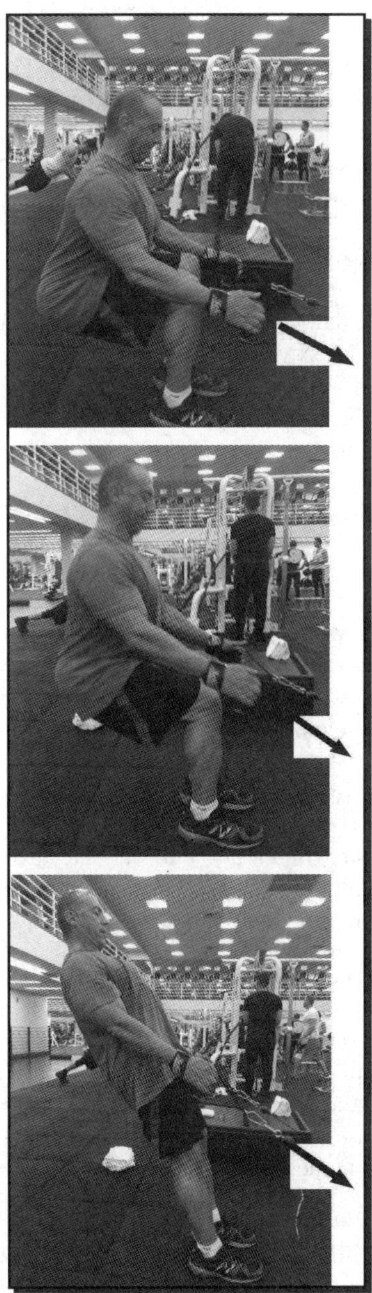

Figure 22-18

Look at the angle of the cable in Figure 22-18 (over which an arrow has been placed, indicating the direction of resistance), relative to the tibia, especially in the fully descended position (top image). This direction of resistance makes the tibia almost fully "active." In other words, it is loading the quadriceps with almost 100 percent of the available resistance.

Since this direction of resistance loads the tibia with a much higher percentage of the weight being used than when you perform regular *barbell squats*, less weight is required. In fact, it is not possible to use as much weight, when doing cable squats, as you could use with *barbell squats*. Getting more load on the quadriceps, with less actual weight being used, as well as the fact that the weight is not bearing down directly on the spine, results in less spinal compression. That's the very definition of efficiency—more benefit with less cost.

While there is still some degree of erector spinae loading (with cable squats), it is much less than with *barbell squats*. The erector spinae is loaded less during *cable squats*, because less weight is being used, but also because the resistance is held with the arms, and the arms are held low (as demonstrated in Figure 22-18). Thus, the arms are used as a secondary lever to reduce the effective length of the torso, thereby reducing the magnification that the full torso length would provide. This exercise is an example of how a secondary lever (the arms) can be used to deliberately reduce the magnification of the primary lever (the torso), in this case, to alleviate an unnecessary load on the erector spinae.

To the dismay of people who like to impress observers by lifting heavy weights, *cable squats* are not as "impressive" to watch as watching someone do heavy *barbell squats*. To someone who doesn't understand physics or biomechanics (which is the vast majority of people in a typical gym), the focus is more on large amounts of weight being used (bars bending with numerous 45-pound plates). More than likely, this is the main reason why some people will stick with standard *squats*, and will reject *cable squats*. Others may be less concerned about impressing observers, but will still have a hard time letting go of an old habit. As such, years of brainwashing and misinformation are often not easily dismissed.

The fact is that the direction of resistance, relative to the angle of the tibia, plays a primary role in determining how efficient a quadriceps exercise is. If a person chooses a quad exercise in which the tibia is mostly "neutral" (i.e., mostly parallel with the direction of resistance), then that person will have to use much more weight in order to provide the quadriceps with enough load. Subsequently, using such heavy weights will surely take its toll on the spine, knees, and hips.

Using a direction of resistance that allows a person's tibia to be more "active" (more perpendicular with resistance) allows a higher percentage of the weight being used to load the quads, while simultaneously loading the spine much less. That's a wise training strategy.

Let us now look at some of the other exercises that are typically used to train the quadriceps, and see how efficient—or not efficient—they are. Keep in mind that "efficient," in resistance exercise, means that a greater percentage of the weight being used is loaded onto the target muscle (the quadriceps, in this case). In turn, "inefficient" means that a lesser percentage of the weight being used is loaded onto the target muscle. In fact, it is the "inefficiency" of some exercises (like *barbell squats*) that allows so much weight to be moved.

❑ Hack Squats

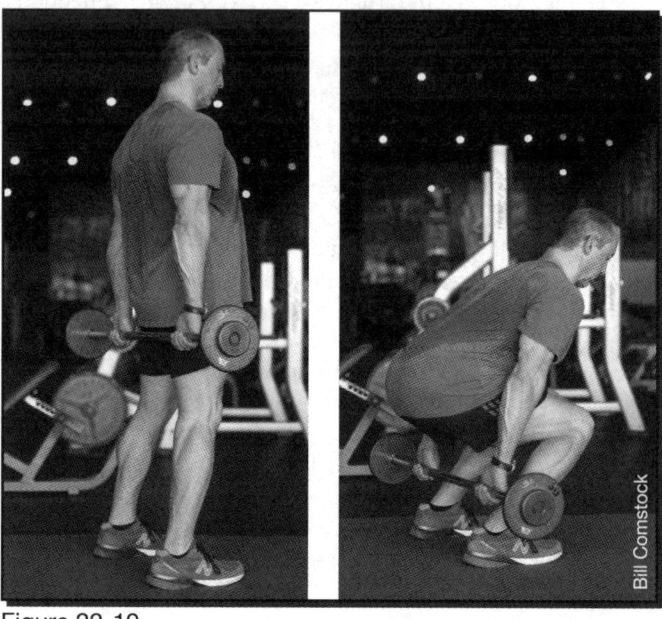

Figure 22-19

The original "*hack squat*" (commonly utilized in the 40s, 50s and 60s) was done by holding a barbell behind the exerciser's buttocks (with the arms straight), and then performing a squatting movement (Figure 22-19).

The intended focus of the exercise was to take the barbell off the spine (which has always been a good idea) and to prevent the torso from leaning forward as much. Holding the barbell lower allows the torso to be more upright, which alleviates the strain on the erector spinae (another good idea). As you can see, even back then, people were trying to find a remedy to the problem of placing a heavy weight on the spine, as well as leaning too far forward during regular *barbell squats*. Although these intentions were good, this exercise was not the solution.

This original, "old-fashioned" *hack squat* was very cumbersome. For starters, it's awkward holding a barbell behind your back. Then, when you get to the descended position of this exercise, the barbell swings underneath your buttocks. Subsequently, in order to rise back up, you have to push the barbell back with your arms, or else it gets blocked by the buttocks. This "pushing the barbell back" is almost impossible, if a heavy weight is being used.

Eventually, the "*hack squat machine*" (Figure 22-20) was invented. Unfortunately, just like *barbell front squats* (Figure 22-21), it only partially solved the problem.

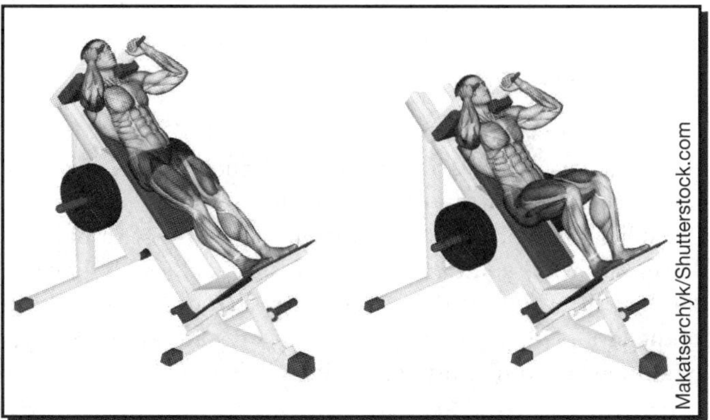


Figure 22-20

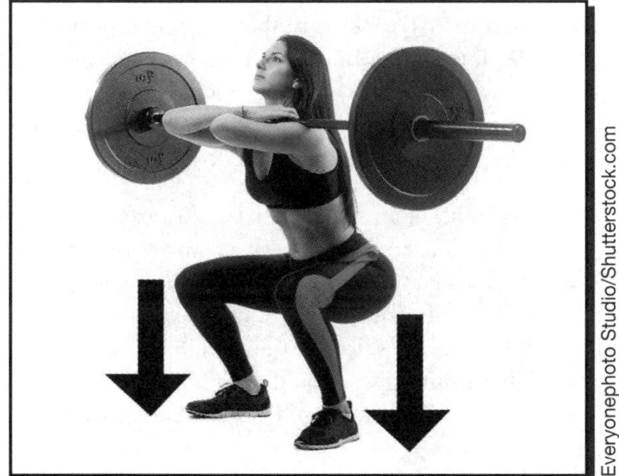


Figure 22-21

The objective of the original *barbell hack squat*, or of a *hack squat* machine, or a *front barbell squat* is to eliminate or reduce the leaning forward of the torso, thereby reducing the stress on the lower back (erector spinae). While that's fine, it does not make any of these exercises more efficient at loading the quadriceps.

The reason these exercises are inefficient is because the operating lever of the quadriceps (i.e., the lower leg) is still mostly parallel with the direction of resistance. This inefficiency then requires that you use more weight, in order to compensate for the fact that the quadriceps are only getting a small percentage of the available resistance. By the time you increase the weight enough to adequately challenge the quadriceps, the downward pull of this heavier weight compresses the spine, and increases the strain on the hip joints and the knee joints.

Notice that the direction of resistance (which is opposite the direction of the trajectory of the movement), on Figures 22-20 and 22-21, and the tibia are very close to being parallel. In both of these exercises, the lower legs are almost "neutral" levers. The tibia are only about 20 to 30 percent "active" (20 to 30 percent away from being completely "neutral"), which means the quadriceps are only getting 20 to 30 percent of the weight that's actually being used.

Go back and look at the *cable squat* photos, for comparison. Notice that the direction of the cable (the arrows) and the tibia are far more perpendicular (i.e., far more "active") than during a *barbell squat*, a *hack squat*, a *front squat*, and the *45-degree leg press* (Figure 22-22), which is why the quadriceps gets a much higher a percentage of the load during *cable squats*.

❑ 45-Degree Leg Press

In Figure 22-22, the arrow indicates the direction of the sled, which represents the direction of resistance. Note that the tibia is almost parallel with the direction of resistance/the arrow. In this instance, the tibia is only about 20 percent "active," which means that, in order to adequately load the quadriceps, a considerable amount of weight must be used. Having to use more weight (being *able* to use more weight) is ONLY due to the inefficient angle of the tibia, during this exercise. If the tibia were more perpendicular with the direction of resistance, a much lighter weight would load the quadriceps more.

*Note: Actually, during a 45-degree leg press, there is also some additional "friction force" that is occurring. The direction of your thrust is not quite parallel with the direction of resistance, because the thrust is originating from the hip joint. If you were to draw an arrow from the hip joint to the feet, it would indicate the actual direction of thrust, which would be slightly more perpendicular with the direction of the sled's movement. This factor, however, is still not enough to qualify the leg press as a "good" (efficient) quadriceps exercise. Other problems with the leg press include a limited range of motion, and "active insufficiency," caused by the piked position of the body (the 90-degree angle of the hip joint).*

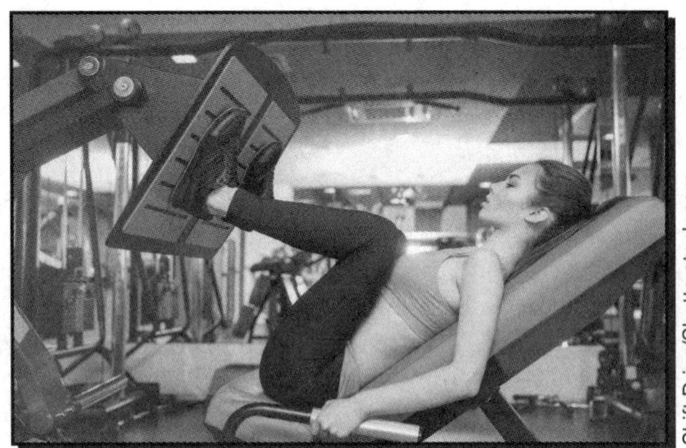


Figure 22-22

It is all-too-common, especially in the (so-called) "hardcore" gyms, to see individuals load up the *45-degree leg presses* with (sometimes) HALF A TON of weight (1000 pounds/more than 20 45-pound plates), wrap their knees, gather a cheering section, and then perform tiny, six-inch repetitions (i.e., very short range of motion), with their mostly "neutral" tibias. Meanwhile, their skeleton (knees, ankles and hips) are near the breaking point. This approach is far from intelligent muscle-building. Rather, it is pure naiveté, exhibitionism, and ego gratification, with very little actual muscle-building reward for the effort and risk involved. You would get much more muscle stimulation with less weight, less wasted effort, and less stress to your skeleton, using a more efficient exercise (one that allows the tibia to interact more perpendicularly with the direction of resistance).

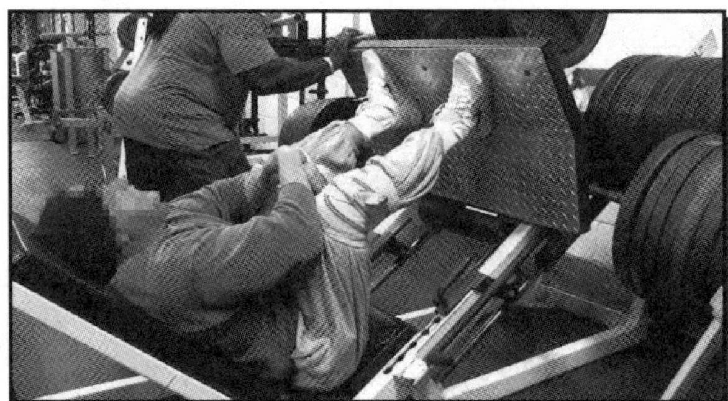

Figure 22-23

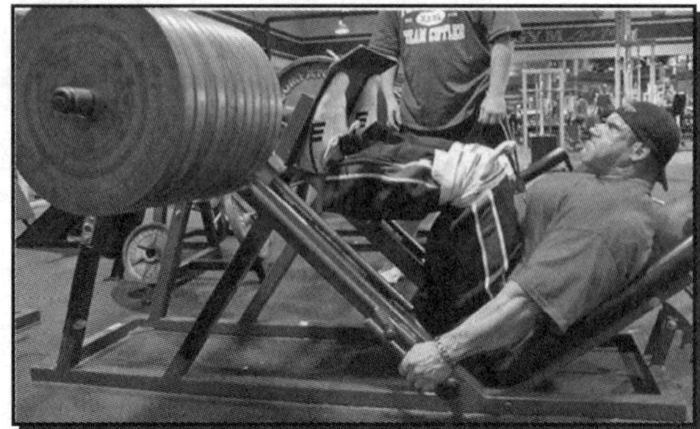

Figure 22-24

If the feet were placed lower on the platform, it would cause the tibia to be slightly more perpendicular with the direction of resistance, as well as cause the knees to bend more (better range of motion). This factor would improve the exercise a bit, even though less weight would have to be used. This adjustment, however, would still not qualify this exercise as "very good."

Most *leg press* machines do not provide a foot plate that allows you to place your feet low enough to adequately improve the efficiency of the exercise (to allow the tibia to be sufficiently perpendicular with the direction of resistance). Furthermore, if you *could* place your feet sufficiently low (for the benefit of the quads), it would cause your heels to lift off of the foot plate, which might make it stressful on the Achilles tendon, when you're using a heavy weight.

In addition, the seated position (i.e., "piked" position) prevents you from using a full range of motion. Note, in Figures 22-23 and 22-24, how the thighs collide with the ribcage, when the exerciser is in the descended position. Note also that the knees may not have even reached a 90-degree bend yet. In other words, getting enough range of motion (sufficient knee bend) on a leg press, is essentially impossible, because of the piked position of the body.

If a person has a large belly (or large ribcage), it's unlikely they'll even be able to reach a 70- or an 80-degree bend in their knees. Ideally, the knees should bend slightly beyond 90 degrees, for full range of motion, when in the descended position. It would help to tilt the seat back as far back as possible. This positioning would give the knees a bit more clearance, although it might still not be enough for an ideal range of motion.

When you perform a *squat* (bodyweight or otherwise), "proper form" requires you to keep your back slightly arched. This positioning is called a "neutral spine." When doing a *leg press*, however, this position is almost impossible to attain, except (possibly) in the starting position, when the legs are extended. By the time the sled is halfway down, your tailbone has begun curling under, thereby "rounding" your lower back. If you're using a heavy weight (as is usually the case with ambitious bodybuilders), this load places a significant strain on the lumbar spine.

As an experiment, try bending over, while standing, so that your torso is nearly parallel with the floor (Figure 22-25, left image). Next, do 20 reps of *squats*, while keeping your body piked in that position (torso nearly horizontal) the entire time, even when your legs are straight. That sequence is essentially what you're doing when you perform *45-degree leg presses* (Figure 22-25, right image). It is basically a "*partial range of motion knee and hip extension*, while bent at the waist." Arguably, no one would consider this a "good exercise," but that is the exact set of mechanics of a *45-degree leg press* exercise.

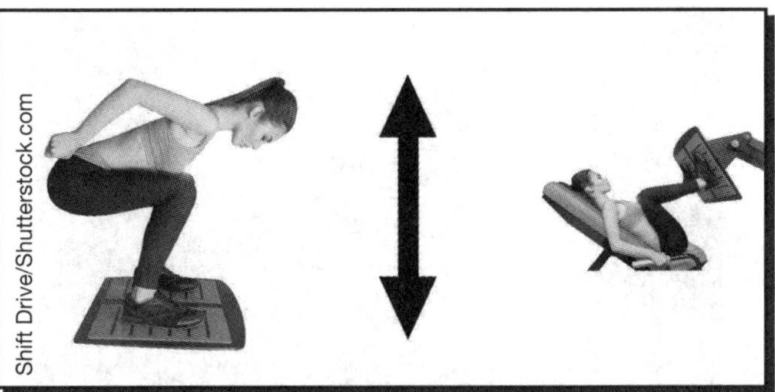

Figure 22-25

As a final cautionary note regarding heavy *leg presses*, take a look at the six photos in Figures 22-26 to 22-28. This person is attempting to perform *45-degree leg presses*, with a very large amount of weight. It appears to be approximately 1,335 pounds. In the first photo, he's completing a repetition (with a very short range of motion), and then suddenly his left knee buckles the opposite direction (second photo). Subsequently, he's left with only his right leg supporting the entire 1,335 pounds and failing, of course. The weighted sled drops down, further bending his left knee backward. Finally, the sled stops at the safety stop of the machine.

Clearly, his left knee joint was severely damaged, probably having ripped all the tendons, ligaments, and muscles that typically attach to the knee. It's possible that veins and arteries were also severed. Knee damage this severe is likely not repairable, possibly requiring amputation from the mid-femur, down. Then, presumably, a prosthetic leg would be put in place.

Fortunately, this type of accident is very rare. It likely occurred, at least in part, because of a genetic tendency for this person's knees to hyperextend. Nevertheless, it was absolutely foolish for him to be attempting to *leg press* (as a verb) this much weight. There was nothing to be gained from it, in terms of muscle development. On the other hand, there was an enormous amount of potential injury risk.

Many people get caught up in this "beast mode" mentality. When you combine that attitude, with knowing nothing about biomechanics or exercise efficiency, you believe that what matters most is lifting extremely heavy weight. In reality, the mantra of "the heavier, the better" is entirely wrong for the pursuit of physique development, and also for general fitness.

The fitness industry, which includes manufacturers of gym equipment, is primarily concerned with revenues. There is a constant need to sell new exercise machines. This is not difficult to do, since consumers typically like whatever is "new"—never mind whether or not a new machine is actually better. With this factor in mind, look at Figure 22-29 and Figure 22-30.

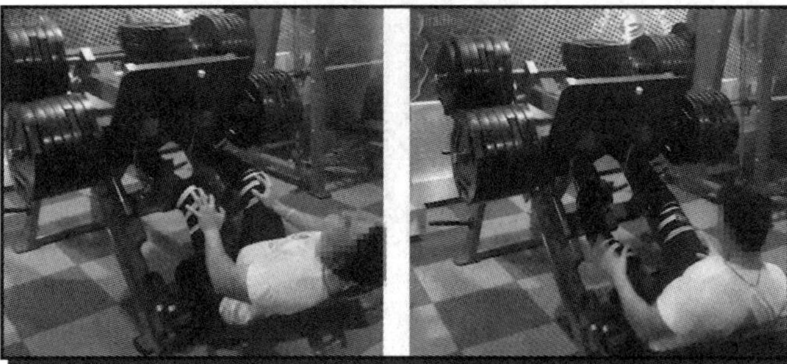
Figure 22-26

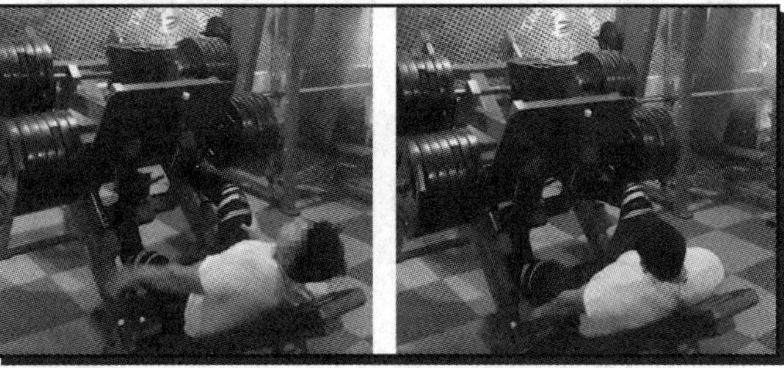
Figure 22-27

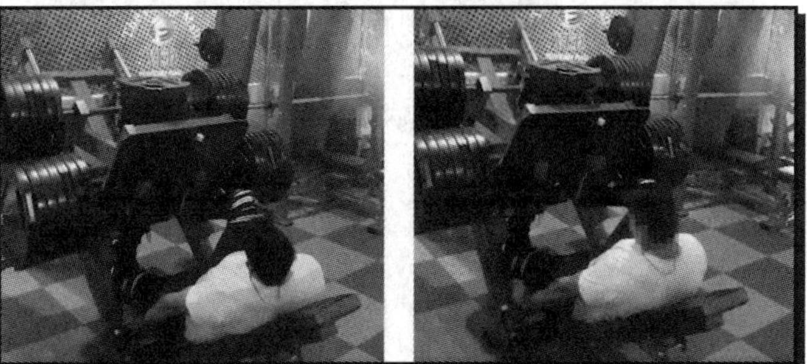
Figure 22-28

Next, imagine that the *lying* exercise represented in Figure 22-29, is "re-created" as a *seated* exercise (Figure 22-30) by the gym equipment industry. The arrows in both images represent the direction of resistance of each version, meaning that the mechanics (the physics) of Figure 22-29 is duplicated in the version represented in 22-30.

The point of this comparison is to demonstrate that the compromised physics shown in Figure 22-29 (i.e., inefficient because the forearm never reaches the perpendicular angle with resistance) is duplicated in a "machine" represented by Figure 22-30, and this happens very often. Gym equipment manufacturers create machines that duplicate the same biomechanical flaws that occur with other machines or with free weight exercises, instead of correcting them. In fact, it does not matter what the position of the body is. What matters is the direction of resistance, relative to the limbs that are operating the target muscle.

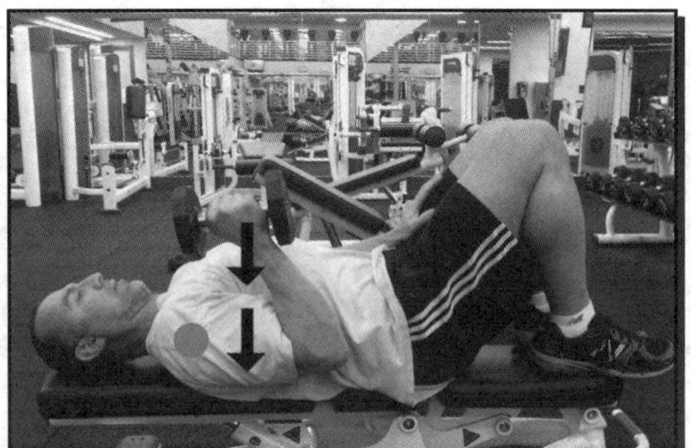
Figure 22-29

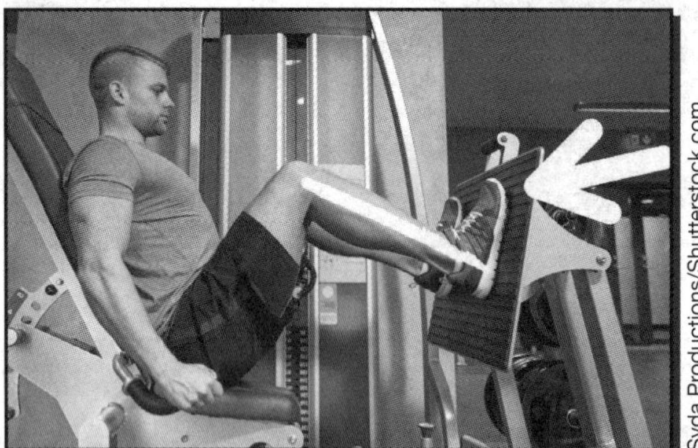
Syda Productions/Shutterstock.com

Figure 22-30

This factor is true, whether the exercise is meant to load the triceps or the quadriceps (or any other muscle). Gym equipment manufacturers have created various *squat* and *leg press* machines, changing the position of the body one way or another, but duplicating the most glaring problem of the standard *barbell squat*: the inefficient angle at which the tibia interacts with the direction of resistance. In Figure 22-30 (meant to represent a *leg press* version of the action shown in Figure 22-29), the exerciser is using the same inefficient angle (of his lower leg), relative to the direction of resistance. The body position is different, and the operating lever is the lower leg instead of the forearm, but the flawed mechanics is the same.

What would improved mechanics look like? It would look like the better version of a triceps exercise, shown earlier (shown again in Figure 22-31), with the forearm (or the lower leg) being more perpendicular with resistance.

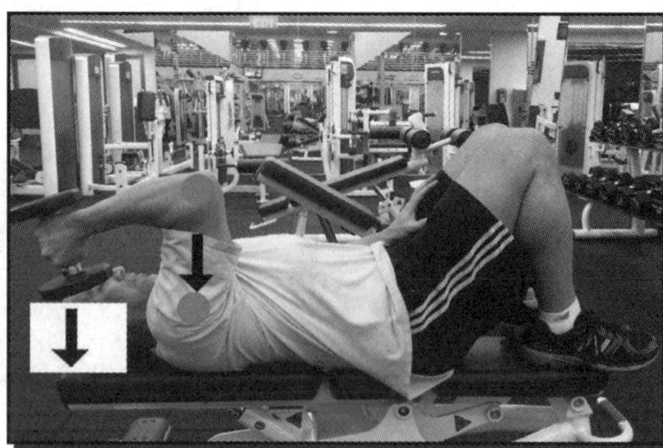
Figure 22-31

The two sets of images in Figure 22-32 show similar actions, with similar physics. The two images at the top show a knee extension (by way of a "*sissy squat*"), being produced by the contraction of the quadriceps, and the lower leg reaching a more perpendicular angle with gravity. The two images at the bottom show an elbow extension, being produced by the contraction of the triceps, with the forearm reaching a mostly perpendicular angle with the cable (which indicates the direction of resistance of this exercise). The elbow extension being performed at the bottom is considered a "standard" method of working the triceps. In contrast, the knee extension being performed at the top is not considered "standard," even though it's the same action with the same physics. Some individuals might even claim that that knee extension is "bad for the knees." Is the elbow extension being performed at the bottom "bad for the elbows?" Of course not. These two actions are exactly the same—and both are good.

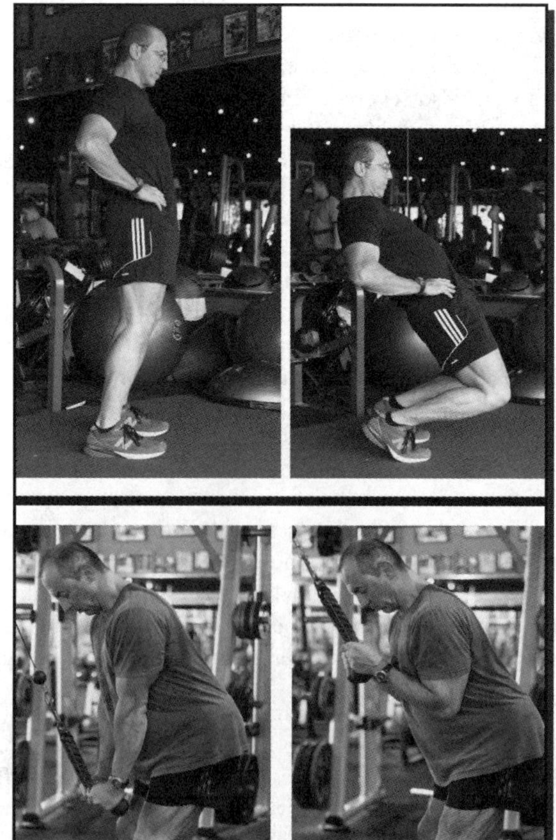
Bill Comstock

Figure 22-32

Allowing the tibia to interact perpendicularly with the direction of resistance benefits the quadriceps much more than doing an exercise that limits the tibia to a mostly parallel angle, relative to the direction of resistance.

Why has the fitness industry continued producing *leg press* machines that inefficiently keep the lower leg mostly parallel (mostly neutral), with the direction of resistance, and limit the range of motion? The reason is simple—it's because people buy *leg press* machines. People like *leg press* machines, because they allow the user to load them with a lot of weight, thereby creating the illusion that it's benefiting their leg muscles more than exercises which don't allow them to use as much weight. In fact, *sissy squats* are significantly better for the quadriceps, and a machine is not needed at all to perform a *sissy squat*. Thus, there is no economic incentive for the equipment manufacturers to acknowledge that a *sissy squat* is better than a *leg press*.

In addition, individuals who want to be regarded as being in "beast mode" (when they're working their legs) prefer using a machine that allows them to use a lot of weight. One way of doing that is by preventing their tibia (their lower leg) from interacting perpendicularly with the direction of resistance—hence, the *leg press*. Conversely, an exercise that allows their tibia to interact perpendicularly with resistance loads their quadriceps with a greater percentage of the weight being used. As a result, a lighter weight feels heavier. This situation is usually considered as less appealing to individuals who want to impress observers, despite the fact that it's simply a more efficient and sensible way to load the quadriceps.

In other words, the industry has taken advantage of the naiveté and validation dependency of the average consumer, and has created ridiculous machines that allow the use of heavy weight, but only because a small percentage of that weight actually loads the target muscle. Part of that naiveté is not understanding that by improving the mechanics in a way that benefits the quadriceps, the participation of the gluteus is reduced, and vice versa. The irrational reverence of "compound exercises," and the irrational disregard of "isolation exercises," has misled consumers into believing that they must do heavy *squats* and heavy *leg presses*, or else they won't develop large quads.

Interestingly, people don't apply quite the same degree of irrational thinking, when they work their triceps. They seem to be more accepting of isolation exercises (exercises that allow their forearm—which is the operating lever of the triceps—to interact perpendicularly with resistance), when working their triceps. The same mechanics should be applied with regard to the quadriceps, because the arm (humerus, forearm, and elbow joint) and the leg (femur, lower leg, and knee joint) are similar mechanisms, and the same physics are at play.

❑ Sissy Squats

The exercise shown in Figure 22-33 is called the "*sissy squat*," believed to have been named (a century ago) after "King Sisyphos," of Greek mythology. This exercise is very challenging, precisely because it's very efficient. In fact, it's often too efficient (too challenging) for many people, even when no additional weight is used. The reason? The tibia is maximally "active." In other words, it goes more perpendicular (relative to the direction of resistance) than most other quadriceps exercises—never mind that nonsense about "not letting the knees go over the toes."

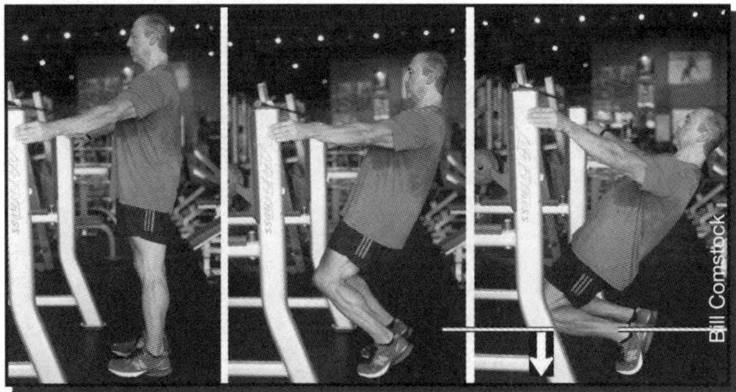

Figure 22-33

In Figure 22-33, far right image, notice how perpendicular the angle of the tibia is, relative to the arrow (indicating the direction of resistance). That's a very "active" lever. Go back and compare THAT degree of "active" (perpendicular with resistance) with the tibia angle of the *leg press*, the *hack squat*, the *front squat*, and the *barbell squat*.

Another way of getting this type of "perpendicular-ness," when working the quadriceps, is shown in Figures 22-34 and 22-35. This exercise—"*cable sissy squats*"—is very similar to a standard *sissy squat*, but with a comfortable way of adding resistance. It's also easier to keep your heels down on the ground, because of the backward lean of the body, which the forward-pull of the cable allows. Note the degree of "perpendicular-ness" that occurs between the cable and the tibia, in Figure 22-35.

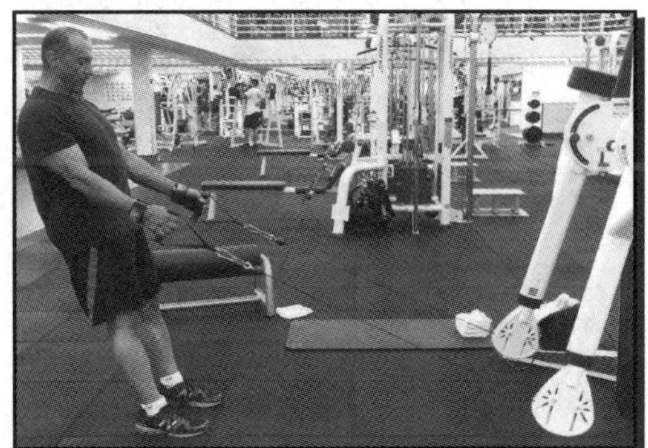
Figure 22-34

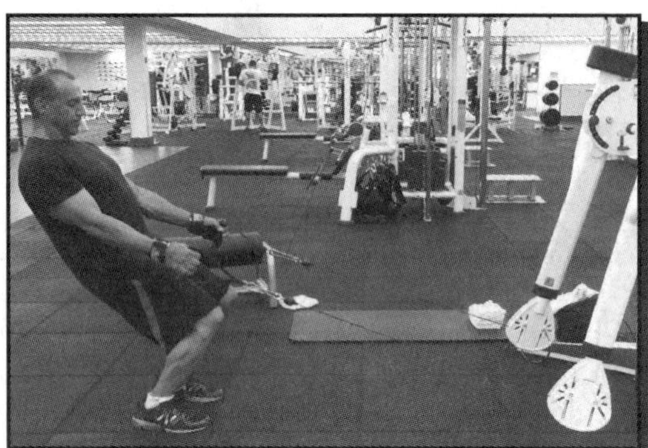
Figure 22-35

❑ Reciprocal Innervation and the Preferred Hip Angle

You'll recall two points discussed earlier in this chapter, when I said—"*...There is one additional reason why it's better to work either the quadriceps OR the glutes, during a given exercise.*" I explained that, "...there are five features that should be considered, when selecting the best exercise(s) for your quadriceps." The fifth feature is *"the avoidance of interference," which refers to "reciprocal innervation" and "active insufficiency."*

In the two images in Figure 22-36, I am doing two different exercises: in the upper image, a "*cable squat,*" using conventional "squat form"; in the lower image, a *cable sissy squat*, during which my pelvis moves forward (instead of back), and my torso leans back (instead of leaning forward).

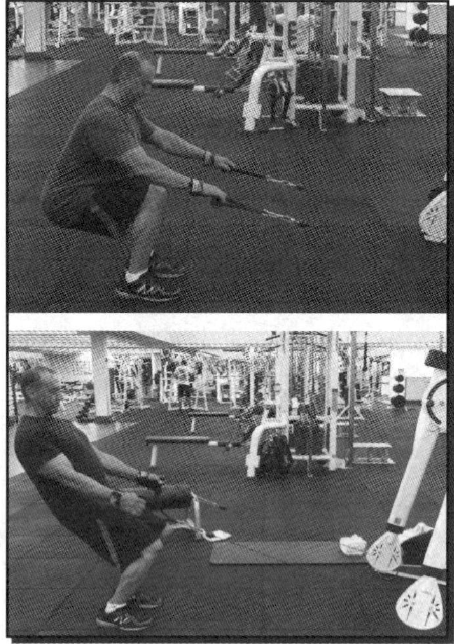
Figure 22-36

You would probably think that the movement shown in the upper image (the more conventional "squat" motion) would feel easier than the movement shown in the lower image, even though the same weight is being used in both. After all, the movement in the upper image involves four muscle groups—the quads, glutes, hamstrings, and adductors—while the movement in the lower image only involves the quads. Yet, the movement shown in the lower image (*cable sissy squat*) feels easier, despite only the quadriceps working, and despite the cable (direction of resistance) being more perpendicular with the tibia, than it is during the movement in the upper image (a standard *cable squat*). Obviously, something interesting is going on here.

Try this experiment yourself, and you'll see that the *cable sissy squat* is easier than the *cable squat*, using the same weight in both instances. One reason for this is that during a traditional "*squatting*" motion (moving the knee joint *and* the hip joint, and engaging the quads, glutes, hamstrings, and adductors *simultaneously*), several neurological conflicts of interest occur, which compromises the strength potential of each participating muscle.

The quadriceps and hamstrings are antagonist muscles, so they cannot both be activated with full force simultaneously, due to reciprocal innervation. Loading and activation of one muscle causes a relaxation synapse to be sent to the opposing muscle, which essentially "weakens" it. The hamstrings plays two roles—knee flexion (primarily) and hip extension (secondarily). Since hip extension is one of the actions occurring during a *squatting* motion, the hamstrings are required to participate. That participation, however, automatically causes the antagonist of the hamstrings—the quadriceps—to be weakened, to a degree. Likewise, the loading and activation of the quadriceps (during a squatting motion), weakens its antagonist—the hamstrings.

In addition, loading and activating the glutes and adductors (as typically occurs when squatting)—which are the primary hip extensors—automatically sends a relaxation synapse to the hip flexors (which are the antagonists of the hip extensors), again due to reciprocal innervation. One of the hip flexors is the rectus femoris muscle, which is one of the four quadriceps heads. In other words, loading and activating the hip extension muscles weakens a primary quadriceps muscle—the rectus femoris. Given that squats are typically used for quadriceps development, this is obviously counterproductive. This neurological compromise was reported in the *Journal of Sports Biomechanics*, Volume 14, 2015 - issue 1, by Megan A. Bryanton, Jason P. Carey, Michael D. Kennedy and Loren Z.F. Chiu.

You'll recall in Chapter 11 that the issue of "active insufficiency" was discussed. This is when a muscle is forced to contract, while it's in a pre-shortened position, resulting in compromised strength. It was established that *leg curls (knee flexion)* performed on a *seated leg curl machine* is "better" than knee flexion performed on the *lying (prone) leg curl machine*, because it avoids "active insufficiency." When knee flexion (leg curl) is performed, while the hip joint is "straight" (i.e., the femur is mostly parallel with the torso), the strength potential of the hamstring is compromised, because the straight hip angle overly shortens the hamstrings (i.e., the muscle insertion is brought too close to muscle origin).

The same weakness that occurs in the hamstrings during supine (hip straight) *leg curls*, happens in the quadriceps during knee extension that is performed while the hip joint is excessively bent. The quads function better (have more strength potential) when the hip is mostly "straight," i.e., mostly parallel with the torso, because the quadriceps (specifically, the rectus femoris) are more elongated, and not prone to active insufficiency.

Notice that during a squatting movement the hip joint bends to approximately 90 degrees (relative to the torso), when it's in the descended position. This degree of hip flexion partially compromises the strength potential of the quadriceps. Conversely—during the *sissy squat* version—the hip angle is more "straight" (more parallel with the torso). When the femur is kept more parallel with the torso, while the quadriceps are loaded/activated, there is less active insufficiency that occurs—less inhibition of optimal quadriceps contraction.

For this same reason, it's good to perform your *leg extensions* the way that I demonstrate in Figure 22-37. Note that the machine's backrest has been moved as far back as possible, and I allow my torso to lean as far back as possible. This positioning allows my femurs to be more parallel with my torso, instead of at the usual 90-degree angle to the torso (as would be the case, if I were sitting perfectly upright).

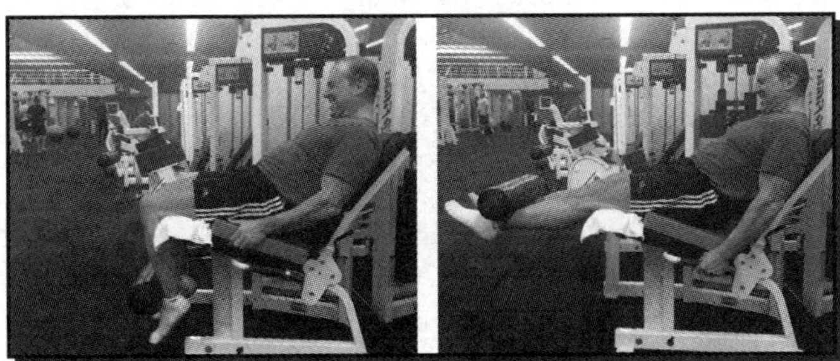

Figure 22-37

You'll be surprised at how this technique allows the quadriceps to be more fully engaged. By allowing the femurs to be more parallel with the torso, the quadriceps experience less active insufficiency (the over-shortening of the rectus femoris). The quadriceps also experience less passive insufficiency (the over-stretching of the hamstrings), which occurs when the knees are fully extended and the hip angle is bent at nearly 90 degrees. Passive insufficiency is another form of interference that would be caused by a less-than-optimal hip angle, when trying to work the quadriceps with maximum efficiency. This same "over-stretching of the hamstrings" occurs during a standard 45-degree leg press, because the hip is bent at approximately a 90-degree angle, and the knees are fully extended to the "leg straight" position. This passive insufficiency and the active insufficiency, that occurs when the hip is bent and the knees are straight, is made worse when the seat back is brought forward as much as possible.

As you can see, several forms of neurological interference (quadriceps weakening) occur, when *squats* and *leg presses* are performed. These include reciprocal innervation—caused by the simultaneous loading of antagonist muscles—and also active/passive insufficiencies—caused by excessive muscle shortening of the working muscle and excessive muscle stretching of the antagonist muscle.

As such, there is no logical reason to believe that combining hip extension (gluteus activation) with knee extension (quadriceps activation) in a single exercise, such as *squats* or *leg presses*, would result in better quadriceps activation, than would result from isolated quadriceps activation. In fact, quadriceps activation is compromised when it is combined with hip extension (gluteus, adductor, and hamstrings loading and activation).

Accordingly, the questions that everyone should ask themselves, when deciding whether or not to do *squats* and *leg presses* (for the purpose of quadriceps/glutes development), are the following:

- Does combining the loading of the quadriceps, at the same time as the loading of the glutes (i.e., by way of *squats* and *leg presses*), produce a better result in each of these muscle groups, as compared with working these muscles with isolation exercises? The answer is "no."
- Does combining the two actions (knee extension and hip extension) produce a benefit that is AS GOOD for the quads and glutes, as it would be if these two actions were performed separately? The answer is "no."
- Does combining the two actions (knee extension and hip extension) produce a compromised benefit to the quads and the glutes, as compared with the benefits that could be achieved by working each set of muscles separately? The answer is "yes."

The benefit to the quads and the glutes, produced by standard *squats* and *leg presses*, is compromised (as compared with working these muscles separately with isolation exercises) due to mechanical inefficiencies—the compromised angle of the tibia, and the reduced moment arm ("effective lever length") of the femur, as well as the neurological aforementioned interferences. Further compromising the value of doing heavy *squats* and *leg presses* is the high risk of injury (spinal compression, as well as hip strain and knee strain), as compared with isolation exercises.

Of course, working the quadriceps with isolation exercises (*leg extensions* and *sissy squats*) means that you'll have to work the glutes separately, which is perfectly fine. *Squats* and *leg presses* work the quads and the glutes simultaneously, but neither muscle group gets optimal stimulation during those exercises. As such, most people are compelled to do isolation exercises in addition to the compound exercise. In fact, isolation exercise is all that is needed.

❑ Best Exercises for the Quadriceps

The best two exercises for the quadriceps are *sissy squats* and *leg extensions*. *Sissy squats* are typically done with just bodyweight, but if additional weight is needed or desired, the best two best ways to apply it are either by way of a weighted vest or by using a pair of downward/frontward pulling cables, as shown in Figures 22-34 and 22-35.

Glutes will be discussed in the next chapter, and you'll see that a dedicated glute exercise is mechanically superior for gluteus development, as compared with compound exercises. A dedicated glute exercise allows more efficient mechanics (use of the full femur), a more complete range of motion, a better (more productive) resistance curve, the avoidance of neurological interference (no reciprocal innervation), and—when performed unilaterally—the avoidance of bilateral deficit and the benefit of unilateral focus.

## Anatomy of the Hamstrings

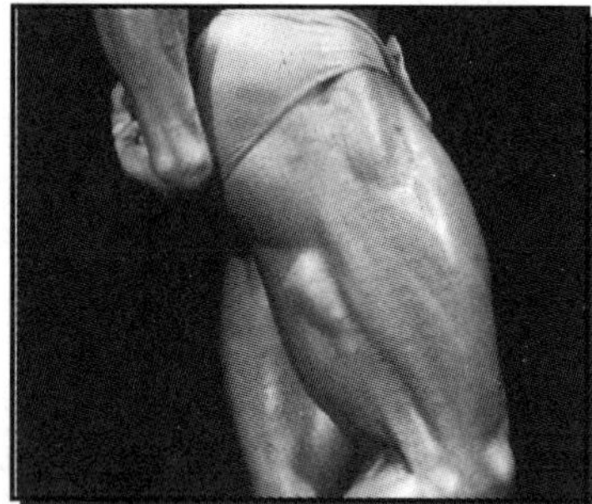

Figure 22-38

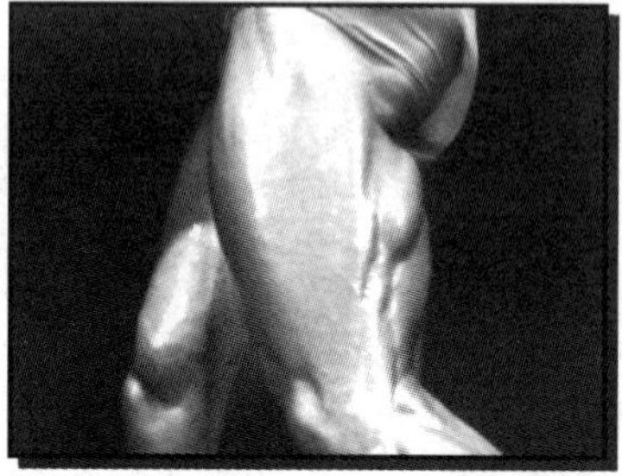

Figure 22-39

"Hamstrings" is the common name used to refer to the group of four muscles that are on the back of the thigh. This muscle group is made up of the biceps femoris short head and biceps femoris long head, as well as the semimembranosus and the semitendinosus (all shown in Figure 22-40).

The Hamstring Group

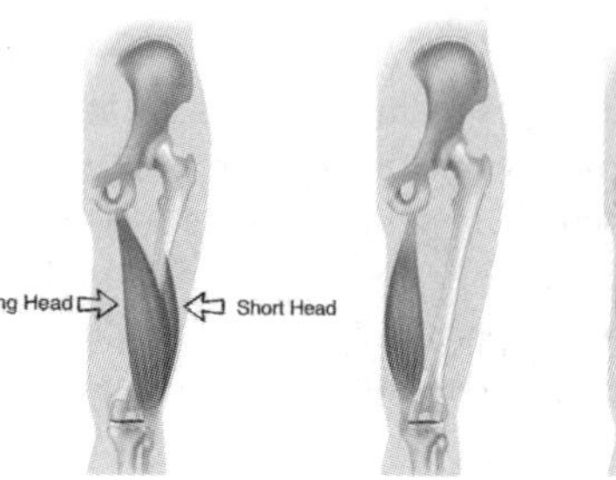


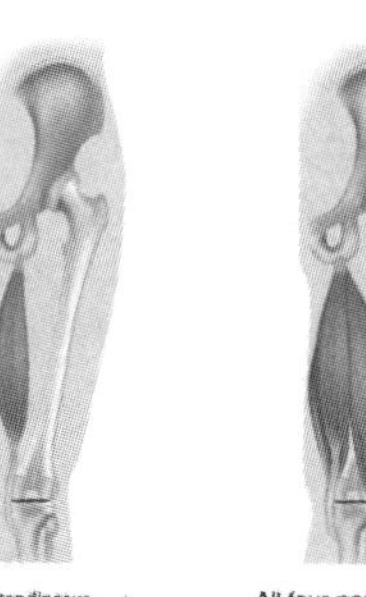


Alila Medical Media/Shutterstock.com

Figure 22-40

In Figure 22-40, you are looking at the right leg, as seen from the rear (posterior view), as if the person is looking away from you. You can clearly see the origins and insertions of each of these four parts of the hamstrings.

The long head of the biceps femoris originates on the pelvis, on the boney loop at the base of the pelvis called the "ischial tuberosity." The short head of the biceps femoris (the smallest of the four heads) originates relatively low on the femur itself. Both of these "heads" then insert onto the head of the fibula, the thinner of the two lower leg bones. Notice that both of these insertions are on the outer side (lateral aspect) of the knee.

The two middle illustrations in Figure 22-40 show the semimembranosus and the semitendinosus. Both of these heads also originate on the ischial tuberosity of the pelvis, and then insert onto the upper end of the tibia (the larger of the two lower leg bones). Notice that both of these insertions are on the inner side (medial aspect) of the knee.

Figure 22-41 and 22-42 show how these hamstring elements look, as part of the whole body musculature. The "A" arrows point to the long head of the biceps femoris, and the "B" arrows point to the semitendinosus.

Figure 22-43 provides a better perspective of the various components of the hamstrings. It allows you to see that the semimembranosus (3) lies partially BENEATH the semitendinosus (2). In turn, the short head of the biceps femoris (4) lies mostly BENEATH the long head of the biceps femoris (1). The more superficial muscles (the ones closer to the surface) are the biceps femoris long head (1, starting on the inside of the femur, but attaching on the outside of the leg, just below the knee) and the semitendinosus (2, starting on the

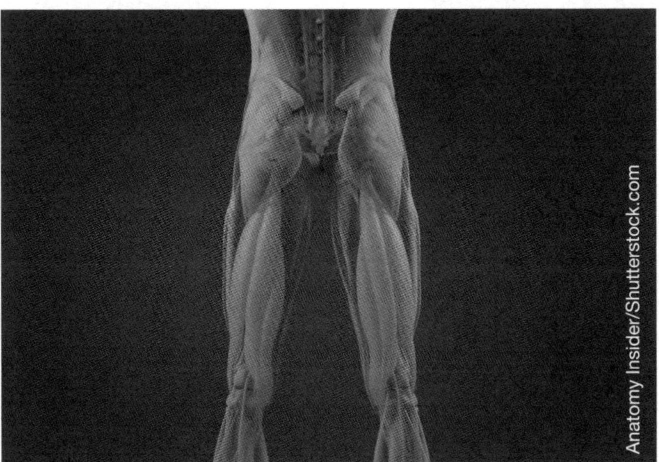

Figure 22-41

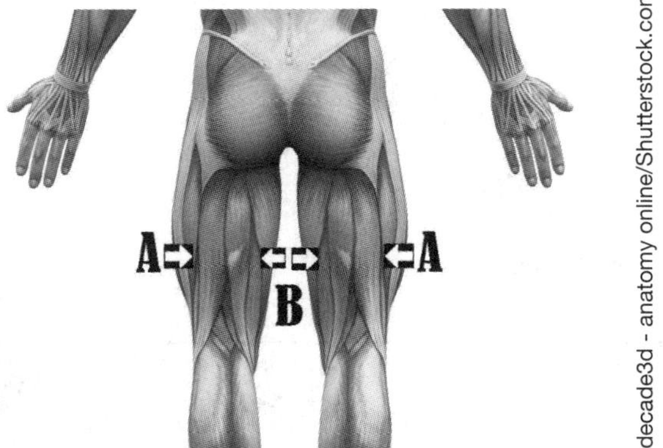

Figure 22-42

inside of the femur, and also attaching on the inside of the lower leg, just below the knee). These are the two muscles that are most visible through the skin, when an individual's level of body fat is sufficiently low.

All four parts of the hamstrings operate in unison, and collectively perform the action of knee flexion, as their primary function, which is illustrated in Figure 22-44—bending the knee/bringing the heel of the foot back and up, toward the buttocks.

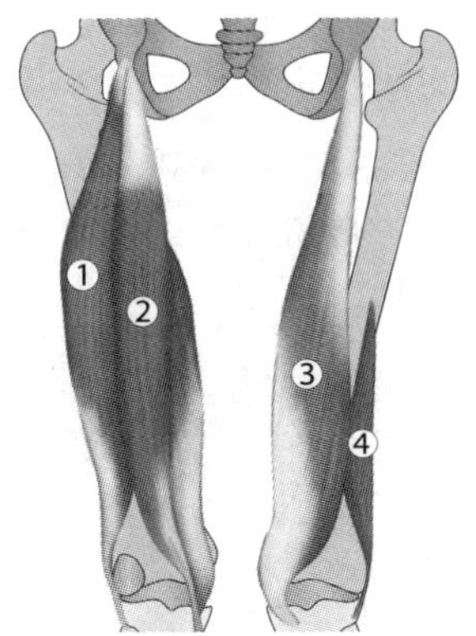

Figure 22-43

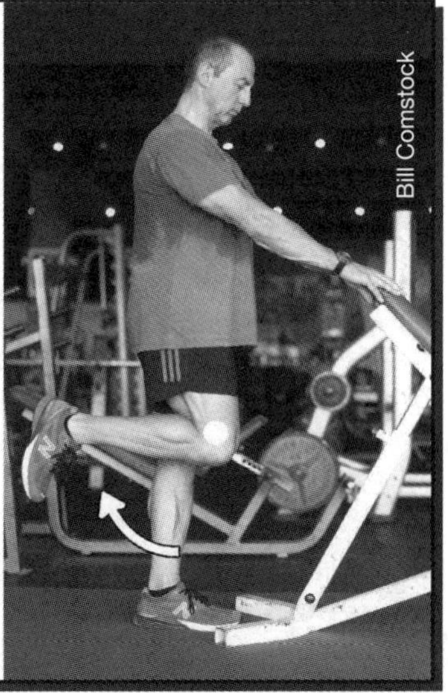

Figure 22-44

The secondary function of the hamstrings is to assist in hip extension, shown in Figure 22-45. Hip extension, however, is performed mostly by the gluteus and the adductors. The hamstrings' role in hip extension is essentially equivalent to the biceps brachii's role in shoulder abduction (the movement more commonly known as a "front deltoid raise"). In other words, the hamstrings' role in hip extension is minor.

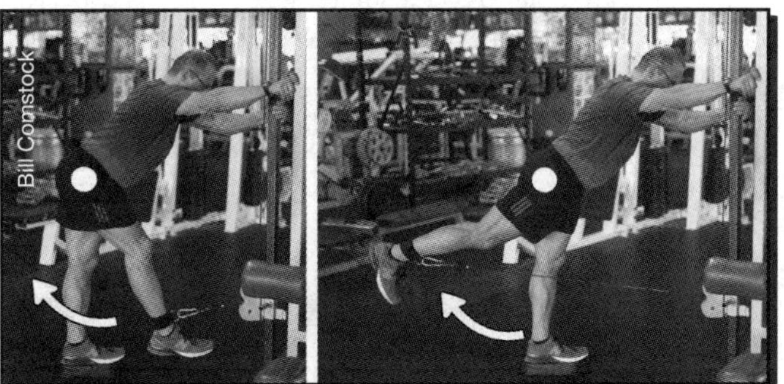

Figure 22-45

The reason that the hamstrings' role in hip extension is minor is because the gluteus (and the adductors) are so dominant in that action. Note that the origin of the gluteus maximus is significantly above the hip joint (Figure 22-46), whereas the origin of the hamstring is actually below the hip joint (Figure 22-7, left image), on the ischial tuberosity. As a result, the hamstrings have much less leverage on the femur, during hip extension, as compared with the gluteus.

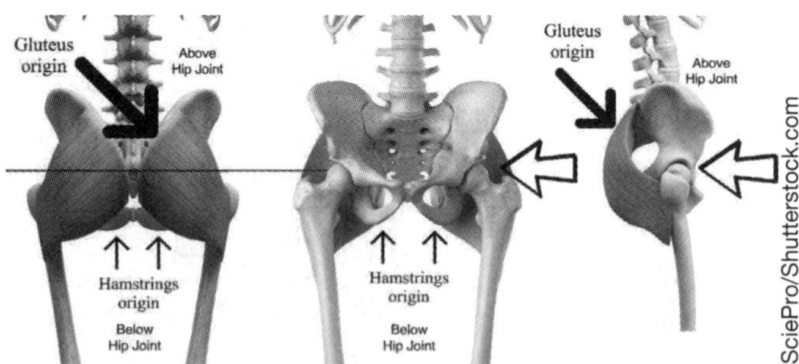


Figure 22-46

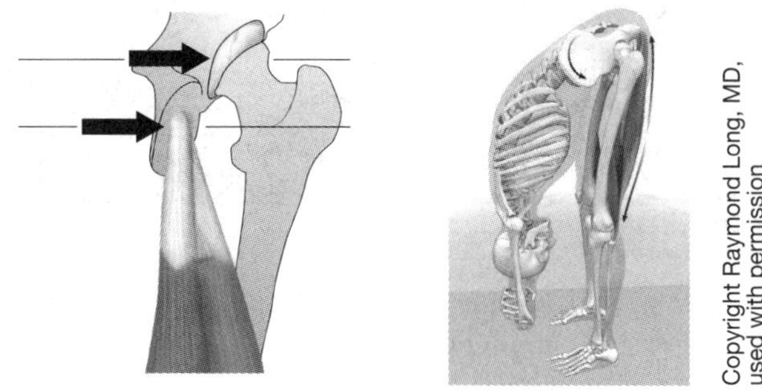


Figure 22-47

Since the hamstrings play such a minor role in hip extension, performing a *stiff-legged deadlift*, for the purpose of developing the hamstrings, is not a good strategy. The only reason you are able to feel a stretch when you bend over, is because doing so causes the posterior part of the pelvis to tilt upward (Figure 22-47, right image)—especially if your spine is arched. On the other hand, the action of raising the torso upward (from the bent-over position) is mostly performed by the glutes and the adductors. The hamstrings are not able to contribute much force in that action.

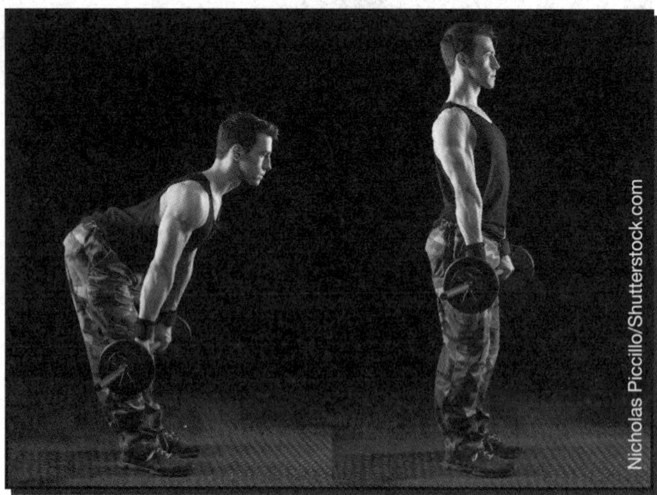


Figure 22-48

By way of comparison, look at the biceps of the arm, which has very similar mechanics to the hamstrings. The origin of the biceps crosses the shoulder joint (Figure 22-49), just like the hamstring crosses the hip joint. In both instances, these muscles play an extremely minor role in the movement of the shoulder (i.e., the biceps) and of the hip (i.e., the hamstrings)—respectively. In both cases, a more primary muscle dominates the movement of those joints—the anterior deltoid (shoulder abduction) and the gluteus (hip extension).

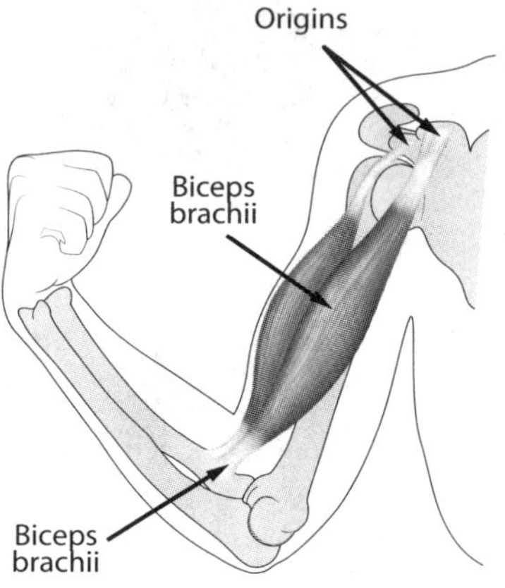


Figure 22-49

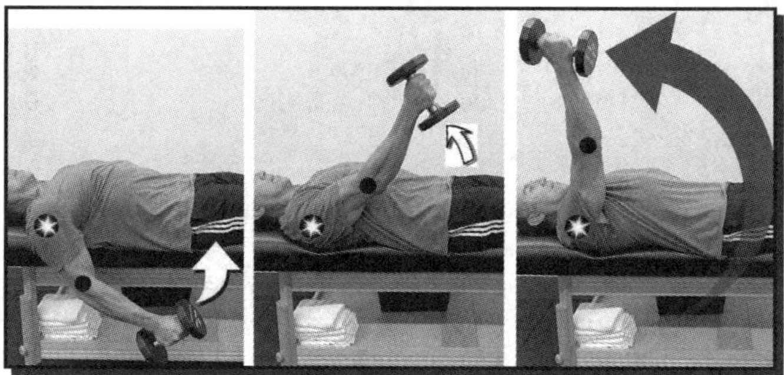

Figure 22-50

If you were to lie flat on your back on a bench, and allow your straight arm to descend below the level of your torso (Figure 22-50), you would feel a stretch in your biceps. If you were to then raise your straight arm upward, the biceps would play an extremely small role in that movement. The primary work would be done by the anterior deltoid.

You would never consider the action represented by the aforementioned example to be a "good" biceps exercise. That action, however, is the mechanical equivalent of a "*stiff-legged deadlift.*" Attempting to develop a muscle by performing an action that is a significantly minor role for that muscle, is simply not a wise strategy.

Muscle development is best stimulated by way of muscle contraction, which implies a substantial degree of muscle "shortening," during which the actin filaments slide sufficiently together to cause the adaptation of hypertrophy (growth). Stretching a muscle, without contracting/shortening it, is not enough to cause much muscle growth, even though loaded stretching can cause a degree of muscle soreness.

There is a functional value in strengthening the "posterior chain" muscles (i.e., which include the glutes and hamstrings), by way of hip extension. The hamstrings do, in fact, contribute to hip extension, as one of several participating muscles. Any good glute exercise, however, already challenges ("works") the hip extension "function" of the hamstrings. This will be discussed in the next chapter.

More importantly, the hamstring shortening that occurs during "*stiff-legged deadlifts*" is insufficient for the goal of hamstring growth. Knee flexion (fully bending the knee) is essential for a hamstrings exercise to be sufficiently stimulating, wherein it results in visible muscle growth.

❑ The Ideal Anatomical Motion for Training the Hamstrings

At this point, it should be obvious that "bending the knee," also known as "knee flexion," is the primary function of the hamstrings. The position of the hip, however, also matters, when you're working the hamstrings. This factor is similar to the mechanics of the arm, where the position of the humerus (the shoulder joint) during a biceps exercise, also matters.

For a number of years, the standard *prone leg curl* machine (lying facing down) has generally been accepted as the best exercise for the hamstrings. There are, however, two other factors, besides knee flexion, which also play a role in determining the ideal action of the hamstrings—"active insufficiency" and "passive insufficiency."

Muscles operate best (i.e., have the most strength potential) when they are at the optimal length, neither overly elongated nor overly shortened. Since the hamstrings crosses two joints (the hip and the knee), the position of the hip influences the "length" of the hamstrings (i.e., the distance between the origin and the insertion). When the hip angle is "straight" (the femur is mostly parallel with the torso), the hamstrings are starting their knee flexion from an overly shortened position.

As the knee is further flexed, and the hamstrings insertion moves even closer to its origin, the actin filaments "run out of room," and are unable to contract with optimum efficiency. They essentially "collide" into each other, and have a reduced capacity to produce contractile force. This is "active insufficiency"—the muscle that is active (in this case, the hamstrings), has an insufficient amount of length (distance between its origin and insertion), with which to optimally contract.

For this reason, it would be better if the hip angle were bent to approximately 90 degrees, thereby allowing more distance between the hamstrings origin and insertion, and avoiding the muscle contraction compromise that is otherwise caused by active insufficiency (over-shortened hamstrings), when trying to optimally load and contract the hamstrings.

Furthermore, the angle of the hip also plays a role in how much a person's quadriceps stretches, when the knee is flexed. As such, when performing a knee flexion exercise with the hip "straight" (i.e., the femur mostly parallel with the torso)—as occurs during the standard *prone leg curl* (lying face down on the bench)—the degree of quadriceps stretch that is produced interferes (to a degree) with the range of motion that could otherwise be produced, if the quadriceps were not being over-stretched, while the knee is bending. This stretching of the quadriceps also triggers a degree of reciprocal innervation (of the hamstrings). The CNS (central nervous system) registers activity/potential danger of the quadriceps (extreme stretching), thereby sending a relaxation synapse to the hamstrings in order to inhibit forceful contraction, in order to protect the quadriceps.

For this reason, it would be better if the hip angle were bent to approximately 90 degrees, thereby preventing the over-stretching of the quadriceps, which occurs when the hip is "straight" and the knee is fully bent.

You'll recall that in Chapter 11, it was discussed that performing a *prone leg curl* with the hip "straight" (with the femur mostly parallel to the torso) causes the hamstrings to over-shorten, and the quadriceps to over-stretch, as the knee progressively bends. A greater hip angle (ideally around 90 degrees) prevents active insufficiency (over-shortening of the hamstrings), as well as passive insufficiency (over-stretching of the quadriceps), when attempting to optimally simulate the hamstrings.

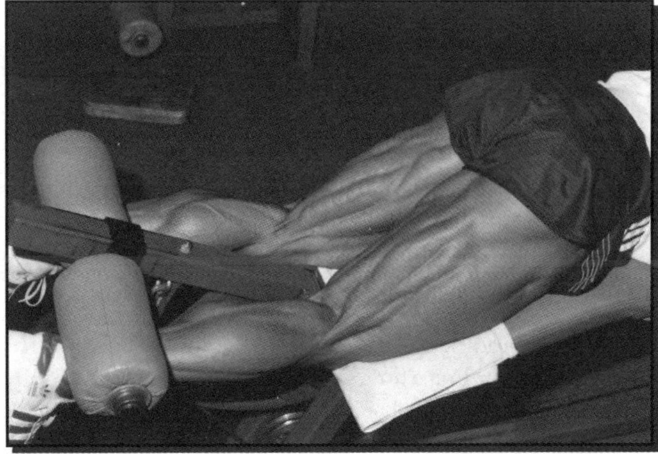

Figure 22-51

*Note: Although my hamstrings in Figure 22-51 appear to be getting a great workout from this prone/lying leg curl exercise, this version of a leg curl is not quite ideal. The seated leg curl is preferable, if it is available.*

The *seated leg curl* exercise (Figure 22-52) is better, because it avoids both active and passive insufficiency of the hamstrings.

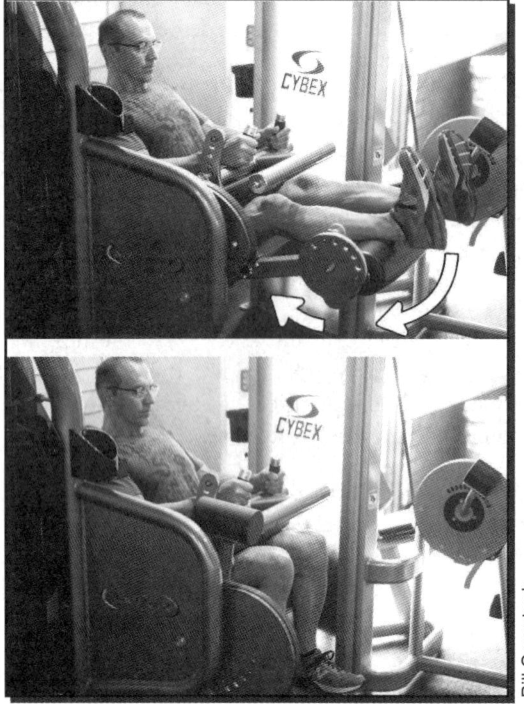


Figure 22-52

You'll recall that the problem with the "stiff legged deadlift," as an exercise for the hamstrings, is that it does not provide sufficient muscle contraction, even though it does provide the stretch. "*Seated leg curls*" satisfy both of these criteria. The seated position allows the hamstrings to get a much better stretch than could be achieved with *prone leg curls*, when the knees are straight, as well as a much better angle with which to get optimal hamstrings contraction, when the knees are fully bent. Furthermore, this "elongation" (stretch) can be made even better, simply by pulling the torso farther forward, when doing *seated leg curls*.

When performing *seated leg curls*, grab the handles that are on the femur brace (in front of you), pull your torso slightly forward (away from the backrest), and raise your chest up (i.e., arch your back a bit). At this point, you'll have the hamstring stretch that occurs at the bottom of the "*stiff-legged deadlift*," as well as the knee flexion that is typically missing from "*stiff-legged deadlifts*."

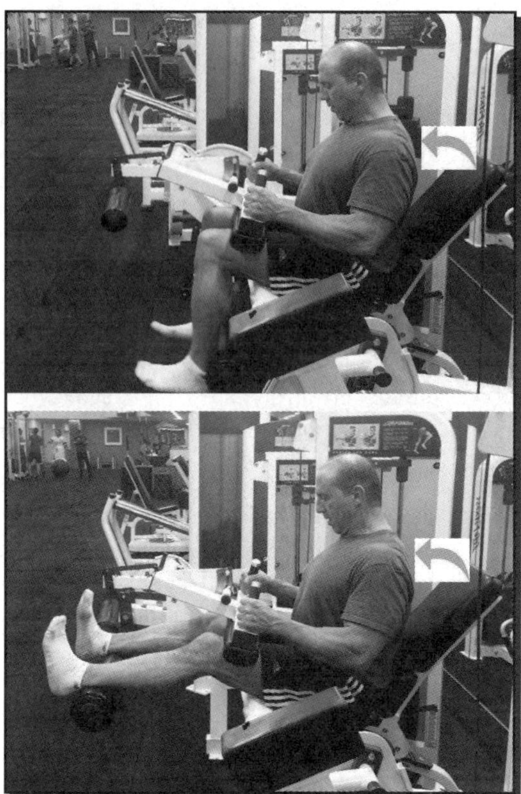

Figure 22-53

There is another bonus that occurs when you perform your *seated leg curls* this way (pulling your arched torso forward). The enhanced hamstrings stretch allows you to fully elongate your hamstrings slightly *before* your knees go all the way straight, which then protects against excessive mechanical disadvantage. You can start the concentric motion with a slight bend in your knee with much less injury risk, because of the reduced mechanical disadvantage. You'll notice that your hamstrings feel stronger, because you are able to start the range of motion with a slight mechanical advantage.

❑ The Ideal Resistance Curve for the Hamstrings

As discussed previously, a muscle's greatest strength potential occurs (generally speaking) when it is mostly elongated, and its least strength potential occurs when it is mostly shortened (contracted). Sometimes, a muscle is "strongest" at the very beginning of the range of motion, and, at other times, it's "strongest" about a third of the way into its range of motion. It seems to differ a bit, from one muscle to the next, in terms of where its peak contractile force occurs in the range of motion. It is clear, however, that a skeletal muscle *always* loses contractile force as it approaches its fully contracted (shortened) phase.

As was noted in Chapter 3, any mechanical disadvantage that may occur during the early part of a range of motion of a "flexion" muscle needs to be factored into the equation of the resistance curve of an exercise. If you're dealing with a muscle that extends a joint (e.g., the triceps, the quadriceps), which does not experience a change in the mechanical disadvantage, it's easy enough to simply load the "early phase" of the range of motion by causing that operating lever to be mostly perpendicular with resistance at the beginning of the concentric movement. On the other hand, it's a bit more complicated, when you're dealing with a muscle that flexes a joint, like the hamstrings.

The hamstrings seem to have a strength curve that is slightly different than the biceps brachii. Not only does it have a bit more strength potential when the knee is straight (as compared to when the elbow is straight), it also has a bit less vulnerability, as compared with the biceps. This factor makes it less necessary to start a *leg curl* with a less "active" tibia (parallel with resistance). It is still preferable, however, to not allow the knees to go fully straight—especially when the hamstrings are heavily loaded.

Remember that the hamstrings is very similar (mechanically speaking) to the biceps brachii, with the primary difference being that you cannot grasp a resistance tool (e.g., dumbbell, cable handle, machine, etc.) with your feet, the way you can with your hands. As such, you need to rely on the roller pad of a machine or an ankle strap with a D-ring (and a cable), as a way of attaching a type of resistance to the distal end of the operating lever—the lower leg. It's the same basic concept as holding a weight in your hand (at the distal end of the forearm), when working biceps.

The easiest and best method is to use a *seated leg curl* machine, given that it has already been established that the best hip position for working the hamstrings is one that allows a 90-degree angle to the torso (approximately). A good *seated leg curl* machine provides a resistance curve that is in sync with the strength curve of the hamstrings, by way of a well-designed CAM (oblong pulley). Ideally, the CAM should allow the resistance to diminish a bit, as the hamstring contraction approaches the end of its range of motion.

It's also important that you adjust the settings on the machine properly, for your height and for the length of your limbs. In that regard, the following considerations apply:

- The position of the backrest adjusts for your femur length and allows you to place your knees alongside the machine's pivot. This alignment allows the trajectory of the machine's lever arm to match the trajectory of your lower leg.
- The setting for the ankle pad adjusts for the length of your tibia. This allows the length of the machine's lever arm to match the length of your lower leg.
- The brace that you lower onto the top of your upper leg (just above the knee) prevents your femur from rising upward. This helps keep your knees alongside the machine's pivot. Be sure to keep your upper leg snuggly against the underside of that padded brace. Do not pull your upper leg (femur) downward, away from that brace.
- There is also (usually) a setting for range-of-motion, which allows you to increase or decrease how far your tibia can travel in either direction. It is not necessary to limit the final part of the range of motion (where the knees are maximally bent), but it is a good idea to limit the final part of the range of motion—the part that determines how straight your knees will go. Unless the weight being used is very light, it's a good idea to not allow your knees go all the way to fully straight.

If the gym you are a member of does not have a *seated leg curl* machine, the *lying/prone leg curl* is a reasonably good "second best choice." On the other hand, it is certainly not the best option.

❑ Exercise Options for the Hamstrings

On a scale of 1 to 10 (with 10 being "best"), I would rate a well-designed *seated leg curl* machine a "10," for effectiveness and safety, and a *prone* (mostly flat) *leg curl* machine a "7." If neither a *seated leg curl* machine nor a *prone leg curl* machine is available, but you have access to an adjustable-height pulley, you might try rigging up a *one leg/seated cable leg curl* exercise, as shown in Figure 22-54.

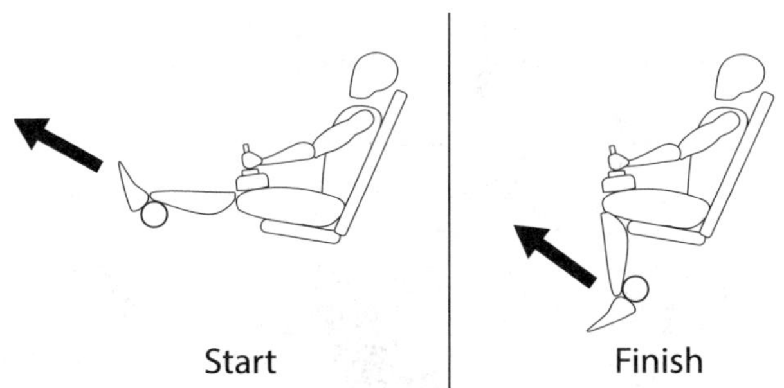


Figure 22-54

To perform a "*seated cable leg curl*" exercise, sit on a "high" bench, facing the pulley. Make sure the bench is high enough, so that your feet do not hit the ground, when your knees fully bend. Attach a strap with a D-ring to your ankle, with the D-ring in front of your ankle. The height of the pulley should be at a level that is about 12 inches (1/3 of a meter) higher than the seat on which you are sitting. As shown in Figure 22-54, imagine that the cable is pulling in the direction of the arrows.

Of course, you won't have the benefit of a femur brace, which would hold down the distal end of your femur. As a result, you'll have to put forth some effort to keep your femur from rising up. On the other hand, since the cable is pulling more forward than it is upward, keeping your femur down should not be too difficult. There will not be much of an increased force requirement—typically caused by the mechanical disadvantage when your knee is straight—because the cable is pulling mostly parallel to the tibia, and the weight of your lower leg (being pulled downward, by gravity) will also offset some of the upward resistance provided by the cable.

When the knee is flexed (fully bent), and the hamstrings are fully contracted, the lower leg will reach a point of being more perpendicular with the cable. This increase of resistance coincides with the hamstrings entering a better mechanical advantage, which results in a relatively good resistance curve for the hamstrings. It is similar to what would occur for the biceps, during *standing cable curls*.

It would be difficult, however, to attempt to do this exercise with both legs simultaneously. For one thing, it might be difficult finding two pulleys that can be set the correct width apart (hip width), as well as at the correct height. In addition, without having the femur brace and the handles (typically provided on a *seated leg curl* machine), it would be more difficult to control the movement of both legs, than to control the movement of just one leg at a time. Therefore, it would be best to do all the reps of a given set with one leg, followed by all the reps of that set with the other leg (isolated unilateral).

Although this exercise is relatively cumbersome to set up, I consider it the third best choice for a hamstring exercise, if neither a *seated leg curl* machine, nor a *lying/prone leg curl* machine, are available.

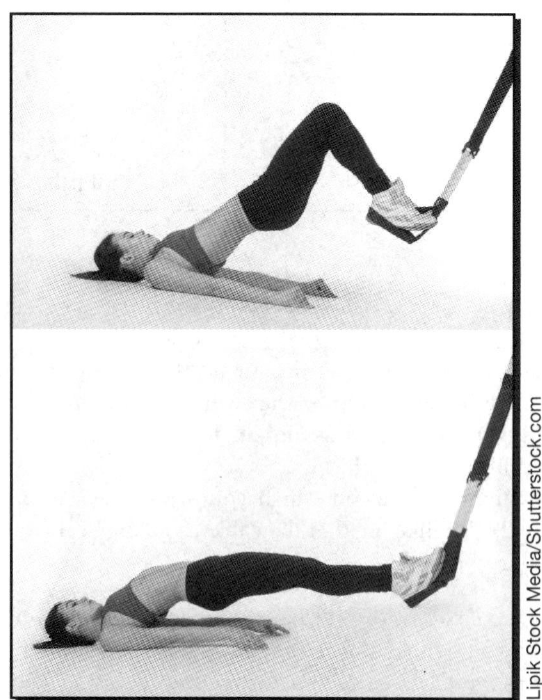
Lipik Stock Media/Shutterstock.com

Figure 22-55

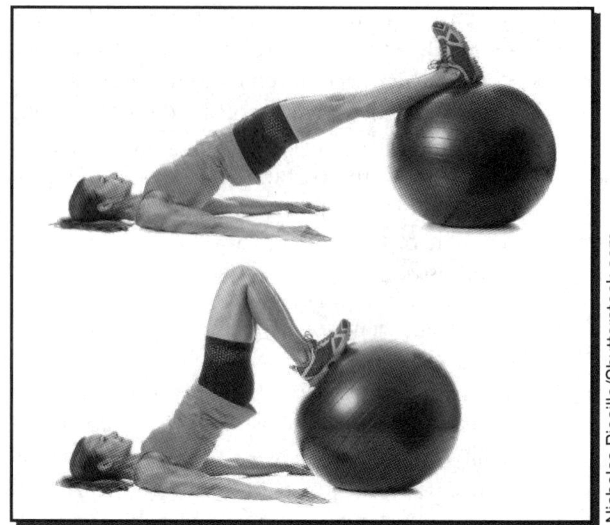
Nicholas Piccillo/Shutterstock.com

Figure 22-56

I would also highly discourage doing either of the two exercises shown in Figures 22-55 and 22-56. While these two exercises might seem perfectly innocuous, there's a hidden danger in both of these exercises. In both instances, when the legs are straight, there is the maximum amount of mechanical disadvantage occurring at the knee/hamstrings, combined with a mostly "active" tibia.

When the knees are straight, the hamstrings can only pull on the lower leg (where the insertion of the hamstrings is located) from maximally parallel angle, which means that the force requirement is about six times greater than it would be if the knees were bent at 90 degrees. At the same time that this situation occurs, the lower leg is mostly perpendicular with gravity. In other words, when the knees are straight, there are two magnifiers of resistance that are loading the hamstrings at the same time. This situation is very similar to the scenario that was discussed in Chapter 3, when the individual performing the heavy *preacher dumbbell curl* tore his biceps.

The combination of maximum mechanical disadvantage and a maximally active operating lever (i.e., the tibia being mostly perpendicular with resistance) could easily cause an injury. To illustrate why, let's do some simplified math.

In Figures 22-55 and 22-56 (knees straight/legs extended position), the women's bodies are mostly horizontal, with their upper body (torso) tilting slightly lower than their feet. This would result in about one-third of their bodyweight suspended by their heels, and about two-thirds suspended on their shoulders/upper back. If the women weigh 150 pounds (for the sake of calculation), it would mean that they are suspending about 50 pounds of weight (at least) by their heels—25 pounds with each leg (at a minimum). That 25 pounds per leg, however, is then magnified by the length of their lower leg (tibia). The average lower leg is 17 inches long.

To be conservative, a factor of 15 can be used. As such, 25 pounds X 15 equals 375 pounds, per leg. That's how much force is "trying" to hyperextend each knee, when the knee is straight. The only factor preventing that from happening is the hamstrings and the knee ligaments.

In order for the hamstrings to produce enough force to prevent the knees from hyperextending, however, it has to produce about six times more force than the 375 pounds, because it is only able to pull from a mechanical disadvantage. That's 2,250 pounds of force, per leg (375 lbs. X 6) that the hamstrings need to generate.

Far more foolish would be attempting to perform either of these exercises with only a SINGLE leg. Not only would it double the load on the knee to 750 pounds, it would also require 4,500 pounds of force to be produced by that one working hamstrings.

Proponents of "bodyweight" exercise tend to view this type of exercise as "better" and more "functional"—somewhat analogous to the concept of "natural ingredients" in food. The suggestion is that because resistance-exercise machines are "synthetic," they would not be as "natural" as bodyweight exercises (as if "natural" and "safe" are synonymous…they are not). This reasoning is nonsense. Plenty of natural ingredients found in food are unhealthful, and quite a few bodyweight exercises have a high level of risk, which could easily be avoided by using a properly designed machine or cables. In fact, with a thorough understanding of biomechanics, every exercise can be assessed, and an informed choice can be made. It's always best to use an exercise that is optimally safe, provides a productive resistant curve, and allows you to select from a wide variety of resistance options.

# CHAPTER 23

# Glutes, Adductors, and Hip Flexors

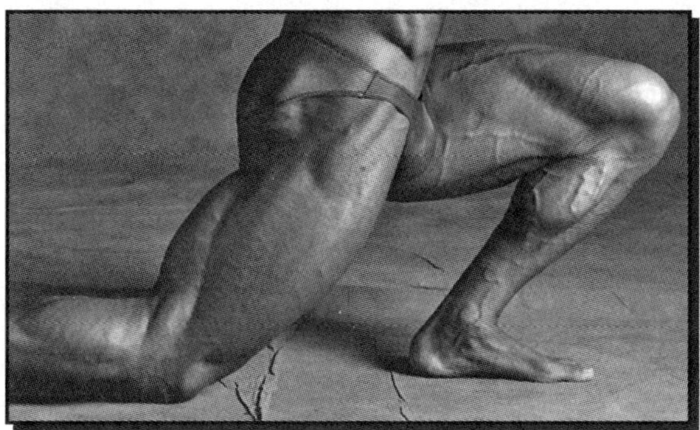

Figure 23-1

The "glutes" are comprised of three individual muscles—the gluteus maximus, the gluteus medius, and the gluteus minimus. The latter two, which lie underneath the gluteus maximus, are therefore referred to as "deep muscles." In Figure 23-2, you can see all three muscles and their location.

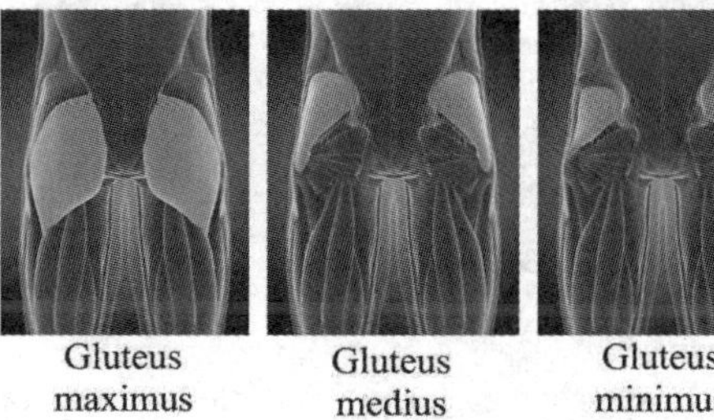


SciePro/Shutterstock.com

Figure 23-2

## Anatomy of the Gluteus Maximus

The muscle that is most significant to the bodybuilder, or any individual pursuing physique development, is the gluteus maximus (Figure 23-3). It is the largest and most powerful of the three gluteal muscles, as well as the one that is most capable of visual improvement. Most of the origins of the gluteus maximus are on the "gluteal surface" of the Ilium—the inside edge on the posterior side of the pelvis, close to the spine (Figure 23-4). Some of the other gluteus maximus fibers originate on the lumbar (spinal) fascia; others on the sacrum (base of spine), and others on the "sacrotuberous ligament" (Figure 23-5).

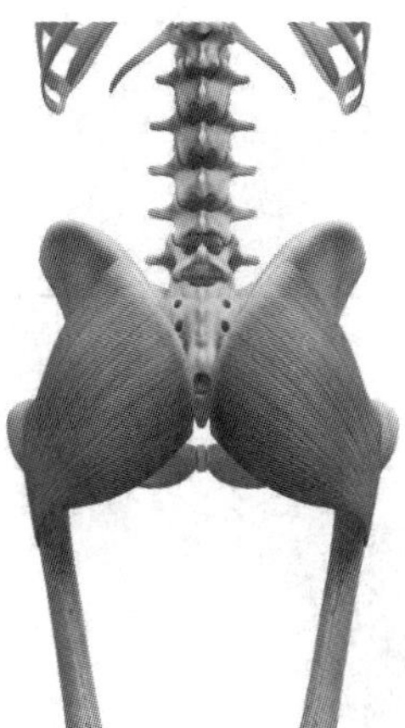

SciePro/Shutterstock.com

Figure 23-3

Notice that all the gluteus maximus fibers originate high and inside ("medial"/close to the center of the body), and then travel laterally and diagonally, attaching low and outside (away from the center of the body). Some of the gluteus maximus fibers then insert onto the gluteal tuberosity of the femur (Figure 23-6, left image)—just below the greater trochanter—while other fibers attach onto the iliotibial tract (Figure 23-6, right image).

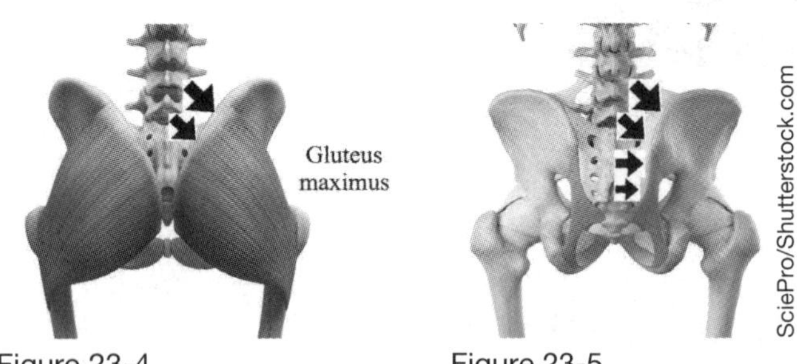


Figure 23-4

Figure 23-5

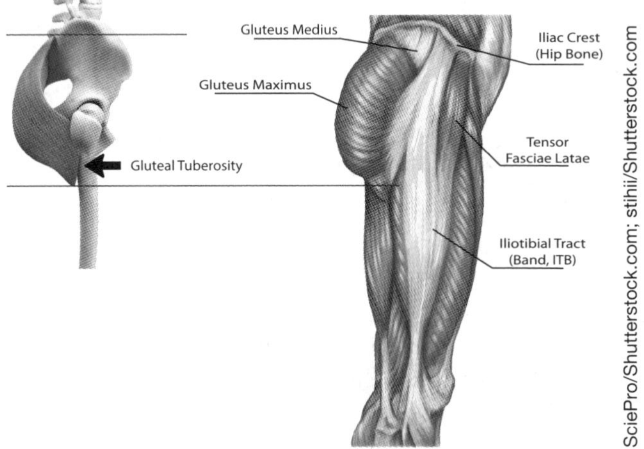


Figure 23-6

The gluteus maximus "extends" the hip joint. In other words, it "opens" (increases the angle of) the hip joint, moving the femur (upper thigh bone, shown as a line in Figure 23-7) downward and back (posteriorly). This "pushing down/back" action, therefore, moves the upper body *upward* from a seated or squatting position, or when you're stepping up onto a step or platform. The gluteus maximus also propels you *forward*, when you're walking or running.

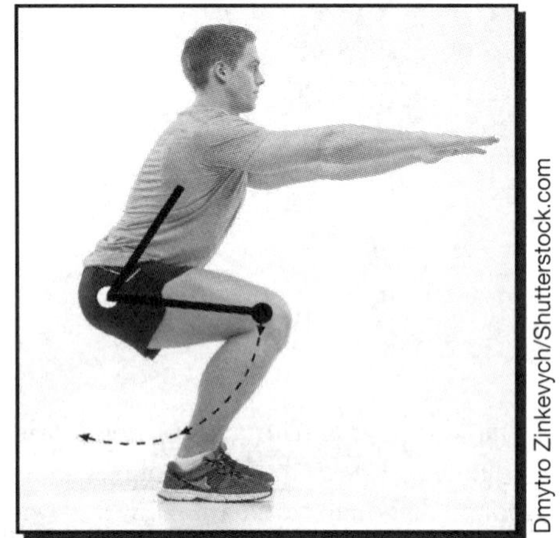


Figure 23-7

In addition to hip extension, the gluteus maximus also externally rotates the femur. This function is apparent by the diagonal direction of the fibers, and the fact that the muscle insertion is lateral to the origin. As such, any time the gluteus contracts, and the insertion moves toward the origin, it naturally tends to rotate the femur externally. Despite this fact, when you walk up a flight of stairs, or stand up from a chair (both of which require gluteus contraction), you don't see or feel your legs (femurs) rotating outward. The reason for this is that there there is an automatic counter-balancing force caused by the contraction of another muscle group, simultaneous to the gluteus contraction.

The action of "hip extension" is never performed exclusively by the gluteus maximus. Another set of muscles—the adductors—also participates in this action. In addition to participating in hip extension, however, the adductors also counter external femur rotation, a factor that will be further discussed shortly.

It's worth noting that performing exercises for the gluteus maximus (or medius or minimus) will NOT directly reduce body fat in that area. This fact extends to bodybuilders, who often try to "etch" gluteal striations in that area.

The fibers of the gluteus maximus only become clearly visible when an individual's percentage of body fat is low enough. A person may have a considerable amount of gluteal development (muscle mass), but the fibers would not be visible until the individual's body fat level is below 5 percent (approximately). Conversely, a person could have very little gluteal development, but—because they are lean enough—their gluteus fibers are clearly visible, as is demonstrated in Figure 23-8.

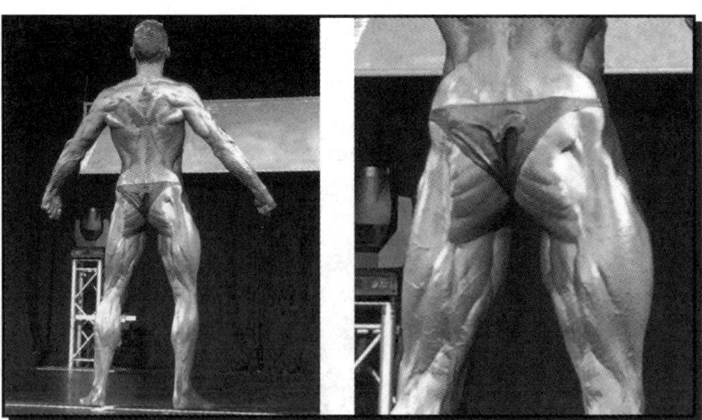

Figure 23-8

Getting lean is a "systemic" (whole-body) process that requires a sustained caloric deficit, over a period of weeks or months, during which adipose tissue (body fat) is reduced from the entire body, including the area of the buttocks. In fact, adipose dissipation (fat loss) cannot be done "locally"—in a specific area of a person's choosing.

It should also be noted that a person's rate of body fat loss is influenced heavily by genetics, as are the areas that lose fat first or last. An individual has no control over which areas of their body diminish their fat reserves first or last. A person can only put their body into "fat loss" mode (via increased caloric deficit/reduced calorie intake/increased calorie spending), and then that person's genetics determines the rate of fat loss and the order of fat loss.

Of course, the degree to which calories are restricted, as well as how intensely and frequently a person exercises, influence the rate of fat loss. The primary point to remember, however, is that exercising a particular muscle will not cause the body fat that covers that muscle to dissipate any more than the loss of body fat from any other area of the body.

## The Ideal Anatomical Motion for the Gluteus Maximus

In resistance exercise, the word "extension"—whether referring to "hip extension," "elbow extension," or "knee extension"—means increasing the angle of a joint. The primary function of the gluteus maximus is "hip extension," which entails increasing the angle of the hip joint, which is the pivot between the femur and the torso. Unlike "elbow extension" and "knee extension, however," where one of the two limbs (the forearm and the lower leg, respectively) is clearly more mobile than the other, "hip extension" can be done by moving either of the two levers (the femur or the torso/spine), while the other is more stationary.

In Figure 23-9, you can see a person performing a "*straight-legged deadlift*." In this instance, the femur is the more stable lever, while the torso is the more mobile lever.

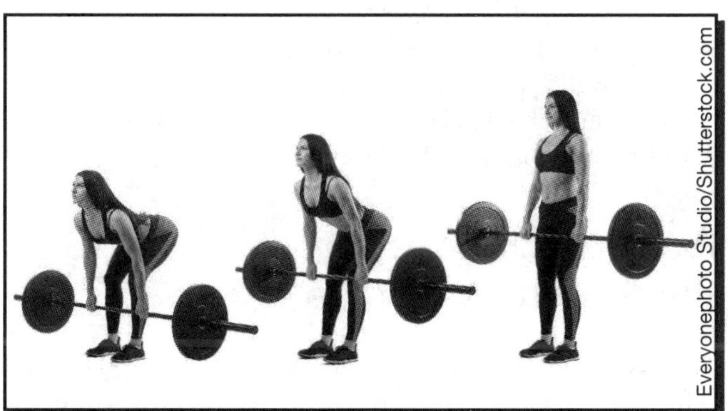

Figure 23-9

The same situation occurs during the exercise shown in Figure 23-10, although with a slightly different resistance curve. The upper legs (femurs) are the immobile lever, and the torso is the mobile lever.

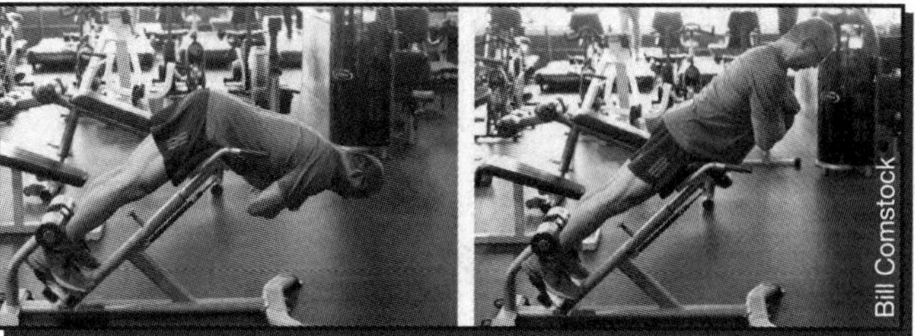

Figure 23-10

In Figure 23-11, a person doing a *squat*, both levers (the torso and the femur) are moving. Although the torso is slightly less mobile, and the femurs are more mobile, both "levers" are moving.

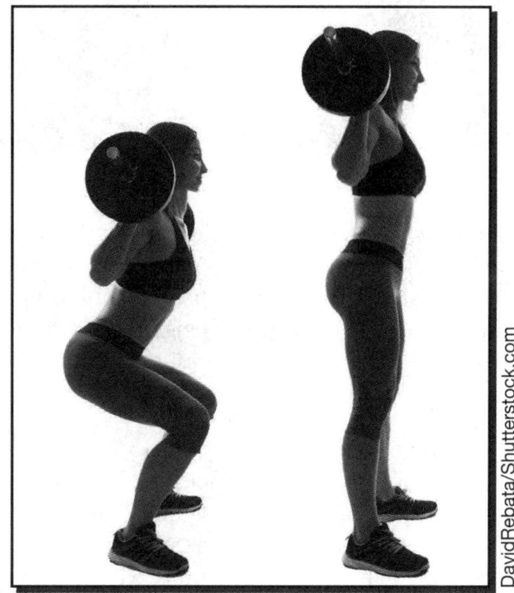

Figure 23-11

In the example shown in Figure 23-12, the torso is completely immobile, and the femurs are mobile—but it's still "hip extension," and the same muscles are causing the action. In all of the aforementioned examples, the gluteus does not "know" which lever is moving, and which is stable. The muscle merely performs its task of "extending" the hip joint, thereby increasing its angle. Even though these exercises all look very different, the same action is occurring in each of them, with regard to hip extension/gluteal contraction.

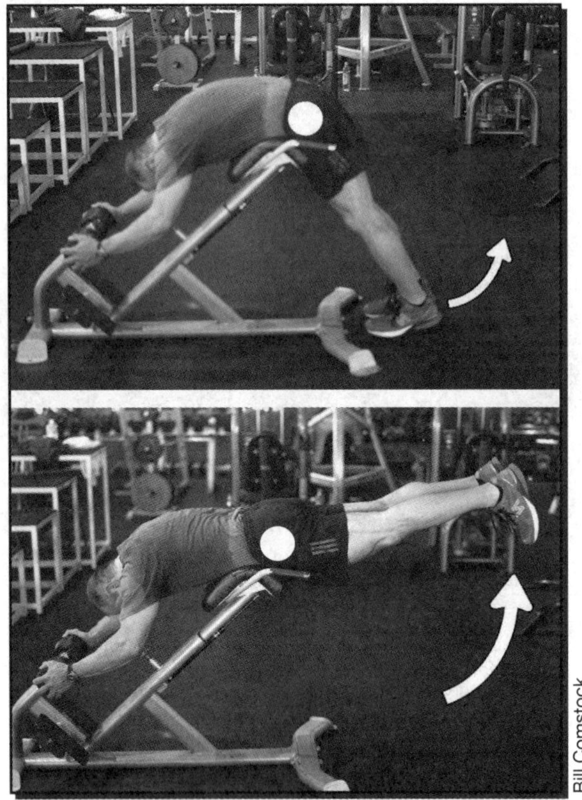

Figure 23-12

There are other factors, aside from the basic "hip extension" movement, that determines which exercise is "best" for the gluteus maximus. These factors include range of motion; a "longer" lever/femur length (not reduced by the tibia, as the secondary lever); the resistance curve; bi-lateral deficit, unilateral focus; and stability.

The exercise shown in Figure 23-13, "*glute extensions*" on the "multi-hip machine," provides the best of all options. The torso is kept still and not "weighted," and the femur is mobile. This avoids having to needlessly load the spine. It is performed with only one leg at a time, which allows you to avoid "bilateral deficit," and employ unilateral focus. As such, you are able to use more weight with the glutes and adductors of one side, than you could, if you attempted to use the glutes and adductors of both sides simultaneously (i.e., more than 50 percent with each side). Plus, you activate cross-over benefits (cross education), when performing unilateral exercise.

This exercise also allows you to use a much greater range of motion than most other gluteus exercises—a full 110 degrees of motion (note the protractor reading). It also avoids straining the erector spinae, as would occur with *squats* and *deadlifts*. Furthermore, by attaching the resistance to the distal end of the femur (instead of at the foot), the quadriceps and the knee are no longer a limiting factor. This allows the avoidance of reciprocal innervation (neurological conflict between the simultaneous loading of the glutes and the quadriceps). It also avoids reduction of the femur's moment arm ("effective length"), which would otherwise be caused by the tibia doubling under the femur. As a result, the full femur length is utilized in the exercise, which allows more gluteus load with less weight used.

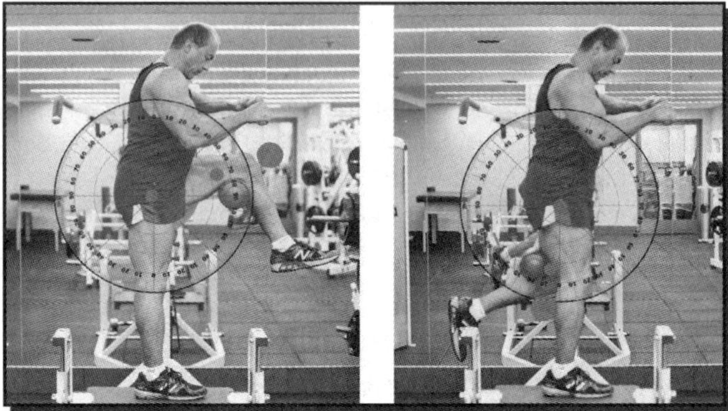
Figure 23-13

This exercise also produces a much better resistance curve than occurs during *squats*. With this exercise, the end of the range of motion still encounters an opposing resistance, whereas in the *barbell squat*, there is zero opposing resistance at the conclusion of the range of motion. Indeed, this exercise is mechanically the best exercise for the gluteus maximus, given the aforementioned reasons.

Unfortunately, the vast majority of gyms do not have one of these machines, which is ridiculous, frankly. The concept of a "multi-hip machine" is elementary—"an exercise that loads the distal end of the operating lever of the target muscle." This concept is utilized in most resistance exercises, for any muscle group (i.e., *dumbbell curls, supine dumbbell triceps extensions, dumbbell side raises,* etc.), and is perhaps most obvious in the standard *leg extension* machine and all *leg curl* machines. It's ironic that most gyms in the world have *leg extension* and *leg curl* machines, yet many gyms do not have a "multi-hip machine," despite the fact that the same method of resistance application is used.

## Exercise Options for the Gluteus Maximus

The following exercises pale in comparison to the glute extensions on a multi-hip machine, discussed above. Nevertheless, they have some degree of merit, although they are all compromised in one or more ways.

The exercise shown in Figure 23-14—*back lunges*—is a fairly good method of working the glutes, especially if you don't have access to a multi-hip machine. Because the torso is held upright, in this exercise, the erector spinae is not loaded, and the spine is not compressed—both of which are good. Furthermore the gluteus on each side is worked unilaterally, which is also good. *Back lunges* can be performed while holding a hand rail (if stability is needed), or while holding a pair of dumbbells for added resistance. It is important to be aware that *forward lunges* (stepping forward, instead of backward) are quite different than *back lunges*. *Forward lunges* load the glutes less, but the quadriceps more.

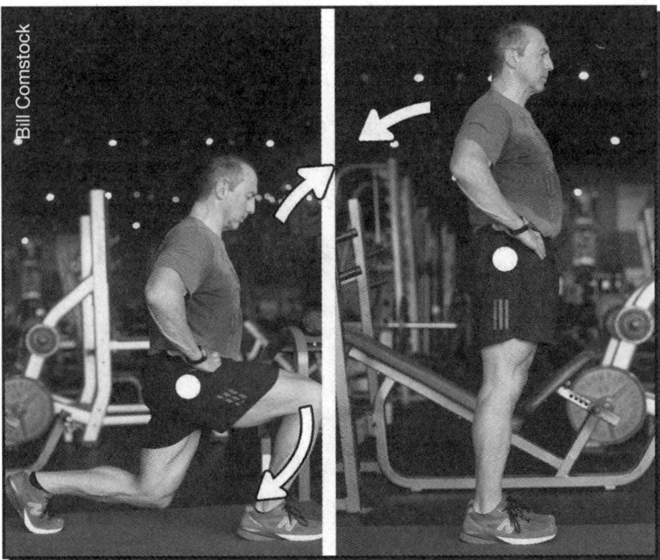

Figure 23-14

Another relatively good exercise for the gluteus maximus is *step-ups* (onto a high step), shown in Figure 23-15. As noted previously, you can choose to use additional hand weights (or a weighted vest), or not. These two exercises (Figure 23-14 and Figure 23-15) provide gluteus load at the beginning of the range of motion, but essentially zero resistance at the conclusion of the range of motion. They are also limited in terms of the amount of load that can be used.

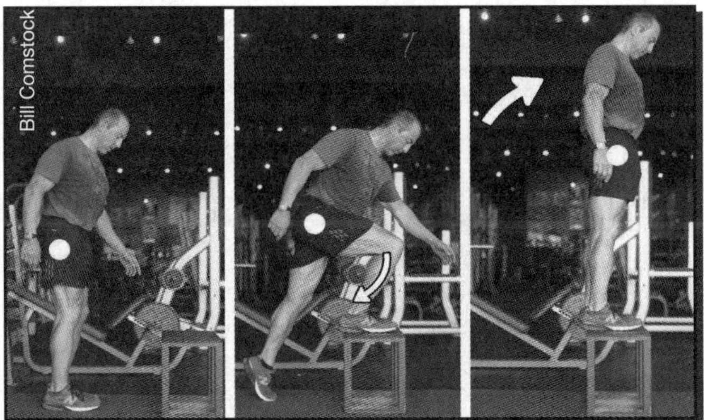

Figure 23-15

The exercise shown in Figure 23-16—"*glute bridges*"—is very popular these days, but it has two compromised components: a limited range of motion (the first 20 percent of the glutes' range of motion is not even used), and it is "late phase loaded," instead of "early phase loaded." Since it is also a bilateral movement, the potential unilateral benefits are lost.

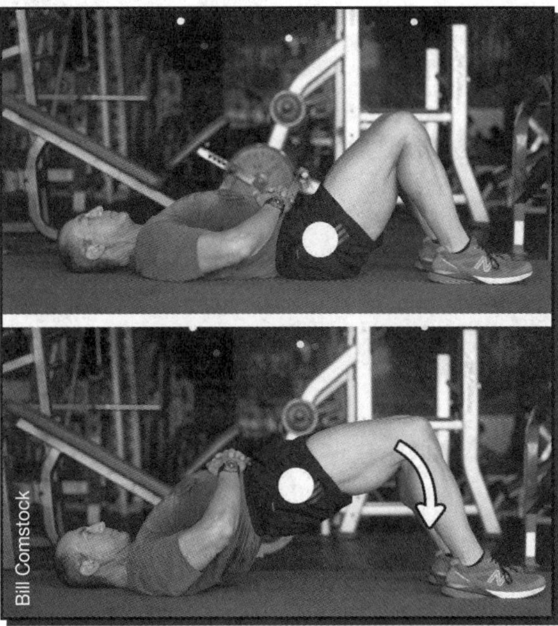

Figure 23-16

The *glute bridge* version shown in Figure 23-17— on a bench and with added resistance—allows a slightly better range of motion, and provides more resistance, but it still has other problems. The resistance curve is still "late phase loaded," rather than "early phase loaded"; it's still bilateral (thereby triggering bilateral deficit); and—because the tibia, and the muscles that move the tibia, are involved—it triggers a degree of reciprocal innervation (simultaneous activation of opposing/antagonistic muscles). These factors compromise the benefit to the gluteus muscle.

As you can see by the protractor that has been laid over the exercise in Figure 23-17, the range of motion of this exercise is only about 45 degrees. In contrast, the range of motion, when using the *glute extension* machine is about 110 degrees. It should also be noted that this is not a comfortable exercise, and situating the barbell on top of the pelvis is very cumbersome. The *glute extension* machine, on the other hand, is much easier to access. It enables a greater range of motion, offers a more productive resistance curve, allows unilateral focus (avoiding bilateral deficit/weakness), and avoids reciprocal innervation (a relaxation synapse sent to the glutes, when the rectus femoris is activated as part of the quad function).

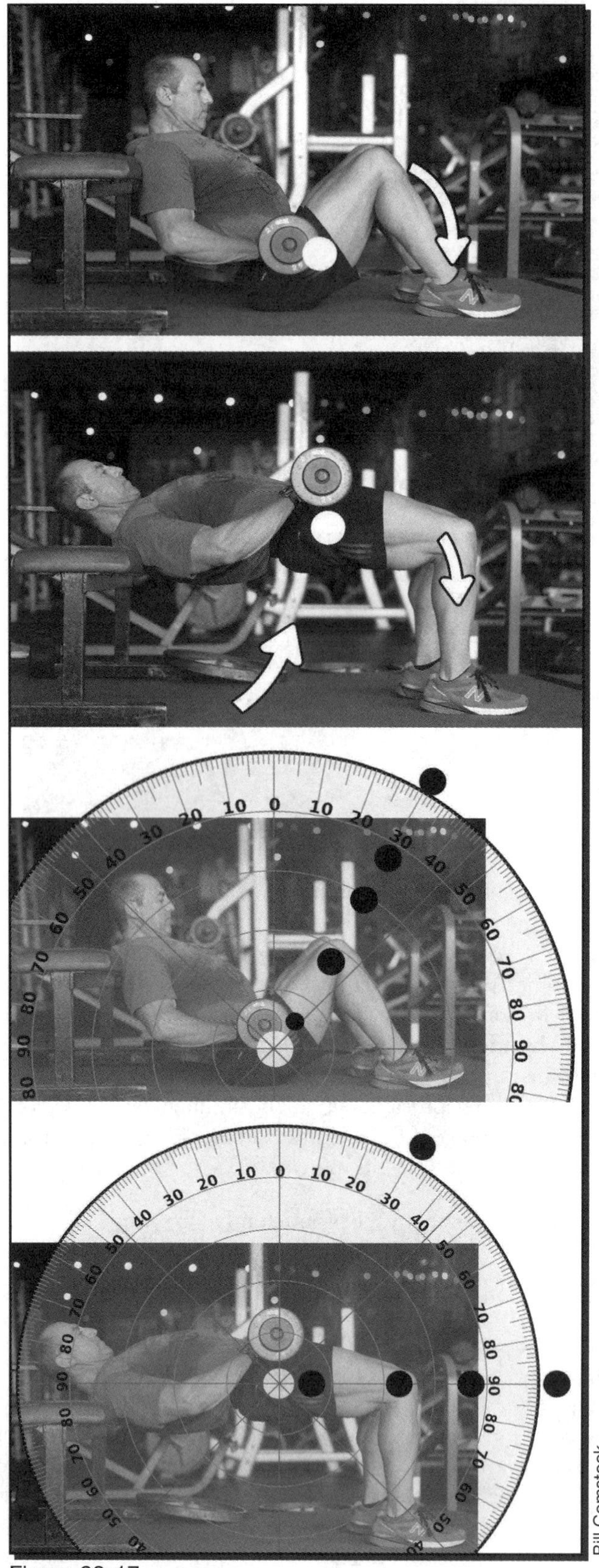


Figure 23-17

Using a *"hip abduction machine"* (moving the femurs outward, laterally), shown in Figure 23-18, also works the gluteus, but with much less emphasis on the gluteus maximus, and more emphasis on the gluteus medius and gluteus minimus. It's difficult to use much weight with this exercise, because of the lesser role that the gluteus maximus plays in this motion, and because the adductors cannot participate at all in this motion. The adductors participate more when the femur is moved straight downward, or pulled inward.

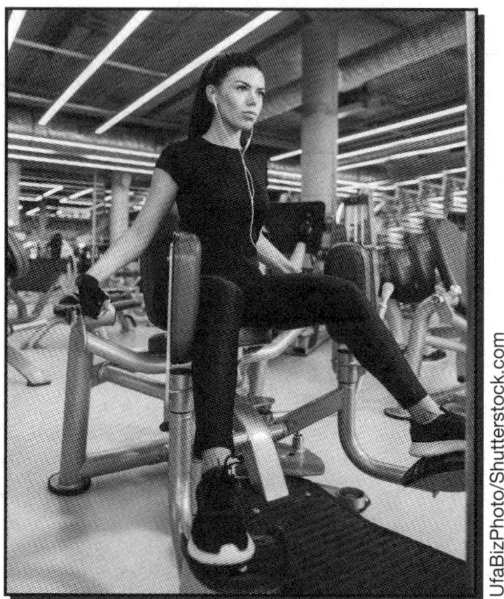


Figure 23-18

The aforementioned exercise is often mistakenly referred to as an "outer thigh" exercise. The "thigh" area, however, is from the hip joint down to the knee, which is actually part of the quadriceps. The quadriceps do not produce "hip abduction" (moving the femur sideways). The quadriceps mainly (almost exclusively) extend the knee joint. "Hip abduction," therefore, does not involve the "outer thigh" at all.

Hip abduction (moving the femur laterally—to the side) is produced mostly by the three gluteus muscles, although with a much greater emphasis on the two smaller muscles—the gluteus medius and gluteus minimus. Because these smaller gluteus muscles do not have much capacity for visible growth—for the competitive bodybuilder—it's not worth investing much energy on "hip abduction." Still, a modest amount of work (three or four sets, every three or four days) is worth doing—primarily for the functional benefit. Hip abduction is helpful for sport-specific training and for rehabilitation purposes, in addition to general fitness.

Hip abduction will NOT produce localized fat loss in the hip and thigh area. It is an unfortunate fact that the majority of people who use this type of machine mistakenly believe that they can reduce fatty deposits on the "upper outer thighs," or they can "firm" the fatty deposits in that part of the body. Both of these beliefs are incorrect.

*Deadlifts* (Figure 23-19) would likely be included in most people's list of "good glute exercises." Certainly, the glutes do play a significant role in this movement. However, the strain on the erector spinae, as well as on the spine itself, should not be ignored when evaluating this exercise. The amount of weight that an individual must use to adequately challenge their glutes—with this exercise—is beyond that which is reasonable for the erector spinae and the spine.

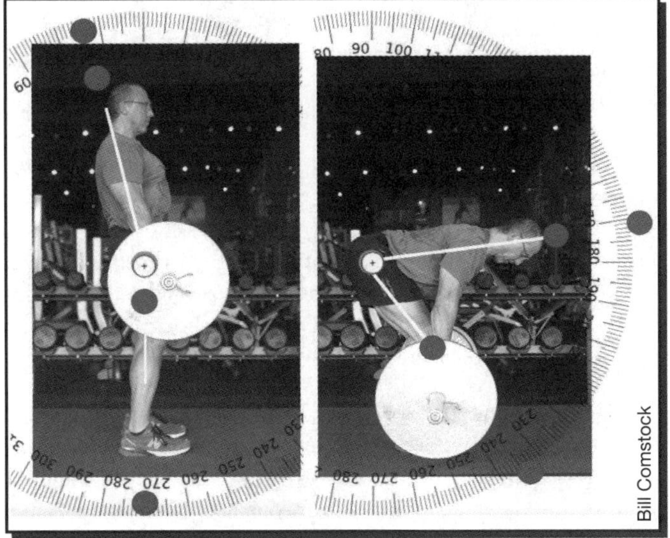

Figure 23-19

If a person uses a weight that is safe for the erector spinae and intervertebral discs, it will likely be insufficient for the glutes. In turn, if a person uses a weight that is productive for the glutes, it will likely be excessive for the erector spinae and will significantly increase the risk of spinal injury.

Causing the torso to become fully ACTIVE (to enter a perpendicular position with gravity) is NOT a requirement for working the glutes. As noted previously, *hip extensions* on the multi-hip machine allow the glutes to be loaded as much, or more (as occurs during heavy deadlifts), without any load on the erector spinae, and without the risk of injuring the spine.

In addition, there is no advantage, in terms of "better" gluteal development, by simultaneously loading the gluteus, the erector spinae and the quadriceps. Each of these three muscle groups can be worked as well, or better, with dedicated exercises, as compared with a compound exercise (e.g., *deadlifts* or *squats*).

## Anatomy of the Gluteus Medius and Gluteus Minimus

In the anatomical illustration in Figure 23-20, you're looking at a posterior view (backside) of the pelvis. The arrows marked "A" are pointing to the gluteus medius. The arrow marked "B" is pointing to the gluteus minimus, which lies underneath the gluteus medius. On the right side of the anatomical illustration, you can see how the gluteus maximus lies OVER the gluteus medius and the gluteus minimus. The medius and minimus both attach onto the greater trochanter of the humerus. The arrow marked "C" shows the attachment point of these two muscles—the greater trochanter on the femur (Figure 23-20, left image).

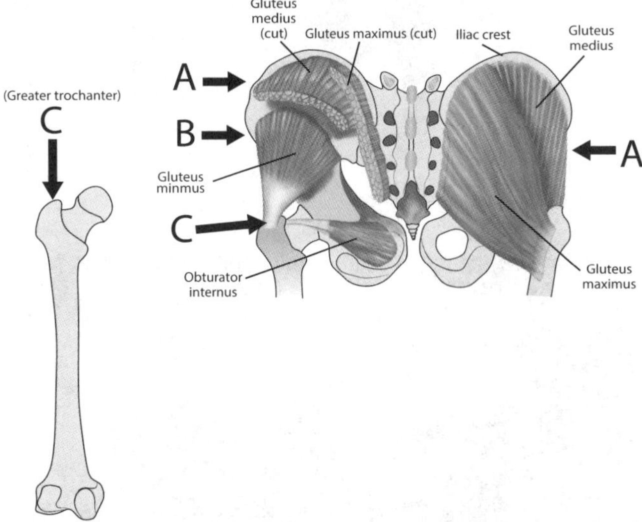

Figure 23-20

The gluteus medius and minimus assist the gluteus maximus in hip extension—moving the femur downward and backward. The gluteus maximus and the adductors, however, are the primary hip extensors because they have better leverage on the femur—and they are larger muscles. Notice that the attachment of the gluteus medius and minimus is higher on the femur than that of the gluteus maximus. The gluteus medius and minimus, however, are primarily responsible for lateral abduction of the femur (moving the leg sideways), a movement that is not dominated by any other muscle.

The obturator internus (Figure 23-20), together with the piriformis, the gemellus inferior, and quadrates femoris (other "deep" muscles that are not shown in the illustration) lie underneath the gluteus maximus, medius, and minimus, and collectively act mostly as "anchors" of the femoral head, in the hip joint. They also assist in rotating the femur, but they mostly ensure that the femoral head stays securely in the hip socket.

The gluteus medius and minimus are generally not considered "physique muscles." These two muscles are relatively small and have very little capacity for growth. Performing a hip abduction exercise (like the ones shown in Figures 23-21 and 23-22) will not result in any noticeable muscle development. It will also not dissipate the adipose tissue (body fat) that has accumulated in that area, because the reduction of body fat only occurs systemically (as a whole-body process), and usually only when there is a caloric deficit.

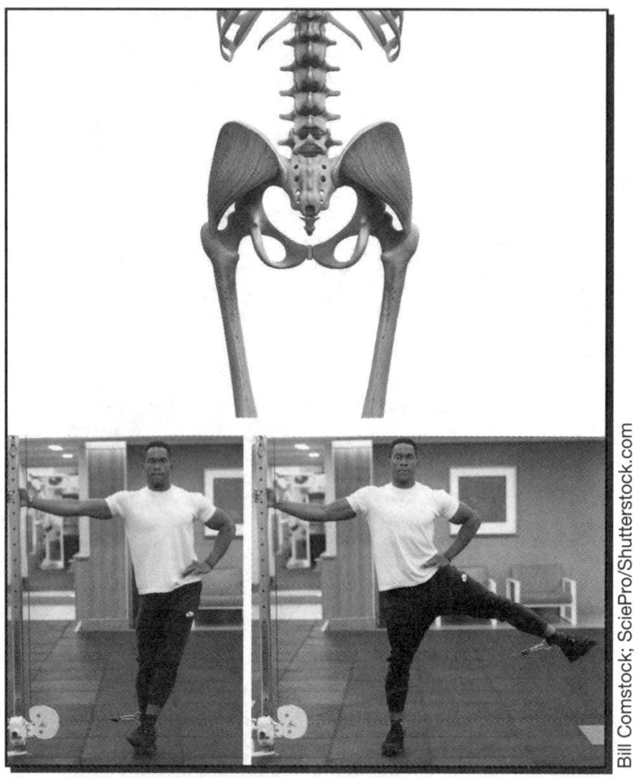

Bill Comstock; SciePro/Shutterstock.com

Figure 23-21

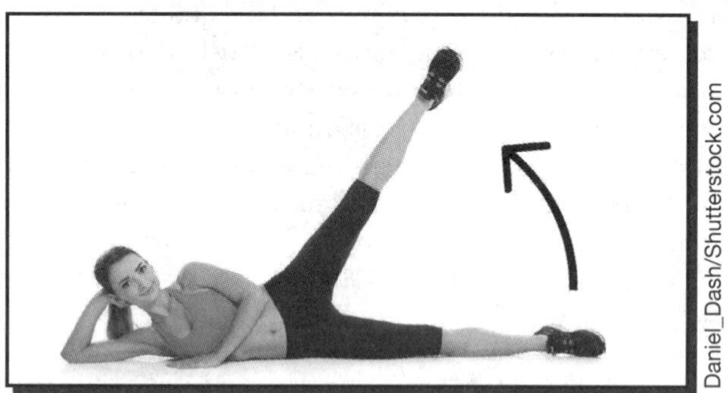

Daniel_Dash/Shutterstock.com

Figure 23-22

## Anatomy of the Femural Adductors

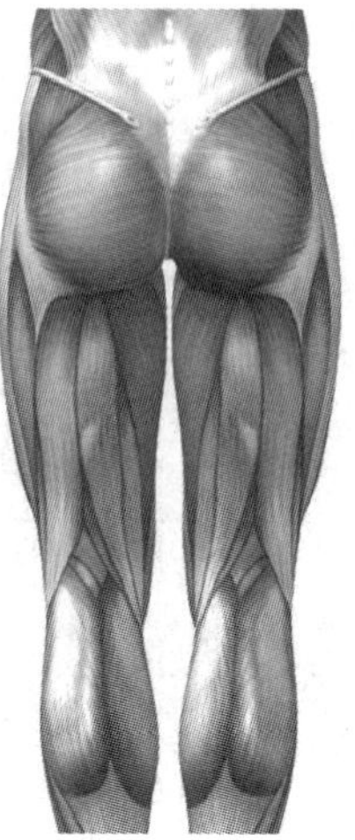

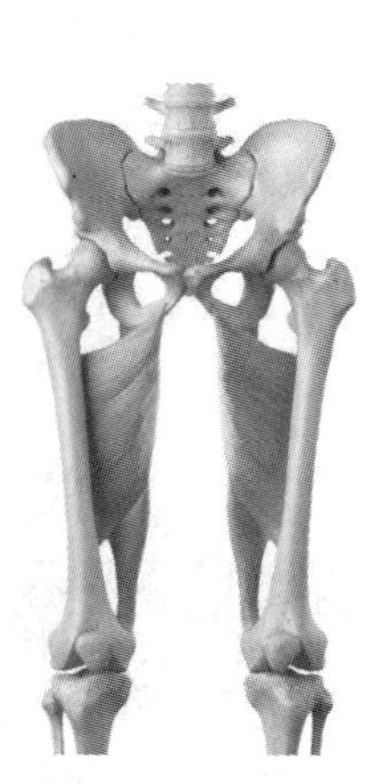

design36/Shutterstock.com; SciePro/Shutterstock.com

Figure 23-23

Figure 23-23, left image, is a posterior view (from the back) of the adductors. Figure 23-23, right image, provides an anterior view (from the front) of the adductors, shown as the only muscles on the skeleton.

The adductor muscle group is relatively misunderstood from the layman's perspective. Most people believe that the adductor's primary function is to bring the femurs together ("adduction"), which is not entirely correct. In addition, many people (mostly women) believe that working this muscle group will dissipate fatty deposits that have accumulated on the inner part of their thighs, which is entirely false.

The adductors do more than just bring the femurs together. They play a significant role in hip extension, as well as counterbalance the external rotation force produced by the gluteus maximus, on the femur. Were it not for the contraction of the adductors during hip extension, the femur would rotate externally, whenever the gluteus maximus contracts. The adductors also play an important role aesthetically, helping to balance the symmetry of the upper legs, when seen from both the front and the back.

In Figure 23-24, the arrow marked "A" is pointing to the adductors of the left leg. The arrow marked "B" is pointing to the gluteus maximus of the left leg. This is meant to show how these two muscles collaborate with each other, in moving the femur downward. Because the insertion of the gluteus maximus is on the outside of the femur, a balancing force is required on the inside of the femur, sharing the task of "hip extension/moving the femur downward." As noted previously, the adductors lend a medial/downward force, counterbalancing the lateral/downward force produced by the gluteus maximus.

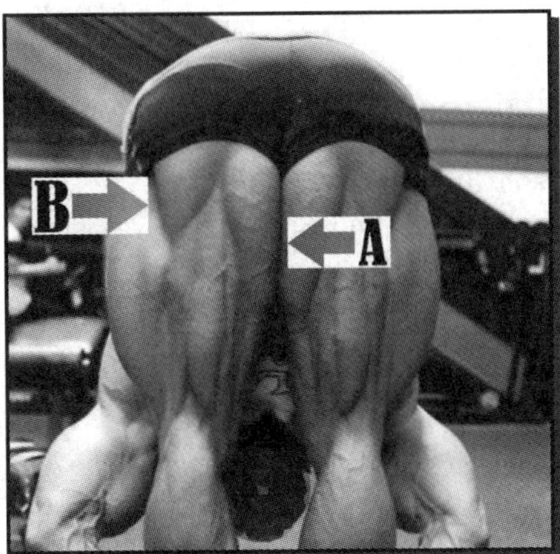

Figure 23-24

Most lay-people (individuals who are not anatomists), looking at Figure 23-24, would probably think that they are looking at a pair of very well-developed hamstrings. In fact, the most impressive aspect of this photo is NOT this man's hamstrings. It is his quadriceps, his adductors ("A"), and his glutes ("B"), that show the most notable development.

There are three parts of the adductor muscle group—the adductor magnus (Figure 23-25, left image), the adductor longus (Figure 23-25, center image), and the adductor brevis (Figure 23-25, right image). The magnus plays the most significant role, given its very low insertion on the femur (giving it the most leverage), followed by the longus, and then the brevis. All three parts originate on the pelvis, and each inserts onto different parts of the femur—low, middle, and high—as you can see in Figure 23-25.

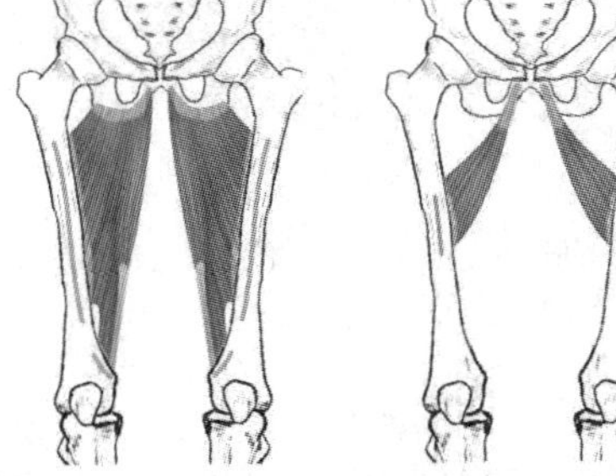

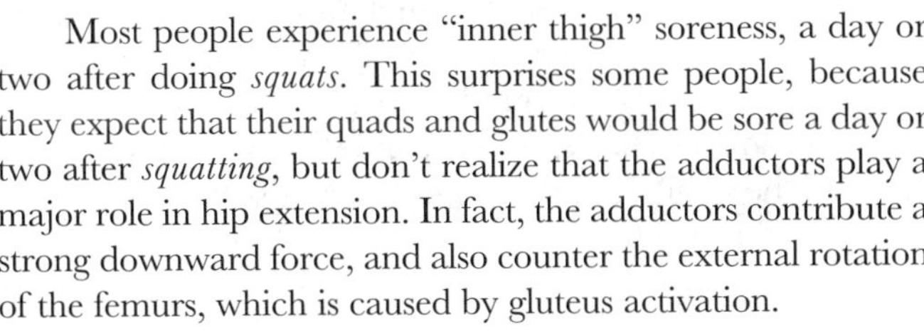

Clint Smith/E2 Systems, Inc.

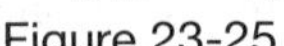
Figure 23-25

Most people experience "inner thigh" soreness, a day or two after doing *squats*. This surprises some people, because they expect that their quads and glutes would be sore a day or two after *squatting*, but don't realize that the adductors play a major role in hip extension. In fact, the adductors contribute a strong downward force, and also counter the external rotation of the femurs, which is caused by gluteus activation.

Thus, the adductors get plenty of stimulation from their participation during *hip extension* exercises, without having to perform a dedicated "inner thigh"/adductor exercise. Using the *hip extension* machine shown in Figure 23-13, or doing some type of *squatting* motion, will satisfy the basic requirement for adductor exercise. On the other hand, performing a dedicated "inner thigh" (adductor) exercise would contribute more to the development of these muscles, and would also be beneficial for certain sports. It could also be used as part of a rehabilitation program that is supervised by a qualified physical therapist.

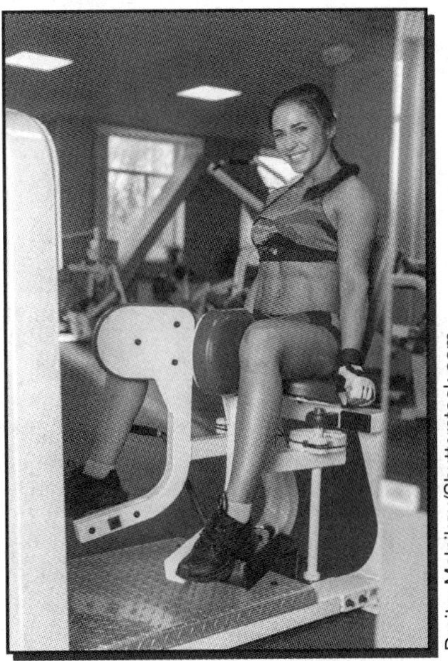

Dmitry Melnikov/Shutterstock.com

Figure 23-26

It's worth repeating that exercises which target the "inner thighs," like the *thigh adduction* machine (Figure 23-26) or "*wide stance squats*," will NOT eliminate or dissipate body fat that is on the inner thighs, nor will it "firm" the fatty deposits that are there. Any burning sensation you feel during an "inner thigh" exercise, or next-day-soreness you experience after having done an "inner thigh" exercise, is NOT proof that localized fat was affected in any way. It is simply proof that the adductor muscles were challenged, prompting them to become stronger.

## Anatomy of the Hip Flexors

There are several muscles that participate in lifting the upper thigh bone (the femur) forward and upward. Lifting the leg/bending the hip joint is called "hip flexion." The primary hip flexors are the psoas major and minor ("A" and "B," in Figure 23-27) and the iliacus ("C" in Figure 23-27). The less primary hip flexors include the sartorius, the rectus femoris, and the tensor fascia lata, which will be addressed in a moment.

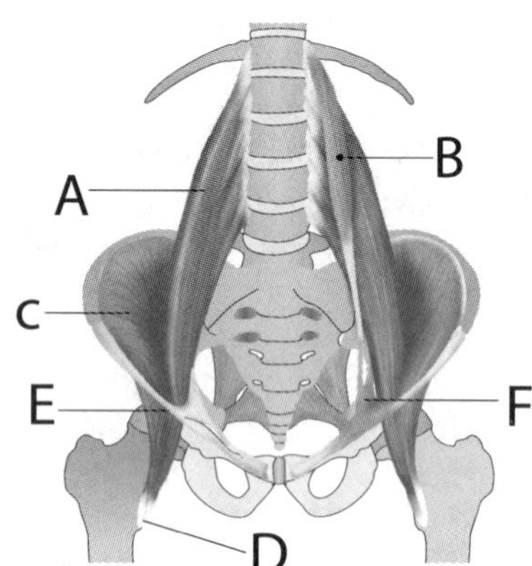


Figure 23-27

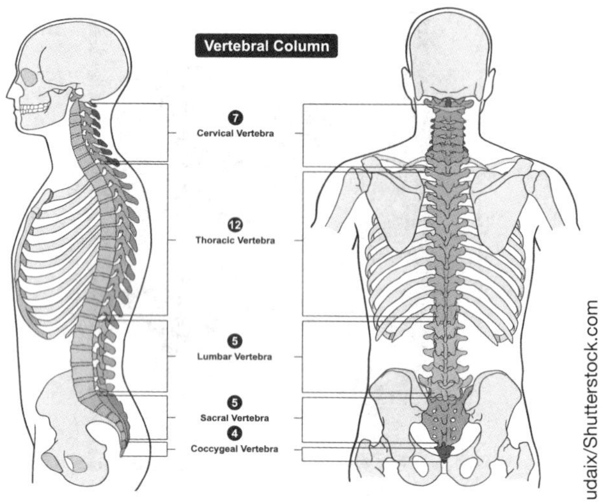




Figure 23-28

The psoas (pronounced "so-as") is technically a two-part muscle, comprised of the "psoas major" ("A" in Figure 23-27) and the "psoas minor" ("B" in Figure 23-27). It's worth noting, however, that since an estimated 40 to 70 percent of people do not have a psoas minor, it is not an essential muscle. Furthermore, even in those individuals who have one, the psoas minor is very small, and hardly a participant in hip flexion. Its point of insertion ("F" in Figure 23-27) is not even on a bone—it's on the "inguinal ligament." The psoas major is the only real hip flexor, between these two. Accordingly, from this point forward in the book, I'll refer to the psoas major, as simply the "psoas."

The psoas originates on the lumbar vertebrae (T12 through L5), which is just above the sacrum and the coccyx (tailbone). This factor is very important to note, as you'll soon see. The psoas then passes by the "inguinal ligament" ("E" in Figure 23-27), and attaches to the "lesser trochanter" ("D" in Figure 23-27).

The second most primary hip flexor muscle, known as the iliacus ("C" Figure 23-27), originates on the upper edge of the iliac ridge, on the anterior (front) side of the pelvis. It then converges with the psoas, and subsequently also attaches onto the lesser trochanter ("D" in Figures 23-27 and 23-29). Collectively, these two muscles are known as the "iliopsoas" (pronounced ILIO-SOAS). The psoas, however, is more dominant than the iliacus, because its higher position of origin gives it better leverage on the femur.

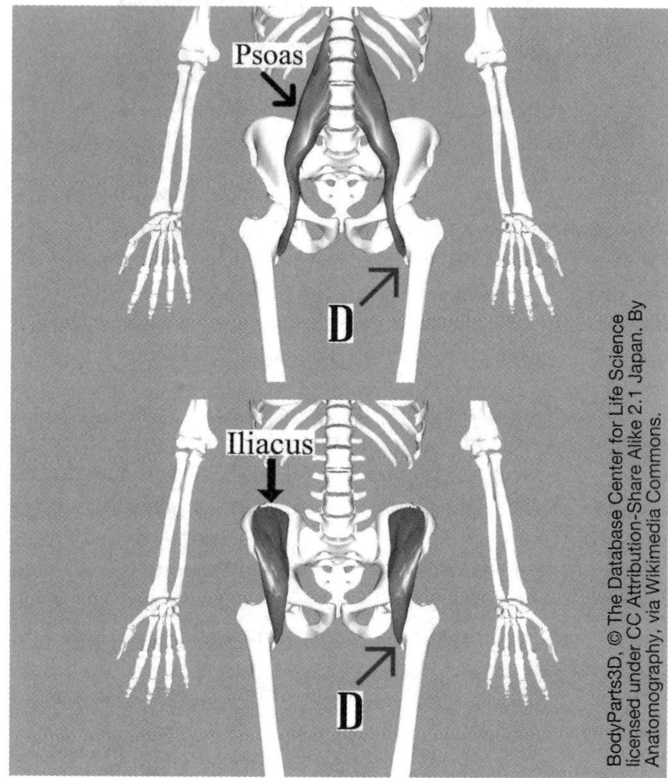




Figure 23-29

When you perform any kind of "leg raise" exercise, the action of raising the legs (pulling the femurs forward and upward) is caused entirely by the hip flexors, mainly by the psoas. Because the abs do not connect to the legs, the abs cannot raise the legs. When the psoas contracts, it pulls from its origin on the lumbar spine. This "tug" on the lumbar spine tends to cause the lower back to arch (upper image in Figure 23-30). Arching the spine—called "spinal extension"—is the opposite of what the abs produce, which is "spinal flexion." The function of the abs (i.e., the rectus abdominis) is to "round" the spine (lower image in Figure 23-30).

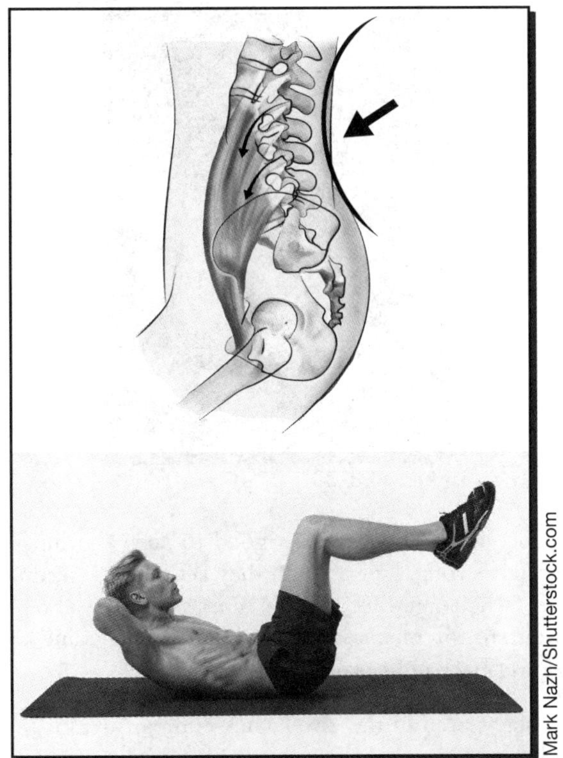

Figure 23-30

It's important to note that contractions of the abs and of the hip flexors produce opposite spinal positions, and therefore interfere with each other, when activated simultaneously. Trying to work the abs by doing *leg raises* presents a significant conflict of interest, given that the abs and the psoas compete for their preferred spinal position. This factor is what often causes lower back discomfort, when doing *leg raises* for the abs. There is nothing wrong with working the hip flexors, but they should not be activated as part of an ab exercise, when the objective is to optimally stimulate the abs, for the purpose of abdominal development.

Activating the psoas, while simultaneously trying to fully contract the abs, is like trying to perform a *standing barbell curl*, with someone blocking the bar and preventing your biceps from fully contracting. Psoas activation interferes with spinal flexion, and thus prevents complete contraction of the abs.

A question you might be asking at this point is "*Why do my abs burn, when I do leg raises?*" The reason is that—during a *leg raise* exercise, the abs participate by trying to prevent the lumbar spine from overarching. The hip flexors, it seems, were designed to be used alternately—one side at a time. Trying to raise both legs simultaneously produces a much greater pull on the lumbar spine than is normal. The combined weight of the both legs is significant, which, when lifted together, produces an enormous forward pull on the lumbar spine. The abs then produce a strong, mostly isometric, contraction, to prevent excessive arching of the lumbar spine. Isometric contraction can certainly be "felt," and can even produce muscle soreness, but it does not produce the strength improvement and muscle development benefits of dynamic muscle contraction.

In reality, it's best to work the hip flexors, without the simultaneous participation of the rectus abdominis, just like it is optimal to work the abs, without the concurrent participation of the hip flexors. Each muscle can be strengthened and developed more efficiently, when worked separately.

In the previous chapter, which addressed the quadriceps, it was established that the rectus femoris is the only one of the four quadriceps muscles that crosses the hip joint. This factor allows the rectus femoris to assist in help flexion, although its role in hip flexion is neither as effective, nor as primary, as that of the iliopsoas.

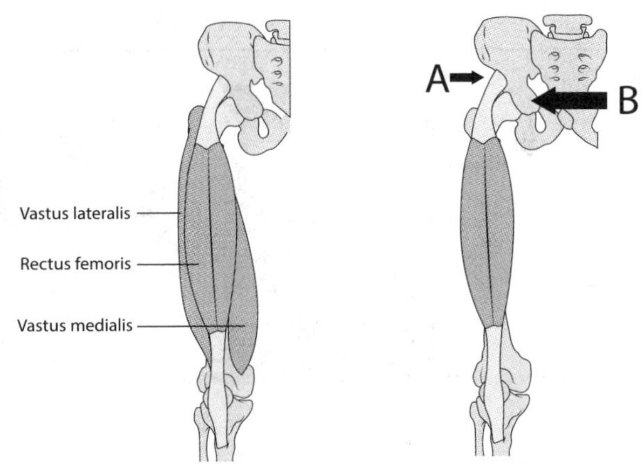

Figure 23-31

In Figure 23-31, left image, you can see the rectus femoris as part of the quadriceps group. In Figure 23-31, right image, you can see the rectus femoris by itself, which allows you to better see that its origin ("A") on the pelvis is slightly above the hip joint ("B"). Since the origin of the psoas is higher above the hip joint, it has better leverage (more power) in hip flexion, than the rectus femoris.

The primary function of the rectus femoris, as part of the quadriceps group, is knee extension. There are two factors, however, that should be noted about the rectus femoris' role in hip flexion: its development can be further enhanced by hip flexion exercise, and its role in hip flexion is opposite the gluteus' role in hip extension. The rectus femoris, therefore is an antagonist to the gluteus maxumus. In other words, either one or the other can be fully activated, in a given moment, due to reciprocal innervation.

When the gluteus maximus is loaded and activated (contracting), a "relaxation synapse" is sent to the hip flexor group, which includes the rectus femoris. In that regard, if you're squatting for the purpose of quadriceps development, the last thing you want is to have part of your quadriceps shutting off—yet this is what happens (when doing *squats*) due to the simultaneous activation of the gluteus maximus. While both muscle groups can, in fact, function simultaneously, there is some degree of compromise in doing so.

The two other muscles that assist in hip flexion are the "tensor fascia lata"—shown in Figure 23-32, left and center images, and the "sartorius"—shown in Figure 23-32, right and center images. The tensor fascia lata is a short muscle that connects to the iliotibial band. The "IT Band" is that long string that runs all the way down the outside of the thigh, and attaches just below the knee (Figure 23-32, left image). The sartorius assists in hip flexion, as well as plays a role in externally rotating the femur. This is apparent by the way it crosses from the outside (lateral side) of the upper leg to the inside (medial side) of the tibia (Figure 23-32, right image).

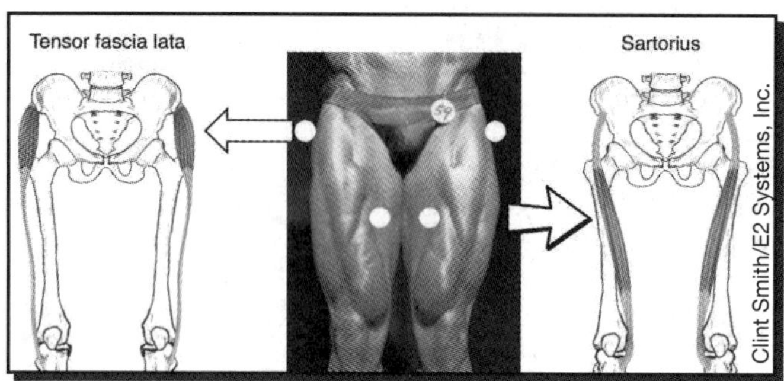

Figure 23-32

## Should You Work Your Hip Flexors?

Assuming you now understand the folly of doing *leg raises*, with the intention of working the abs, you might, at this point, ask the following question: "Is there a benefit to working the hip flexors, for their own sake?" The answer is "yes," but *not* at the same time as working the abs.

Ideally speaking, the two muscles should be worked separately, in order to achieve optimal development in both areas, and to avoid lower back discomfort. You should also avoid raising both legs simultaneously. As such, it's much better to work the hip flexors unilaterally. The only exception to this recommendation would be if you are training for a particular sport, which requires that both legs be lifted simultaneously. An example of this objective would be the gymnastics move shown in Figure 23-33. Even in this instance, however, it's important to understand that this movement should not be considered a "good" ab exercise. If anything, it should be considered a challenging, but unnatural, movement, the performance of which is judged in gymnastics, but is neither a "good" ab exercise, nor a "good" hip flexor exercise.

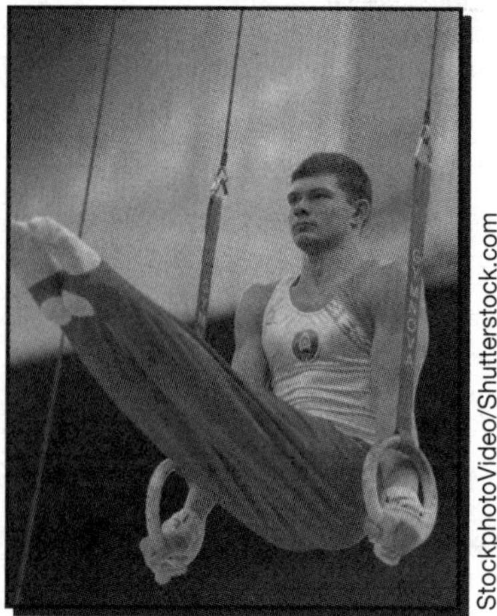

Figure 23-33

Functionally speaking, it's good to keep the hip flexors moderately strong. Not only do they keep you from dragging your feet when you walk, hike, or climb stairs, they also play an important role in maintaining good posture, including keeping your lower back in its proper position.

A slight arch in the lower back (lumbar area) is normal; it's called "lordosis." Maintaining this position is assisted by the hip flexors. Strong hip flexors help you maintain a neutral spine ("A" in Figure 23-34). Weak hip flexors could lead to a flattening of that lordotic curve ("B" in Figure 23-34), which could cause lower back discomfort or pain. It could also eventually lead to the typical "old person shuffle"—dragging the feet when walking, instead of lifting the leg and extending it forward with each step.

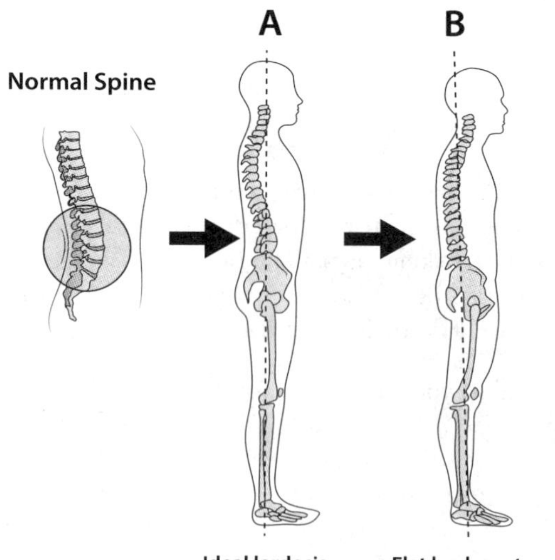

Figure 23-34

The simplest way to keep the hip flexors adequately strong is by simply raising the femur, with the knee bent and the spine slightly arched, up to a point where the femur is perpendicular with the torso. This movement can easily be done at home, while standing in a doorway, holding onto a doorframe for balance. First raise and lower one leg, and then the other leg—alternating the left leg and right leg. For basic maintenance, performing three sets of 15 repetitions would be adequate. A light ankle weight (5 to 10 pounds) could be used for added benefit.

Full range of motion for the hip flexors requires that the femur be raised at least to the point where it is perpendicular to the torso (parallel to the ground), if not a few degrees higher. That would allow full muscle contraction. It is important, however, that the spine be maintained in the normal, lordotic (slightly arched) position, during this action. Therefore, the goal is to raise the femur as high as comfortably possible (slowly and deliberately—not with momentum), but not beyond the point where the arch in the lower back becomes a spinal flexion (the tailbone shifts forward).

The other end of the range of motion—muscle elongation— requires that the femur be allowed to reach the point where it is parallel with the torso. Taking the femur farther back, posteriorly, would provide more stretch of the hip flexors, but is not necessary for optimal stimulation from the exercise. Furthermore, if the hip flexors are taken to an extreme stretch while loaded, it greatly increases the risk of injury. This is due to the mechanical disadvantage that occurs in this situation—similar to what occurs with fully extended elbows, when the biceps are loaded. In general, stretching the hip flexors is good, but it should not be done when the hip flexors are loaded. The hip flexors should be stretched separately, during unloaded, dedicated stretching.

Another way of exercising the hip flexors, while alternately exercising the gluteus, is by doing "*high steps*" (shown in Figure 23-35). Lifting the leg up to the level of a high step requires hip flexors contraction. Then, pushing the leg downward (thereby lifting you upward on to the step) requires glutes and adductors contraction. In addition to exercising the hip flexors and hip extensors, this exercise has the added benefit of providing cardiovascular stimulation. This exercise could also be done on a staircase, or by walking up a flight of stairs, stepping up two or three steps at a time.

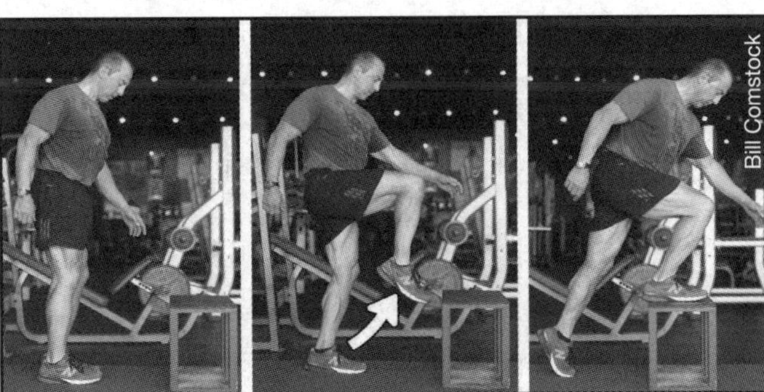

Figure 23-35

If your goal, however, is optimal physique development, you'll need to work your hip flexors with a bit more intensity than simply climbing stairs or doing high step-ups. There are visible advantages to well-developed hip flexors, even though only three of the five hips flexors are superficial (visible). The visible advantages, as well as the method for their development, will be discussed very shortly.

Some people think that, "as long as hip flexion is good, it's better to lift both legs simultaneously, and save time." On the surface, that may seem logical. Part of the appeal behind traditional *leg raises* has been that it's a "compound exercise"—the belief that it works the abs and hip flexors simultaneously. Several versions of traditional *leg raises* are shown in Figures 23-36 to 23-38.

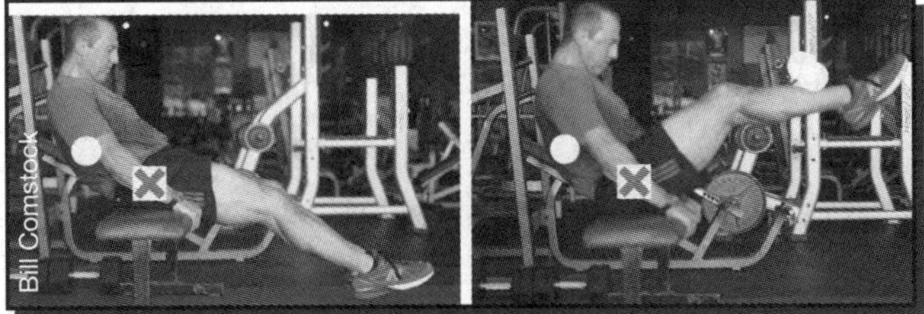

Figure 23-36

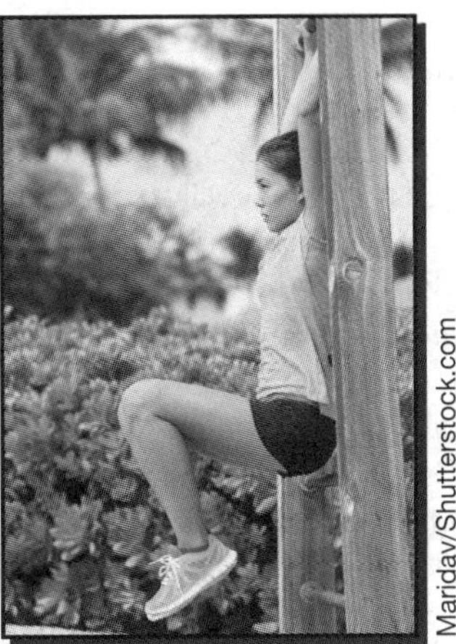

Figure 23-37

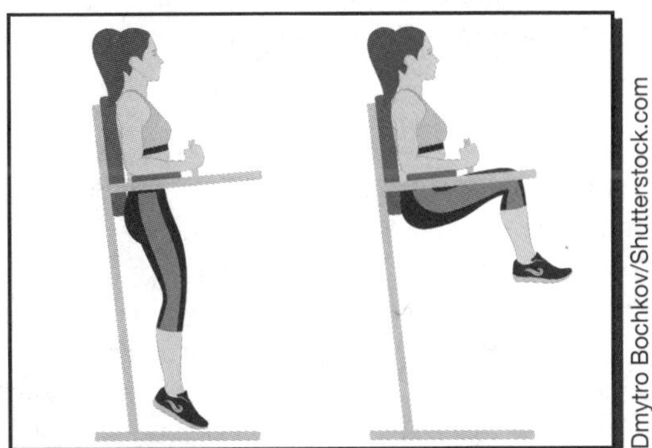

Figure 23-38

There are often significant compromises, however, associated with doing compound exercises. The idea of working two or three muscles in a single exercise is appealing, of course, until the tradeoffs are fully understood. It would be sensible to work several muscles at one time, provided each participating muscle gets as much benefit as it would, if it were worked individually, and as long as there is no risk of injury or discomfort, in combining two or three functions in one exercise. That's the problem, however, with many compound exercises—they usually do not provide "as much benefit" to each participating muscle. They often strain one muscle, while another muscle is not loaded enough. Furthermore, there is frequently some risk of injury, or at least orthopedic discomfort, involved.

A savings of time is not worth an injury (or pain) during an exercise. It is also not worth a compromised benefit, at least not in my view. While other people may be willing to accept such a trade-off, the underlying purpose of this book is to identify the exercises that work best, and to explain why those exercises work best.

As discussed previously, lifting (raising) the weight of both legs simultaneously, during a *leg raise* exercise, often creates a significant amount of lower back discomfort, as compared with lifting one leg at a time. This is obviously due to the fact that activating both psoas muscles (the left side and right side) simultaneously—with the weight of both legs—pulls on the lumbar spine with twice as much force.

Furthermore, there may be a central nervous system mechanism at play that "dislikes" both legs being raised simultaneously. It seems very UN-likely that early humans needed to lift both legs simultaneously, very often. There were no "chin-up bars," nor other readily available method—nor survival purpose—for hominins to simultaneously lift both legs off the ground. Accordingly, early humans would not have had to develop an evolutionary adaptation to lifting both legs simultaneously. This is probably the reason why doing so today creates an unnatural strain on the lumbar spine.

It is preferable to maintain a slightly arched ("lordotic") lumbar spine when performing hip flexion, and it's easier to do that when raising only one leg at a time. After all, this is how a person walks or runs—alternately using the left hip flexors and then the right hip flexors.

At this point, it would be helpful to do another experiment. Go back to the doorway, and hold onto the doorframe with both hands. Then, put all your bodyweight on your left foot, and raise your right leg (flex the right hip), with your knee straight. Next, do the same thing, but with your knee bent. Notice how much more difficult it is to raise your leg, with your knee straight? That's reciprocal innervation and passive insufficiency (two separate neurological factors) at play.

You might think that the straight leg feels heavier, because the leg (as a lever) is longer when the knee is straight. After all, the weight of the leg would be magnified more. On the other hand, if you attach a 20-pound weight to your ankle, and lifted your leg with your knee bent, it would STILL be easier than lifting the leg straight, even without the ankle weight. It is not, therefore, the heavier weight of the leg that makes raising the leg with the knee straight more difficult.

You will also discover that you cannot raise your leg as high, when your knee is straight. Your quadriceps (actually, the rectus femoris, of the quadriceps) will feel like it's cramping long before you get to the point where your femur is perpendicular with your torso. Conversely, you can raise your leg much higher (flex your hip with a greater range of motion), when your knee is bent, and you will not get that cramping sensation at all.

The reason for this is that lifting the leg (the femur) forward with knee straight, stretches the hamstrings. This is perceived as "activation" by the central nervous system, which triggers a "relaxation synapse" (an inhibition message to contract with less force) to the rectus femoris, as well as to the sartorius (another hip flexor), both of which are antagonists (opposite direction function) of the hamstrings. You are likely to feel a cramping sensation in both of these muscles, when you attempt to perform hip flexion with a straight-knee hip.

In addition, the limits of hamstring flexibility further "interfere" with an individual's ability to raise the femur with the knee straight. This is passive insufficiency at work.

Interestingly, you'll notice that when a straight-knee *leg raise* (hip flexion) is attempted, you have a tendency to round your back (Figure 23-39). This reaction is the body's effort to minimize the hamstring stretch that occurs when raising the leg with a straight knee. The hamstrings always stretch more when the lumbar spine is arched. The hamstrings stretch less

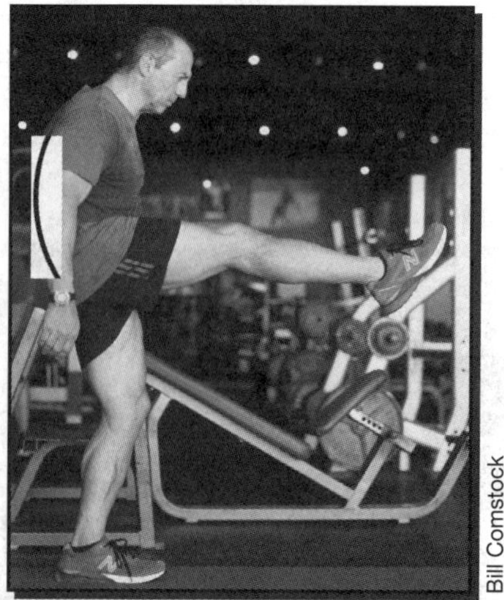

Bill Comstock

Figure 23-39

when a straight leg is raised forward, while the lumbar spine is allowed to round. When the leg is raised forward with a bent knee (Figure 23-40), it is easy to keep the lumbar spine in the neutral/arched position.

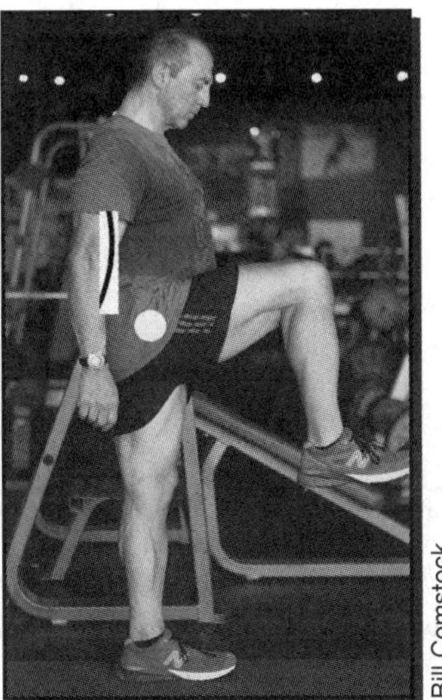
Bill Comstock
Figure 23-40

In fact, raising the femur forward and up, with your knee straight, seems to violate the way the body was designed to operate in nature. Therefore, it is best to work the hip flexors one leg at a time (or alternating between right leg and left leg), with the knee bent (note: the knee can be straight before the hip is flexed, but it needs to bend as the hip is flexed).

This factor also underscores how "unnatural" a *leg raise* is, when performed as an abdominal exercise, because it is typically done with both legs being raised simultaneously, often with straight legs. Frankly, I've never met anyone who didn't "hate" *leg raises*. As such, their disdain for the movement is understandable, given the aforementioned conflicts. Intuitively, people know it doesn't feel natural. It's not so much that a *leg raise* is "difficult"—"challenging" in the way moving a heavy weight is challenging). The movement itself is awkward, and it is also compromised, in terms of benefit.

## Developing the Hip Flexors for Physique Display

In terms of "visible development," the rectus femoris, the sartorius, and the tensor fascia lata are the only three of the five hip flexors that can be seen on a person who is very lean. These are the muscles that are closer to the surface. Because the iliacus and the psoas are "deep" muscles (beneath layers of other muscles), they are never visible.

In bodybuilding (physique display), there are two ways the frontal thigh muscles can be "flexed." One is a straight leg, locked-knee contraction, shown in Figure 23-41. The other is with a slight "upward pull" on the femur (knee slightly bent), which tenses the rectus femoris and the sartorius, shown in Figure 23-42. As you can see in Figure 23-42, my right knee is not locked. Rather, I am flexing my right leg by pulling it slightly upward, deliberately flexing the rectus femoris and the sartorius.

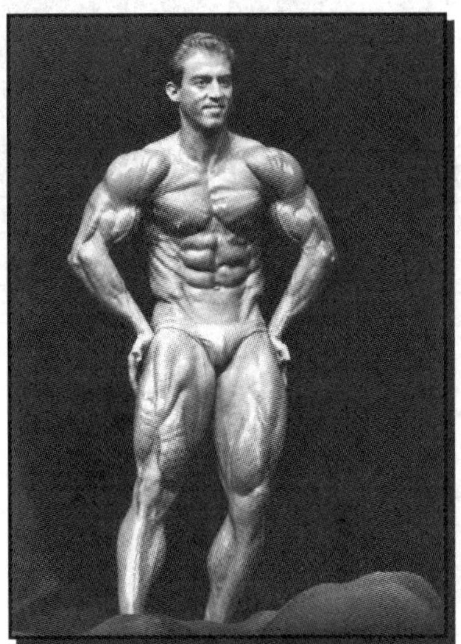
Figure 23-41

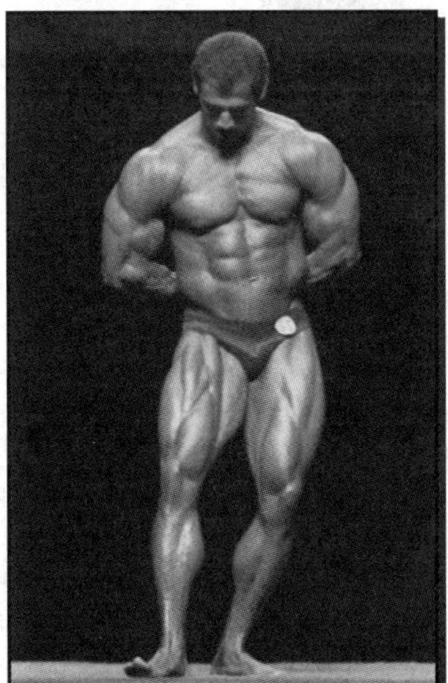
Figure 23-42

The tensor fascia lata is a small muscle at the top/side (lateral) aspect of the thigh, which can be mainly be seen from the side (the arrow in Figure 23-43). Despite the fact that it is situated only at the top of the outer thigh, however, it often plays a role in the appearance of the entire thigh (when viewed from the side), because it pulls on the iliotibial band. In Figure 23-44, left image (photo taken at a 2016 competition, at the age of 56), you can see a deep groove running down the entire side of my right thigh. That is the precise path of the iliotibial band, as you can see in Figure 23-44, right image.

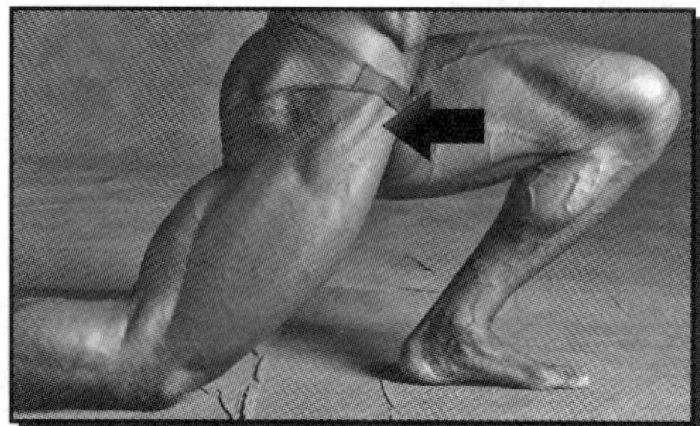

Figure 23-43

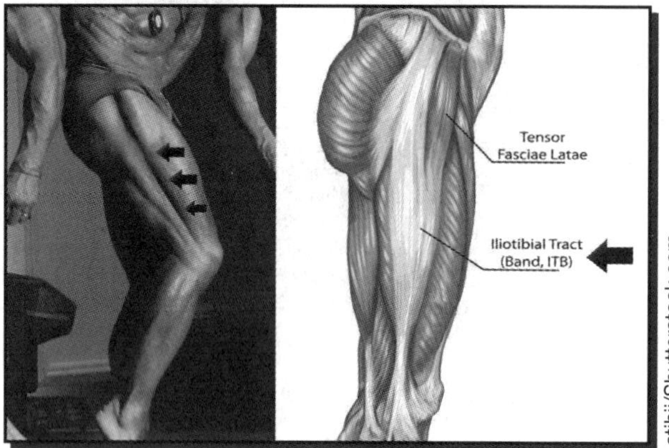


Figure 23-44

As you can see there are benefits—both functional as well as visible—for exercising the hip flexors.

## Exercise Options for the Hip Flexors

The following are the biomechanical factors that an exercise should provide for the most un-compromised engagement of the hip flexors:

- Do not use hip flexion as part of an "ab workout." Do not attempt to flex the spine, while performing hip flexion, as this creates a competing force for spinal position.
- Perform hip flexion one leg at a time, ideally, as an alternated unilateral exercise, as this prevents excessive pulling on the lumbar spine.
- Do not perform hip flexion with a straight knee. You can start the movement with a straight knee, but it's best to bend the knee (of the leg that's being raised), because this avoids reciprocal innervation and passive insufficiency (hamstring stretch limitations).
- Perform hip flexion with your spine arched, as this is the preferred spinal position for psoas engagement.
- Use a resistance curve that takes into consideration the mechanical disadvantage that occurs when the femur is parallel with the torso. In other words, the exercise should provide less resistance at the beginning of the movement, and more resistance toward the middle and end of the movement.

Hip flexion is similar to elbow flexion, in the sense that both movements experience mechanical disadvantage at the beginning of the range of motion. The hip flexors (the psoas, iliacus, tensor fascia lata, rectus femoris, and sartorius) all pull on the femur from a mostly parallel angle when the femur is in line with the torso. This is exactly like the biceps, pulling on the forearm from a mostly parallel angle, when the elbow is straight.

Therefore, just like with the biceps, the ideal exercise for the hip flexors should provide less resistance at the beginning of range of motion (offsetting the mechanical disadvantage), and more resistance toward the middle of the range of motion, when the muscles gain mechanical advantage.

In Figure 23-45, imagine that this individual is wearing an ankle weight. The arrow indicates the direction of resistance (gravity), pulling straight down on that ankle weight. As you can see, that direction of resistance would be "zero/neutral" (parallel with the femur) at the beginning of the range of motion. Then, as the femur is raised, it becomes more perpendicular (more "active") with the direction of resistance. This factor compensates for the mechanical disadvantage at the beginning, and provides an increasing level of resistance when mechanical advantage improves. This scenario is exactly like what occurs with the biceps, during a *standing dumbbell curl*, and it's a very good resistance curve. Simple as it may be, this would be a good exercise for the hip flexors (alternating left leg, then right leg), although I would suggest holding onto either a doorway or the handles of a *parallel bar dip* station, for balance.

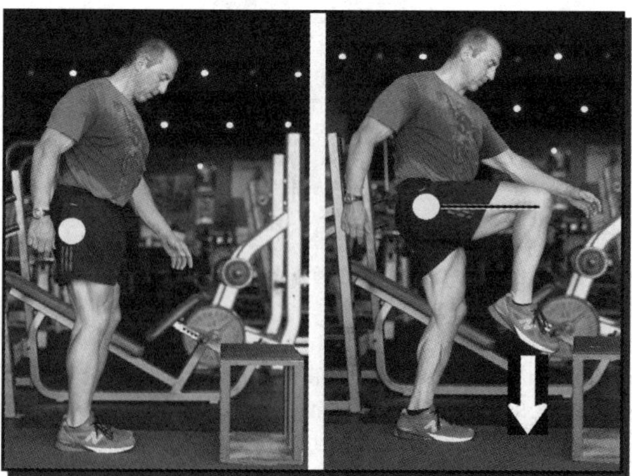

Figure 23-45

While doing this exercise, you should keep your torso upright with a slight arch in the lumbar spine. Raise the leg (the femur) up to the point where you begin feeling it difficult to maintain the slight arch in the lumbar spine—no farther. It would be best to keep the lower leg (i.e., the tibia of the leg being lifted) as vertical as possible, as it is being lifted.

You might be surprised to discover that performing this movement, with a full range of motion (bringing the leg as high as possible, without losing the arch in the lower back), for 15 or 20 repetitions, is very challenging, even with only the weight of the leg. You can make it significantly more challenging, and thus more effective, by adding an ankle weight. It doesn't take much added weight to make a big difference—5 lbs., 7 lbs. or 10 lbs. is more than enough.

The exercise shown in Figure 23-46 is NOT a good option. With this lying version, the legs are perpendicular, with gravity at the beginning of the range of motion, which consequently loads the hip flexors the most during the early part of the range of motion—precisely where the mechanical disadvantage of the hip flexors is at its worst. Notice the arrow, indicating the direction of resistance, acting perpendicularly upon the horizontal femur—where mechanical disadvantage (of the hip flexors) is at its worst. Then, as mechanical advantage is gained—when the legs are raised and the hip flexors can pull on the femurs from a more perpendicular angle—the resistance is diminished, because the legs would be more vertical (parallel with gravity). In other words, this exercise provides more resistance when your hip angle is at its "weakest," and the least amount of resistance, when your hip angle is at its "strongest."

Doing this exercise with both legs simultaneously places a tremendous amount of stress on the lower back (lumbar spine), because the psoas must pull the weight of both legs simultaneously. This is because the psoas originates on the lumbar spine, and the force required of them—given the mechanical disadvantage that occurs in the early phase of the range of motion—is significantly more than would occur while in the upright position. In addition to the lower back strain, this exercise is also very compromised (very unproductive) for the "abs."

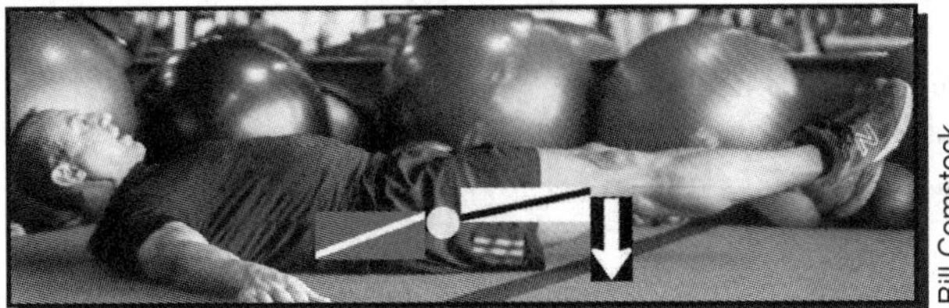

Figure 23-46

The exercise shown in Figure 23-47—"*hip flexion* on a multi-hip machine"—is a fairly good option. Notice that the roller is in front of my femur now, and I am PULLING upward against it—I am not pushing downward against the roller, as I would when performing hip extension, for the gluteus. This exercise provides more resistance in the flexed-hip position (where mechanical advantage is gained), as compared with the aforementioned exercise. Arguably, however, it provides a bit more resistance at the beginning of the range of motion than is ideal (i.e., due to the mechanical disadvantage that occurs at that point). On the plus side, it allows unilateral movement (one leg at a time), and it also facilitates keeping the lumbar spine arched, because you can use the hand rail to help lift the chest up and keep the tailbone back.

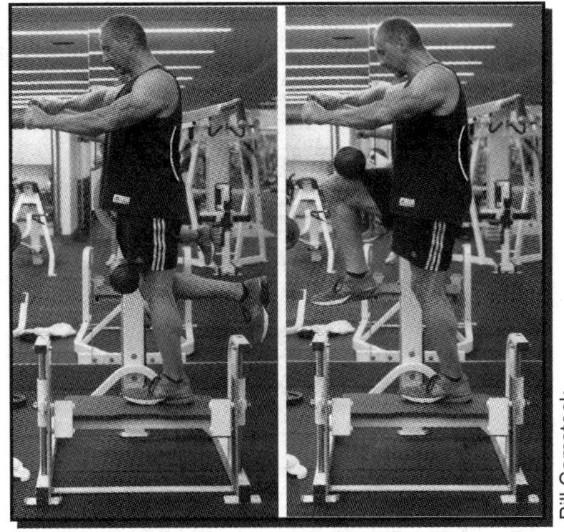

Figure 23-47

In my opinion, the "best" hip flexor exercise, if you want to use more resistance than a 10 lb. ankle weight can provide (however, more than 30 lbs. is *not* necessary), is the one shown in Figure 23-48, "*lying alternating cable hip flexion.*" Its components are all biomechanically "ideal." If you are fortunate enough to have access to a pulley machine that allows this type of adjustability, this exercise is worth doing, because of the following factors:

- It allows the unilateral motion (one leg at a time, alternating or single leg).
- It provides "hands free" stability (lying flat on the ground).
- It allows the lower back to be arched, a positioning that can be further assisted by placing a pad under the tailbone, as shown in Figure 23-48.
- It allows an individual to select the exact weight that feels appropriate
- It allows the direction of resistance (pulley height) to be set for a perfect resistance curve (less challenging at the early phase, and more challenging toward the latter phase, compensating for the mechanical disadvantage).
- It allows the knee to be bent, as the hip is being flexed.

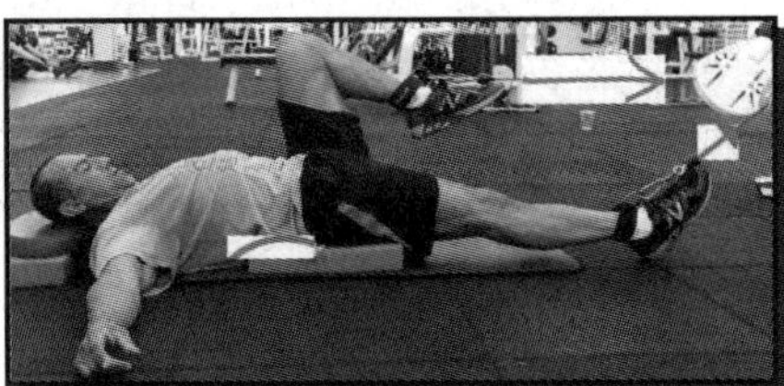
Figure 23-48

Note that the pulley height is set at the same height as where the distal end of the femur (i.e., the point where the femur and the tibia meet) is positioned, on the raised leg. That position is when the femur is perpendicular with the cable, which makes the femur most active, precisely when the hip angle is at mechanical advantage (which is good). This positioning also allows the cable to pull slightly upward on the leg when it's at the beginning of the movement, thereby compensating for the weight of the leg, when the hip angle is at the mechanical disadvantage position.

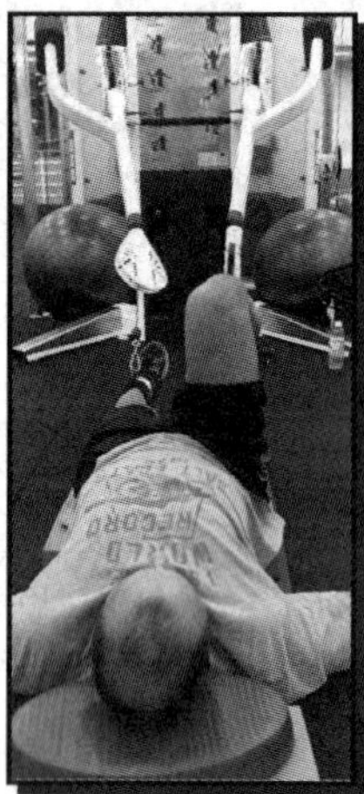

Figure 23-49

Figure 23-49 shows that the distance between the two pulleys is approximately the same as the width of the hips. This factor helps meet the criteria of proper alignment, between the direction of the motion, the direction of resistance, and the origin and the insertion of the target muscle(s).

If you only have access to a single adjustable pulley, you could do a one-legged version of this exercise, which would require you to shift left and right, so that the pulley is aligned with the leg that's working. In either case (whether alternating between right leg and left leg, or doing all your left leg reps, and then all your right leg reps), once you've attached the cable(s) to your ankle cuffs, you need to scoot back (away from the pulleys), so that the selected weights are lifted up off the remaining weights (on the weight stack), when your legs are straight.

As an interesting experiment, try doing this exercise, while deliberately focusing on the arching of your lower back. Then, try it without arching your lower back, perhaps even with the abdominals contracted (spine slightly flexed/tailbone tucked forward). You'll quickly realize that it feels much more "natural"/more comfortable, when the lower back is arched. This factor demonstrates the conflict of trying to flex the abs and the hip flexors, at the same time. When performing this exercise, I suggest using between 20 and 30 pounds (with each leg), for 15 to 20 repetitions per leg, per set, for three or four sets, with a minute or two between sets.

The range of motion during this exercise is influenced by the arch of your lower back. There is a point where the femur cannot be raised any farther, without releasing the arch of the lower back. That is the point where the range of motion should stop. The spine must be kept in its normal "lordotic" (slightly arched) position, through the entire range of hip flexion. You should resist the temptation to pull the femur "higher" (closer toward your chest), by rounding the lumbar spine.

A misconception exists that working the hip flexors causes them to be "tight." As such, some trainers discourage their clients from working their hip flexors, mistakenly believing that most people's hip flexors are already "too tight," and working them will just make them more so. This advice is ridiculous.

Do you walk around with "tight" biceps (elbows bent), simply because you exercised your biceps? Of course not. Strengthening a muscle does not cause it to be in a constant state of contraction. In fact, a muscle that is exercised regularly is LESS likely to be tight, due to the process of muscle elongation, which occurs between dynamic contractions, with each repetition. Of course, stretching is always helpful.

Incidentally, "muscle soreness" is not the same thing as "muscle tightness." They are very different conditions. A muscle can be tight, without being sore. Furthermore, a muscle can be sore, without being tight. In fact, individuals often stretch a sore muscle, and it feels good to do so. Soreness, however, does not mean that a muscle is excessively "short," or that it is in a constant state of contraction, restricting normal skeletal movement.

Finally, you are encouraged to conduct one more experiment. This experiment will allow you to have some context for the chapter (25) involving the abs and the transverse abdominis, which is upcoming.

While lying on the floor with your lumbar slightly arched, notice that your abdomen naturally tends to fall inward. With just a little bit more effort, you can even pull your abdomen further inward, drawing it toward your spine, essentially creating a "vacuum." Next, instead of arching your lumbar spine, round it, by pulling your tailbone upward and pushing your lumbar spine toward the floor. At this point, try pulling your abdomen inward.

What you'll discover is that pulling your abdomen inward, i.e., doing a "vacuum," is impossible, if your tailbone is pulled upward/forward (spinal flexion). Yet, this combination of two actions is what trainers often tell their clients to do, when they are performing abdominal crunches. It is impossible to combine a flexed spine and an abdominal vacuum, at the same time. You cannot "hold your abdomen in," while simultaneously contracting your "abs" (rectus abdominis). The reason for this fact will be discussed at greater length in Chapter 25.

# CHAPTER 24

# Calves, Abs, and Lower Back

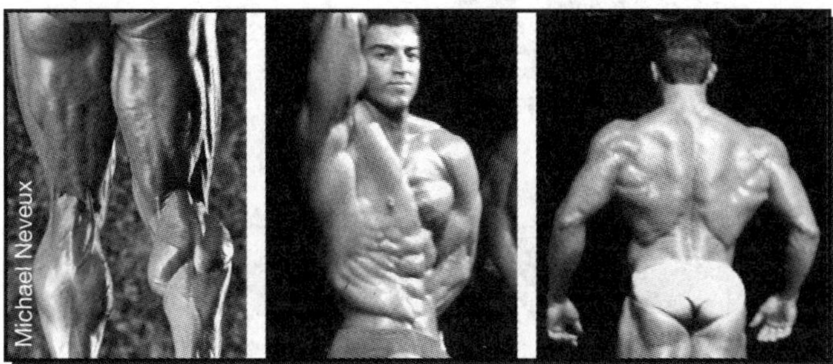

Figure 24-1

## Anatomy of the Calves

The "calves" are generally thought to be comprised of two separate muscles—the gastrocnemius and the soleus. Some anatomists, however, consider the two as just one muscle, because the two parts converge at the single Achilles tendon and produce one single function—plantar flexion (i.e., extension of the ankle). This situation is similar to the triceps, which has three separate "heads," and three origins, but one single insertion. The triceps is generally considered "one muscle."

Although the "gastroc" and the soleus produce the same anatomical function, some individuals believe these two parts can be separately targeted in the weight room. The reason you might hope for this to be true, is to optimize hypertrophy (growth) of the calves. The soleus, however, appears to have extremely little capacity for growth. Furthermore, there is evidence that, if these two parts have different functions, it is not based on anatomical movement, nor the degree of knee bend. Rather, it is based on the degree of effort (amount of resistance), or the intensity of force required of any particular movement, a factor which will be addressed shortly.

Figure 24-2 shows the anatomy of the "calf" from both the back and the side. The side view shows that the soleus lies underneath the gastrocnemius. Note that the soleus is a very flat muscle, which suggests that it has very little capacity for growth. In fact, "calf" growth is due mostly to hypertrophy of the gastrocnemius.

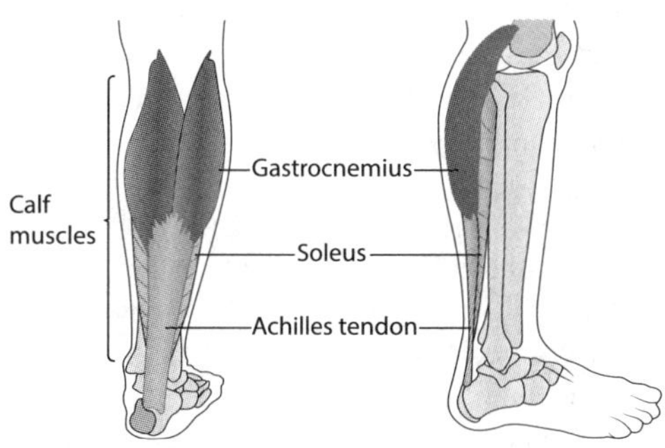

Figure 24-2

The more detailed illustrations in Figure 24-3 (lower image) show a posterior view of the right lower leg. In the image on the far left, you can see that the gastrocnemius is made up of two parts, referred to in gym jargon as "the inner head" and the "outer head." The inner part, which is technically called the "*medial head*," originates on the medial condyle of the femur ("A"). The outer part, which is called the "*lateral head*," originates on the lateral condyle of the femur ("B"). Both of these origins are just above the knee joint.

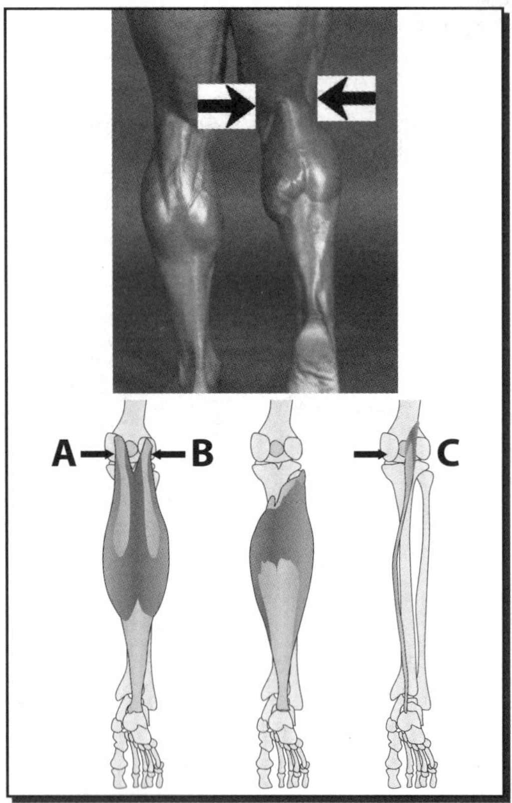

Figure 24-3

The center figure in Figure 24-3 shows the soleus. As you can see, it originates just below the knee. Its origin spans both the tibia and the fibula (the two lower leg bones), but it is still considered as one single origin.

The gastrocnenius and the soleus (both) then converge into the one single "Achilles" tendon, as it's commonly known. Technically, it's called the "calcaneal tendon." This tendon then connects to the heel bone, which is called the "calcaneus." When the calf muscle contracts (shortens), it pulls upward on the heel bone by way of the Achilles tendon, which causes the forefoot to extend downward.

The far right image in Figure 24-3 shows a muscle that is not commonly known, which is called the "plantaris" ("C"). Only the highest part is the muscle (5 to 10 centimeters long), and the rest of it is tendon. In fact, it is considered the longest tendon in the human body. Interestingly, 8 to 12 percent of modern humans do not have a plantaris at all, which has led some experts to speculate that it may be a remnant from the early primate days of humans, when "grasping" with the feet was necessary. In fact, the plantaris may be evolving out.

This tiny muscle originates just above the lateral condyle of the femur. Its tendon then crosses the ankle joint, and attaches onto the calcaneus (heel bone), adjacent to the Achilles tendon (it does not merge with the Achilles tendon). It participates, although weakly, in plantar flexion.

## The Function of the Gastrocnemius vs. the Soleus

Some people believe that performing straight-leg calf exercises (e.g., like the *standing calf raises* shown in Figure 24-4) will work the gastrocnemius more than the soleus, and that performing bent knee calf exercises (like the *seated calf raises* shown in Figure 24-5) will work the soleus more than the gastrocnemius.

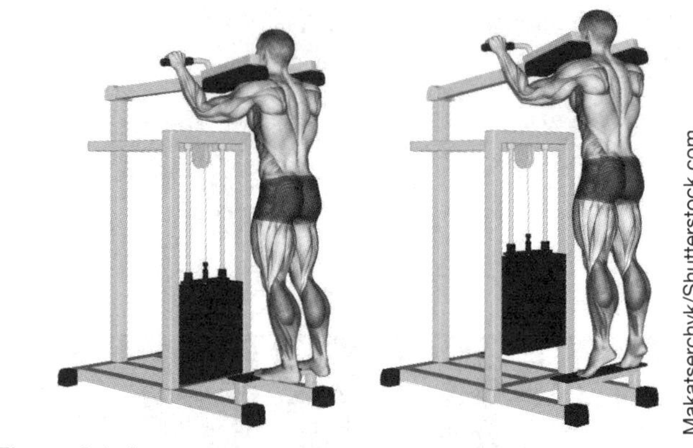
Makatserchyk/Shutterstock.com

Figure 24-4

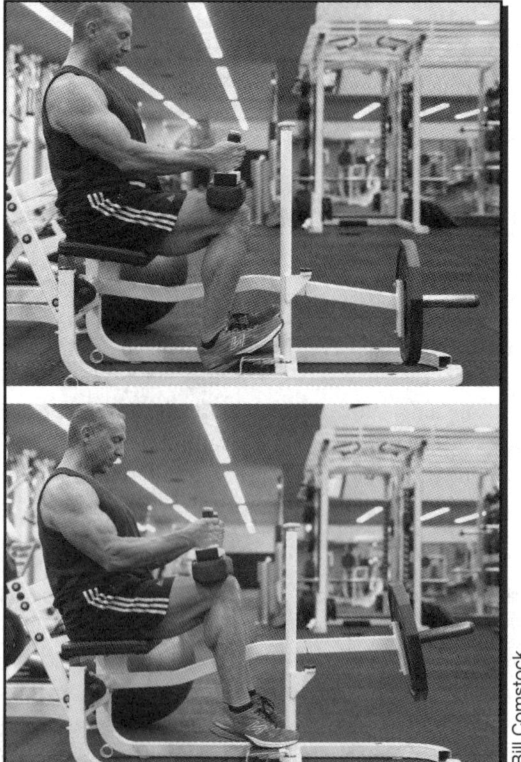
Bill Comstock

Figure 24-5

This *theory* is based on the fact that when the knee is straight, the gastroc is more elongated (stretched) than it is when the knee is bent. Since the origin of the gastrocnemius is above the knee, rather than below it, bending the knee causes the origin to move closer to the insertion, thereby shortening the distance between the two. It is assumed, therefore, that since the gastroc is less able to stretch (during *seated calf raises*), the soleus will be forced to work more, because the soleus gets more stretch (in the heel-descended position), than does the gastrocnemius, when the knees are bent at 90 degrees.

It's true that the gastrocnemius does not benefit as much from a *seated calf raise* (a calf exercise with the knees bent at 90 degrees), as it does from a calf exercise performed with straight, or nearly straight knees. On the other hand, this does not automatically cause the soleus to benefit more, in terms of activation or development.

What appears to be more influential in determining whether the gastroc works more or the soleus works more is the speed and/or the intensity of the movement (i.e., plantar flexion). Both muscles participate to a degree any time plantar flexion is activated, but it appears that the *effort, speed,* or *intensity* required by the activity determines which "muscle/ part" (gastroc or soleus) is activated more.

Apparently, the gastrocnemius is comprised of mostly "white" (type II/fast-twitch) muscle fibers, while the soleus is comprised of mostly "red" (type I/slow-twitch) muscle fibers. As a result, the gastroc tends to work slightly more when called upon for speed, or during high-load/high-intensity efforts. Examples of this would be running or performing loaded-resistance exercise. The soleus tends to work slightly more when called upon for low-speed or low-load/low-fatigue efforts. Examples of this would be walking or simply standing.

This conclusion is not merely theorized. The pathway for this preferential activation (gastrocnemius versus soleus), which has been researched, is explained in the following passage (https://en.wikipedia.org/wiki/Gastrocnemius_muscle):

> *"Along with the soleus muscle, the gastrocnemius forms half of the calf muscle. Its function is plantar flexing of the foot at the ankle joint and flexing the leg at the knee joint. The gastrocnemius is primarily involved in running, jumping and other 'fast' movements of leg, and to a lesser degree in walking and standing. This specialization is connected to the predominance of white muscle fibers (type II fast twitch) present in the gastrocnemius, as opposed to the soleus, which has more red muscle fibers (type I slow twitch) and is the primary active muscle when standing still, as determined by EMG studies."*

The reason that the gastroc benefits less from a *seated calf raise* (i.e., ankle extension performed with knees bent at 90 degrees) is because of "*active insufficiency.*" In Chapter 11, it was discussed that a muscle that crosses *two* joints (instead of just one joint) must have sufficient length in order to operate with full strength. When an individual performs a *seated (bent-knee) calf raise,* the length of the gastrocnemius is excessively shortened, because the origin of the calf muscle is brought closer to the insertion of the calf muscle. As a result, active insufficiency (muscle weakness) is triggered as the muscle contracts, because it over-shortens. This weakness is typically accompanied by a cramping sensation in the operating muscle.

For this reason, it is more productive to perform a calf exercise with the knees straight or nearly straight—either by way of "*standing calf raises*" or some type of calf extension performed on a *leg press* machine—if the goal is optimum development of the calves.

*Seated calf raises* can be used a nice warm-up for the ankles and calves, before moving to a straighter-leg version a calf exercise, using heavier weight. It would be unwise, however, to expect much (calf) muscle growth from doing *seated calf raises.*

It should also be noted that attempting to use a heavy weight on the *seated calf raise* is potentially dangerous. This risk occurs because, since there is less gastroc stretch in the bent-knee position, there is less ankle protection. When the knees are mostly straight, the gastroc essentially prevents the ankle from bending beyond its safe limit. When the knees are bent at 90 degrees, however, the soleus is left with the entire burden of preventing overflexion of the ankle, which it is much less capable of doing than the gastrocnemius. For this reason, it would be wise to not go very heavy, or avoid descending into the excessive ankle flexion position (deep stretch range) using heavy weight, when doing *seated calf raises.*

## Impossible to Emphasize "Inner" Calf vs. "Outer" Calf

Some bodybuilders feel dissatisfied with the shape of their calves, as their calves are developing. As a result, they assume that they can alter the shape of their calves by modifying the way they perform their calf exercises. This assumption is misguided.

Over the years, many individuals have heard (erroneously) that they can preferentially activate the medial (inner) head of the gastrocnemius or the lateral (outer) head of the gastrocnemius, simply by angling their toes IN or OUT, during a calf exercise. This is absolutely not true, however. It is simply gym lore (like folklore)—wishful thinking.

Nothing, based on individual preference, can influence whether the medial head or the lateral head works harder. The reason for this fact is that both the "inner" and the "outer" calf heads pull on the one single Achilles tendon, and the ankle bends/extends (mostly) in one direction. When the calf muscle contracts, both "inner" and "outer" heads of the gastroc (along with the soleus, to the degree required) collaborate in unison, and pull straight upward on the heel bone. This collaborative effort of upward-pulling on the heel bone produces plantar flexion/ankle extension.

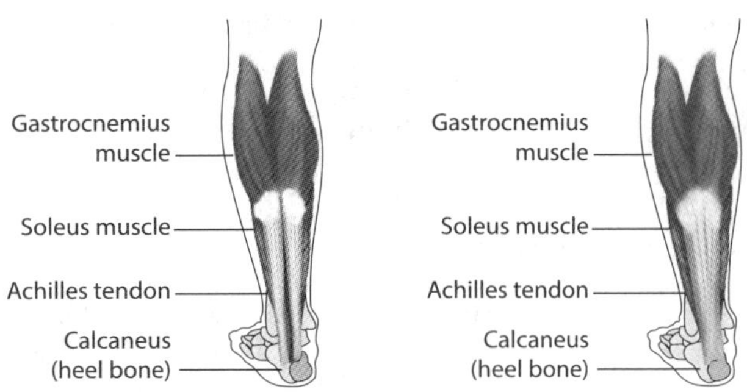


Figure 24-6

Figure 24-6, left image, includes two separate "make-believe" Achilles tendons. Hypothetically, consider, for just a moment, that this is the actual anatomy of the gastrocnemius. If it were possible for the "inner calf" to work separately from the "outer calf," each head would have to have its own separate tendon, and separate attachment to the heel bone. Each of these tendons would then have the ability to pull the calcaneus in a different direction, which would allow the inner or the outer head to act separately, based on separate ankle movements.

Figure 24-6, right image, illustrates reality. The inner and outer heads of the calf muscle can only pull straight upward on the one single tendon, and cannot be separately isolated.

Examine what happens when you turn your toes inward or outward. It is obvious that turning the toes inward or outward cannot possibly alter the direction of ankle movement, and cannot possibly preferentially load the inner or the outer head of the gastroc. Rather, angling the toes inwardly or outwardly requires rotation of the entire leg at the level of the hip. It does not change the mechanics of how the calf pulls upward the Achilles tendon, and on the heel bone.

It's impossible to rotate the foot without rotating the lower leg. It is also impossible to rotate the lower leg without rotating the femur. As such, the orientation of the calf muscle, relative to the ankle and the Achilles tendon, is the same, regardless of whether the toes are pointing inwardly or outwardly.

The shape of your calves is determined by your genetics. We have no control over the shape of our calves, other than simply increasing and decreasing their size. In fact, I have never seen anyone change the shape of their calves as a result of exercise selection, or as a result of having turned their toes in or out, during *calf extensions*, in the 40-plus years I've spent in bodybuilding. It has never been demonstrated empirically, nor does it make sense mechanically.

## Ideal Foot Position, When Training the Calves

Since the angle of the foot (during a calf exercise) does not influence the shape of the calves, you are left with the question of whether there is an ideal foot position, for the sake of comfort or "grip." People are often seen in the gym, doing their calf exercises, with ONLY their toes on the block. This technique would be like trying to do *dumbbell curls*, while holding the dumbbells ONLY with your fingertips. In fact, the wisest approach would be to use the most secure grip (or footing) possible, so that there is no "weak link" in the chain.

The "ball" of the foot refers to the large, bony pad that is just behind the "big toe." That part of your foot is the podiatric equivalent of the first knuckle on your hand, otherwise known as the "sesamoid" bone (Figure 24-7). In fact, that entire part of your foot should be on the block, because it is much more solid than are your toes. That is the part of the foot from which you can best push resistance, and from which you can achieve the best calf stretch, while loaded.

As you can see in Figure 24-7, the sesamoid bones do not form a perfect horizontal line across a vertical foot. They line up diagonally, along that line that has been placed there. As a result, in order to place the more solid part of your foot on the block, while the rest of the foot is OFF the block, you should angle your toes inward (heels outward). This positioning would give you the most secure grip on the foot plate, of whichever apparatus you're using for your calf exercise.

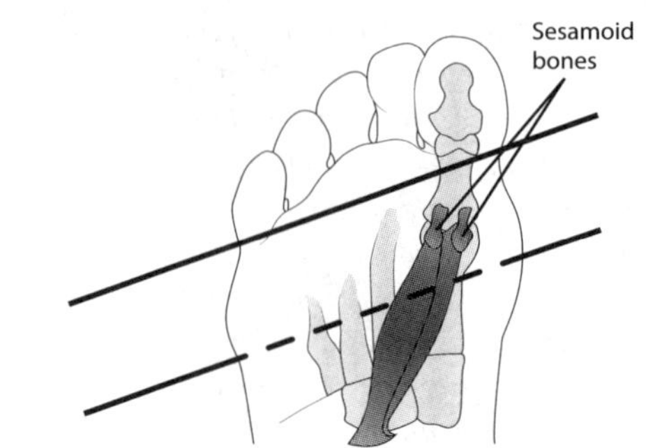


Figure 24-7

In Figure 24-8, you can see how your feet would be placed on the "block," during a calf exercise, given the aforementioned rationale. The two bold lines indicate the firmest part of the forefoot, while the thin line at the top indicates where the top edge of the block may be. What's important is that the area shown between the bold lines be fully on the block.

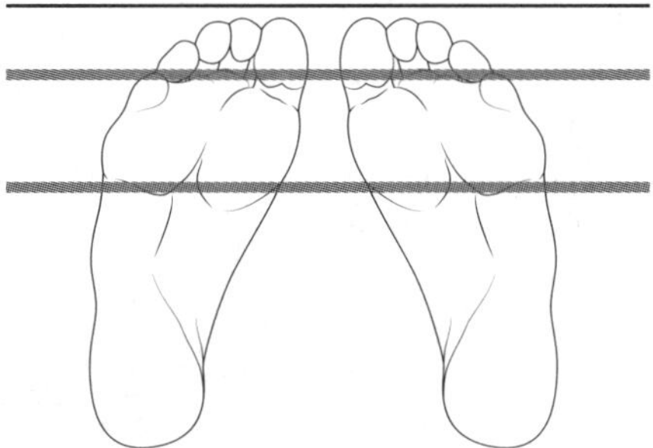

Figure 24-8

Your goal should be to employ the most secure footing, thereby allowing you to avoid fatiguing the toes before the calf muscle is thoroughly fatigued. I am not suggesting that positioning the feet straight (parallel to each other), or that "toes out" are not productive alternatives. Rather, I am suggesting that placing your feet on the block with a "toes-in" position provides a more secure footing, from which you can best perform plantar flexion with resistance.

It should also be noted that during most calf exercises, the feet usually slip off the foot block, little by little. When this situation happens (usually every 5 to 10 repetitions, or so), you should briefly pause, bring your feet back up to their original position, and then continue the set. If your feet are barely hanging onto the block by the toes, it will be impossible to enter into a full calf stretch position, or a full calf contraction position, which then compromises the effectiveness of the exercise.

## Range of Motion, When Training the Calves

The most common "mistake" that occurs, with regard to calf training, is people using an extremely short range of motion during their calf exercises. In fact, it's amazingly pervasive—individuals using a range of motion that is very abbreviated, often just a short "bouncy" movement, completely failing to bring their heels low enough for a full stretch, nor high enough for any sort of legitimate muscle contraction. As a rule, this situation usually occurs because people are trying to use too much weight, although it could also happen as a result of laziness or a lack of awareness.

"Range of motion" was addressed extensively in Chapter 9. Clearly, it was pointed out that a "repetition" is not just a twitch. It is a motion that represents a significant percentage (70 to 80 percent, if not 100 percent) of the full range of skeletal movement that a given muscle is able to produce. Unfortunately, individuals often sacrifice range of motion in favor of using a very heavy weight, either believing that it's a worthwhile trade, or not even realizing that they've reduced the potential range of motion by as much as 80 percent. In that regard using a very heavy weight for a range of motion that only represents 10 or 20 percent of a muscle's full range capability is hardly more effective than an isometric contraction, which is almost entirely unproductive for the purpose of muscle growth.

The reason we place only our forefoot on a calf block—allowing the heel to hang off the block—is so that the heels can (and do) drop lower than the balls of your feet. More often than not, however, people do not allow their heels to drop even to the same level as the block, which defeats the purpose of placing only the forefoot on a block.

In fact, it is far more productive to use less weight and a full range of motion. The weight you select should challenge you, but still allow a full calf stretch and a full calf contraction, on every single repetition. If the weight you select does not allow you to get a full calf stretch (complete flexion of the ankle) and a full calf contraction (complete extension of the ankle), then it is too heavy.

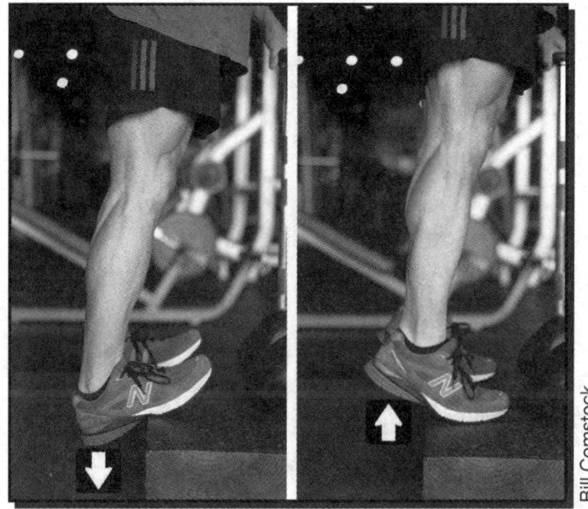


Figure 24-9

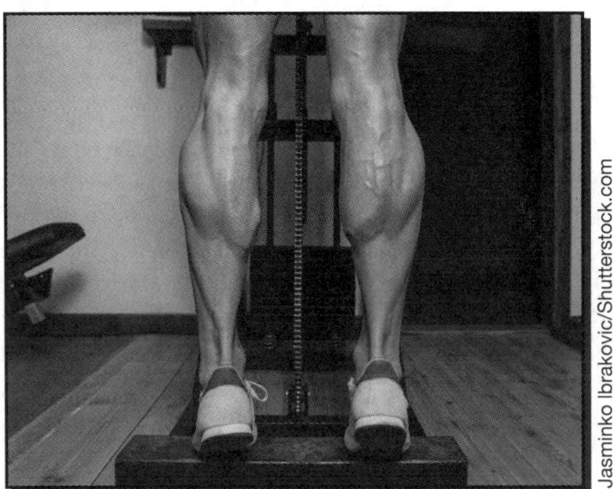


Figure 24-10

Keeping the knees completely straight, when performing either *standing calf raises* or *leg press calf extensions*, may cause some discomfort in the area behind the knee, for some (if not most) people. This factor depends (to a degree) on whether an individual's knees tend to hyperextend, as well as on how much weight is being used. In reality, even a small degree of hyperextension of the knee (the knee bending beyond "straight") will place a significant degree of stress on the knee joint, when a heavy weight is being used.

The solution to this situation is to maintain a very slight bend in the knee during the entire set of *calf raises/calf extensions*, when the weight being used is "heavy."

Keeping the knees perfectly straight is fine, when utilizing a light weight, assuming your knees do not naturally hyperextend. Achieving a "very slight knee bend" (as shown in Figure 24-11) may be difficult to coordinate in the beginning, but it will eventually become "second-nature" (habit).

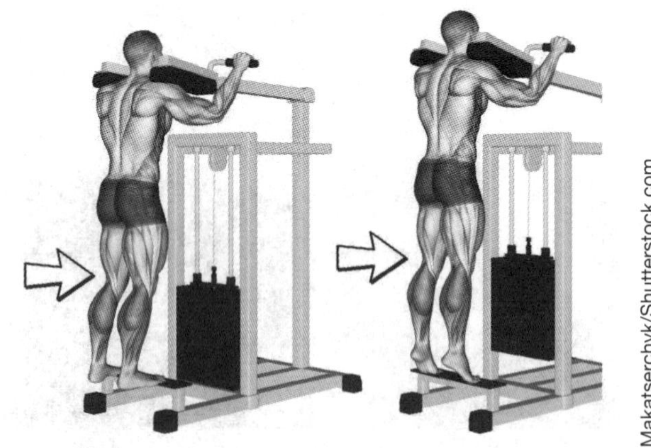


Figure 24-11

## The Proper Amount of Resistance, When Training the Calves

In order to build/develop a muscle, it must be sufficiently challenged. A "sufficient challenge" requires a significant percentage of maximum effort. "Maximum effort" can be achieved two different ways—either by total muscle fatigue, after having performed high repetition (20 to 50 reps), or by using a weight that is heavy enough to represent 80 percent to 90 percent of maximum effort, for low repetitions (4 to 10 reps), even if that set is not to total fatigue. Either of these situations results in a high percentage of muscle fiber recruitment, which results in optimal muscle growth.

*Note: Optimal muscle growth is also influenced by genetics, proper nutrition, adequate rest, and recovery. Furthermore, it's important to warm up a muscle with lighter weight and higher reps, before "heavy" weight is used, in order to minimize risk of injury and to maximize strength potential.*

For a more detailed explanation of the adaptive effects of high repetition resistance training versus low repetition resistance training, you should consult the following articles in the NCBI—the National Center for Biotechnology Information/NLM ; U.S. National Library of Medicine:

- "Effects of different volume-equated resistance training loading strategies on muscular adaptations in well-trained men," Schoenfeld BJ, Ratamess NA, Peterson MD, Contreras B, Sonmez GT, Alvar BA
- "Effects of low – versus high – load resistance training on muscle strength and hypertrophy in well-trained men," Schoenfeld BJ, Peterson MD, Osborn D, Contreras B, Sonmez GT)

The amount of weight that a person "should" select for a given exercise, whether you're discussing calf training or any other skeletal muscle, is different for every person. As such, for the goal of muscular development, it should be based on the following five factors:

- The number of reps intended
- Using full (or mostly full) range of motion
- Deliberate muscle force/no momentum used
- Proper exercise form (exercise performed correctly)
- Represents maximum (or almost maximum/95 percent) effort, given the number of repetitions selected

The aforementioned criteria requires a degree of thoughtfulness, as well as the ability to feel/identify compliance. It also requires you to keep your ego in check, e.g., to not be influenced by self-deception or unrealistic ambitions.

It is a mistake to select a resistance level that is based on the amount of weight someone else uses. The weight you select for any exercise must take into consideration each of the aforementioned five factors. If you are unable to comply with these five factors, because the weight you've selected is too heavy, your results will be compromised.

Very often, either when training the calves or another muscle group, people feel compelled to use the entire weight stack (on a standing calf machine, for example, shown in Figure 24-12), or as much weight as the *leg press* will accommodate, and then perform the set using 10 – 20 percent of the possible range of motion. This approach is foolish.

The amount of weight that is provided on a given machine is arbitrary (i.e., in reference to "selectorized" machines, which have a weight stack, from which a weight is selected by moving the "pin" from plate to plate). The size of that weight stack has not been calculated using actual testing of people performing that particular exercise, using proper exercise form/complete range of motion. It is simply an amount of weight that is likely to satisfy the greatest number of people, commercially speaking.

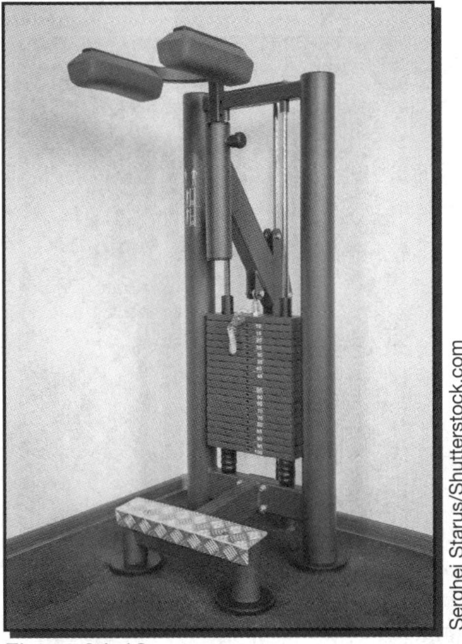
Serghei Starus/Shutterstock.com

Figure 24-12

If you are honest with yourself, and you use the aforementioned five criteria, you will likely discover that your calves can be worked very well, using much less weight than is typically available on a machine's weight stack. Your goal should be to work the calf muscle—not to focus on lifting an "impressive" amount of weight, without regard to the quality of the repetitions.

Consider the fact that a 180-pound person, who is performing a *standing calf raise* with only his bodyweight, already loads EACH calf muscle (right side and left side) with well over 540 pounds (approximately). This amount of load is due to the physics involved, as the following calculation shows: *180 pounds of bodyweight divided by two legs = 90 x the magnification provided by the length of the foot lever...a factor of approximately six ... 90 x 6 = 540 per calf)*. Accordingly, a "*one-legged bodyweight calf raise*" would load each calf muscle with over 1,080 pounds (two x 540 pounds), without using any additional resistance.

Personally, I find that "bodyweight" is already a bit too much for an initial high-repetition, warm-up set (e.g., usually 30 repetitions), if the exercise is done properly (full range of motion, with deliberate stretch and contraction on each repetition). What's needed, with regard to gym equipment, is NOT a calf machine that has a heavier weight stack. Rather, what's needed is a calf machine that allows a person to use LESS than their full bodyweight, at least for their warm-up/higher rep sets. Ideally, it would also offer the option to use as much as two or three times the exerciser's bodyweight, and every option in between.

For this reason, I find it very practical to use a type of *leg press* (like the one shown in Figure 24-13), where I can use a weight that is equivalent to about half my bodyweight (e.g., 100 pounds) for the warm-up sets. In fact, some individuals might only need 50 pounds (when using both legs), which is perfectly acceptable, if that's what their strength level requires. It is misguided for anyone to assume that they "must" use the heaviest weight possible for calf exercises (or for any other

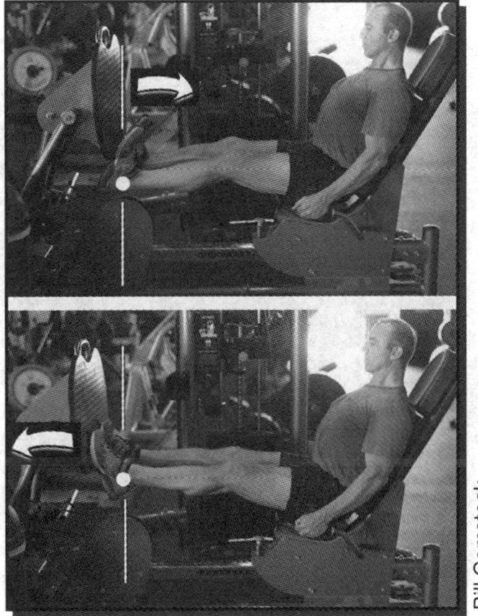
Bill Comstock

Figure 24-13

skeletal muscle), or to be influenced by what other people use, or to be "challenged" by the entire amount of weight that is provided on the average *standing calf* machine. In reality, you should allow the "feeling" of the exercise to help you determine how much weight to use, while performing the repetitions properly.

In the absence of a *leg press*, like the one above, consider starting on the *seated calf* machine (Figure 24-14) using 30 or 40 pounds to comfortably perform 20 or 30 repetitions. After a few sets of that, you can then move to a *standing calf* machine, or a *leg press* machine, using a heavier weight. I've trained (prepared myself) for State, National, and International competitions, using high intensity, and have never needed more than 400 pounds (200 pounds of added resistance, plus my 200 pounds of bodyweight). This level of resistance has provided me with more than enough "challenge," and my calf development, using this method, has been very good (Figure 24-15).

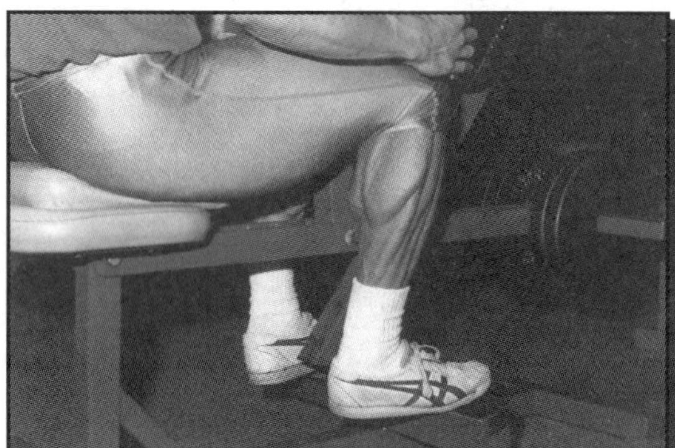
Figure 24-14

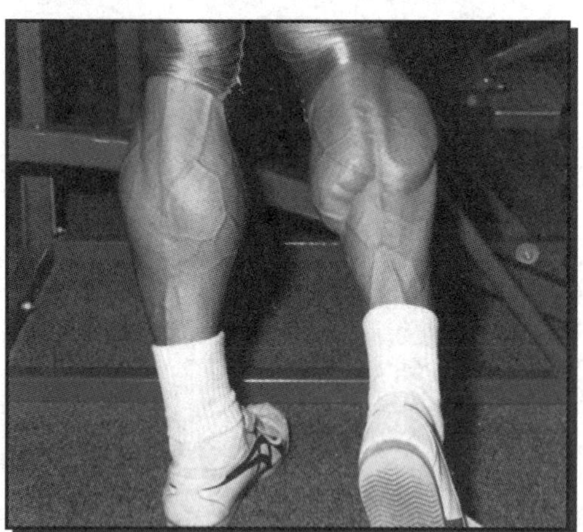
Figure 24-15

## Anatomy of the Rectus Abdominis

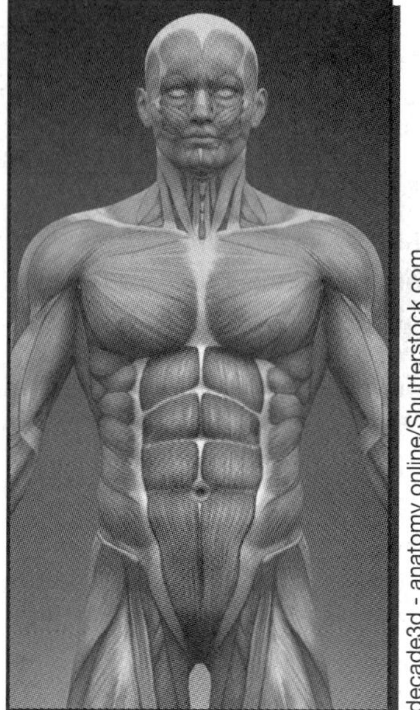

Figure 24-16

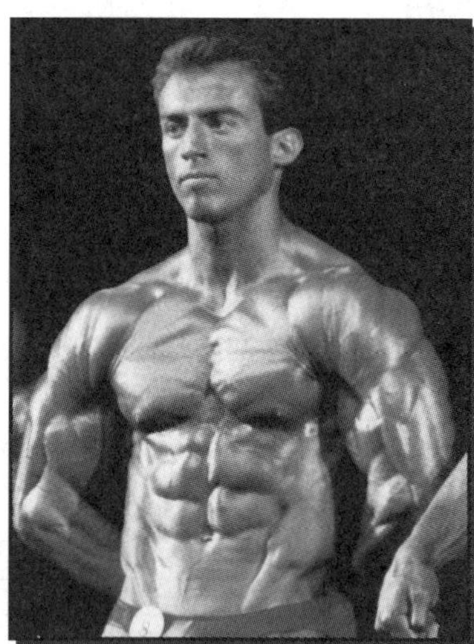
Figure 24-17

This section addresses the rectus abdominis—the muscles that are sometimes referred to as "the six pack," or just the "abs." Ironically, the abs may be the most misunderstood of all the muscles of the body, and yet one of the simplest to develop. In fact, it's one of the greatest ironies in the fitness industry.

The anatomy of the rectus abdominis is very simple and straightforward, simpler even than that of the biceps brachii. Yet, people are much more confused about how to work their abs, than how to work their biceps. As such, far more "mistakes" are made when attempting to develop the abs, than when attempting to develop the biceps.

This confusion is due to the enormous amount of misinformation that is typically circulated, regarding how to train the abs. "Wishful thinking," myths perpetuated by misguided "gurus," false advertising, and the industry's overcommercialization, have all contributed to the problem. Everyone has been led to believe that it's better to use three or four different exercises for training the abs, when (in fact) the abs only perform one simple function—spinal flexion.

❑ The Most Common Misunderstanding Related to Getting "Good Abs"

Before we get into the anatomy of the rectus abdominis, it is necessary to address the biggest misconception related to getting great abs: abdominal exercise will NOT diminish the fat that is on your midsection. And yet, the most common reason that many people do "ab" exercises is to reduce the FAT that is in that area. More often than not, people's rationale for performing ab exercises is clear from the language they typically use when expressing their goal—"I want to tone my abs." Body fat, however, cannot be "toned." It can only be reduced or increased.

In reality, people often conflate "abdominal definition" (i.e., the ability to clearly see the ab muscle, because there is little or no fat between the muscle and the skin) and the strengthening/development of the muscle itself. These are two separate concepts, and they occur by way of two separate processes.

Exercising a muscle will strengthen and develop that muscle, but it will not reduce the layer of fat that covers that muscle. Furthermore, until that fat layer is reduced or eliminated, you will not have "abdominal definition," regardless of how strong and developed the muscle is, underneath that layer of fat.

The layer of body fat that obscures the clarity of the abdominal muscle can only be reduced or eliminated as a "whole-body process." You cannot diminish fatty deposits (technically known as "adipose") in only one area, and you also cannot choose the anatomical area where the fat would be reduced. In reality, body fat is dissipated (reduced) as a whole-body process, when the calorie demand exceeds that calorie intake, thereby forcing the body to use its body fat reserves.

The type of exercise that you perform (aerobic versus anaerobic) and the types of foods that you consume (high-glycemic carbs versus low-glycemic carbs) also play a role in the reduction of body fat—separate from the quantity of calories eaten, the amount of exercise performed (measured in number of minutes/hours per week), and the intensity of exercise performed (heart rate/respiratory rate). In any case, performing "ab" exercises will absolutely not result in localized fat loss in the abdominal area (i.e., improved abdominal definition/muscle clarity).

Most people who hear the aforementioned description of how body fat is reduced typically nod in agreement, and claim they know all about the myth of "spot reduction." Yet, they still perform ab exercises every single day, often with very high reps—a mindset that they would not apply to any of the other muscles of their body. In other words, while logically they understand that body fat cannot be reduced locally, they still "feel better"—psychologically—treating their ab workouts, as if they MIGHT produce localized fat loss. Unfortunately, it simply does not work that way.

The process of losing body fat—whether from the waistline or from any other place on the body—is relatively straightforward:

- When you eat more calories than we you expend, you store the "extra" calories as body fat. That body fat is distributed all over your body, more in some areas than in other areas. This distribution of body fat is determined by your genetics.
- You cannot choose where (on your body) body fat will accumulate, and you also cannot choose where (on your body) body fat will be reduced. All you can do is put your body into "fat loss mode" by eating fewer calories than you are spending. This can be done by simply eating fewer calories, or spending more calories by increasing exercise time and duration). When you arrive at the point where you are burning more calories than you are eating, body fat will diminish in the reverse order in which it accumulated.
- When you perform abdominal exercise, you are strengthening and developing the abdominal muscle, which is underneath a layer of body fat. As such, any muscle development that occurs will not be visible, unless/until the layer of fat that covers the muscle is reduced to a total "body composition" (percentage of body fat) that is approximately 10 percent or lower.
- When the calories you expend (by way of exercise or other physical activity) exceed the calories you consume (possibly by way of reduced calorie intake), you lose body fat—but only as a whole-body process.

*Note: Body fat loss is a complex process that involves caloric deficit, food selection, and a person's individual genetics, which includes hormone production. This is why the type of food you consume is important. Certain foods cause negative hormonal effects, while others cause positive hormonal effects, and the degree to which this happens depends partly on a person's individual genetics. Since this book is about biomechanics, and the subject of diet is an entirely different field of science, it is not sensible to delve into the details of dieting in this book. It is important to understand, however, that an individual's diet plays a much more significant role in "abdominal definition" (the visibility/clarity of the rectus abdominis) than does abdominal exercise.*

Now that that misconception has been cleared up, the next step is to examine the anatomy of the abs—the "rectus abdominis." Figure 24-18 shows the abs from the front and the side. These two illustrations allow you to see where the muscle originates and where it attaches.

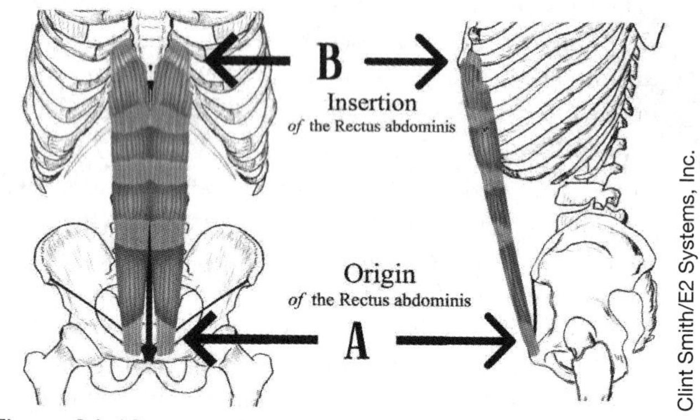


Figure 24-18

This flat muscle originates on the pubic bone ("crest of the pubis"—Figure 24-18, "A") of the pelvis, and inserts onto the front of the ribs (the costal cartilage of the fifth, sixth, and seventh ribs, and the xiphoid process—Figure 24-18, "B"). When the muscle contracts (shortens), it pulls the origin and the insertion closer together, thereby producing "spinal flexion," a forward curving of the spine. This function is very simple and straightforward.

It is important to note that the rectus abdominis ("the abs") is one muscle; it is not two muscles. There is no separate "upper abs" and "lower abs." The rectus abdominis has one origin, one insertion, and one primary function—spinal flexion.

The "dividers" you see in the muscle sheath—the vertical line that runs down the center and the ones that run horizontal to the muscle—are similar to "tendons." In fact, they are called "tendinous intersections." They have been there since birth. Their configuration and how many of them you have are determined by your genetics and cannot be changed. You can only improve the clarity of what is already there (by way of fat loss), and the apparent depth of those "grooves" (by enhancing the muscle fiber thickness between the "grooves"). You cannot, however, change the shape of the "grooves," nor add any additional "grooves" (dividers).

In other words, you cannot convert a "four pack" into a "six pack," no matter how hard you try, or which exercises you do. The configuration of each person's abs (shape and number) is unique. As such, it is as permanent as are a person's fingerprints.

In Figure 24-19, you can see that the vertical divider that runs down the middle is called the "linea alba." The horizontal dividers are called "tendinous intersections." The linea alba and tendinous intersections are technically "fascia" and similar to tendons, in the sense that you can no more add another "ab tendon," than you can add another Achilles tendon. This is why it is impossible to add another "row" of abs in the lower part of your midsection. It is foolish, therefore, to think that targeting the "lower abs" would be productive. It is impossible to add tendinous intersections, and it is also impossible to "spot reduce"—to reduce the fat of the lower region of the midsection.

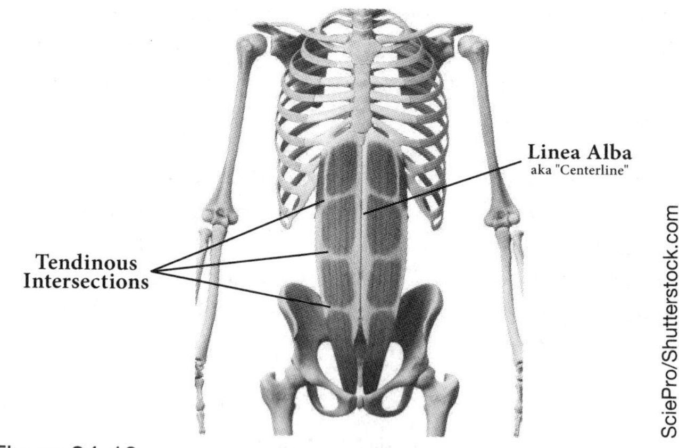


Figure 24-19

❑ The Myth of the "Lower Abs"

Chapter 10 (the "All or Nothing" Principle) briefly discussed how a muscle pulls all the way from origin to insertion, with evenly distributed tension through the entire length of the muscle, if it contracts at all. As such, the rationale that compels people to attempt to work their "lower abs" is entirely without merit. The abs contract for the purpose of bringing its origin and insertion points closer together, thereby flexing the spine.

It is very common for people to want to lose body fat in the lower region of their abdomen, and for them to think they can add more "notches" to their abs (convert a four-pack into a six-pack). Neither option, however, is possible.

Although there is no separate "lower ab" muscle, there does appear to be a small degree of difference in the muscle activation that occurs in the upper part of the rectus abdominis, versus the lower part of the rectus abdominis. This difference is constant, however. It occurs the same way, anytime the abs contract, regardless of the exercise used to contract the abs.

The muscle fibers that are between the upper two tendinous intersections, contract with a tiny bit more force than do the fibers between the next two tendinous intersections. The lower the location of the fibers (moving toward the pubic bone), the less the degree of activation, with the least contractile force occurring in the fibers of the lowest part of the rectus abdominis. As noted previously, this factor is constant, regardless of the exercise used. The "upper" fibers always contract with a tiny bit more force than the "lower" fibers.

Most importantly, this fact is meaningless, since neither the function, nor the appearance, of the lower part of the abdomen can change—even if you could activate the lower part of the abs more than the upper part. Any effort to work the "lower abs" would be unrewarded, not only because localized fat loss is impossible, but also because adding another row of "notches" (tendinous intersections) is impossible.

In the early 2000s, Dr. Eric Sternlicht and his colleagues examined this very factor. The results of their study were published in the February issue of the *Journal of Strength and Conditioning Research* (2005; volume 19, issue 1). In their investigation, the degree of rectus abdominis activation—upper versus lower—was evaluated by way of EMG (electromyography) analysis, during seven different exercises. The results are shown in Figure 24-20. As such, none of the exercises that were tested showed more activity in the lower part, as compared with the upper part, even though each exercise produced a different degree of overall stimulation of the rectus abdominis.

A device called the "Ab-ONE" showed a slightly higher degree of activity than a standard *crunch*. The difference between the upper and lower activation, however, was relatively the same (percentage-wise), as it was with all of the other exercises. You should note that all the other exercises registered lower activity than the *standard ab crunch*, which demonstrates that a basic movement (producing simple spinal flexion) is all that is necessary to stimulate optimal muscle activity in the rectus abdominis.

**Mean electromyographic values (mean ± *SD*) for the 7 exercises tested (*N* = 46).**

| | *Muscle (volts)* | |
|---|---|---|
| *Device* | *Upper rectus abdominis* | *Lower rectus abdominis* |
| Ab-ONE (supine position) | **1.72 ± 1.01** | **0.76 ± 0.38** |
| Ab Scissor | 0.87 ± 0.59* | 0.35 ± 0.15* |
| Ab Swing | 0.47 ± 0.27* | 0.25 ± 0.11* |
| 6SecondAbs | 0.86 ± 0.68* | 0.30 ± 0.14* |
| Perfect Abs Roller | 1.30 ± 0.72 | 0.54 ± 0.26 |
| Torso Track | 0.95 ± 0.63* | 0.45 ± 0.24* |
| Crunch | 1.36 ± 0.79 | 0.58 ± 0.28 |

* Indicates significantly lower muscle activity relative to a traditional crunch. **Bold** indicates significantly higher muscle activity relative to a traditional crunch. $p < 0.05$, using Dunnett's test to hold α at 0.05.

Reprinted by permission from Wolters Kluwer Health, Inc: *Journal of Strength and Conditioning Research*, Electromyographical analysis and comparison of selected abdominal training devices with a traditional crunch, Eric Sternlicht et al, 2005, 19(1), 159, https://journals.lww.com/nsca-jscr/toc/2005/02000

Figure 24-20

A logical assumption as to why there is always more muscle activity in the upper part of the rectus abdominis, as compared with the lower part of the rectus abdominis, is that the spine does not bend (flex) evenly. Rather, it tends to bend more in the area that is slightly above the lumbar region, due to the natural curvature of the spine. That area—approximately T6 through T12—is directly across from the upper part of the rectus abdominis (Figure 24-21).

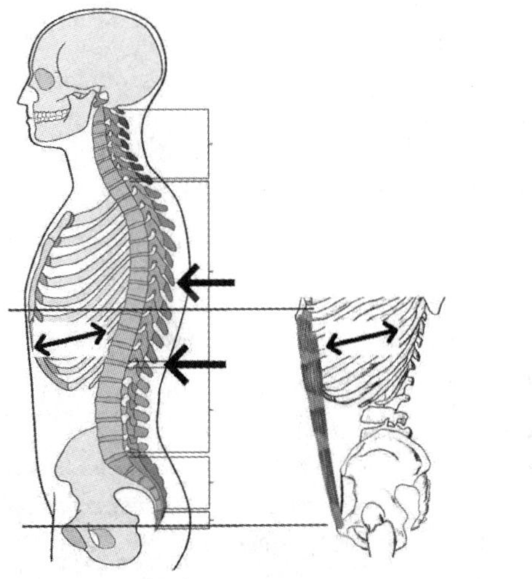

udaix/Shutterstock.com; Clint Smith/E2 Systems, Inc.

Figure 24-21

The degrees of most and least muscle fiber activation appear to coincide with the areas of the spine that bend most and least, during spinal flexion. The spine naturally bends more in the area that is across from the "A" portion of the abs (Figure 24-22). As such, it bends a bit less in the area that is across from the "B" portion of the abs, while it bends a bit less in the area that is across from the "C" portion of the abs. The lowest portion of the spine, which is across from the "D" area of the abs, flexes the least (because it naturally curves the other direction, at that point).

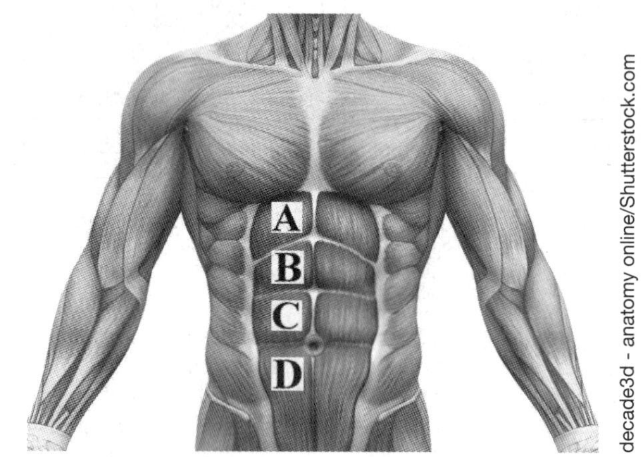


Figure 24-22

To reiterate, regardless of how much muscle activation is achieved in the lower portion of the rectus abdominis, the appearance of that lower area cannot be selectively improved. You cannot add more tendinous intersections, nor can you increase the dissipation of adipose tissue (body fat) that has accumulated precisely in that area.

Consistent with the "all or nothing principle of muscle contraction," whenever the rectus abdominis is activated, the entire muscle is activated—both the upper and lower sections—each to the degree that is anatomically normal, regardless of the exercise used. In that regard, whenever you see a person with a very impressive "six-pack" or "eight-pack," you can be assured that this person did not achieve that abs configuration by way of some "magical" exercise or "advanced" technique. That individual is just more genetically fortunate (aesthetically speaking), and therefore derives a "better" outcome (from any exercise) than do others who are genetically less fortunate.

*Note: The "Ab-ONE" was a prototype product that was apparently never brought to market. The exercise that I believe is biomechanically best for the rectus abdominis—the "seated cable crunch,"— is also better than the standard ab crunch, performed on the floor.*

❑ Function and Range of Motion for Training the Abs

Figure 24-23, upper-left image, shows a side view of how the rectus abdominis originates on the pubic bone of the pelvis, at its lower end. The upper end of the abs attaches onto the anterior inferior (front/lower part) of the ribcage. When the ab muscle contracts (shortens), it brings the two ends toward each other. This contraction produces "spinal flexion"—a rounding of the spine (Figure 24-23, upper-right image). "Optimal muscle contraction" results in a maximally shortened distance between the origin (pubic bone/pelvis) and insertion (lower anterior ribs) of the muscle, which results in a maximally flexed (rounded) spine.

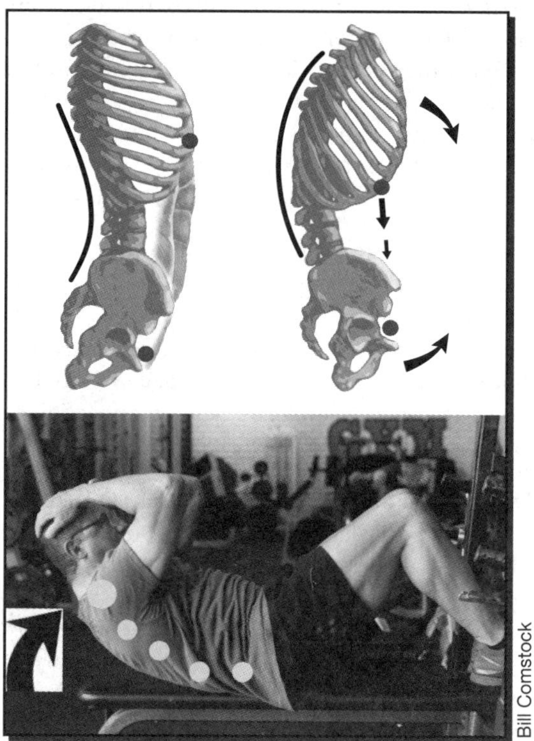


Figure 24-23

When the spine is at its normal "straight" position (Figure 24-24, upper image), the abs (rectus abdominis) are sufficiently elongated. That position can be considered the "start" of the full range of motion of a good abdominal exercise. Arching the spine more than this (Figure 24-24, lower image) is not necessary for optimal development of the rectus abdominis, even though it does elongate the abs (rectus abdominis) more. In reality, excessive arching of the spine (attempting to maximally stretch the rectus abdominis) increases the risk of intervertebral (spinal) disc distortion, and provides little or no additional value to the exercise.

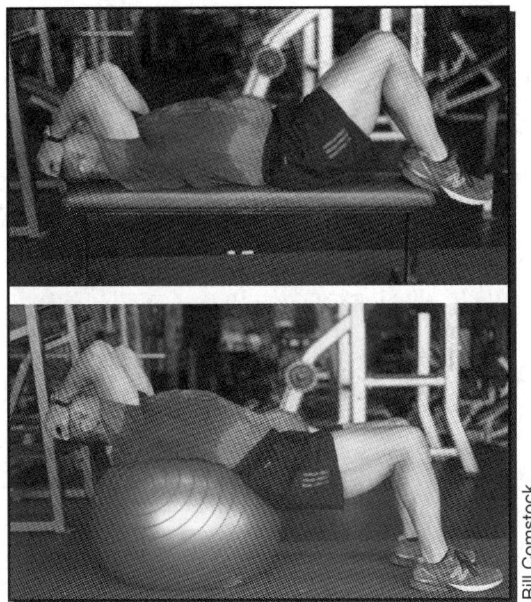


Figure 24-24

Both of the images in Figure 24-25 show a fully contracted rectus abdominis. Either of these is fine. In both cases, the spine is fully flexed (curved), thereby bringing the base of the ribcage as close as comfortably possible, to the front of the pelvis.

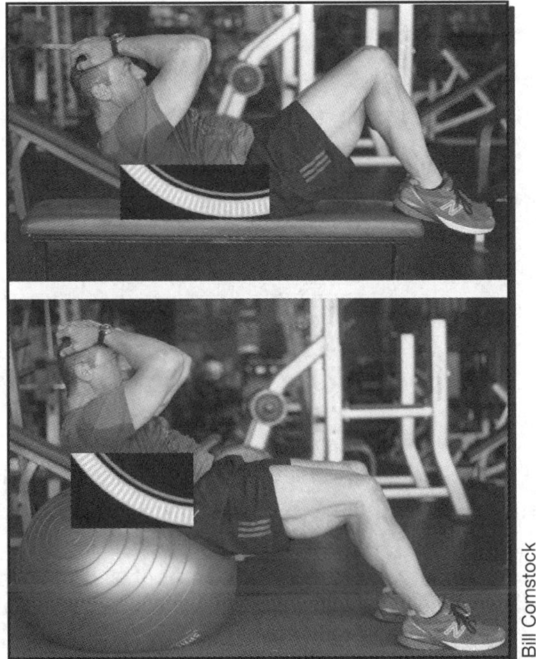


Figure 24-25

The generally accepted "safe" ranges of spinal movement are 40 to 60 degrees of flexion (forward bending), as measured from the straight spine position, and 20 to 35 degrees of spinal extension (back arching). In fact, the spine has significantly less back-arching (spinal extension) mobility, as compared with forward bending (spinal flexion) mobility.

The degree of spinal mobility varies greatly from person to person. Some individuals have very little spinal mobility in either direction, while others could practically be circus performers. Everyone, however, should be careful to not hyper-extend nor hyper-flex their spine beyond what is comfortable.

It should also be noted that arching the spine by way of deliberate erector spinae contraction (known as "active" extension) is more safe than arching the spine assisted by gravity (known as "passive" extension), as demonstrated in the *Swiss ball crunches* (Figure 24-25). Likewise, forward flexion of the spine by way of deliberate contraction of the abs ("active" flexion)—like when performing either of the *crunch* exercises in Figure 24-25—is more safe than forward flexion of the spine that is assisted by force ("passive" flexion), as would be the case when doing *bent-over barbell rows, deadlifts*, etc.

❑ Exercise Options for the Abs

Some people, knowing that the abs do not actually pull the legs upward, rationalize their belief that *leg raises* work the "lower abs" by stating that the pelvis is pulled upward toward the ribcage (during *leg raises*), instead of the ribcage being pulled downward toward the pelvis. They appear to think that bringing the origin of the abs (on the pubic bone) toward the insertion (on the base of the ribcage) will emphasize the fibers that are closer to the origin, a belief that is entirely wrong.

As was discussed in Chapter 10 ("The All or Nothing Principle of Muscle Contraction"), a muscle does not "know" which end is moving toward which end. The muscle only "knows" that it's contracting, which brings the two ends closer together. This concept is like a tug-of-war, mentioned in Chapter 10. It doesn't matter who's "winning" (which direction the rope is moving)—either way, the tension is distributed throughout the length of the rope.

There is a reason why the attachment of the rectus abdominis on the pubic bone is deemed as the "origin," and the attachment on the ribcage is deemed as the "insertion." The "origin" of any muscle is classified, as such, because it is the more stable (less mobil) of the two ends. In contrast, the "insertion" end of a muscle is attached to the more mobile part of the skeleton.

It is much easier to hold the hips (the pelvis) still and move the ribcage "downward" toward the pelvis (e.g., as in a standard "*crunch*" movement), than it is to hold the ribcage still and move the pelvis "upward" toward the ribcage (e.g., as in a *leg raise/hip thrust* movement). There is also no developmental benefit— no muscle stimulating advantage whatsoever—in attempting to move the pelvis toward the ribcage.

In fact, there is a significant disadvantage when you do *leg raises* (when intending to work the abs), because of the tremendous load on the hip flexors. The weight of the legs is significant (given the strength capacity of the hip flexors). As a result, a tremendous amount of effort is required on the part of the hip flexors, in pulling the legs upward.

The primary hip flexor—the psoas—originates on the lumbar spine. Heavy-load activation of the psoas naturally causes the origin of the psoas to be forcefully pulled forward, thereby causing the lumbar spine to arch. Spinal arch is the opposite of what the abs are trying to do, which is to flex (forward bend) the spine. As a result, the abs are unable to reach full contraction (shortening), because the psoas is preventing it. This is one reason why basic *ab crunch* movements are always better—for working the abs—than any *leg raise* movement. *Ab crunches* allow the insertion of the rectus abdominis (on the lower part of the ribs) to move toward the origin (on the pubic bone of the pelvis)—which is the most natural function of the abs—without interference from the hip flexors.

The most common exercise for the abs is the standard "*abdominal crunch*," shown in Figure 24-26. As stated previously, this movement is correct. For most individuals, however, this version is too difficult. Specifically, the position of the torso, relative to gravity, maximizes the resistance beyond most people's strength level. While this factor typically results in an inability to use proper form, it also leads to an inability to perform enough repetitions, which is why individuals are often seen doing what appears to be "head lifts" (moving mostly the neck)—hardly lifting their shoulders and upper back off the ground.

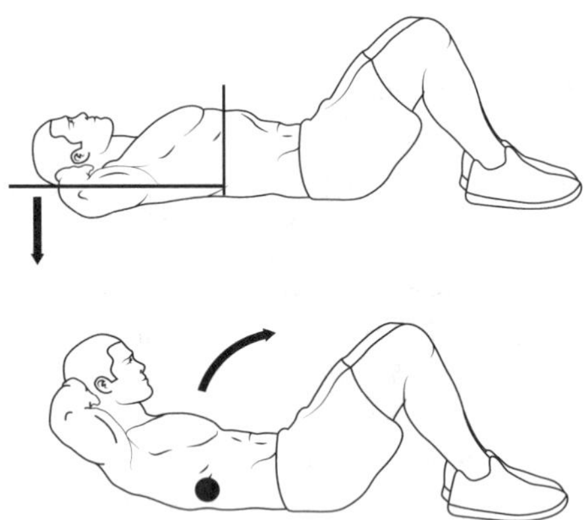

Figure 24-26

As was discussed in Chapter 2, a lever that is perpendicular with resistance is a 100 percent lever. It is "maximally active." In the version shown in Figure 24-26, the upper half of the torso (the area to the left of the vertical line) is the operating lever the abs, and it is 100 percent perpendicular with resistance in that starting position. For most individuals, this factor results in too much resistance. It would be like trying to do a *standing barbell curl* with a barbell that is too heavy to perform a full range of motion. It prevents you from doing enough repetitions, and makes you hate the exercise.

That type of scenario is precisely what often happens when people try to do *ab crunches*, while on a flat surface. It results in an incomplete range of motion (i.e., often only a neck lift), insufficient repetitions, lower back discomfort, and causes the person to hate the exercise. In reality, all of these negative outcomes are due to the simple fact that the resistance (at this particular angle) is "too heavy." It is not that the exercise itself is too hard. It is only the level of resistance—with the torso at this particular angle—that is excessive.

The good news is that it's very easy to reduce the resistance, simply by changing the angle of the torso, relative to gravity. In Figure 24-27, the starting angle of the torso has been changed from being horizontal (perpendicular with gravity) to one that starts with an angle of approximately 20 degrees. At this point, the torso is no longer perpendicular with gravity (arrow), which causes the torso (lever) to be about 78 percent "active," instead of 100 percent "active." This effectively reduces the resistance by about 22 percent.

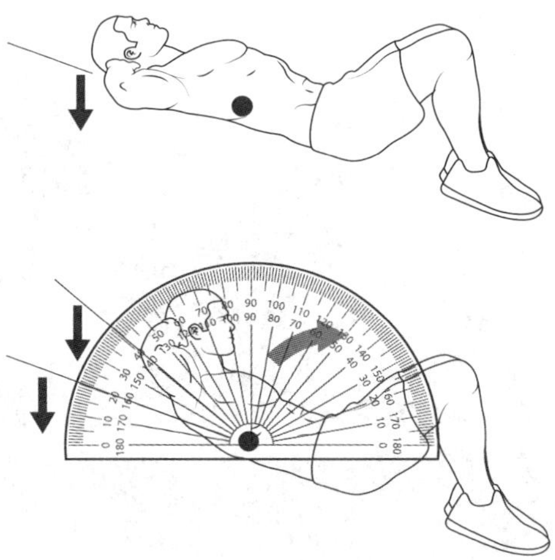

Figure 24-27

This angle could be achieved either by using an adjustable massage table or a standard incline bench set at this angle, or by propping up a piece of plywood against a low stool. Ideally, it's good to have about a 45-degree angle of hip bend (i.e., the femur would be at 45 degrees, relative to the torso). As such, you may need to elevate your feet to accommodate this positioning.

Of course, you could use a higher (more steep) incline angle, if you need a greater reduction of the resistance. That adjustment is entirely acceptable, if that is the level of resistance that matches your current strength level. It's perfectly appropriate to choose the proper resistance level for this exercise, just as you do with all your other exercises. The resistance level should allow you to do 20 repetitions with full range of motion, yet challenging enough so that 20 repetitions represents about 70 to 80 percent of your maximum effort.

The resistance curve of this version of an *ab crunch*, which is called "*incline bench ab crunches*," is also very good. It is "early phase loaded," and the resistance diminishes as the muscle contracts, which matches the strength curve of most skeletal muscles.

Using an incline angle like this allows you to reduce the resistance enough so you can do the exercise with proper form, which means using full range of motion, and achieving a deliberate contraction of the rectus abdominis at the conclusion of each repetition. This factor is no different than the goal of every other exercise, for any other muscle group you typically exercise. The biomechanical requirements for the abs are no different.

Doing *crunches* on a flat surface (e.g., a floor mat) usually prevents using proper form. The horizontal angle of the torso (i.e., the resistance that this angle produces) usually disallows using full range of motion, and disallows deliberate contraction of the rectus abdominis.

If you've never tried doing *ab crunches* using a slight incline angle, you'll be pleasantly surprised by how much better it feels than doing *crunches* on a flat surface. Not only will you discover that you can achieve full and deliberate contraction of the abs with each repetition, you'll also feel no strain on your neck and lower back.

In Figure 24-28, I am demonstrating a "*seated cable ab crunch.*" As you can see, I am sitting mostly upright on a back-supported bench. The reason this exercise can be done from an upright position (instead of lying on a floor mat) is because the resistance is coming from a cable, instead of from "free-weight-gravity."

Note that the height of the pulley has been set so that the direction of the cable is fairly perpendicular with the torso in the starting position. The primary advantage of using cable resistance is that you can choose precisely the amount of resistance that feels appropriate for 20 or 30 repetitions, using full range of movement, at your current strength level. All you need to do is move the pin on the weight stack to adjust the resistance.

A dot has been placed at mid-spine to illustrate the primary pivot point of this movement (actually, of any ab exercise). In reality, the spine bends at multiple vertebrae. It doesn't actually "jackknife" the way an elbow does, but "mid-spine" should be the focal point of a good ab exercise. It is best to keep the lower back (everything below the dot) GLUED to the backrest of the seat, as the upper half of the torso curls forward. If you were to continue moving the torso forward (e.g., pulling the lower back forward off the backrest), you would engage the hip flexors, which would compromise the movement.

In Figure 24-29, I'm doing the same exercise, but with the pulley set slightly higher than in the aforementioned example. This adjustment changes the resistance curve a bit, reducing it at the beginning of the movement, and increasing it at the end. This isn't necessarily better or worse. In fact, both versions are good. You can (and should) try them both. You might favor one over the other, in terms of your ability to feel the muscle contraction.

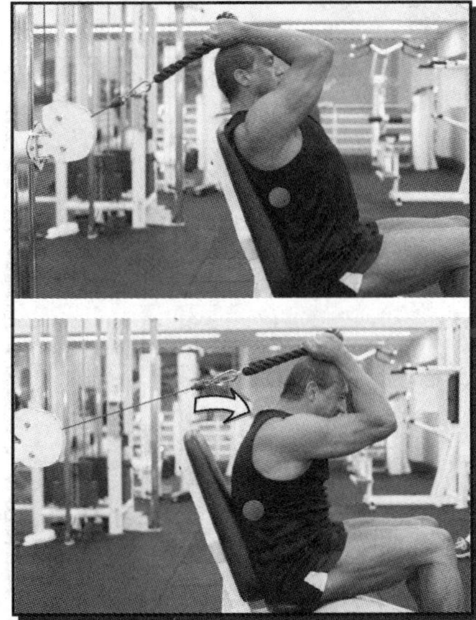

Figure 24-28

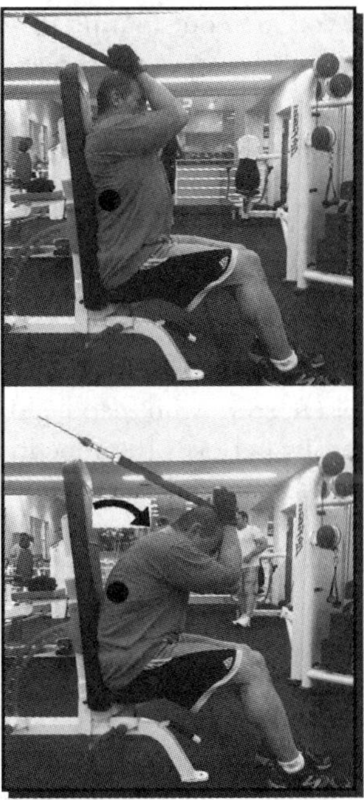

Figure 24-29

Keep in mind that this particular exercise also deals with the issue of a "secondary resistance," which was discussed in Chapter 6. The farther forward you bend your torso (from the upright position), the more that your own torso weight "falls" forward, because you're on the "downside" of the apex. As such, the weight of the torso progressively subtracts from the opposing cable resistance, the farther forward you move the torso. Of course, you easily compensate for this factor by selecting a slightly heavier weight on the pulley. In fact, you would likely do this, without even being aware of why you're doing it. You would simply sense that you are capable of using a heavier weight, and would automatically increase it.

## Best Number of Reps for Training the Abs

It's very common for individuals to do very high repetitions, when performing an abs exercise. As noted previously, the reason most people tend to do this is because they subconsciously equate a high degree of localized fatigue/"burn," with localized fat loss. In fact, they might misinterpret the "burn" as *evidence* that their abdominal fat is becoming "firm," or somehow converting into muscle. All three of these concepts (localized fat loss, fat becoming more "firm," and fat transforming into muscle) are entirely unrealistic.

The underlying problem with such a mindset stems from the fact that many people think of their entire midsection as "the abs." In reality, the midsection is not "one thing." It is two things: the muscle and the fat that covers the muscle. Each must be addressed separately—by different means.

When you perform ab exercises, you are only working the muscle. Although you are contributing to "calorie spending" when you work the abs, it does not preferentially cause the fat on the midsection to be reduced. When you perform ab exercises, you should regard it in the same manner as when you do a biceps exercise, or any other exercise for any other muscle on your body. In fact, the same bio-mechanical and physiological principles apply when working (exercising) any skeletal muscle.

It is foolish to do a set of 100 reps of "partial range of motion"—as is often seen with people doing *ab crunches*. People do not typically perform 100 repetitions of *biceps curls*, nor of any exercise for any other skeletal muscle, when the goal is physique development. Some individuals may enjoy the challenge of seeing if they can perform 100 repetitions of a particular exercise (sit-ups or push-ups, for example), but that is not the best approach for physique development, nor even for optimal health.

The resistance level you use during abdominal exercise should be light enough to allow at least 15 full range-of-motion repetitions, but heavy enough (challenging enough) so that muscle fatigue forces you to stop at 20 to 30 repetitions. In terms of the proper resistance level and number of repetitions (per set), you should treat the abs like most other muscles on your body.

The only caveat to the aforementioned is that, since the rectus abdominis does not have the force capacity of a pectoral muscle, or a quadriceps, it would be unwise to use a resistance level that limits you to performing only six repetitions. In reality, 10 repetitions is the minimum number of repetitions you should perform for an abs exercise, and only if those repetitions are full range, deliberate, and with full contraction (shortest distance between muscle origin and insertion). Doing more than 30 repetitions is not more productive. Arguably, it's less productive, because—just like any other muscle—once a muscle is fatigued, it loses its ability to contract.

In my opinion, the two aforementioned exercises—*ab crunches on an incline bench* and *seated cable ab crunches*—are the two best ab exercises. These two movements are anatomically correct; the resistance curve is optimally productive; their range of motion is good (as long as you perform them correctly). In addition, the amount of resistance can be adjusted/moderated to your specific level of abdominal strength.

In reality, all other ab exercises seen in the gym are usually "inferior" to these two, in terms of efficiency, comfort, efficacy, and/or safety. Let's look at some of these "less than ideal" exercises, and identify their inefficiencies:

❑ "Reverse Crunch"

The "flat" version of this exercise (Figure 24-30), as well as the "incline" version (Figure 24-31), is sometimes called a "*reverse crunch*" because it attempts to bring the pelvis upward toward the ribcage, instead of the ribcage down toward the pelvis.

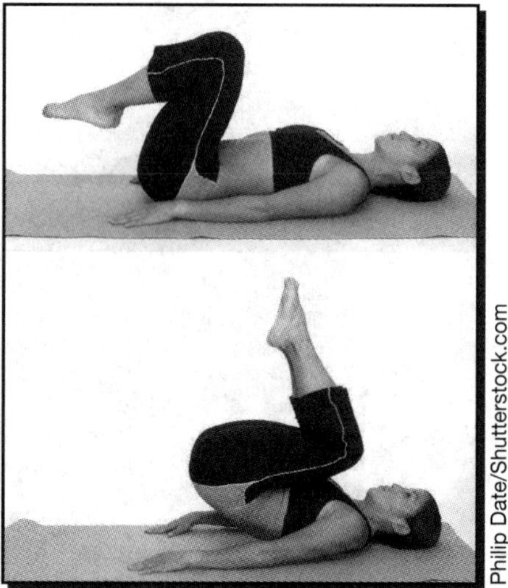

Figure 24-30

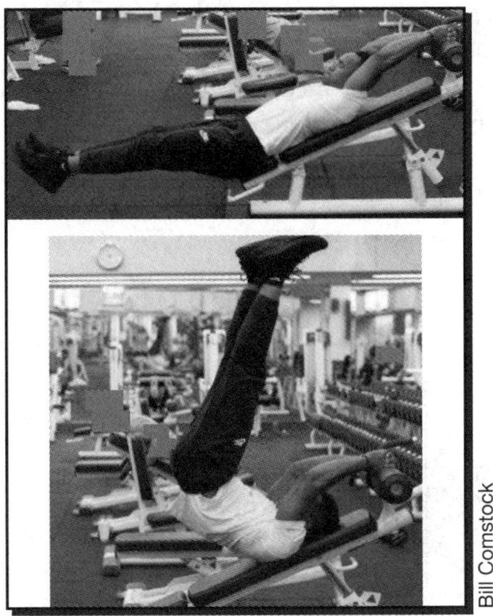
Figure 24-31

Bill Comstock

As was discussed earlier in this chapter, because the rectus abdominis does not "know" which end is moving toward which end, there is no advantage in bringing the pelvis toward the ribcage, as compared with bringing the ribcage toward the pelvis. It requires a much higher energy cost, without any "bonus" benefit, nor any difference in terms of which part of the rectus abdominis is emphasized (works harder). Furthermore, the engagement of the hip flexors *interferes* with the efficient contraction of the rectus abdominis.

❑ "Knee Tucks"

During *knee tucks* (Figure 24-32), the dynamic work is done almost entirely by the hip flexors, which are pulling the legs (the femurs), causing the hip to bend. The abdominals are working mostly isometrically, by holding the flexed spine position.

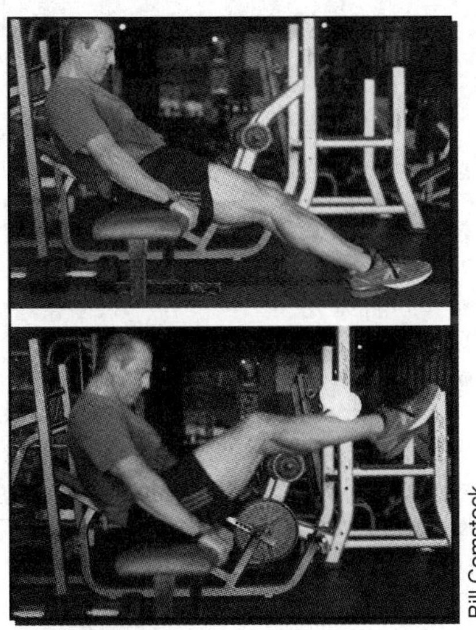
Figure 24-32

Bill Comstock

Isometric contraction is an inferior form of muscle contraction, in terms of strengthening and visible development. The rectus abdominis (the "abs") only moves the spine, and—it's important to note—there is almost no postural change (movement) whatsoever in the flexion/extension (bending) of the spine, during this exercise. The abs do not bend the hip joint, which is where most of the movement is occurring.

❑ "Planks"

The *planks* exercise is completely isometric. There is no rectus abdominis elongation or shortening during this exercise—no dynamic muscle contraction. To grasp how unproductive this exercise is, consider the following: If isometric tension is optimally productive for muscular development, everyone would be using isometric tension (static/no movement/no repetitions) on ALL their exercises, for all of their muscle groups. Obviously, they don't—and for good reason. Isometric tension is not optimally productive.

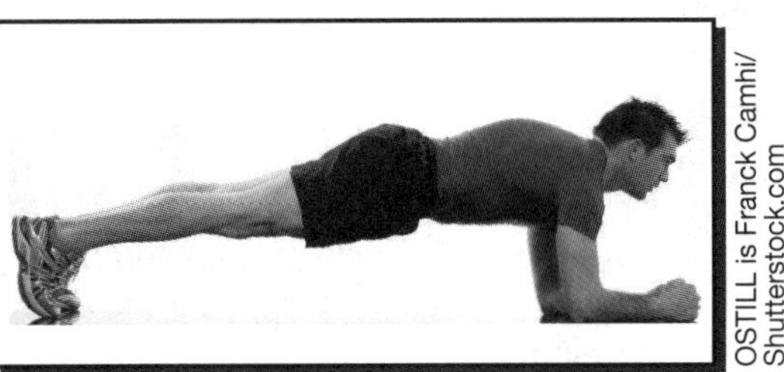
Figure 24-33

OSTILL is Franck Camhi/ Shutterstock.com

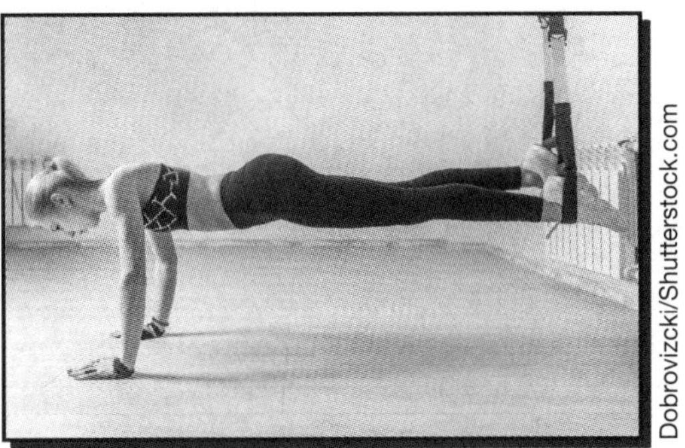
Figure 24-34

Dobrovizcki/Shutterstock.com

In addition to the rectus abdominis being engaged isometrically (during *planks*), there is also isometric engagement of the quadriceps and hip flexors. All three of these muscle groups demand energy and effort, despite the fact that isometric muscle tension is not as productive as dynamic muscular contraction. In other words, when doing *planks*, the "cost" (i.e., effort and energy required) is much greater than the "benefit" (i.e., strength increase through the full range of motion, and visible development), as compared with the "cost/benefit" of dynamic exercise (i.e., *ab crunches, leg extensions* and a *hip flexion* exercise).

The other issue that cannot be ignored is the fact that, as a bodyweight exercise, *planks* do not provide the ability to adjust the resistance level, based on a person's individual strength. Ironically, people who are overweight tend to be weaker (because, very often, they've been inactive), yet they are forced to use more resistance (i.e., their heavier body mass). Meanwhile, the person who is more slim, and may actually be stronger than the overweight person, is able to use less resistance (i.e., their lighter body mass). Furthermore, forcing an overweight person to place a large percentage of their body mass onto their elbows, which then causes their humerus to be pushed upward into their shoulder joint, is not prudent. It is neither comfortable nor entirely safe.

There is one caveat, however, in terms of doing *planks*. This exercise would be an acceptable alternative if you are a boxer, and your objective is to develop strength mainly in that one "stiff spine" position, in order to better tolerate punches to your belly. Otherwise, *planks* are simply not as productive (for abdominal conditioning), as an exercise that employs dynamic movement, like *ab crunches*.

❑ "Knee Tucks on a Swiss Ball"

The *knee tuck on a Swiss ball exercise* (Figure 24-35) is sort of a combination of *planks* (Figure 24-33) and *knee tucks on the bench* (Figure 24-32), with the difference being that it involves much more quadriceps and hip flexor loading. While the energy cost is greater with this exercise (than with standard *knee tucks*), the reward to the abs is still not great, because the abs are working mostly isometrically. The quadriceps and hip flexors are working dynamically, which is better than if they were only working isometrically, but the benefit to the quadriceps and hip flexors is less than could be achieved with dedicated exercises for these muscles (e.g., *cable squats, leg extensions, hip flexion with cables,* etc.).

Note that the spinal position doesn't change (from beginning to end), which means the abs are simply holding contraction. This would be like keeping your elbows bent at 90 degrees (while holding a pair of dumbbells), then moving the shoulder joint (instead of the elbow joint), and believing that that is a good biceps exercise. Needless to say, that would not be a good biceps exercise, for the same reason any isometric exercise is not good—the absence of dynamic muscle contraction.

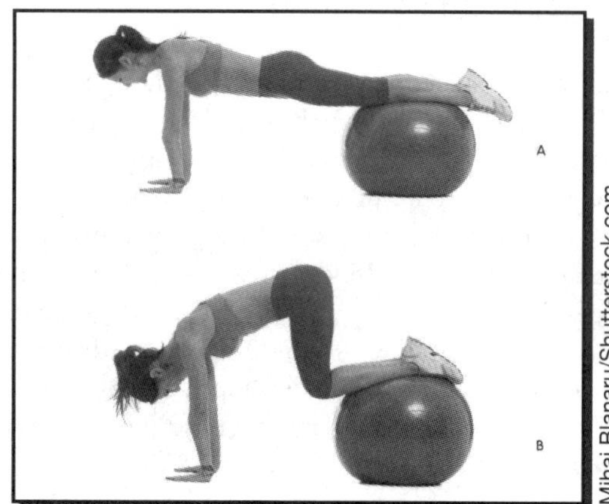

Mihai Blanaru/Shutterstock.com
Figure 24-35

❑ "Hanging Leg Raises" and "Roman Chair Leg Raises"

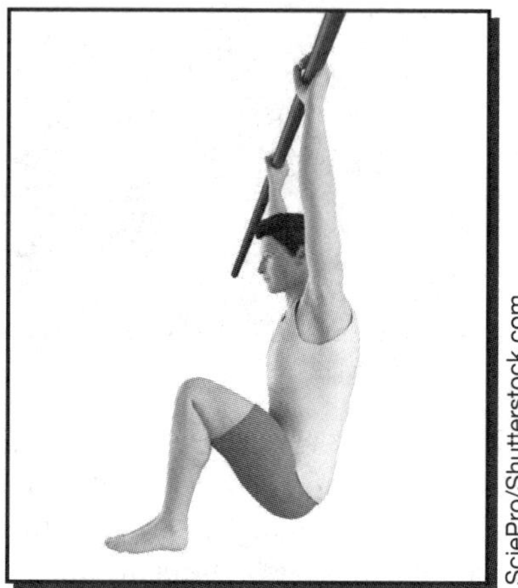
SciePro/Shutterstock.com
Figure 24-36

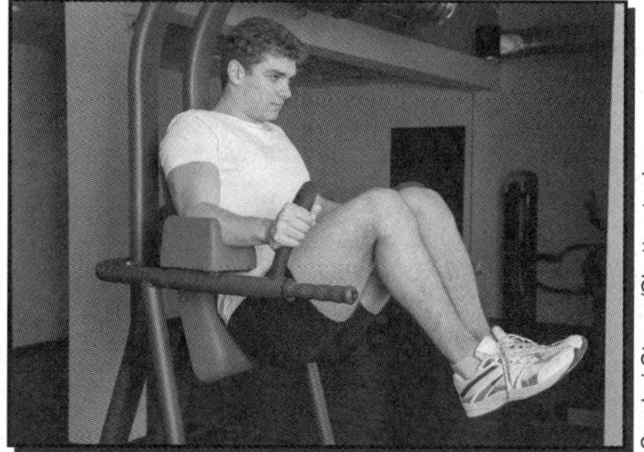
Serghei Starus/Shutterstock.com
Figure 24-37

Any kind of *leg raise* exercise works the hip flexors much more than the abs, as noted previously. The abs do not connect to the legs, so they cannot raise the legs, which is the primary action of any *leg raise* exercise.

The participation of the abs, during a *leg raise* exercise, is limited to mostly isometric contraction, preventing the tailbone from kicking back as a natural response to the legs being raised forward/upward. The harder, dynamic work (muscle elongation and shortening) is done by the hip flexors. Furthermore, the engagement of the hip flexors—most notably, the psoas muscle—actually interferes with spinal flexion (i.e., exerting an opposite, spinal arching force), thereby preventing complete contraction of the abs.

Not only is there absolutely no advantage to the abs by involving the muscles that raise the legs, there is a tremendous disadvantage to the abs in doing so. In addition, the other muscles that must work to hold the body in a suspended position only work isometrically. This requires more effort and energy, but without any benefit to the abs, nor even much benefit to these assisting muscles, due to the absence of dynamic muscle contraction.

*Leg raises*, with the intention of working the abs, is among the most foolish (i.e., least efficient) of all the exercises typically performed for general fitness or physique development. They require a tremendous amount of effort, but bestow very little benefit to the abs.

❑ "Kneeling Cable Crunches"

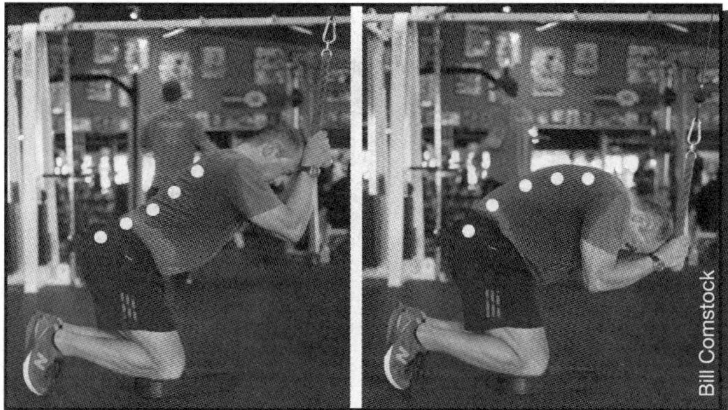


Figure 24-38

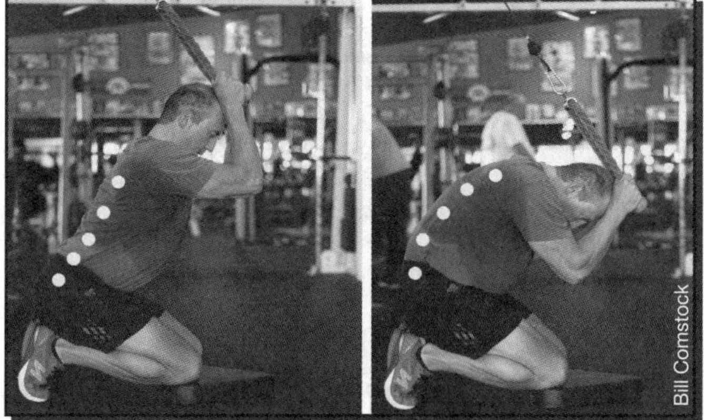


Figure 24-39

The standard *kneeling cable crunch* exercise (Figure 24-38) is fairly good, if performed correctly (i.e., flexing the spine). Unfortunately, most people do not perform it correctly (emphasizing hip flexion, instead of spinal flexion). In addition, the direction of resistance is not quite ideal. The standard version (Figure 24-38) has the direction of resistance (the angle of the cable, relative to the torso) coming from in front of the torso, whereas it would be much better if the resistance came from behind the torso (Figure 24-39). This would provide more resistance at the beginning of the range of motion, and a bit less at the end (i.e., a better resistance curve).

By facing away from the pulley, as shown in Figure 24-39, the direction of resistance is made more perfect. Note that the cable is now more perpendicular (i.e., more "active") with the torso, at the beginning of the range of motion. The problem with this version, however, is that—without a brace against your back—the cable resistance will pull you backward, off balance (assuming the resistance is sufficiently heavy). Note that this direction of resistance starts to resemble that which occurs during the *seated cable crunch*, shown in Figures 24-28 and 24-29.

The best way to perform a kneeling cable crunch, is to position your torso as horizontally as possible (bend as far forward as possible), in order to cause your torso to be more perpendicular with the cable. Then, ensure that the movement occurs mostly at the mid-spine, as shown in Figure 24-40. Try to minimize (or eliminate) much movement at the hip joint. This will provide a better resistance curve, and will emphasize contraction of the rectus abdominis (i.e., the abs), and minimize contraction of the hip flexors. This is the best version of this exercise, but it's still a bit compromised, as compared with *seated cable crunches*, because the absence of a back support allows (essentially "invites"/encourages) hip movement and use of momentum, i.e., swinging the torso up and down.

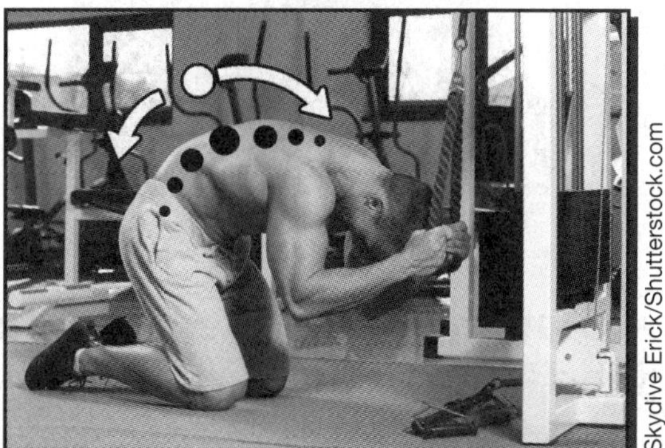


Figure 24-40

If this exercise is performed well, as shown in Figure 24-40, it could be considered one of the better exercises for the abs. On the other hand, if it is not performed correctly, because the body is positioned too far away from the pulley, or because the torso is held "too high" (diagonally instead of horizontally), or if you fail to emphasize spinal flexion (flexing mostly at the hip joint instead), or if momentum is used, then the exercise quickly loses most of it potential benefit.

To be clear, I'm not suggesting that the aforementioned exercises do not work at all. To a degree, they do work. In fact, there is plenty of evidence of that.

The issue is efficiency—the amount of effort and energy that an exercise requires, as compared with the amount of benefit it produces. The ratio of "cost/benefit" of a compromised ab exercise is not nearly as good as that of an exercise that provides better biomechanics, such as *ab crunches on an incline bench*, or *seated cable crunches*. As such, performing inefficient ab exercises requires more time, more sets, more effort and more discomfort, to get a result that could otherwise be achieved by performing one highly efficient ab exercise, for fewer sets, with less discomfort, and less wasted effort.

My investment of time and energy to produce the abdominal development you see in Figure 24-41, was just six sets of one single abdominal exercise (*seated cable crunches*), 10 to 30 reps per set, performed once every five days. Of course, this condition also required me to adhere to a strict diet, but it did not require any additional abdominal exercise, beyond that which I described.

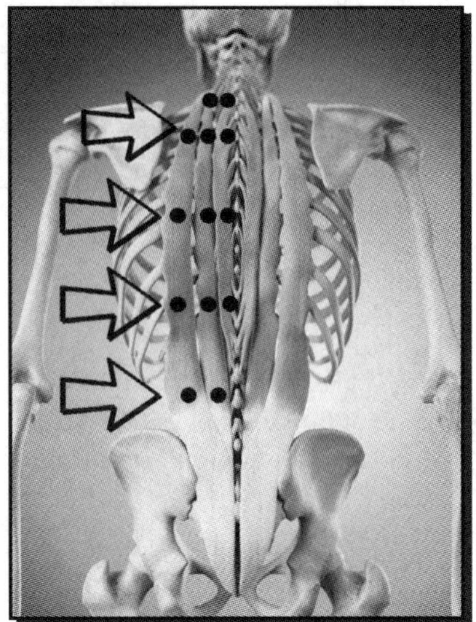

Figure 24-42

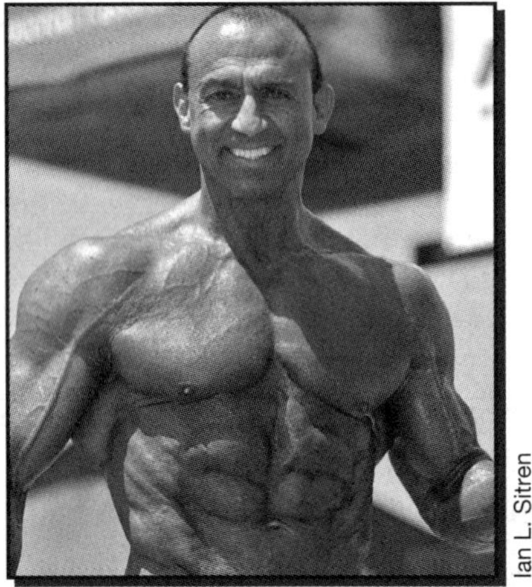

Figure 24-41

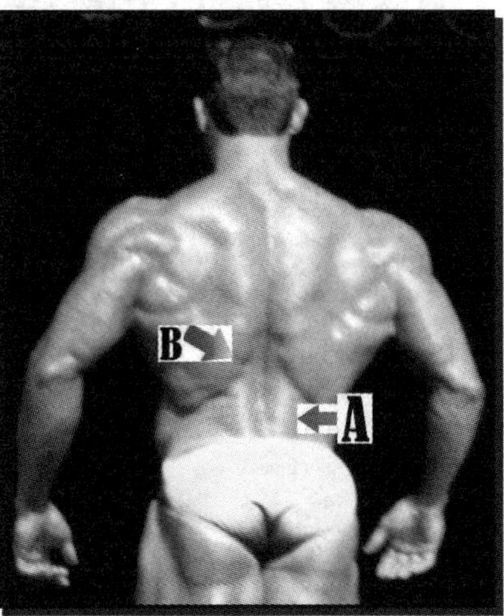

Figure 24-43

## The Anatomy of the Erector Spinae and the Myth of the "Lower Back"

The first thing that needs to be established is that there is no "lower back" muscle, per se. While some people can be heard saying, "...XYZ is a good exercise for the lower back," that statement is technically incorrect. The muscle that many people assume is "the lower back muscle" is actually the lower part of the erector spinae, which starts at the back of the pelvis, but then goes ALL the way up to the neck (Figure 24-42). Only the lowest part of the erector spinae—that which is closest to the pelvis (Figure 24-43, the "A" arrow)—is visible on an individual who is sufficiently lean. In fact, the majority of the erector spinae is hidden behind layers of other back muscles (latissimus, trapezius, etc.).

Some people mistakenly assume that the line that is formed by the lower part of the latissimus dorsi (indicated by the "B" arrow in Figure 24-43) is part of the "lower back." It is not. In fact, that is the where the latissimus muscle meets the latissimus fascia. The "lats" is an entirely different muscle, with an entirely different function.

The origins of the erector spinae group are on the back/upper portion of the pelvis, the sacrum, and the lumbar (lower) spine. Its insertions are on various parts of the thoracic and cervical (mid and upper spine) spine, as well as most of the ribs and even the base of the skull.

The erector spinae "group" actually consists of three separate muscle columns:

- The "spinalis" (closet to the spine; seen on Figure 24-44, uppermost image)
- The "longissimus" (next column, lateral from the spine; seen on Figure 24-44, middle image)

- The "Iliocostalis" (farthest column, lateral from the spine; seen on Figure 24-44, lowermost image)

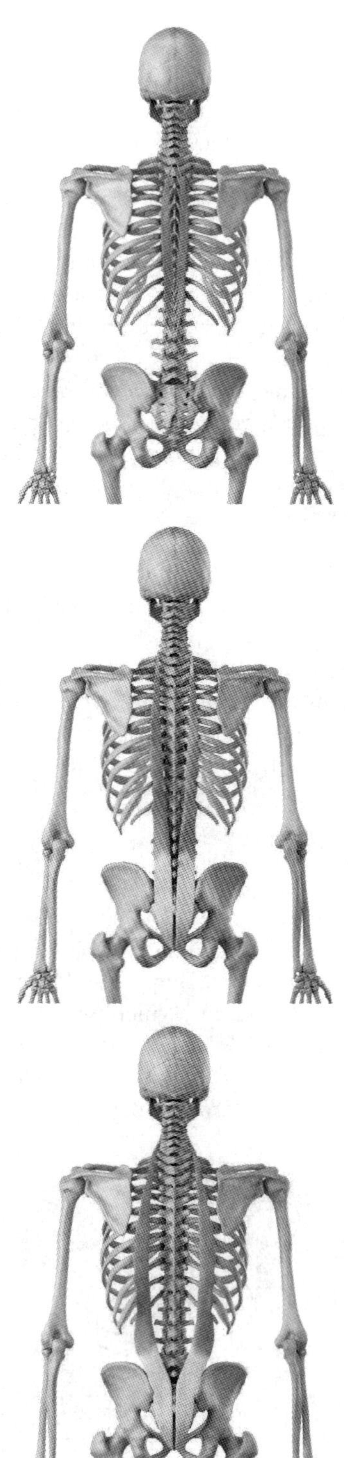

Figure 24-44

SciePro/Shutterstock.com

The primary function of the erector spinae is to "extend" the spine—to pull it back (to arch the spine) posteriorly, and to prevent the spine from being pulled (flexed) forward. The most lateral of the three columns (the one farthest out to the side from the spine) also assists in rotating the spine, although torso rotation is primarily caused by the internal and external obliques.

❑ Erector Spinae Weakness: Lower Back Pain and the Rationale for Training the Erector Spinae

There are two likely reasons why the "lower back" has been mistakenly regarded as an individual muscle—at least by bodybuilders. One reason is that only the lower part of the erector spinae is visible (i.e., not covered by the latissimus or trapezius). Another likely reason is that people often feel pain and/or discomfort in their "lower back" area, which has led to the belief that the pain is somehow related to weakness of the "lower back." This has led to the assumption that there must be a way to strengthen that specific area. These assumptions are incorrect.

There are various reasons a person could be feeling pain in their lower back, but "weakness" is not likely one of them. In reality, there are many people whose entire body is weak, but they don't necessarily have pain everywhere. Weakness does not itself cause pain, and lower back pain does not necessarily indicate muscle weakness in the lower back region.

A person could be having lower back pain, because they have been performing exercises that strain that region, and have developed a type of injury. As was discussed in Chapter 22, there are a number of potential spinal injuries that could occur either as a result of excessive spinal compression, or from inappropriately "rounding" the back (flexing the spine), while it's heavily loaded, which might cause an intervertebral disc to "herniate."

The first step to take (to prevent further injury) is to stop doing the exercises that stress the spine (including barbell squats, deadlifts, and any unsupported rowing exercise), and to ensure that proper form is being used during exercises that require a neutral spine. The next step might be to have your spine examined by a qualified orthopedic doctor—perhaps a spine specialist. If it is established that your spine and the intervertebral discs are not damaged, you can proceed with a biomechanically correct exercise program. On the other hand, if your spine or any intervertebral discs are injured, you should not perform exercises that load the erector spinae, nor any exercise that compresses the spine, or requires any kind of spinal movement (forward, backward, lateral or rotation), even if the exercises performed are anatomically correct.

If you have lower back pain, you should not assume that doing an exercise that strengthens your "lower back" will resolve the problem. Personal trainers are not qualified to diagnose back pain, and they are also not qualified to prescribe "remedial exercise" for lower back pain or spinal injury. Improper exercise can make an existing lower back injury worse. Exercising the erector spinae is generally good, provided you do not have a spinal injury.

❑ Misunderstood Exercises for the "Lower Back"

To demonstrate how misunderstood the concept of "lower back exercise" is, it can be helpful to examine the following hypothetical situation. Let's say that you have structured your workouts as a four-way split program (your muscle groups divided into four groups/four separate workouts), and on day four, you're supposed to work your "lower back." So, on this fourth day, you perform two common "lower back" exercises—*deadlifts* (Figure 24-45) and *"low back extensions"* (Figure 24-46).

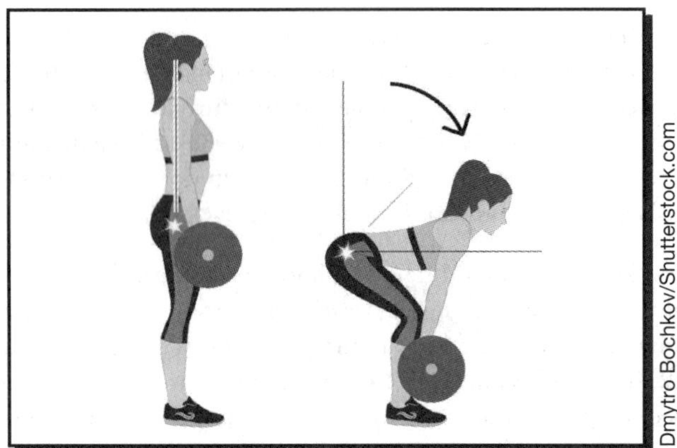


Figure 24-45

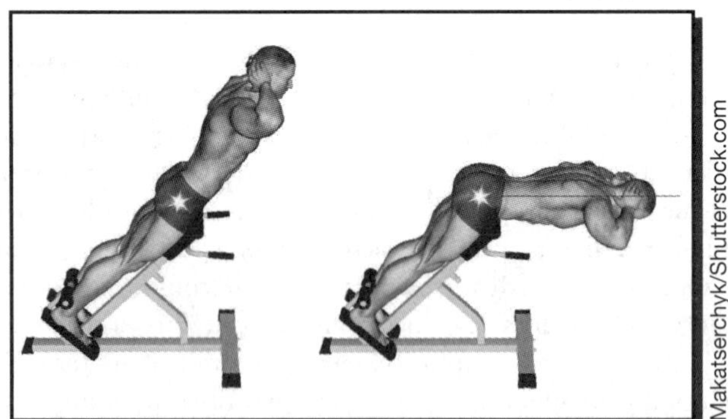


Figure 24-46

A dot has been placed on the hip joint of the two exercisers (Figures 24-45 and 24-46) to show that that is the primary joint that is moving, during both exercises. Given that the gluteus is the primary muscle that crosses the hip joint, it is the gluteus that primarily produces that movement—hip extension (with some help from the adductors and hamstrings)—during these two exercises. As such, it is the gluteus muscle that is doing the "dynamic" (the more productive) work in these two exercises.

The erector spinae is maintaining rigidity in the spine, isometrically preventing the torso from collapsing forward, while the gluteus does the harder work of producing skeletal movement. So, although you may be doing these two exercises with the intention of targeting the erector spinae, that is not the muscle that is doing most of the work in either of these two exercises. Dynamic (concentric) contraction of the erector spinae would produce movement in the spine—extension/arching the spine, from a rounded/flexed position—but there is obviously very little of that type of movement occurring during these two exercises.

The first discovery, therefore, is the realization that specific exercises which are typically believed to be "lower back exercises," actually work the glutes more than they work the erector spinae. The next surprise is that many *other* exercises (as well as various activities), which are *not* considered to be "lower back exercises," load the erector spinae (although isometrically) as much as exercises which are designated as "lower back exercises."

For example, in Figure 24-47 (left image), you see a *low pulley rowing* exercise, which many people do as part of their "lat and upper back" workout. In Figure 24-47 (right image), you see a *barbell squat*, which people typically perform as part of their "legs" workout. In Figure 24-48 (upper image), you see a *standing barbell front raise*, which people often do as part of their "anterior deltoids" workout. In turn, Figure 24-48 (lower image) shows a *standing barbell curl*, which people often perform as part of their "arms" workout.

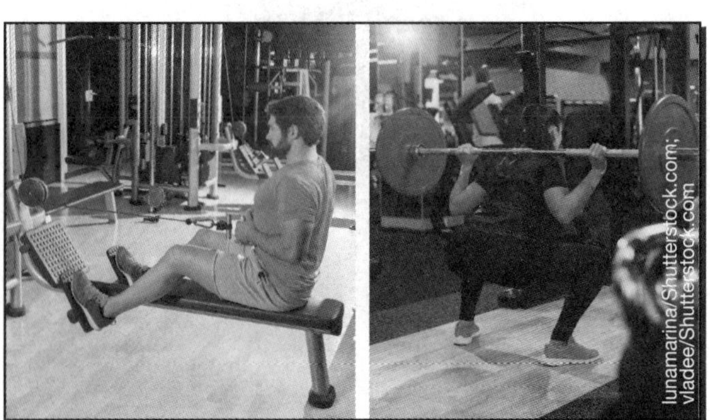


Figure 24-47

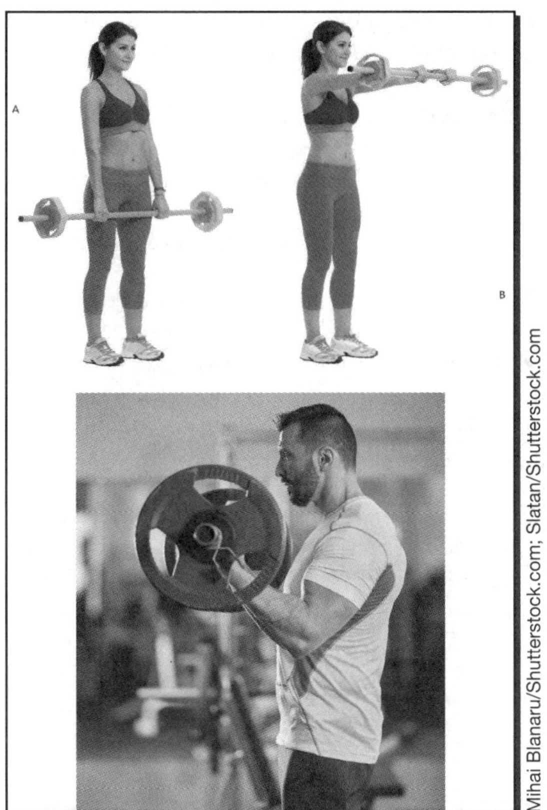


Figure 24-48

These four exercises all have something in common—with each other, as well as with the first two exercises previously shown (*deadlifts* and *low back extensions*). They all involve isometric activation of the erector spinae, while other sets of muscles work dynamically.

In Figure 24-47 (left), the erector spinae are preventing the torso from folding forward, while the target muscles (ostensibly, the lats and "upper back") work dynamically. In Figure 24-47 (right), the erector spinae are preventing the torso from folding forward, while the glutes and quads work dynamically. In Figure 24-48 (upper image), the erector spinae are preventing the torso from folding forward, while the deltoids dynamically produce movement of the shoulder joint. Finally, in Figure 24-48 (lower image), the erector spinae are preventing the torso from folding forward, while the biceps dynamically bend the elbows.

The point is that, although the first two exercises (*deadlifts* and *low back extensions*) are generally considered "lower back" exercises, the erector spinae is not working much more productively—during these two exercises—than it does during other exercises which are not intended for the erector spinae. The same type of isometric contraction of the erector spinae occurs during many other exercises. In fact, even putting your weights away (Figure 24-49) causes the erector spinae to be isometrically loaded—they hold the torso rigid as you lean forward to place weights on a rack. In addition, many daily tasks—like carrying the trash out, carrying groceries, and any other activity that front loads the torso or requires bending over— isometrically loads the erector spinae.

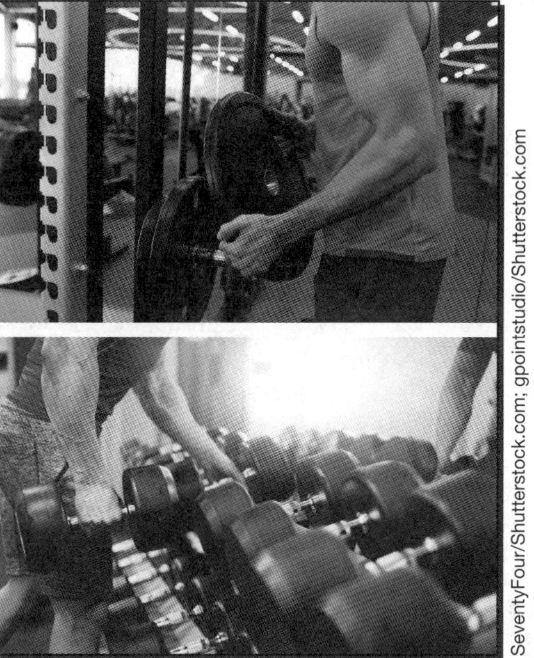


Figure 24-49

Accordingly, when you perform *deadlifts* and "*low back extensions*" (sometimes referred to as "*hyper extensions*") as part of your "lower back" workout, you are unwittingly doing more of the same thing for your erector spinae that you've done during your other workouts—*isometric* loading of the erector spinae. Very few exercise enthusiasts realize this redundancy. In fact, a reasonable argument can be made that the erector spinae of most people is already "overworked," simply by doing all of the exercises that typically load it.

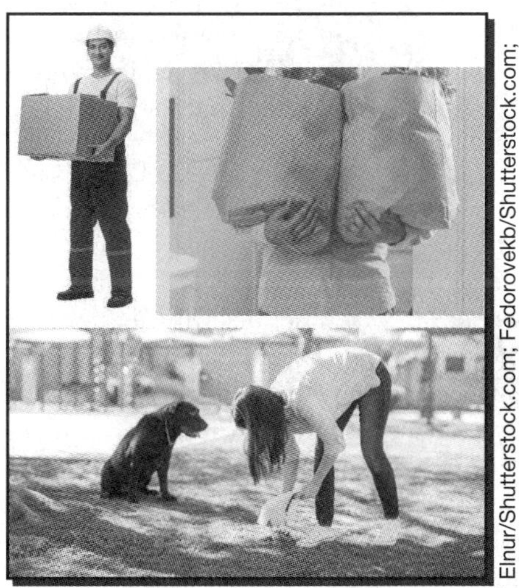


Figure 24-50

It's likely that your erector spinae does not need any additional *isometric* loading, beyond that which is required as "peripheral recruitment," during many other exercises and activities performed in the gym. What your spinal erector is likely not getting, however, and which may provide some additional benefit, is a *dynamic* exercise. At a minimum, it would provide the muscle with a type of stimulation that is different than the usual isometric contraction.

❑ Ideal Movement for Training the Erector Spinae

In Figure 24-51, I am performing a *seated torso extension*. You'll notice that the "pivot" (the dot) is now mid-spine. It is not at the hip, as was the case with the *deadlift* and the "*low back extension*." This mid-spine pivot causes the erector spinae to lengthen and shorten, which means that the erector spinae is now working dynamically. The muscle is now elongating and shortening, rather than merely working to maintain rigidity in the spine, isometrically.

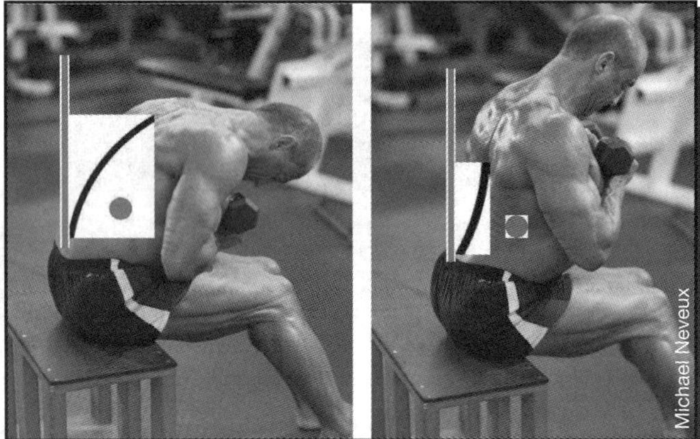


Figure 24-51

This *seated torso extension* exercise may look like it would not be very challenging, especially compared to the thought of doing a *deadlift* with 200 pounds or more, but you'd be surprised how much fatigue you'll feel in the erector spinae, when doing this exercise. There is a big difference between working a muscle isometrically, and working it dynamically.

As you can see in Figure 24-51, I first round my spine forward (left image), thereby elongating the erector spinae. Then I arch my back (right image), thereby contracting the erector spinae. This spinal movement is a similar to what occurs during a good abs exercise, but with the resistance (gravity) pulling the torso from the opposite side, and the concentric movement occurring in the opposing direction. During this exercise, the concentric movement arches (extends) the torso posteriorly, whereas during an abs exercise, the concentric movement curls (flexes) the torso anteriorly, but the pivot point at mid spine is the same. This is like the biceps and triceps, where the elbow joint is the common pivot point.

In the aforementioned example, I am holding a 10-pound weight, but this is hardly necessary. This exercise is usually challenging enough without using any additional resistance, when it is done correctly. Once you have mastered this spinal motion using only torso weight, you can add 10 or 20 pounds, if you feel capable of doing so. Given that the emphasis must be on spinal movement, however, it would be foolish to add resistance and then minimize spinal movement.

Notice that I am keeping my torso on the frontside of the vertical line. That line represents the apex. Keeping the torso on the frontside of the apex will load the erector spinae. If you allow the torso to tilt to the backside of the vertical line, you would load the rectus abdominis, a factor that was discussed in Chapter 5, "Opposite Position Loading."

In Figure 24-52, I am performing a different version of a "*torso extension*" exercise. It is the same spinal motion, but with a different resistance curve. Since my torso is more horizontal in this version, i.e., more perpendicular with gravity, it is more "active." In other words, in this version, a higher percentage of the torso's weight loads the erector spinae. Accordingly, this exercise would be considered "more advanced" than the *seated torso extension*.

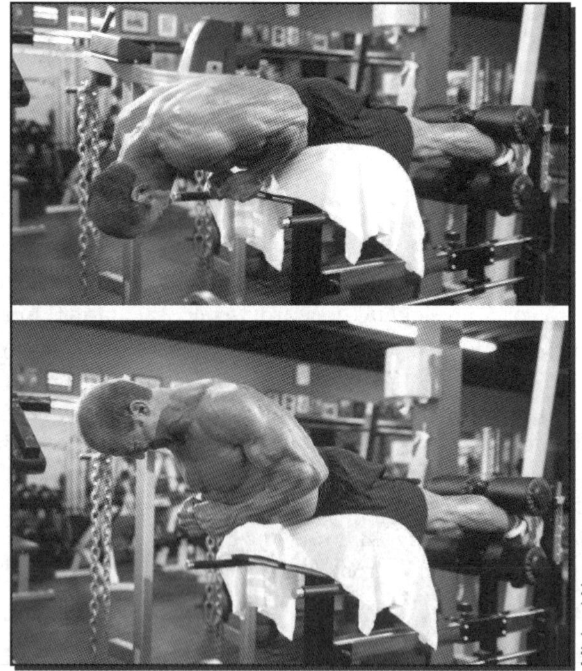


Figure 24-52

Note that the emphasis is still on spinal extension—not on hip extension. The hip joint is held perfectly still, while the torso (spinal) movement occurs.

As mentioned previously, if you perform most of the usual bodybuilding/fitness exercises, in addition to moving weights off and onto various racks at the gym, you probably don't need any additional exercise for your erector spinae. It's likely your erector spinae is already getting more than enough exercise for functional strength. On the other hand, if you feel you need some additional stimulation for your erector spinae, the two dynamic aforementioned exercises would be more productive than doing either *deadlifts* or *"low back extensions."*

There is one caveat, however. If you have a spinal injury, a herniated disc, for example, any type of spinal movement may be contraindicated. If you are experiencing back pain, it would be wise to be examined by an orthopedic doctor/ spine specialist, before performing exercises that involve any kind of spinal flexion or extension—to the front, back, or sides. Even with a healthy (uninjured) spine, it's always wise to avoid overflexing or overextending the spine beyond its comfortable limits.

❑ Realistic Expectations for "Lower Back" Development

Three young, amateur bodybuilders are shown in Figure 24-53, while three seasoned, professional bodybuilders are shown in Figure 24-54. If you focus your attention on the "lower back" area of all these athletes, you'll notice that there is very little difference in that area—amateur bodybuilders versus high level pro bodybuilders—despite a tremendous difference in the development of their other muscle groups.

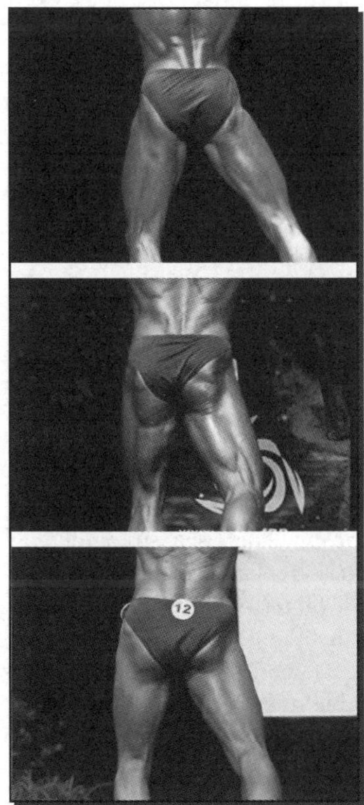

Figure 24-53

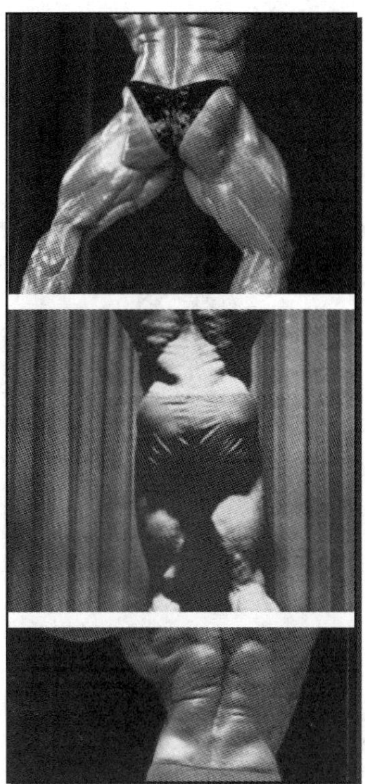
Figure 24-54

What this comparison demonstrates is that the erector spinae does not have much capacity for growth. Of course, the lats, middle trapezius, deltoids, biceps, triceps, etc., have a significant capacity for growth, which is what makes the veteran pro bodybuilders look so impressive in this pose. The "lower back" area of the veteran pro bodybuilders, however, is not much "better" than that of their younger, more novice counterparts.

It's also worth noting that Arnold Schwarzenegger began his bodybuilding career as a powerlifter. In fact, he spent a considerable amount of effort and years doing heavy *deadlifts*, heavy *barbell squats*, and heavy *rowing*. He obviously loaded his erector spinae quite a lot, yet his "lower back" was not significantly more developed (deeper) than other bodybuilders, including amateurs.

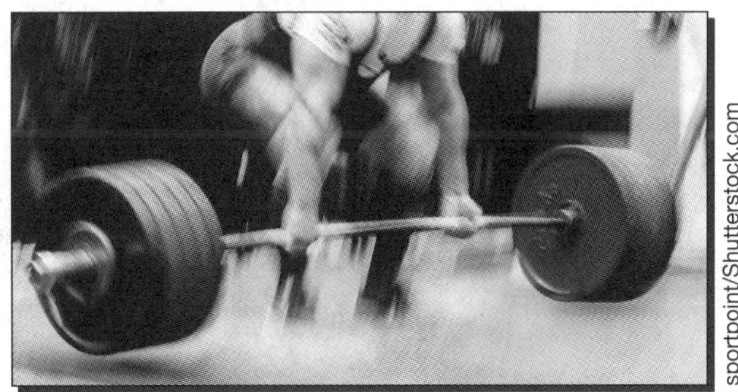
sportpoint/Shutterstock.com
Figure 24-55

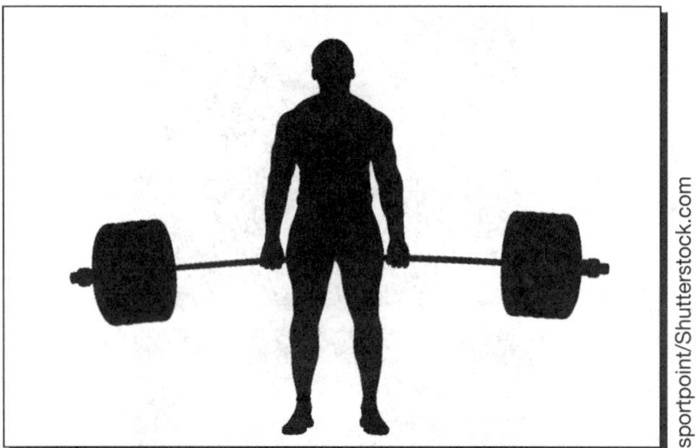
sportpoint/Shutterstock.com

Figure 24-56

What could account for this lack of "lower back" advantage, despite having done so much "lower back" work? Consider the two illustrations in Figures 24-57 and 24-58. The lower part of the erector spinae, which is visible (not covered by the latissimus), is mostly connective tissue—fascia. Tendons and connective tissue have almost no capacity for growth. Even the actual muscle fibers of the erector spinae (above the connective tissue) don't have much capacity for growth (because they are flat muscles, like the soleus), as compared with other skeletal muscles, such as the pectorals, latissimus, biceps, triceps, quads, etc.

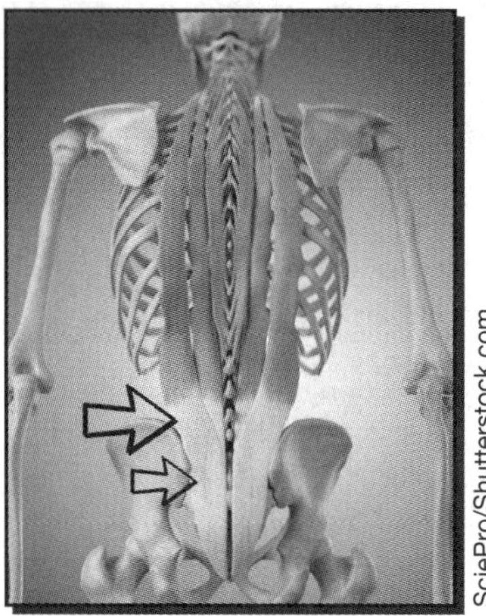
SciePro/Shutterstock.com

Figure 24-57

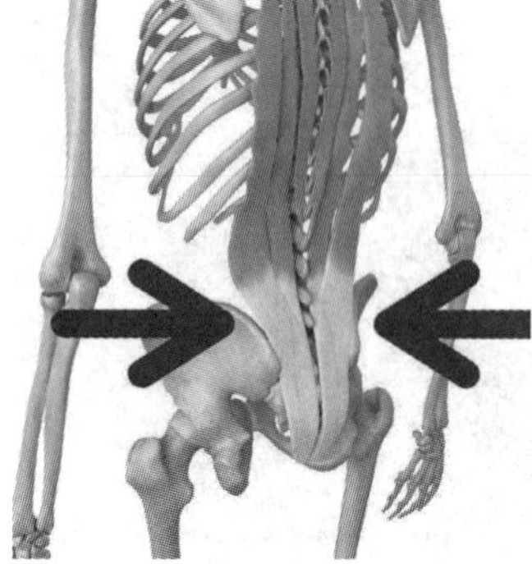
SciePro/Shutterstock.com

Figure 24-58

The point is that it's unwise for you to expect much visible development from working the erector spinae. It's especially foolish to *deadlift* 300 pounds, thereby risking the health of your spine, when the potential reward is almost insignificant, in terms of visible "lower back" development.

Keep in mind that the "Christmas tree" appearance you see on some bodybuilders is not part of the erector spinae. Rather, it is part of the latissimus development. That part of the musculature can still be developed, even if you don't perform any "lower back" (erector spinae) exercise. In fact, most of the depth and thickness that is seen on the backs of advanced bodybuilders is latissimus and middle trapezius development—not erector spinae development.

On occasion, we do see an individual with an unusually deep crevice between the two columns of their lower back area. This development is mostly due to genetics. Some people are genetically fortunate to have a very deep muscular groove down the center of their back (including the lower back), even if they don't do any type of bodybuilding workout. Personally, I've seen basketball players who have that type of "depth" in their lower back area, despite them not doing any heavy lifting, and despite the rest of their body not being very muscular. When these genetically fortunate individuals pursue bodybuilding, observers mistakenly assume the "lower back" musculature of these individuals is due to *deadlifts* they're doing, not knowing those people had some of that musculature even before they started doing resistance exercise. Most of us are not so genetically fortunate.

## Summary

The erector spinae gets a significant amount of loading as part of the "peripheral recruitment" that occurs when you are working other muscle groups, as well as when you are moving weights around the gym and doing daily tasks at home. As such, any standard (non-torso-supported) *rowing* exercise loads the erector spinae, as do most types of *squats*, some deltoid exercises, and most standing biceps exercises—especially *barbell curls* (this is due to both arms being extended in front of the body simultaneously).

This type of muscle activation (of the erector spinae) is mostly isometric, which has a strengthening effect (in that one position) but is generally regarded as less productive than dynamic exercise (in terms of full range of motion strength and muscle development). Still, as noted, the amount of loading the erector spinae gets "peripherally," every day, is significant. As such, a reasonable argument could be made that the erector spinae does not necessarily need any additional exercise.

Performing *deadlifts* and *"lower back" extensions*, with the belief that they target the "lower back" better than any of the other exercises (which also load the erector spinae isometrically) is misguided. In fact, it's just more of the same kind of isometric muscle contraction. Performing a dynamic exercise for the erector spinae, such as the *seated torso extension*, provides a different (arguably "better") type of muscle contraction, as compared with an isometric muscle contraction.

Because the appearance/visible development of the erector spinae ("lower back") does not have much capacity for change, it's likely that even a dynamic exercise will not make much of a difference, in terms of visible development. It may, however, improve spinal mobility, as well as enhance the level of erector spinae strength through its entire range of motion, as compared with isometric erector spinae contraction.

As noted previously, it is important to remember that excessive degrees of spinal extension or flexion (or lateral movement) should be avoided. All joints have their limits of mobility, and, since the spine includes soft (gelatinous) intervertebral discs, and nerves that run alongside them and affect the whole body, it's especially important to not bend the spine beyond its natural limits.

## References

Berger W, Dietz V, Quintern J (1984). Corrective reactions to stumbling in man: Neuronal co-ordination of bilateral leg muscle activity during gait. J Physiol, 357:109–125.

Burke RE, Jankowska E, Bruggencate G ten (1970). A comparison of peripheral and rubrospinal synaptic input to slow and fast twitch motor units of triceps surae. J Physiol, 207:709–732.

Capaday C, Stein RB (1987). Difference in the amplitude of the human soleus H reflex during walking and running. J Physiol, 392:513–522.

# CHAPTER 25

# Internal and External Obliques, Transverse Abdominis, and Shoulder Rotators

## Anatomy and Function of the Obliques

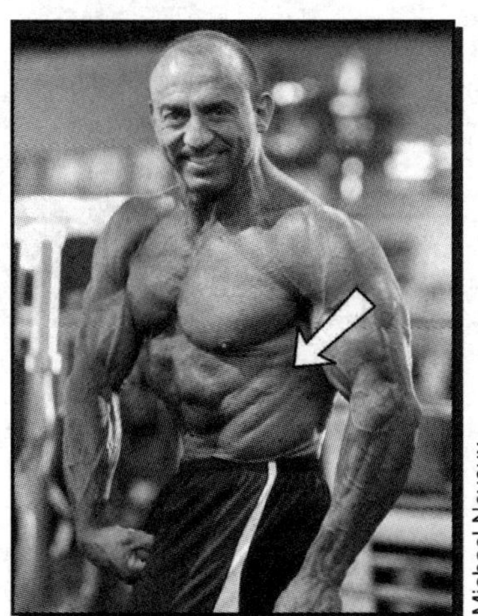


Figure 25-1

The "internal obliques" and "external obliques" are two sets of muscles located on each side of your midsection. The external obliques are the more superficial (closer to the surface) of the two muscles. For this reason, only the external obliques fibers are visible to an observer, and only when the person's body fat level is low enough (usually below 6 percent body fat). The internal obliques lie beneath the external obliques, and cannot be seen by an observer, regardless of how lean the person is.

The primary anatomical function of the obliques is lateral flexion of the spine ("side bending"), as well as torso rotation. These two movements (side bending of the torso and rotation of the torso) are indicated by the direction of the fibers of these two muscles. Naturally, torso movements that combine lateral and rotational movements, would engage the external and internal obliques simultaneously—each assisting the other. In fact, these two muscles always work in tandem, although to different degrees, during any kind of lateral flexion of the torso, and rotation of the torso. They even participate during forward flexion of the torso, which is primarily a function of the rectus abdominis.

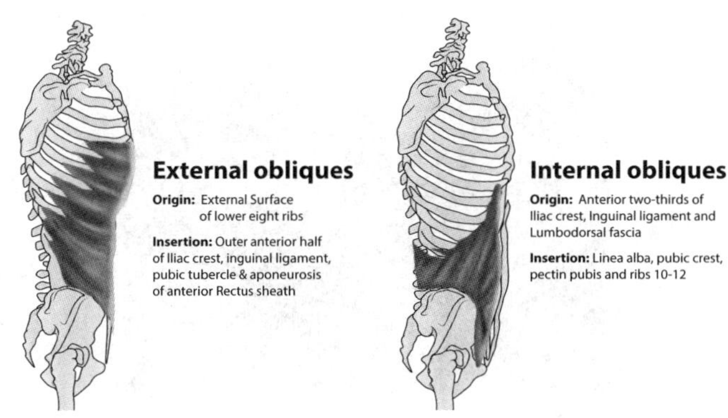


Figure 25-2

Figure 25-2 shows the origins and insertions of the external obliques (left image) and the internal obliques (right image), in addition to the direction of their fibers. Their attachments are on the ribs, the iliac crest (sides of the pelvis), the pubic bone (front/center of the pelvis), and the fascia of the rectus abdominis.

## Ideal Direction of Resistance for Training the Obliques

With regard to "physical fitness" or "physique development," there is no benefit in attempting to distinguish between the function of the external obliques versus that of the internal obliques, since they work together. As such, in order to keep things simple, this text is going to collectively refer to these two muscles singularly, i.e., as "the obliques" or the "oblique muscles."

In addition to the skeletal functions—lateral torso flexion, torso rotation, and assisting the abs in forward flexion—the obliques also provide support for the internal organs, and assist in breathing. The primary anatomical movement, however—the movement that best allows individuals to visibly develop this muscle, is lateral torso flexion, also known as "*side bends.*"

The *side bend* movement is the best way to "stretch" (elongate) and contract (flex) this muscle. If you are competing in a bodybuilding competition or otherwise displaying your physique, you would bend your torso laterally, in order to flex your obliques (Figure 25-3), such that they become more visibly pronounced. This muscle contraction can be felt between the side of the ribcage and the hip bone on the lateral side of the pelvis, which is also where a *side bend* exercise typically concludes its range of motion.

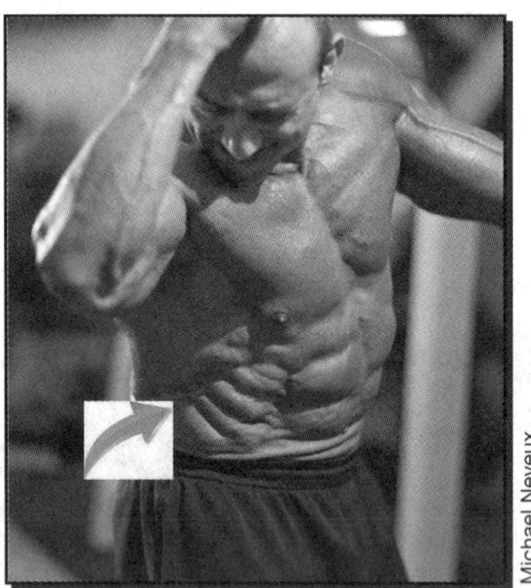


Figure 25-3

There are several versions of *side bends*, each of which has a different degree of productivity,* ranging from "mostly not productive" to "very productive." It can be helpful to review each of them, and ascertain what makes the difference between the productive and the unproductive versions.

**Note: "Productivity," in this context, refers to the successful development of the obliques muscle. Side bends do not reduce or diminish body fat deposits that have accumulated in that area. As such, "productivity" does not refer to the loss of body fat in that area.*

In Figure 25-4, you can see a man performing a "standard" *side bend*, while holding a dumbbell in his left hand. His other hand is on his head, although it doesn't matter where that hand is placed. It could be on his waist, or just hanging straight down.

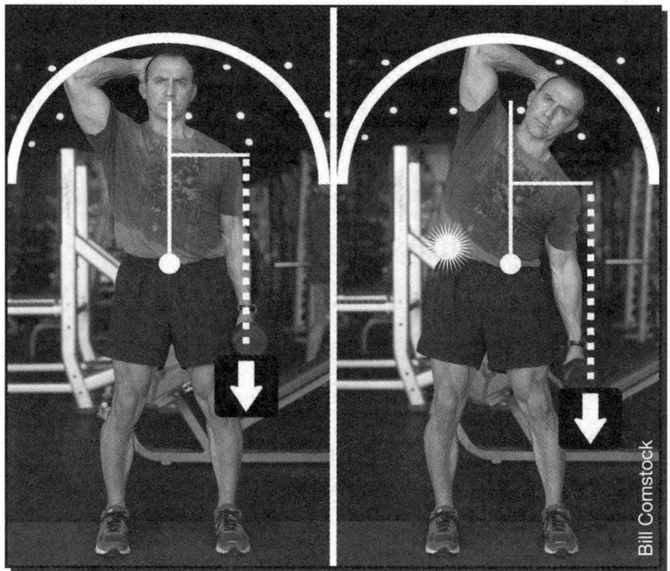


Figure 25-4

The "operating lever" of the obliques is the torso itself, just like the operating lever of the biceps is the forearm. Instead of the elbow (i.e., the pivot for the biceps), however, the "pivot," when working the obliques, is the thoracic and lumbar vertebrae (i.e., middle and lower spine/multi-pivotal). In Figure 25-4, the individual is challenging the obliques on his right side, because the load is coming from his left side. As the resistance pulls the torso to the left, the right oblique muscles pull the torso to the right, against the opposing resistance.

It has already been established that, ideally, the operating lever of a target muscle should cross resistance perpendicularly, somewhere in the range of motion. As you can see here, however, that does not happen very well in this version.

In Figure 25-4, left image, a line has been placed in the center of the torso to show that it is parallel to the arrow (pointing down from the dumbbell), which indicates the direction of resistance. Clearly, those two lines are not perpendicular to each other.

You might think that the torso (as a lever for the obliques) is in the neutral position (parallel to resistance). The resistance is not "zero," however, because the two lines are not on the same plane (overlapping each other). They are, nevertheless, fairly close to each other. In other words, the resistance that is loading the right oblique, in this scenario, is not quite zero, but it's also not much more than that.

Then, in the photo in Figure 25-4, right image, you can see that the torso has moved to about 20 degrees from the vertical position. This movement would load the target muscle (the right obliques) with only about 25 percent of the load being held in the left hand, due to the angle between the torso and the vertical pull of gravity. The other 75 percent of the weight being held is essentially wasted. This version of a *side bend*—using a straight downward direction of resistance (while standing)—is extremely inefficient.

What's needed is a better (more efficient) direction of resistance, as indicated in Figure 25-5. As you can see, an arrow has been placed, showing what would be a better direction of resistance—more perpendicular with the torso. This resistance would be provided by a cable, coming from a pulley that is set at about the height of the knee.

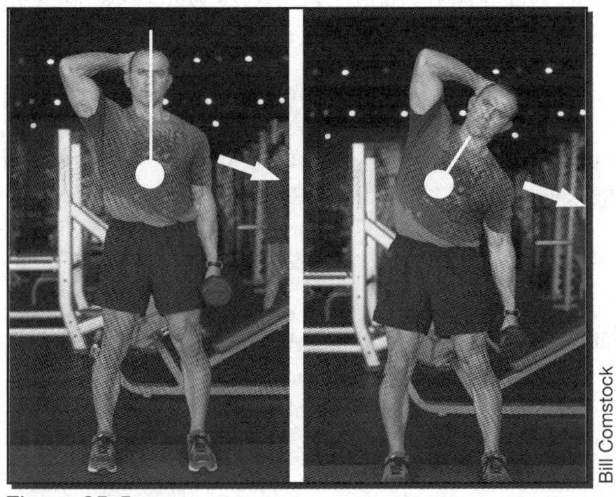

Figure 25-5

A left-lateral direction of resistance (coming from the left side)—perpendicular to the torso—would load the right obliques with a significantly higher percentage of the weight being used, as compared with the straight-downward direction of resistance provided by a "free weight" dumbbell. This direction of resistance would result in more load on the left obliques, even if the same amount of weight is used in both versions of the exercise. This is because a greater percentage of the resistance loads a muscle when it pulls perpendicularly on that muscle's operating lever (i.e., in this case, that is the torso).

In Figure 25-6, the pulley has been set at about the height of my hip. This slightly higher setting causes the resistance to pull on the torso-lever from a more perpendicular angle, which loads the obliques with an even higher percentage of the load being used, than if the pulley had been set at the level of my knee. The more perpendicular to the torso, the higher the percentage of the load being used that loads the obliques. As such, a lighter weight can be used while still optimally loading the obliques.

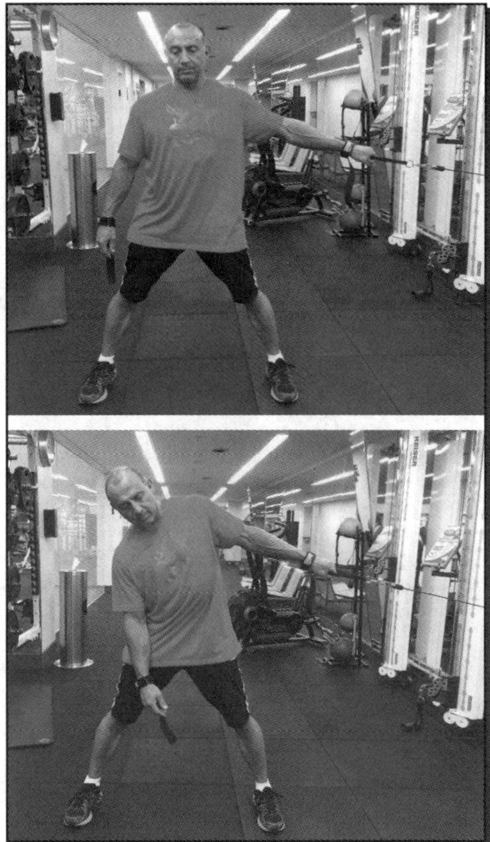
Figure 25-6

*Note: You'll need a slightly wider foot stance—for stability—when you use a lateral resistance like this, because if the stance is too narrow, the resistance will pull you off balance.*

The least efficient version of a *side bend* is holding two dumbbells simultaneously—one in each hand (Figure 25-7), a point that was explained in Chapter 6. Performing a *side bend* like this is analogous to putting the same amount of weight on each side of a balance scale—each side neutralizing the other side. When *side bends* are (foolishly) done like this, the downward force loads the trapezius (both sides, although not enough to benefit them), and results in unnecessary downward compression of the intervertebral discs of the spine (which increases spinal injury risk). The obliques, however, get no more opposing resistance than they would if no weight (in either hand) were used at all—because the two weights simply counterbalance each other.

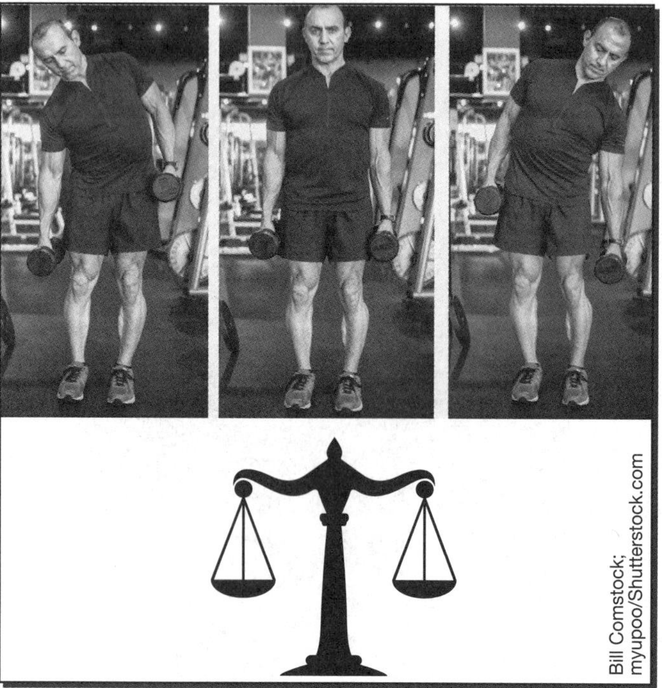

Figure 25-7

When doing *cable side bends,* with a *lateral* resistance (pulling perpendicularly to the torso), there is very little spinal compression—almost zero—and it also does not load the trapezius. *Cable side bends* result in more of what you want (efficient loading of the obliques) and less of what you don't want (spinal compression and trapezius loading).

In fact, it is NOT possible to load both obliques (left side and right side) simultaneously, because they are agonist/antagonist to each other. Each side requires an opposite direction of resistance, originating from the opposite side of the working muscle. When working the right side obliques, a left-lateral resistance must be used. Similarly, when working the left side obliques, a right-lateral resistance must be used.

## Range of Motion and Limitations of Spinal Mobility

The recommended "safe" range of motion for lateral torso (spinal) flexion, as per orthopedic/physical therapy guidelines, is 15 to 20 degrees. Compare this limit to the safe range for forward flexion (40 to 60 degrees) and backward extension (20 to 35 degrees).

The spine has less lateral (sideways) mobility, than it does either forward or backward mobility. This factor is worth noting. As such, it is unwise to use an extreme range of motion when bending sideways. More lateral stretch is not more productive, and it increases the risk of damaging one or more intervertebral discs.

When performing *side bends* with resistance, there is more risk in bending too far toward the resistance (the eccentric phase), than there is when bending away from the resistance (the concentric phase). If you excessively bend your torso toward the resistance (the eccentric phase), it is the resistance that is pulling on your spine. This factor, which is called "passive stretch," has a much higher injury risk. When you bend your torso away from the resistance (the concentric phase), it is your oblique muscle that produces that degree of bend, and the body naturally limits self-imposed excessive joint movement.

As such, the part of the range of motion that should be avoided, during *side bends*, is the excessive stretch during the eccentric phase of the range of motion. It's perfectly safe to utilize the full range of motion on the contraction side, during the concentric phase of the range of motion. Personally, I would recommend avoiding the first 20 to 30 degrees, on the stretch side. Then, I suggest taking the range of motion all the way to full contraction, on the other side.

Furthermore, I also recommend trying to bend your spine as a rounded "curve," rather than "jackknifing" your spine only at the base. "Curving" the spine produces a very slight lateral bend at each vertebrae. "Jackknifing" places all of the bend at just one point near the lumbar spine, and also fails to adequately engage the obliques through their full range of motion.

In the composite photo/illustration in Figure 25-8, a "stiff spine" *side bend* is shown, bending only the base of the spine, on the left. The right image shows the correct "curved spine" *side bend*, which evenly distributes the movement through multiple vertebrae of the spine.

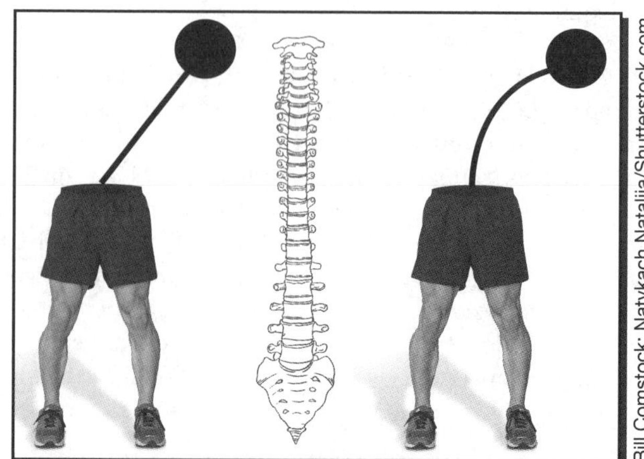

Figure 25-8

It's somewhat common for people to lean sideways, while their spine is still straight. The spine is not like an arm or a leg, both of which have only one pivot. The spine is multi-pivotal, like a chain link. It is designed to bend at all its pivots. In essence, therefore, the obliques are meant to cause the spine to move at multiple vertebrae.

## Commentary About Other Exercises for the Obliques

❑ Diagonal Side Bends

The exercise shown in Figure 25-9 is another version of a *side bend.* The position of the torso is more perpendicular to gravity than that of the standing version—halfway between vertical and horizontal. This exercise is a reasonably good substitute for the *standing cable* version, eliminating the need to add a secondary resistance (body weight is more than enough, in this version). There are a couple minor problems with this version, however.

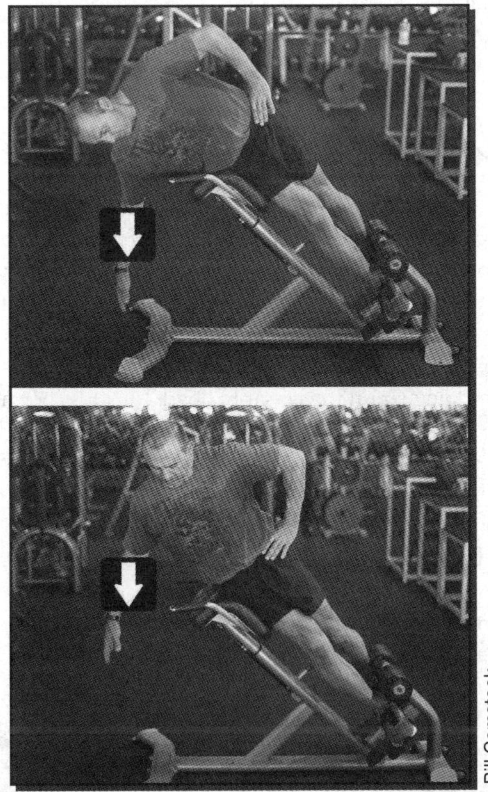

Figure 25-9

The main problem with this exercise is that it requires the use of "bodyweight"—actually, torso weight—which is actually too much for most people, using this angle. When the torso is vertical, and you're using a pulley, an appropriate resistance would be between 30 and 50 pounds. The weight of the average torso is usually around 80 pounds. Using too much weight on any *side bend* movement makes it difficult (possibly dangerous) to produce that "curving" of the spine.

As a result, people tend to do this version of the exercise with a mostly straight spine, which is not ideal. It's especially risky in the stretch phase (Figure 25-9, upper image), because the spine is most "active" (perpendicular with gravity) at that point, and it's simultaneously entering its stretch (eccentric) phase. Forcing the spine to bend laterally, while using excessive weight, is not prudent. As such, adding additional weight to this version (i.e., holding a dumbbell) is completely unnecessary, and further increases the risk factor of this movement.

People often think—mistakenly—that using a very heavy resistance on *side bends* will be more conducive to reducing the body fat that has accumulated around the waistline. That reasoning is entirely incorrect. Nothing (other than liposuction) will selectively reduce body fat from the place of an individual's choosing. Using heavier resistance during a *side bend* won't change that fact—it only increases the likelihood of injury.

This version of this exercise, shown in Figure 25-9, is also very uncomfortable. The feet must be crossed in order to "fit" into the small space that is typically provided on this type of bench. This bench is not designed to be used this way. Furthermore, the hip placement on the pad is usually very uncomfortable, because it's designed for the front of the pelvis to be placed on it, not the side of the hip. In addition, the thighs are squeezed together, because of the required foot placement.

If no pulleys are available (for performing a *standing cable side bends*), this version might be a reasonably good alternative. On the other hand, if an adjustable pulley is available, *standing cable side bends* is a much better choice. It provides a lateral-pulling resistance, similar to this horizontal side bend, but also allows you to stand more comfortably. More importantly, it allows you to use the resistance level of your choosing—one that is most comfortably challenging, given your particular strength level. It does not force you to use your body weight, however much that happens to be.

❑ Side Planks

The exercise shown in Figure 25-10, known as the "*side plank*," is commonly seen in gyms. It has, however, the same drawbacks as the standard *planks* described previously—it's an isometric exercise (lacks dynamic muscle contraction), as well as a bodyweight exercise (does not allow variations of resistance, based on individual strength capacity), plus two additional drawbacks.

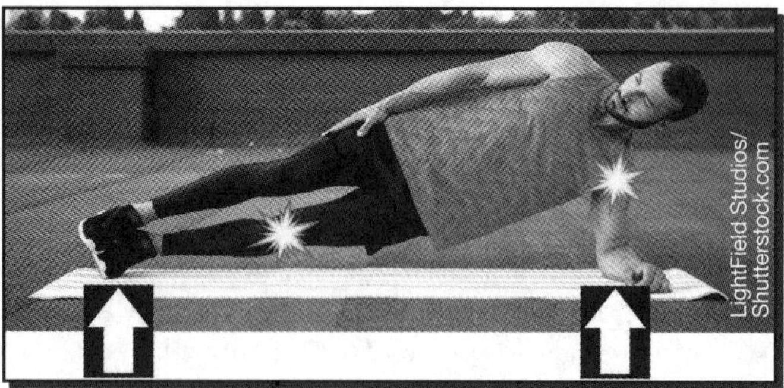

Figure 25-10

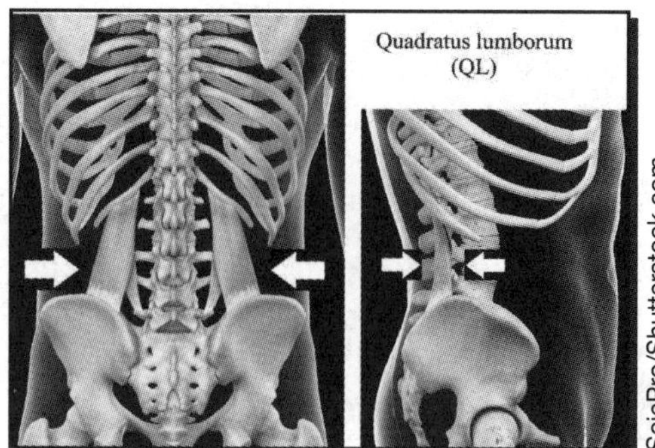

Figure 25-11

During this exercise, approximately one-third of your bodyweight is loaded onto the shoulder joint of the supporting arm. This forces the humerus inward, against the glenoid socket, with about 60 pounds of force (for a 180-pound person). A young, healthy shoulder joint might easily tolerate this. An older, arthritic or previously injured shoulder joint, however, would NOT do well with this amount of inward force.

In addition, there is also a significant amount of sideways force that is placed on the knee that is closest to the ground—"trying" to bend the knee sideways. Approximately two-thirds of your bodyweight is loaded onto the side of that foot, a load which is then magnified by the length of the lower leg. In other words, a force that could be as much as 2,400 pounds (120 pounds of bodyweight magnified by a factor of approximately 20, for tibia length), is attempting to bend your knee in a direction it does not naturally bend—sideways.

Frankly, it's extremely foolish to perform this exercise, given that it causes discomfort and risk of injury to the shoulder and knee joints, and forces you to use bodyweight (i.e., more resistance than is necessary, thereby making it psychologically burdensome), but then provides a compromised benefit due to the lack of dynamic muscle contraction.

In contrast, you could perform *standing cable side bends*, with the amount of resistance that you've selected, based on your individual strength capacity, without any shoulder and knee strain, while achieving dynamic muscle contraction (range of motion). This would produce more benefit, with less discomfort and less risk of injury—a greater reward for less cost.

❑ Additional Comments About *Side Bends* and Obliques

Lateral torso flexion (*side bends*) is assisted by a muscle called the "quadratus lumborum," also known as the "QL" (shown in Figure 25-11). The QL is a small muscle—one on each side at base of the spine. People often have pain in this area, which is another reason why it's not wise to use excessive resistance, when doing *side bends*. There is more risk, than there is benefit, in using a heavy weight when doing *side bends*.

If you are experiencing lower back pain, and you are under the care of an orthopedic physician or a physical therapist, ask them if your particular condition allows you to do "lateral spinal flexion," before you attempt to perform any kind of *side bends*, with resistance. Depending on their response, it may be necessary for you to abbreviate (shorten) the range of motion, or to use no motion at all ("isometric"), if you have a condition/injury that precludes you from moving your spine laterally. If that is the case, you could do an isometric version of the *side cable raise*, using that same type of lateral cable resistance, but without any motion. Just hold the cable resistance, with your torso in a stationary position, for a count of 30 to 60 seconds.

❑ Torso Rotation

*Torso rotation* (shown in Figure 25-12) is another movement that is produced primarily by the internal and external obliques. From a functional standpoint, this is a good movement, provided the direction of resistance is correct (i.e., it should be pulling in the opposite direction as your concentric motion). There is no need to angle your *torso rotation*—either upward or a downward—although doing so isn't necessarily "bad." It's just not necessary, nor is it much more advantageous. Simply rotate horizontally, like you're swinging a baseball bat, but slowly and deliberately, without initiating momentum. Also, do not overrotate (excessively twist) your spine, especially on the eccentric phase. Try to stay in the middle 80 percent of the range of motion of *torso rotation*.

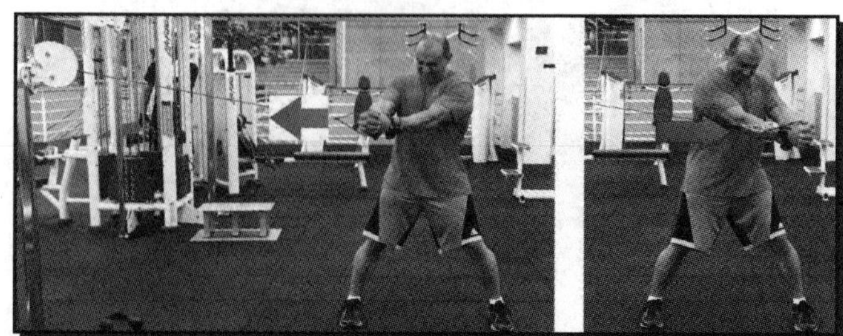
Figure 25-12

The resistance curve of this exercise (Figure 25-12) can be easily varied, simply by adjusting where you stand, in relation to the pulley. If you are standing with the pulley slightly behind you (but still to the side), the resistance will feel "heavier" at the beginning of the movement, and "lighter" at the end of the range of motion.

On the other hand, if you stand with the pulley slightly in front of you (but still to the side), the resistance will feel lighter at the beginning of the movement and heavier at the end of the range of motion. This latter option is better, because it prevents overrotation of the spine in the early (stretch) position.

As noted, *torso rotation* (as an exercise), performed with a moderate resistance, is functionally useful. The strength gained from this movement can be applied to any activity that requires a similar movement, such as golf, baseball, tennis, and martial arts. Unfortunately, this movement is not likely to produce much (if any) visible development of the external obliques. For this reason, it is not commonly used in physique development.

To test this conclusion, simply compare the ending position of a *side bend*, with the ending position of a *torso rotation*. The ending position of a *side bend* results in a deliberate and obvious contraction of the obliques. The ending position of a *torso rotation* does not end with any kind of obvious muscle contraction ("flex"), the way a *biceps curl*, a *triceps pushdown*, an *ab crunch*, or *a leg extension*, etc. does.

## Anatomy of the Transverse Abdominis

The transverse abdominis is located three layers down from the surface. It lies beneath the internal obliques, which lie beneath the external obliques (Figure 25-13, upper image). The two illustrations in Figure 25-13, middle and lower images (from the front and from the back), show that the fibers of this muscle are mostly on your sides, running horizontally to the torso. The transverse abdominis originates on the thoraco-lumbar fascia (on the lower back), and connects to the fascia of the posterior rectus abdominis (the sides of the abs) as well as to the inguinal ligament (Figure 25-14, right image).

This muscle mostly connects to and from fascia (connective tissue). It does not connect (much) from "bone to bone," like most other skeletal muscles do. There are some peripheral connections to boney areas, but since the fibers run horizontally, and those horizontal connections are from fascia to fascia, it does not produce any actual skeletal movement.

Rather, it acts as a sort of "girdle" for the abdomen, provides spinal support, and assists in breathing. It also participates in torso *coordination*—proprioceptively and kinesthetically. In other words, it provides "feedback" to the brain, as it relates to torso position.

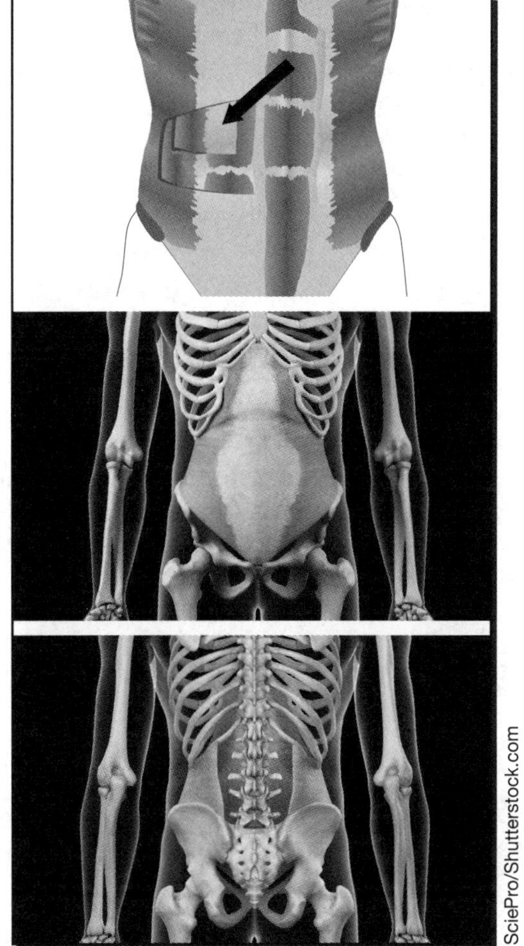


Figure 25-13

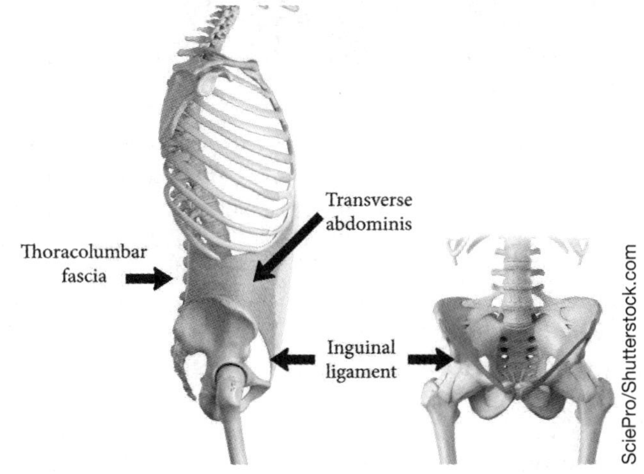


Figure 25-14

Because the "TVA" (transverse abdominis) is three layers deep and cannot be seen, you might wonder whether it's worth exercising this muscle. It is, however, one of the muscles associated with "the core," along with the rectus abdominis, the obliques, and the erector spinae. For this reason (primarily), it does have some functional importance.

The transverse abdominis participates in activities that could be characterized as "athletic"—helping facilitate coordination during activities, such as tennis, volleyball, basketball, and dancing, in which the body moves spontaneously in a variety of directions. In fact, performing these types of activities helps improve the TVA's ability to provide the coordination required for activities such as these. This type of proprioceptive coordination is sometimes referred to as "core" training, although I think this reference is ambiguous. I believe it should be regarded as "coordination" or "athletic" exercise.

There is one specific exercise that can be used to directly strengthen the transverse abdominis—an "abdominal vacuum." In this exercise, the abdomen is drawn inward (toward the spine) and held for a few seconds. The best way to learn how to do this exercise is by first lying on your back, on a floor mat (Figure 25-15, left image). It might be helpful to elevate your tailbone with a pad. Allow your lumbar spine to arch upward. Then exhale and—without inhaling—try to pull the abdomen inward, toward your spine. The more you attempt this, the more your coordination to do this will improve. A partial vacuum can be achieved without a full exhale, but a full vacuum requires a full exhale.

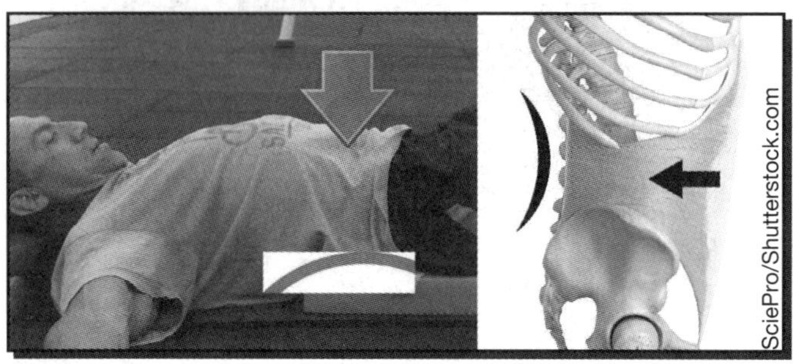

Figure 25-15

Once you have mastered doing this exercise while lying on your back, you can then attempt it while standing. To do this exercise while standing, I suggest you place both hands on a shelf or other firm surface in front of you, about the height of your chest. Gently push downward with your hands on the shelf (which helps you lift your chest upward, and arch your lumbar spine). Then, draw your abdomen inward, and hold it for about five seconds. You may feel a slight muscle contraction in your lower back, on each side of your spine. That is where the TVA originates. That sensation you feel is the transverse abdominis pulling the front part of the abdomen posteriorly—toward the spine (the arrow in Figure 25-15, right image)—toward the origin of the transverse abdominis.

The "vacuum" can also be used as a pose on the bodybuilding stage. The bodybuilder who is most famous for this particular pose is the great Frank Zane (three-time Mr. Olympia winner in 1977, '78, and '79), whose vacuum pose is still considered iconic. He is pictured in Figure 25-16, far left. The center photo in Figure 25-16 is of me at the age of 22, attempting to do that same vacuum pose. The photo on the far right in Figure 25-16 is of me at the age of 54, coming a little closer to replicating the perfection of Frank Zane's pose.

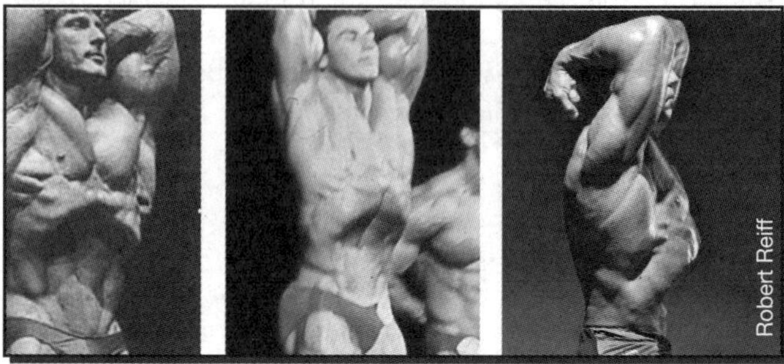

Figure 25-16

Practicing the vacuum pose, regularly—either while lying down or while standing—will help keep the transverse abdominis strong.

As noted previously, it's virtually impossible to do a "vacuum," if your lower back is not slightly arched (tailbone back). Yet, it's common to hear trainers tell their clients to pull their abdomen inward, while the individual is doing *abdominal crunches*. *Ab crunches* require spinal flexion (tailbone under), which is the opposite spinal position.

In fact, it is impossible to contract the rectus abdominis (to flex your abs), while simultaneously pulling your abdomen inward. These two functions are mutually exclusive. Either you contract your abs with your tailbone tucked under (your spine rounded), or you pull your abdomen inward (vacuum) with your tailbone back (arched spine). You cannot do both at the same time.

## Shoulder Rotators (AKA the Rotator Cuff Muscles)

This group of muscles has been saved for last in this chapter, because they are not normally considered "physique muscles." Understanding these muscles, however—when they participate, when they should not participate, how and why they are so often injured during weight training—is extremely important in the application of resistance exercise for physique development, in order to prevent injury.

The four muscles that constitute the "rotator cuff" are the supraspinatus, the infraspinatus, the teres minor, and the subscapularis. These muscles hold the humeral head in the glenoid fossa (shoulder socket), and they rotate the humerus (upper arm bone) internally (forward) and externally (posteriorly).

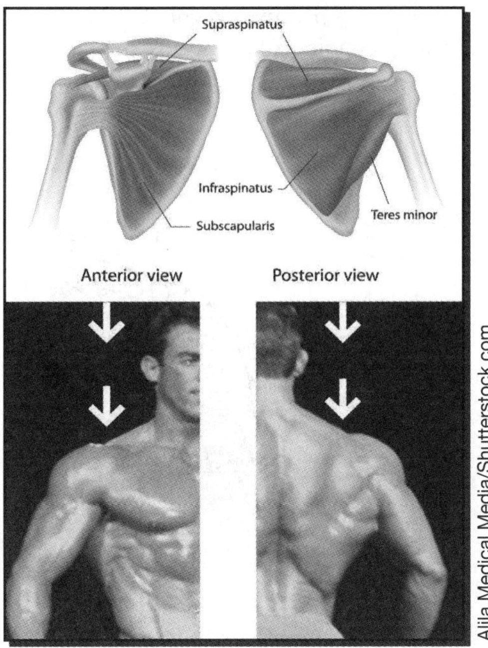

Figure 25-17

The upper left image in Figure 25-17 shows the perspective you would see, if you were looking at someone from the front, and could see through their chest cavity (through their ribcage), at the frontside of the right scapula. In contrast, the upper right image in Figure 25-17 shows the perspective you would see if you were looking at someone from behind, and could see through their skin, at the backside of their right scapula.

❑ Anatomy of the Supraspinatus

The supraspinatus is a small muscle that runs along the top of the scapula. It originates on the inside edge of the top of the scapula, and then passes under the acromion process, before attaching onto the upper/outer part of the humeral head.

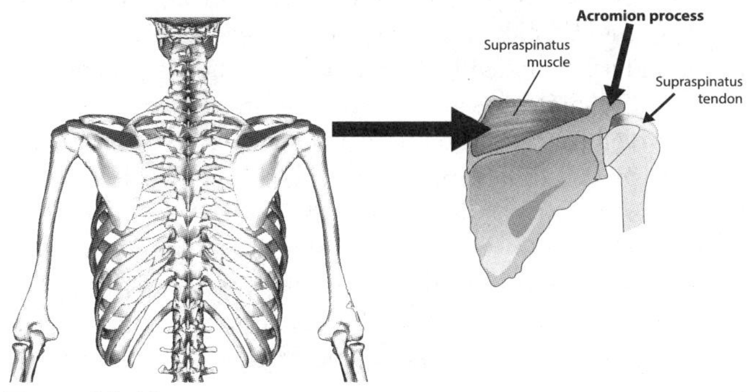

Figure 25-18

Of the four rotator cuff muscles, this is the only one that does not participate in rotation of the humerus. Rather, it mainly helps hold the humeral head in the glenoid socket. In addition, when it contracts, it pulls the upper outer part of the humeral head inward, thereby assisting in the first 10 degrees of lateral abduction (side raise) of the humerus (Figure 25-19).

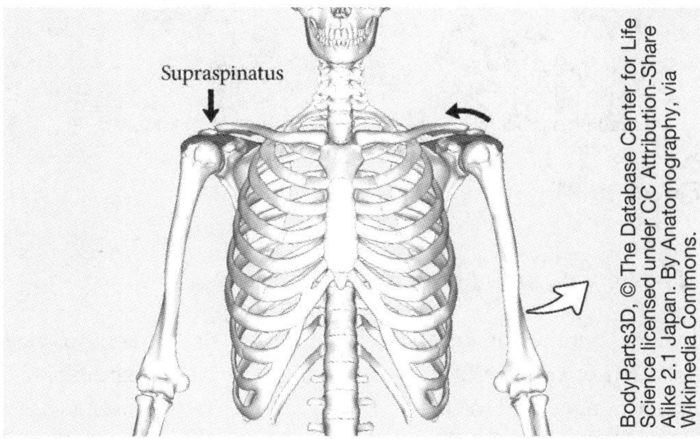

Figure 25-19

In Figure 25-20, you can see that the "acromion" is a bony protrusion (part of the scapula), which is situated just above the head of the humerus. You can also see the end of the supraspinatus, as well as its tendon, as it comes out from under the acromion, and attaches onto the top of the humeral head.

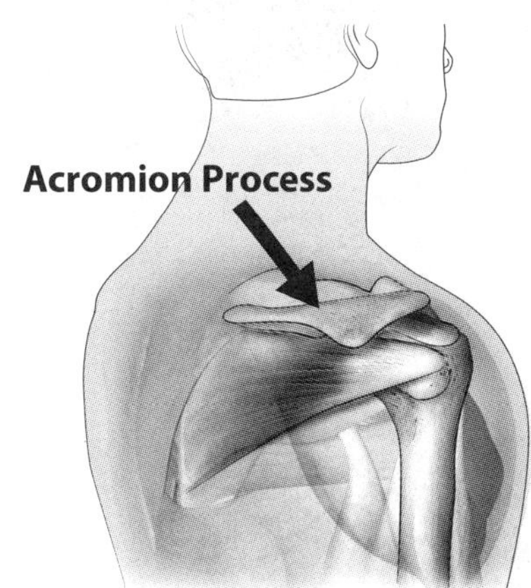

Figure 25-20

Figure 25-21 shows an even better perspective of how the acromion process is positioned directly over the supraspinatus tendon, like a guillotine waiting to clamp down on that tendon, when the humerus is elevated too high. In other words, the humerus should not often be elevated higher than the acromion process, or else that tendon will get squeezed between the two bones.

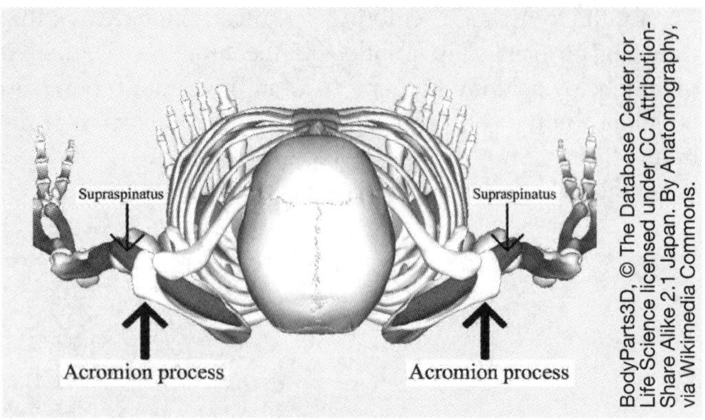


Figure 25-21

❑ Avoiding "Impingement Syndrome"

In fact, one of the most common causes of shoulder pain is irritation or rupture of that supraspinatus tendon (Figure 25-22, upper image), and/or of the bursa (Figure 25-22, lower image), caused by repeatedly pinching the tendon and the bursa between the humerus and the acromion process. This is referred to as "impingement syndrome," and it happens as a direct result of repeatedly raising the arms overhead.

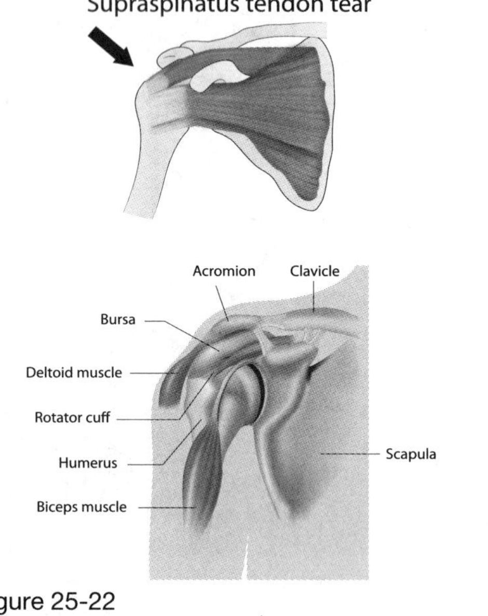




Figure 25-22

The purpose of the bursa sac is to provide a cushion between the humerus and the acromion—helping to reduce the friction that occurs when the humerus pushes against the acromion. The bursa, however, is not designed to withstand the frequency and the pressure that occurs when heavy *overhead presses* are performed regularly. That type of abuse often leads to a condition known as "subacromial bursitis," which is a sub-category of "impingement syndrome."

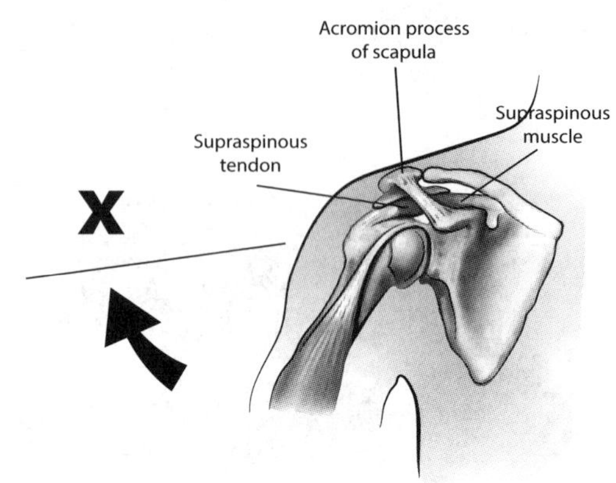


Figure 25-23

In Figure 25-23, a semi-horizontal line has been placed at the level of the acromion process. The curved arrow below that line indicates the limit of safe humeral movement. The "X" above that semi-horizontal line indicates the range of humeral movement that is beyond perfectly safe. Moving the humerus beyond that point will inevitably result in the supraspinatus tendon and the subacromial bursa being compressed. The higher the arm is raised, the more compression of the tendon and the bursa that occurs.

Squeezing the supraspinatus tendon and the subacromial bursa, as happens occasionally during normal day-to-day activities, does not cause a problem. Squeezing this tendon and bursa repeatedly, however, with heavy weight bearing downward, for months or years (as happens when various types of *overhead presses* are performed regularly) often causes irritation, inflammation, and/or rupture of the tendon or bursa, or both.

As you can see, it's very obvious why *overhead presses* can be injurious. Frankly, it is truly perplexing how it is that the fitness industry—individuals charged with the task of ensuring that exercise guidelines are keeping consumers safe—has failed to inform all trainers who are seeking trainer certification that *overhead presses* should be discouraged. It is also ironic that the fitness industry "warns" consumers (by way of personal trainers) about other movements that are demonstrably *not* dangerous (e.g., *leg extensions*, and allowing the knees to go over the toes when *squatting*), but then fails to acknowledge the dangers of *overhead presses*, and "neglects" to discourage their use.

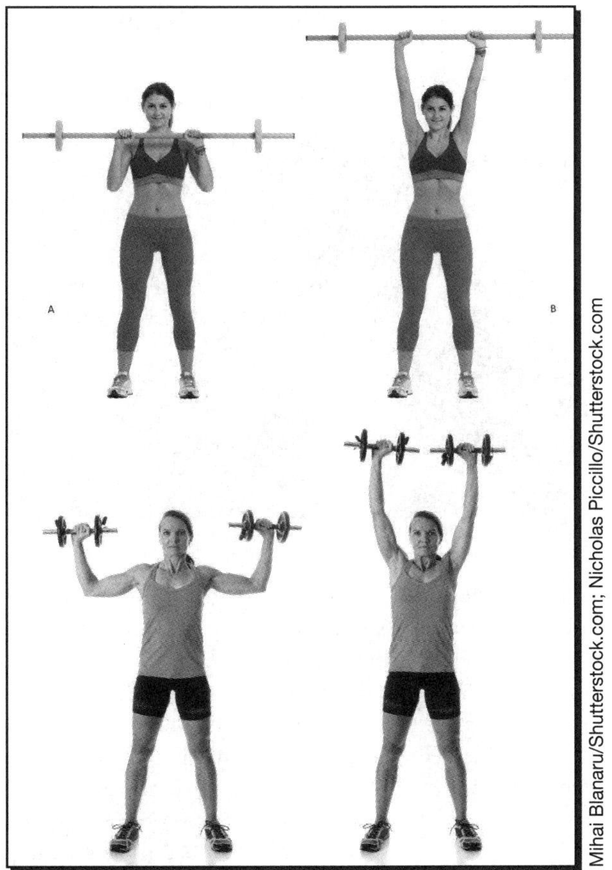


Figure 25-24

In addition to *overhead presses* being relatively unsafe, it is also important to be aware of the fact that this exercise is not a "necessary" movement for complete deltoids development. Although the deltoids participate during an *overhead press* movement, it is absolutely not the best anatomical movement for the anterior deltoids, lateral deltoids, or the posterior deltoids. The "ideal" anatomical motion for each of these three muscles has been defined (Chapter 20), and none of those motions resembles that of an *overhead press*.

As such, the *overhead press* is an unnatural movement (not consistent with the evolutionary design of the shoulder anatomy), and was simply "grandfathered" into bodybuilding by former powerlifters and individuals who performed "strength exhibitions." Subsequently, it was naively embraced by early bodybuilders who did not understand biomechanics, in the late 1800s and early 1900s.

Individuals seeking optimal muscular development, while simultaneously trying to maintain the integrity of their shoulder joints, should be aware that *overhead presses* are not only very inefficient for developing the deltoids, they also have a high probability of causing impingement syndrome—irritation, inflammation, or rupture of the supraspinatus and/or of the subacromial bursa. Overhead presses can also strain the infraspinatus, as will be explained shortly.

The supraspinatus cannot be isolated during exercise, and does not need any additional exercise, beyond that which occurs peripherally anytime the lateral ("medial") deltoid head is engaged. If the supraspinatus is injured, it is typically due to its tendon being repeatedly impinged—not as a result of muscle strain.

## ❑ Anatomy of the Infraspinatus

The infraspinatus is the second-most vulnerable muscle of the rotator cuff group, especially for bodybuilders and those individuals who do traditional weight lifting. This muscle covers a significant portion of the posterior side of the scapula. It originates on the inside ("medial") edge of the scapula (Figure 25-25, "A"). It then stretches across the shoulder joint, wraps around the backside of the humeral head, and connects onto the "greater tubercle" on the humeral head (Figure 25-25, "B").

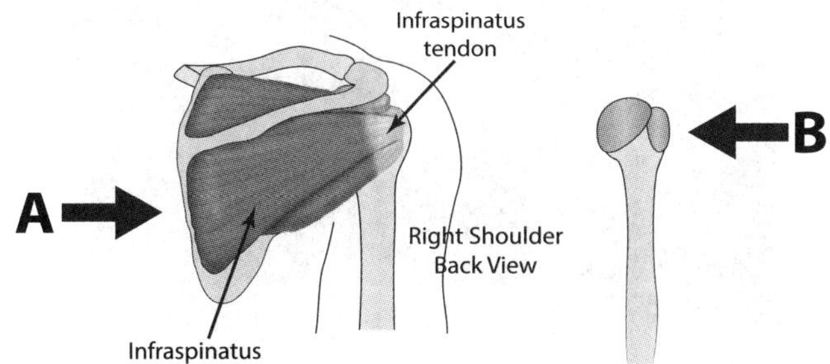


Figure 25-25

Like all muscles, when this muscle contracts, it pulls its insertion point toward its origin. As you can see in Figure 25-26, this results in "external rotation of the humerus." As such, it pulls the humerus around, "posteriorly," rotating it toward the rear.

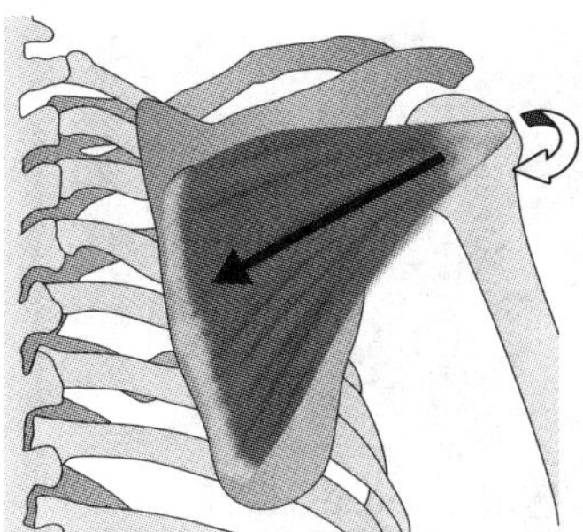

Figure 25-26

The exercise shown in Figure 25-27 (*external rotation of the humerus/with elastic band*) is typically performed for the purpose of exercising and strengthening the infraspinatus. Although "external rotational of the humerus" can be isolated during an exercise like this one, contraction/activation of the infraspinatus rarely occurs as an isolated movement, in day-to-day life or in sports. It usually occurs in conjunction with a "backhand" type of action, which also engages the posterior deltoids and teres major.

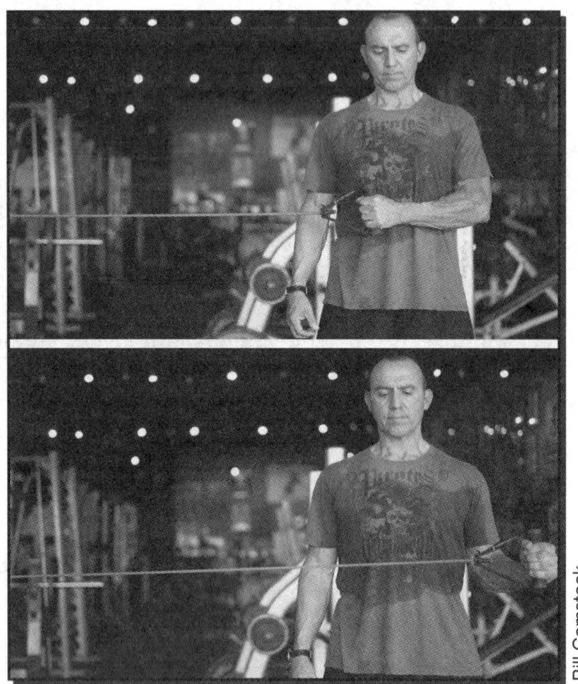


Figure 25-27

For example, in Figure 25-28, you can see that this tennis player's (Roger Federer) elbow is bent, which allows the forearm to act (potentially) as a rotational mechanism for the upper arm. In other words, in this move, two motions typically occur at the same time—a backward swing with the upper arm (which engages the posterior deltoid), as well as an external rotation of the upper arm (which engages the infraspinatus).

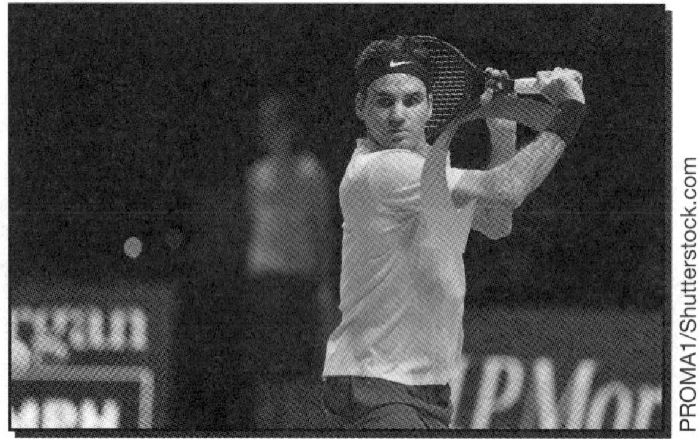


Figure 25-28

By way of comparison, in Figure 25-29, you can see that Roger Federer's elbow is nearly straight, which virtually eliminates the possibility of engaging the infraspinatus much, because the forearm is now on the same plain as the upper arm. When the arm is straight, the forearm is unable to act as a "rotational mechanism" of the humerus. Therefore, there can be no load on the infraspinatus.

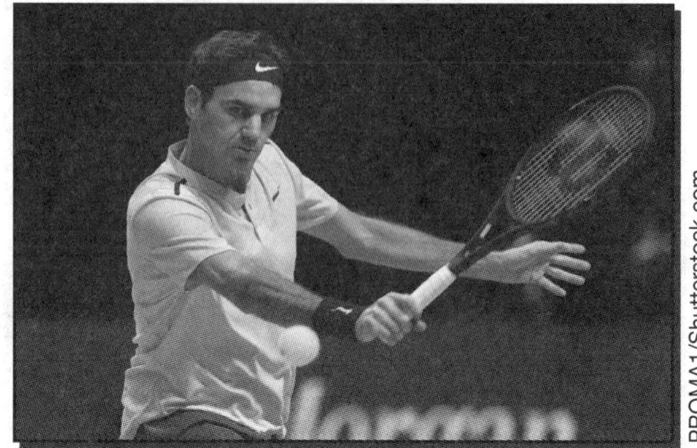


Figure 25-29

The following examples show how you may unintentionally, as well as dangerously, engage your infraspinatus—even though you may be entirely unaware of it. In the two images in Figure 25-30, you can see an individual doing *overhead presses*. Notice how he inadvertently allows his forearms to tilt forward, during the motion. His forearms (when viewed from the side) should be perfectly vertical, in order to not produce any rotational force on his humerus. A vertical line (starting at his elbow) has been placed, showing where his forearms should be (theoretically), in order to keep it from straining the infraspinatus.

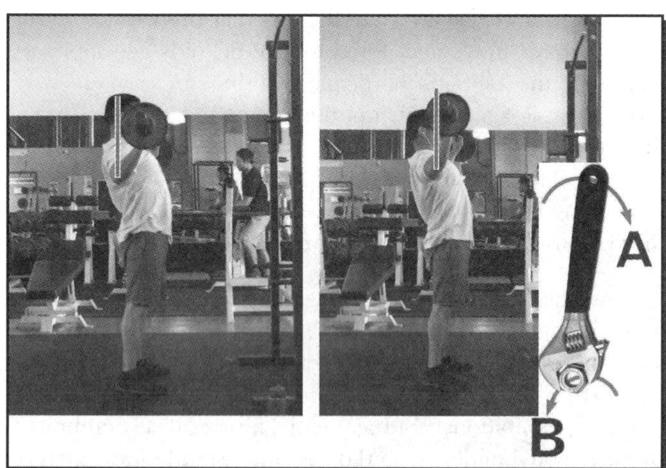


Figure 25-30

A forearm that is tilted forward (as is happening in this scenario) acts like a wrench handle, trying to rotate (twist) the humerus forward. In order to prevent the forearm from falling farther forward, the infraspinatus must work very hard to resist this forward rotation.

In the inset image of the wrench, "A" represents the forward force caused by the weight and gravity, trying to rotate the forearm forward, while "B" represents the force required by the infraspinatus, trying to resist that forward pull. The farther forward the forearm tilts (away from the vertical/ neutral position), the greater the percentage of load that is shifted onto the infraspinatus.

While this exercise is intended to work the larger deltoid muscles, it often ends up loading and straining the infraspinatus muscle as much, if not more, than the deltoids. The infraspinatus is not nearly as large, nor as strong, as are the deltoids. As a result, this forward tilt of the forearm creates a significant risk of injuring the infraspinatus.

It should be noted that this forward tilt of the forearm occurs frequently, generally for two reasons. First, when a barbell is used, the person must move the barbell forward to prevent hitting themselves on the head. Furthermore, most people are unable to externally rotate their upper arms enough to cause their forearms to be vertical. Even when dumbbells are used (thereby eliminating the concern about hitting their head with the bar), people's forearms are often STILL tilted forward, when doing *overhead presses*, and also when performing *incline presses* or *flat bench (supine) presses*.

In Figure 25-31, you can see how I've allowed my forearm to tilt *forward*. This tilt happens unintentionally, but when it does, it results in a forward rotation of the humerus, against which the infraspinatus must struggle to prevent. In Figure 25-31, one arrow represents the forward pull of gravity on the forearm, trying to rotate the upper arm forward, within the shoulder joint. The other curved arrow represents the effort of the infraspinatus, trying to rotate the humerus "externally" (backward), to prevent that forward pull, or to bring the forearm back up to the vertical position.

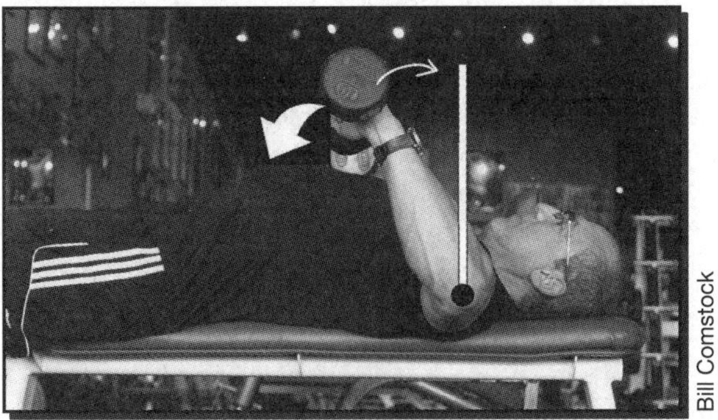

Figure 25-31

❑ When Improper Alignment Combines With Mechanical Disadvantage

As you'll recall, "alignment" was discussed in Chapter 7, where it was established that, in order to have proper alignment, the direction of resistance, and the direction of anatomical motion, as well as the origin and insertion of the target muscle, must all be on the same plane. The following is an example of what happens when improper alignment meets mechanical disadvantage.

When the forearm tilts *forward* during any *pressing* motion, the alignment is disrupted, which causes a percentage of the weight that is being used to shift onto the infraspinatus.

What makes this situation so dangerous is that, when the humerus is operating from a position that is perpendicular to the torso (instead of alongside the torso), the force which the infraspinatus must produce is enormous (relative to its limited strength capacity), due to mechanical disadvantage.

In Figure 25-32, the image of both (left side and right side) infraspinatus, with scapula, has been placed on this person's back. Focus your attention on his right infraspinatus, with his upper arm extended away from the side of his body. Keeping in mind that "muscles always pull toward their origin," notice what happens when the right-side infraspinatus tries to rotate this man's RIGHT humerus, while his humerus is perpendicular to his torso.

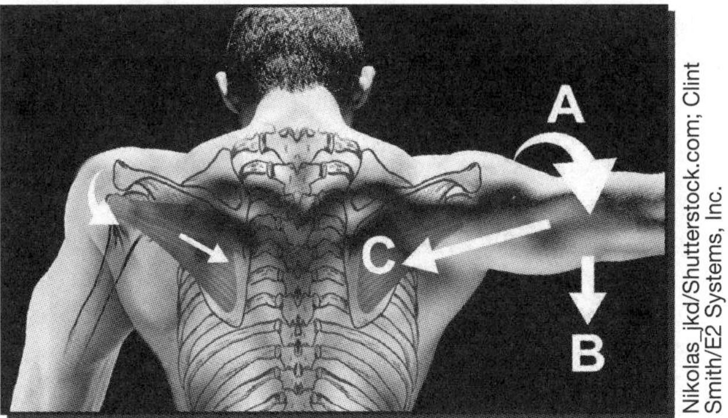

Figure 25-32

Imagine that this individual is doing a press of some kind (e.g., an overhead press or a supine dumbbell press), and that he has inadvertently allowed his RIGHT forearm to tilt forward from the neutral position. In order to prevent his humerus from rotating farther forward, his infraspinatus must exert an (opposite) "external rotation" force on his humerus, like that which is represented by the arrow marked "A." However, the infraspinatus can only pull FROM its point of origin, which is located on the medial edge of his right scapula, labeled as "C."

Obviously, that rotating "A" arrow is NOT pointing toward the origin of the infraspinatus ("C"). The man is trying to rotate his humerus in the direction of "B" (because he's trying to prevent forward rotation), but his infraspinatus cannot pull in the "B" direction, because its origins are not situated there.

As a result, his infraspinatus must generate an enormous amount of "extra" force—most of which will be pulling in the "C" direction. Only about 10 percent of the force produced by the infraspinatus can be used in the "B" direction, when it pulls from his angle. This is a classic example of mechanical disadvantage—a muscle trying to move a lever in a direction that is not directly toward its origin. In this particular scenario (which is quite common), the infraspinatus could easily be overloaded, strained, or torn, while the individual is doing *overhead presses*, or any other type of press, during which their forearm tilts forward.

By comparison, look at what happens on the LEFT side of this person's body, when the humerus is down alongside the torso. From this position, rotating the humerus externally allows the infraspinatus to pull directly toward its origin on the inner edge of the scapula. In this instance, the infraspinatus is able to pull on the humerus from a mechanical advantage. Since all of its effort can be utilized productively (i.e., the infraspinatus pulling in the same direction as the desired direction of humeral rotation), it doesn't have to produce as much effort to get the job done. Not only is this scenario much more efficient, it creates little (if any) risk of injury. Conversely, when the infraspinatus tries to externally rotate the humerus, and the humerus is perpendicular to the torso, the force required may be as much as 8 to 10 times more than when the arm is down alongside the torso.

How often does the forearm tend to tilt forward, during any kind of press (either dumbbell or barbell)? It happens most often during *overhead presses*; a bit less often during *incline presses*; and a bit less often during *flat presses*. It is least likely to happen during *decline presses*. This is because it is more natural (easier) to internally rotate the humerus, and less natural (more difficult) to externally rotate the humerus. As such, the more an exercise "requires" the humerus to be externally rotated, the more difficult it is achieve, the more likely it is that there will be a forward tilt to the forearm, and the higher the injury risk is.

In other words, the more you need to externally rotate the humerus, in order to accommodate a particular exercise, the more strenuous it is for you to externally rotate the humerus far enough. The farther you move away from the decline angle of *pressing* (in terms of external humeral rotation), the farther you are from "normal anatomical shoulder movement." The more upward the angle of the *pressing* movement, the more difficult it is for the humerus to accommodate that degree of external rotation, which causes many people to unintentionally tilt their forearms forward (internal rotation of their humerus)—mostly during *overhead presses*, secondarily during *incline presses*, and thirdly during *flat (supine) presses*.

It would be enlightening for you to observe individuals in the gym (from a side view), as they perform *pressing* movements. As such, you'll notice this factor for yourself. Anytime you see a person (from the side) tilting their forearm forward during any kind of *pressing* movement, you can be assured that they are straining their infraspinatus, especially if they are using a heavy weight.

The aforementioned is why the infraspinatus is the second most vulnerable muscle of the rotator cuff, during traditional "weight lifting." It is a fact that many people commonly perform *incline presses* and *overhead presses* (and sometimes *flat presses*) with a slightly forward-titling forearm, because they are unable to keep it vertical (neutral), due to limited shoulder mobility, which results in the infraspinatus being greatly overloaded (strained).

When you consider the risk of straining the infraspinatus during *overhead presses*, as well as the risks of shoulder impingement and subacromial bursitis, which also occur when performing *overhead presses*, you can understand how these risks must be factored into the decision of whether to perform *overhead pressing* motions. These undeniable risks, combined with the compromised benefits of *overhead pressing* exercises, should logically compel you to forego this antiquated exercise, in favor of exercises that are more bio-mechanically efficient and safe.

It should be no surprise that many people who routinely perform these lifts with heavy weight often have achy shoulder joints and rotator cuff injuries. In fact, a number of the leading bodybuilders from the 80s and 90s (and before that, of course) have had shoulder surgeries or shoulder replacement, due to this unnecessary abuse.

To those individuals who have been lucky enough not to have had shoulder injuries, despite doing heavy *overhead presses* for many years, remember this: Some people live their entire lifetime smoking cigarettes, yet somehow never get lung cancer or heart disease. They are the rare exception to the rule. That is not "proof" that cigarette smoking is "safe." *Overhead press* exercises are like smoking cigarettes—they have considerable downside and very minimal upside. Cigarette smoking and doing *overhead presses* are both unwise choices.

❑ Training the Infraspinatus

Having established that external rotation of the humerus with the arms down alongside the torso, is the ideal humeral angle for the infraspinatus, the exercise shown in Figure 25-33 would obviously not qualify as one of the better exercises for the infraspinatus. Yet, you often see people doing this in the gym.

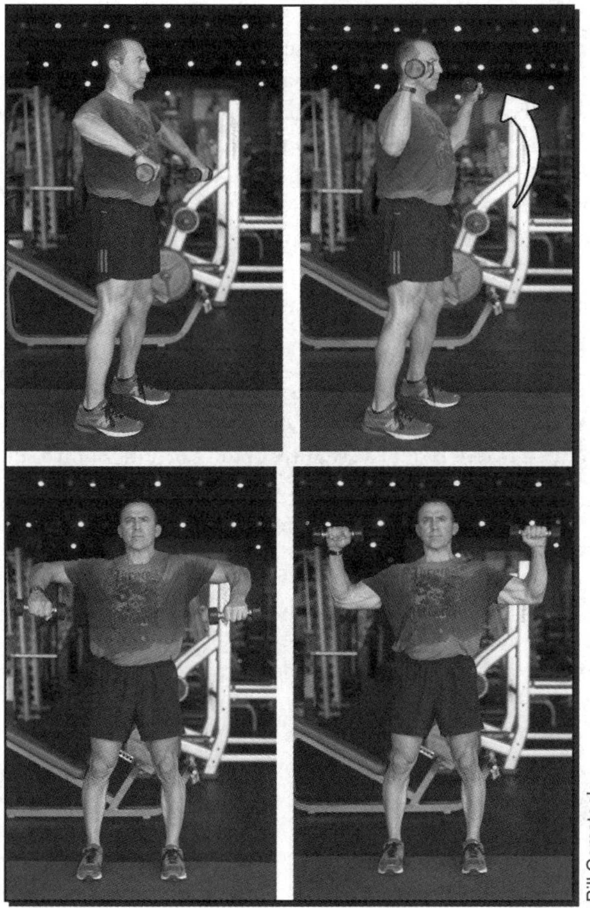

Figure 25-33

Ironically, people who do this exercise usually do so in an effort to either "heal" or strengthen (in order to protect) their infraspinatus, but the exercise itself invites an injury. If this exercise is performed with a very light weight (like two or three pounds), the risk is low. A better option, however, would be to do an exercise that allows the infraspinatus to work from a mechanical advantage—with the arms down alongside the torso—using a slightly heavier weight.

Of course, if a person participates in a sport that requires this exact movement, then it would be advantageous for him to perform this particular exercise, provided the weight he uses is not too heavy. Remember that the humeral angle of this exercise (relative to the torso) produces a dramatically increased force requirement, due to the mechanical disadvantage. For this reason, this particular exercise is not the wisest way to strengthen or to develop the infraspinatus, for the average fitness enthusiast, or an individual pursuing physique development.

The two exercises shown in Figure 25-34 "A" (left side) and "B" (right side) are better options, because the humerus is held alongside the torso, as it's being rotated. These two exercises are better, but still not quite ideal, however. Each can be improved by using a better direction of resistance, as well as by modifying the range of motion.

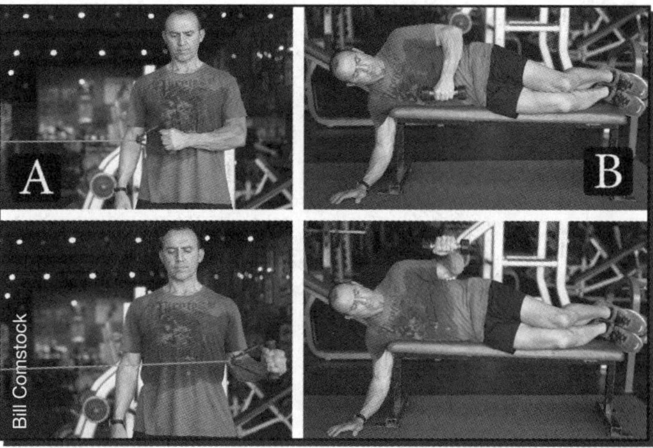

Figure 25-34

In order to get a better understanding of what might be a better range of motion and a better resistance curve, it can be helpful to do a little experiment. Stand in front of a mirror, with your right arm alongside your torso. Next, bend your right elbow to 90 degrees, as if you are halfway into a *biceps curl.*

Now, ensuring that your elbow is held tightly against your side, allow your humerus to rotate "internally," as far as possible. You'll find that you can easily bring your forearm all the way IN, so that it touches your abdomen (Figure 25-35, "A"). Then, rotate your humerus externally, as far as is comfortably possible, while keeping your elbow tightly against your side. You'll notice that you do not have the same degree of mobility rotating "externally" (toward the outside), as you do "internally." You may only be able to rotate externally to the point where your forearm is pointing straight ahead, or barely 10 to 15 degrees past that "straight forward" point (Figure 25-35, "B").

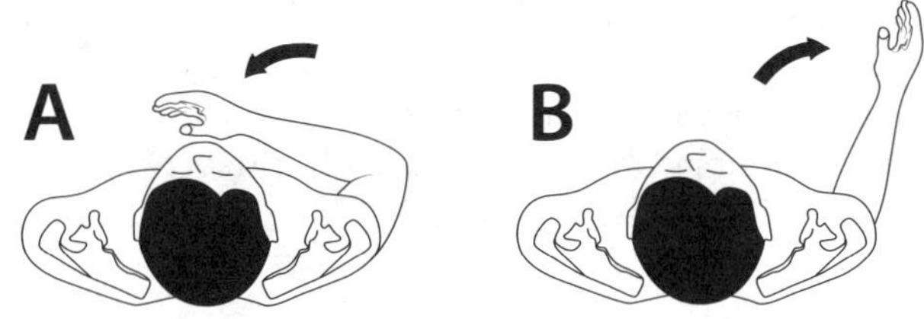

Figure 25-35

Most people who perform an "external humeral rotation" exercise rotate their humerus much farther than is safe and comfortable. You may also notice that rotating the humerus farther to the outside requires you to move your elbow away from your side, which then misrepresents your actual degree of shoulder mobility.

An infraspinatus exercise that incorporates the ideal range of motion (Figure 25-35)—more range toward the inside and less range toward the outside—represents a normal, natural, safe range of humeral rotation. Forcing the humerus to rotate farther out (externally) than the range described here, will likely cause shoulder joint irritation.

There is an irony, given the fact that individuals who perform "shoulder rotation exercises" typically do so because they are trying to reduce their shoulder pain. They then overrotate (externally) their humerus, when performing the exercise, which further aggravates their shoulder pain. They are unaware that the exercise they've been doing (i.e., the way they've been doing it) has been exacerbating their shoulder problem.

Most importantly, however, is the fact that shoulder pain is not caused by weakness of the shoulder rotators. Shoulder pain is caused by an irritation or injury, which is typically caused by having performed heavy, biomechanically "unnatural" or improper exercises for the deltoids, arms, latissimus, and pectorals. Performing shoulder rotation exercises cannot possibly reduce or eliminate pain that is caused by a damaged muscle (i.e., the infraspinatus), tendon (i.e., supraspinatus), or bursa. The only way to reduce or eliminate that pain is to allow the injured muscle, tendon, or bursa to heal, which requires the elimination of the exercises that typically cause that injury.

Attempting to strengthen a muscle that is injured is foolish. It's is like attempting to heal a sunburn by lying in the sun. The injured muscle needs rest and recovery—not more load. Once the injured muscle has healed, you can perform shoulder rotation exercises, using the ideal anatomical motion, a reasonable amount of resistance, and the proper range of motion.

❑ The Ideal Resistance Curve for the Infraspinatus

Let's suppose you are attempting to strengthen an UN-injured infraspinatus. We've already established the ideal anatomical position of the humerus, as well as the "ideal" range of motion for external shoulder rotation and the infraspinatus. The next step is to determine the ideal direction of resistance, which will provide the ideal resistance curve.

In the previously illustrated exercise—*external rotation* using the elastic band (Figure 24-34, "A")—there are two issues affecting the resistance curve. One is the direction of the resistance, i.e., where the elastic band is anchored. The other is the fact that using an elastic band causes the resistance to increase (become more difficult) the farther the band is outstretched. As mentioned in Chapter 4 ("The Resistance Curve"), this aspect of using elastic bands is somewhat problematic.

When an elastic band is being used for an exercise, the resistance increases toward the end of the range of motion, just as the muscle gets weaker (i.e., loses muscle contraction potential). Ironically, the elastic band resistance diminishes during the early part of the range of motion, precisely where the muscle is strongest (i.e., has the most strength potential). Therefore, using an elastic band for resistance will always overwhelm the muscle toward the end of the range of motion, and deprive (underwhelm) the muscle of resistance during the early part of the range of motion. As such, while using an elastic band for external humeral rotation is better than doing nothing, it's not nearly as productive as it would be to use either a dumbbell (free weight/hand weight) or a cable/pulley, attached to weights.

The other "external shoulder rotation" exercise previously illustrated—the person lying on his side, using a dumbbell (Figure 24-34, "B")—is a slightly better version, but it's still not ideal. The issue of an elastic band's increasing resistance (as it stretches) has been resolved, but the direction of resistance is still not ideal.

Due to this person's body position (relative to gravity), the movement is still "lightest" at the beginning of the range of motion (because the forearm is mostly parallel with gravity)—where the infraspinatus is strongest—and "heaviest" at the end of the range of motion (because the forearm is mostly perpendicular with gravity)—where the infraspinatus is weakest.

Ideally, an infraspinatus exercise should provide more resistance at the beginning of the range of motion, and less resistance at the end of the range of motion—thereby matching the strength curve of most skeletal muscles. This scenario is precisely what occurs with the exercise shown in Figure 25-36.

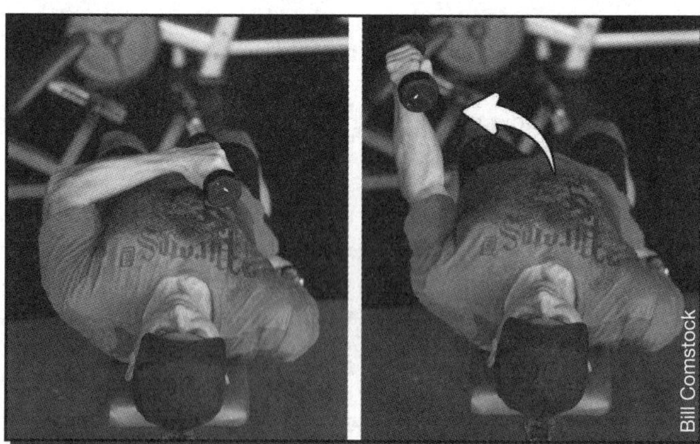


Figure 25-36

In this exercise, you can see that the forearm, in the starting position, is very close to horizontal (almost fully perpendicular with gravity), which would make the forearm about 90 percent "active," at that point. This factor is good, because it means that the infraspinatus is getting about 90 percent of the available resistance, in the early phase of the range of motion, where it's strongest. As the forearm arcs upward, ultimately reaching the vertical position, the resistance progressively lessens, finally becoming "neutral" (when the forearm is vertical), precisely when the infraspinatus is fully shortened and, therefore, weakest.

Keep in mind that when performing a humeral rotation exercise, the forearm is acting as the secondary lever to the humerus. The infraspinatus connects to the humerus, but requires the forearm as the "tool" for loading humeral rotation. This is why you need to focus your attention on the angle of the forearm, relative to gravity or whatever other source of resistance (e.g., cable) is being used.

When I perform this exercise (*"lying supine external humeral rotation,"* with dumbbell), I start with a three-pound dumbbell for 50 repetitions—first one arm, then the other arm. I then move to a five-pound dumbbell for 40 repetitions; then a seven-pound dumbbell for 30 reps, a nine-pound dumbbell for 20 reps, and a 12-pound dumbbell for 15 reps. That's a total of five sets, every four or five days.

You'll recall that during the discussion of the muscles of the "upper back" (Chapter 19), you looked at the photo in Figure 25-37, which highlighted the infraspinatus. The infraspinatus is the only muscle, of the four rotator cuff muscles, that is actually visible in a "back double biceps" pose. The other three rotator cuff muscles lie beneath/behind other more superficial muscles and bones. As such, the exercise—*"lying supine external rotation with dumbbell"*—is not only good for shoulder joint integrity, it's also good for physique display.

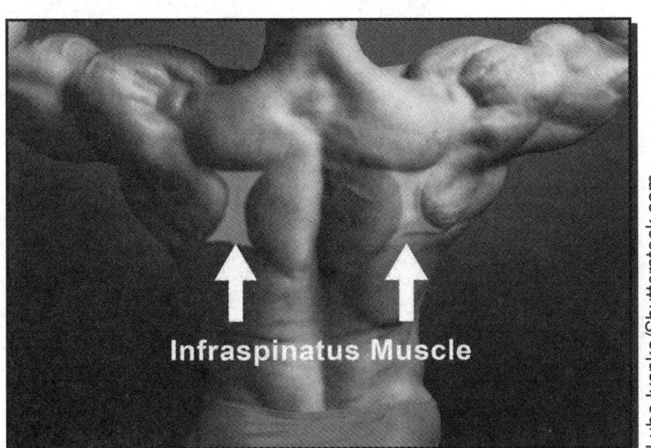


Figure 25-37

❑ Anatomy of the Teres Minor

The teres minor is positioned alongside the infraspinatus. Its origin is closer to the outer (lateral) edge of the scapula, whereas the origin of the infraspinatus is on the inner (medial) edge of the scapula. Their insertion points, however, are side-by-side, on the humeral head. Like the infraspinatus, the teres minor is also an external rotator of the humerus—although a smaller, weaker assistant to the infraspinatus, in that task.

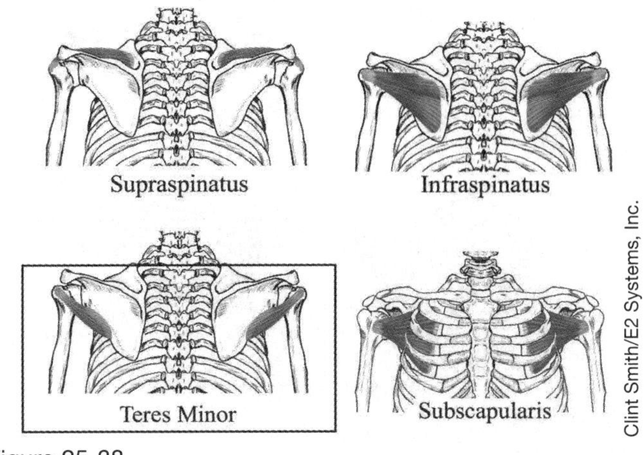


Figure 25-38

Anytime the infraspinatus is activated/loaded, the teres minor (Figure 25-39, left image) participates as well. Since the teres minor's origin is slightly lower on the scapula than that of the infraspinatus, it is slightly better positioned to help rotate the humerus, when the humerus is perpendicular to the torso. On the other hand, because it is small and can be easily overwhelmed, it is also more prone to injury, when that type of situation (forward tilting forearm during *overhead* or *incline presses*) occurs.

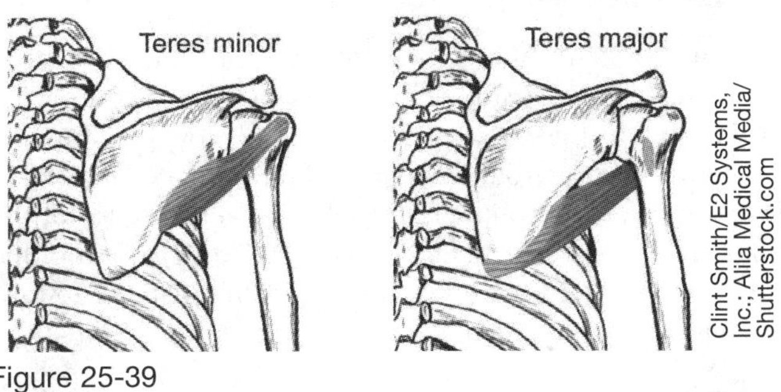


Figure 25-39

❑ Anatomy of the Teres Major

The teres major (shown in Figure 25-39, right image), is situated just below the teres minor. It is not formally considered part of the rotator cuff group, because its role in humeral rotation is very minor. Its insertion is lower on the humerus, which gives it better leverage for pulling the humerus downward, backward and inward. These are its primary functions. It engages whenever the latissimus dorsi or the posterior deltoids are activated. It also assists, however, during internal humeral rotation, because its insertion is on the *anterior* side of the humerus and its origin is on the *posterior* side of the torso, on the scapula.

❑ Anatomy of the Subscapularis

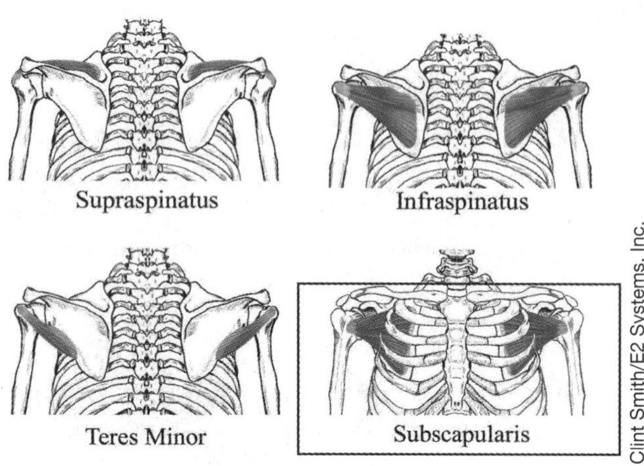




Figure 25-40

The illustration of the subscapularis (Figure 25-40, lower right image) is a view from the front, as if you could see through the chest cavity of a person's right shoulder. It is the only "front view" in this line-up of shoulder rotators. The illustrations of the other three rotator cuff muscles in Figure 25-40 are "posterior views" (from the rear).

The subscapularis is on the anterior (front) side of the scapula. It originates on the medial edge (closest to the spine) of the anterior wall of the scapula (small arrows in Figure 25-41) and attaches onto the lesser humeral tuberosity ("B" arrow, in Figure 25-41).

Figure 25-41 shows how the subscapularis is tucked between the anterior wall of the scapula and the posterior side of the ribs. In this view, you can also see how this muscle's attachment wraps around the front of the humeral head ("B"). When this muscle contracts, it pulls that outside edge of the humeral head, forward and around, toward the origin of the subscapularis. This rotates the humerus "internally"—toward the midline of the front of the torso.

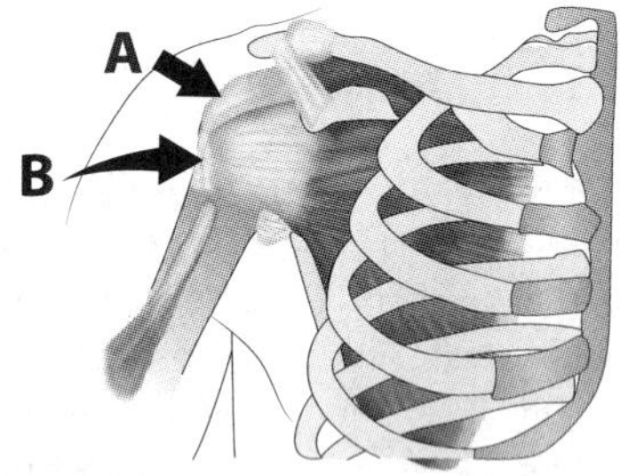


Figure 25-41

In Figure 25-41, you can also see the supraspinatus tendon ("A"), as it comes out from under the acromion, and attaches onto the top portion of the humeral head. The other two rotator cuff muscles (infraspinatus and teres minor) would not be visible from this view, because they are both on the backside of the scapula.

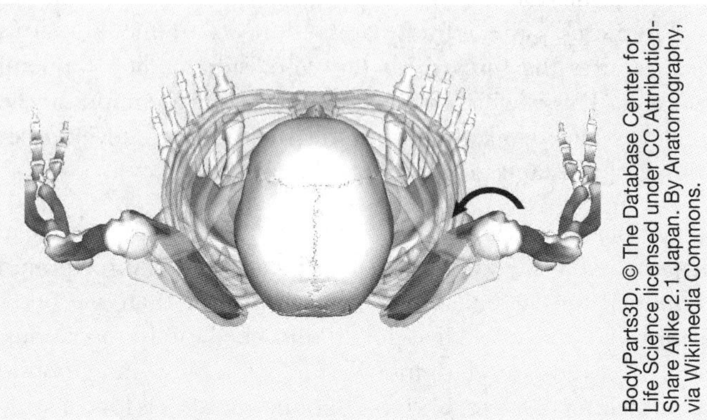



Figure 25-42

Figure 25-42 provides an overhead view, showing how the subscapularis muscle originates on the medial edge of the anterior wall of the scapula, and then attaches onto the front of the humeral head. A curved arrow has been placed in front of the shoulder joint, showing the action that occurs when the subscapularis contracts—internally rotating the humerus, as the subscapularis pulls its insertion toward its origin.

Just as occurs with the infraspinatus (but in the opposite direction), rotation of the humerus occurs most naturally when the upper arm is down alongside the torso. In Figure 25-43, you can see that rotating the humerus, when it's in this position, allows the subscapularis to pull from a mechanical advantage.

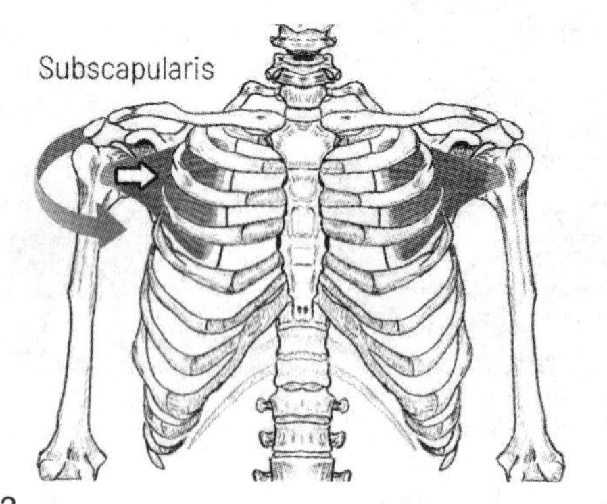




Figure 25-43

Conversely, you cause your subscapularis to pull from a mechanical DISadvantage, when the upper arm is perpendicular to the torso. When internal humeral rotation is performed, while the upper arm is held away from the side of the torso, the subscapularis must pull with significantly more force. Arm wrestling (Figure 25-44) is one example of this scenario. There is a very high degree of injury risk that occurs when great force is exerted in this way (internal rotation of the humerus while in mechanical disadvantage, with humerus horizontal to the torso).

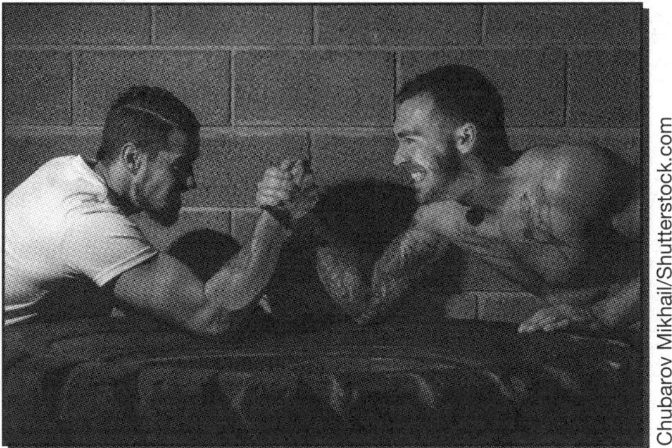
Chubarov Mikhail/Shutterstock.com

Figure 25-44

The photo of the tennis player in Figure 25-45 (Novak Djokovic) shows another example of this scenario, although this move has a much lower risk of injury, as compared with arm wrestling. Hitting the ball forward, with a bent elbow, creates a sudden external rotational force on the humerus, against which the subscapularis must brace. Concentric contraction of the subscapularis then produces a forward thrust of the forearm, which helps propel the racket forward.

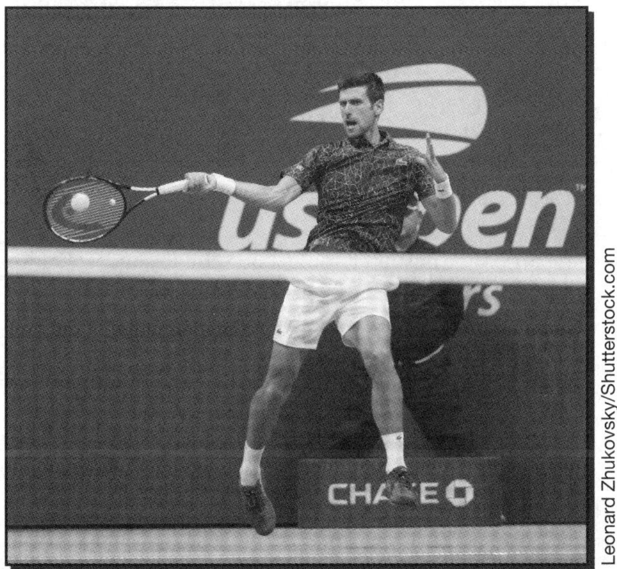
Leonard Zhukovsky/Shutterstock.com

Figure 25-45

In Figure 25-46, you can see two baseball pitchers in the early part of a forward throw. This scenario is forceful activation of the subscapularis, producing internal humeral rotation. Baseball pitching requires a significant amount of force by the subscapularis, because of the mechanical DISadvantage of having the humerus perpendicular to the torso. There is also an extreme degree of external (backward) rotation of the humerus in the "wind-up," with which the pitch begins. This factor greatly exacerbates the mechanical DISadvantage of the subscapularis, and also strains the limits of external (toward the rear) humeral rotation.

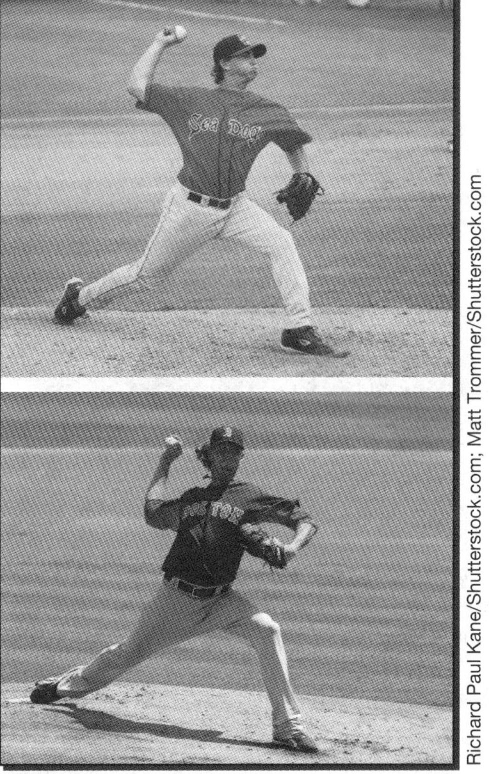
Richard Paul Kane/Shutterstock.com; Matt Trommer/Shutterstock.com

Figure 25-46

In day-to-day activities, you engage the subscapularis anytime you squeeze your hands together with your elbows bent, as you might when picking up a heavy box (Figure 25-47). If, for any reason, you are unable to "hook" your hands under the box with your hands, thereby allowing you to keep your elbows straight, you would have to squeeze your hands against the sides of the box, which would require force from the subscapularis. This internal rotation of the humerus, combined with additional inward force provided by the pectorals, and upward force provided by the deltoids, would allow you to apply sufficient pressure against the sides of the box, in order to prevent it from falling. The less the elbows are, the less engaged the subscapularis is. If the arms are straight, there is little or no engagement by the subscapularis.

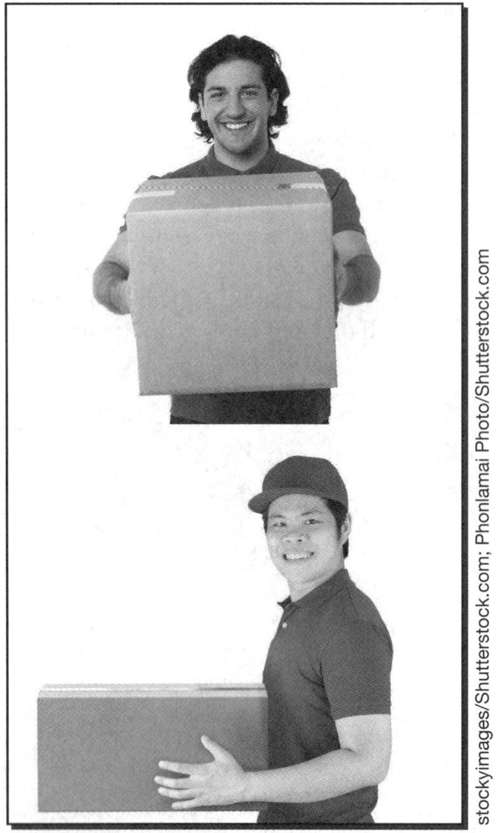

Figure 25-47

This scenario is why most people usually prefer grabbing a box by putting their hands under it, or grabbing it by a handle or strap, which would reduce the need to engage the subscapularis. The heavier the box, the more inward force you would have to use to keep the box from slipping. The more inward force you must use, the more you load the subscapularis, which is not an especially strong muscle.

The subscapularis only engages when your elbows are bent, and an inward force is applied. Most of the time, when you engage the subscapularis, you also engage the pectorals.

Because the subscapularis is obviously never visible, this is not a muscle that needs to be worked for the purpose of physique display. The rationale for working this muscle would be strictly functional—to maintain the strength and integrity of the shoulder joint, as well as to perform sport-related movements that specifically involve forceful inward rotation of the humerus. This would include most "throwing" sports, as well as "grappling"/wrestling.

❑ Training the Subscapularis

The exercise shown in Figure 25-48 (overhead view) is good for strengthening the subscapularis, although using a cable (pulley with weights) would be better than using an elastic band. Note that the movement starts with the forearm pointing straight forward ("A"). There is no need to begin with a more external rotation than this. Doing so would increase the risk of straining the shoulder joint, and would not add any significant advantage. Even stretching the joint beyond this point, without resistance, would have questionable merit.

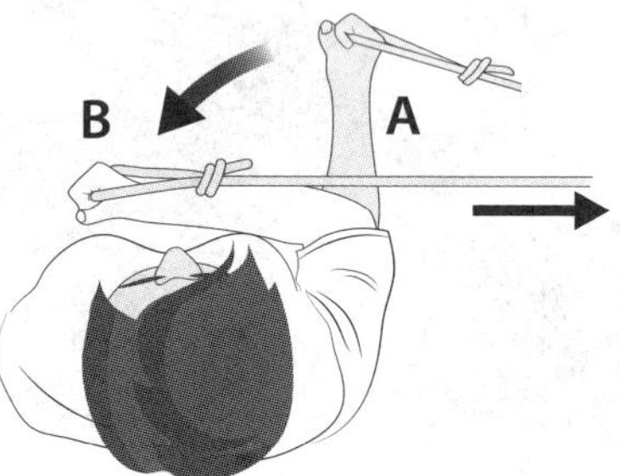

Figure 25-48

Note that the direction of resistance (indicated by the straight arrow pointing to the right in Figure 25-48) is lateral to the torso (originates from the side). This factor allows the forearm to be perpendicular with that direction of resistance at the beginning of the movement, thereby providing "early phase loading." Then, at the conclusion of the movement ("B"), the forearm is parallel with the elastic band, which results in the subscapularis experiencing a lesser resistance as it enters the weaker part of its range of motion. As a result, the resistance curve of this exercise matches the strength curve of the muscle.

The resistance curve can also be altered, simply by stepping slightly backward (but still facing the same direction). This adjustment would place the origin of the resistance slightly more in front of you (although still to the side), which would cause the resistance to be a little bit less at the beginning of the range of motion ("A"), and a little bit more at the end of the range of motion ("B").

Ideally, using a cable is the best option for this exercise, with the pulley set to about the height of your elbow, as measured by standing alongside the pulley. This setting would provide alignment between the direction of resistance and the direction of movement. You should select a weight that permits you to perform approximately 20 or 30 repetitions, with a moderate amount of challenge. While an elastic band is acceptable, it is much less ideal. It would still provide some degree of benefit, but the fact that the resistance increases as the band stretches produces a resistance curve that is the opposite of the muscle's strength curve.

# CHAPTER 26

# In Conclusion

As you have come to learn throughout the past 25 chapters, resistance exercise is all about mechanics (physics)—the levers of your body, working against external forces that are acting upon your levers (limbs) from certain angles, which results in various outcomes of more or less efficiency. It's also about natural versus unnatural anatomical motions, as well as selecting exercises that avoid physiological conflicts of interest, such as reciprocal innervation, bilateral deficit, active/passive insufficiency, and instability.

Every resistance exercise has a unique biomechanical profile, which affects its "value." "Value" is determined by three attributes of an exercise: its efficiency (the amount of effort/amount of weight used versus the amount of muscle loading); its productivity (ideal resistance curve); and its safety (ideal anatomical motion and alignment, as well as the avoidance of combining mechanical disadvantage and a maximally active lever/limb).

Determining an exercise's value demonstrates that some exercises are clearly "better" than others, in terms of efficiency, productivity, and safety. All exercises have some degree of benefit—even the exercises that do not rate highly on the aforementioned factors. The wisest approach, however, is to select only the exercises that have very high value—the ones that are most efficient, most productive, and have the least risk of injury. Performing only high-value exercises allows you to reap the greatest amount of benefit, with the least amount of wasted effort and the least risk of injury.

The following criteria determine the biomechanical value of a given resistance exercise:

- An exercise that allows the operating lever of the target muscle to move directly toward that muscle's origin is better (more efficient) than an exercise that moves the operating lever of a target muscle in a direction other than toward that muscle's origins. The more "directly toward the muscle origin," the more efficient the movement is. The less "directly toward the muscle origin," the more inefficient the movement is, in terms of that muscle's percentage of participation in that action.
- Dynamic muscle contraction is better than isometric muscle contraction, with regard to visible muscle development, and also with regard to strength improvement throughout that muscle's entire range of motion. In contrast, isometric contraction only tends to improve strength in that one place where the isometric contraction is held.
- More range of motion is always better than less range of motion. Generally speaking, "the more, the better"—although the earliest 5 to 10 percent of the range of motion, as well as the final 5 to 10 percent, seem to cause more risk and bestow less benefit than the middle 80 percent of the range of motion.
- Unilateral exercise (independent limb resistance) is generally better than bilateral exercise (shared-instrument resistance). Bilateral exercise tends to cause "bilateral deficit"—a slight weakness in the muscle of both sides—as compared with unilateral exercise. Furthermore, unilateral exercise is likely to produce "cross education"—a small percentage of benefit to the muscle of the non-working side. This benefit is not likely to occur when bilateral exercise is performed. In addition, there seems to be a distinct advantage in performing unilateral exercise (one side at a time), when training a muscle that produces motion in opposite directions (e.g., lateral deltoids, latissimus dorsi, etc.).

An exercise that requires simultaneous bilateral participation of opposite facing muscles is compromised because, it seems, each opposite-side muscle requires slightly different posture, bracing, leaning, peripheral action, innervation, and mental focus. Doing one side at a time (e.g., left side only, then right side only) allows one to use "unilateral focus," thereby optimizing the strength potential, coordination, and benefit to each side.

- Exercises that provide alignment between the direction of the resistance and the direction of the motion, as well as the origin and insertion of the target muscle, are generally better (more efficient) than exercises that do not provide this alignment. Proper alignment automatically implies that the direction of resistance and the direction of your concentric motion be directly opposite each other—although on the same plane. If an exercise lacks alignment, instead of fully loading your intended target muscle, the resistance will be diluted, as a percentage of the load is diverted to other non-target (often weaker) muscles (like the rotator cuff). Improper alignment may also produce joint strain.

- Exercises that allow your target muscle to be positioned directly opposite the direction of resistance (i.e., the line of force/"opposite position loading") are better (more efficient) than exercises in which the target muscle is not positioned directly opposite the direction of resistance. Whichever muscle is positioned directly opposite resistance will be the most loaded, whether you intend it to be so, or not. A muscle that is not positioned directly opposite the line of force will receive diminished percentages of the actual weight being used. The farther away a muscle is from the line of force, the less percentage of load it receives.

- Exercises that avoid 1] reciprocal innervation (the shutting-down of that muscle caused by the activation/loading of the opposing muscle) are better than exercises that trigger reciprocal innervation. Likewise, exercises that allow the anatomy to function without competing interests, e.g., 2] two different muscles inhibiting each other, because they are battling for an opposite spinal position, as occurs with *leg raises*, and 3] "active/passive" insufficiencies (over-shortening a target muscle and over-stretching an opposing muscle), are better than exercises that present these conflicts of interest.

- Exercises that allow the operating lever of a target muscle to cross resistance perpendicularly (i.e., to be a mostly "active" lever) are better (more efficient) than exercises that cause the operating lever to be mostly parallel with resistance (i.e., mostly an "inactive" lever).

- Exercises that allow the operating lever (limb) of a target muscle to work with its full length are better (more efficient) than are exercises in which the operating lever (limb) is effectively shortened by a secondary lever (e.g., forearm or lower leg).

- Exercises that avoid combining mechanical disadvantage (i.e., a muscle pulling on its operating lever from a mostly parallel angle) with an operating lever that is too "active" (too perpendicular with resistance, given the mechanical disadvantage) are better (less risky) than are exercises in which those two force magnifiers are combined.

- Exercises that are early phase loaded are generally better than are exercises that are late phase loaded. If mechanical disadvantage occurs during an exercise, it would need to be factored into this analysis. This process could be referred to as "finding the optimal resistance curve for your target muscle."

- Exercises that do not strain a joint (by unnecessarily twisting or distorting it) are better than exercises that strain (twist/distort) a joint. This "rule" of thumb actually does not need to be stated, if the aforementioned 10 criteria are met. Any exercise that moves the target muscle's insertion toward that muscle's origin, and has proper alignment, will automatically operate its corresponding joint in a way that is natural and consistent with human musculoskeletal design.

- Exercises that are performed with deliberate muscle contraction are generally better than exercises that are performed with momentum. Given that efficiency is defined as "getting the most benefit with the least cost," using momentum causes loss of efficiency because it reduces the resistance to a target muscle, while more weight must be used. Using more weight, while simultaneously using momentum, is like "paying more" for "equal or less" benefit.

The aforementioned 13 criteria allow you to separate high-value exercises from exercises that have varying degrees of lesser value. It is misguided to believe that all exercises have the same degree of value or benefit. They do not. Therefore, exercises are not equally interchangeable, as many people believe. Certainly, someone can choose to change exercises for the sake of variety, or perhaps convenience, but changing from a highly rated exercise, to an exercise that is biomechanically compromised—for the same target muscle—would not be beneficial.

It is misguided to believe that "varying exercises is essential," or that different exercises allow you to alter the shape of a muscle. The shape of your muscles is genetically determined. Exercises differ primarily in terms of mechanical efficiency and in terms of how closely they mimic the "most natural"/most ideal anatomical function of your target muscle and its corresponding joint.

Understanding these concepts allows you to realize that much of what we have all been "taught" about resistance exercise is false. This realization should lead you to several questions:

- Why have individuals been given incorrect information about resistance exercise?
- Why have individuals embraced certain exercise recommendations, even when it's not logical to do so?
- Why individuals should not always believe what they are told, even when told to them by people whom they might assume are knowledgeable about that subject.
- Why do individuals often select (prefer) certain exercises which are not necessarily good exercises, and why do they often use more weight than is necessary, safe, or practical?

## The Causes of "Bad" Choices Related to Exercise

In fact, humans have natural psychological tendencies, which often cause them to make improper choices with regard to exercise. As such, it's important to know what those tendencies are, and why individuals often refuse to change their preferences and habits, despite more logical alternatives being offered.

Many people select exercises, largely on the basis of whether that exercise allows them to use a lot of weight—which is not a good strategy. Individuals often have this mindset, under the misguided belief that using more weight loads the target muscle better—regardless of exercise mechanics. Frequently, however, an exercise that allows you to use more weight, actually loads a target muscles less—as compared with "better" exercises for the same muscle group—due to the mechanical profile of that exercise.

In addition, people often make the mistake of being influenced by the opinions of their peers, in terms of how much weight they select for a given exercise, or they select an exercise that allows them to use a "heavy" weight. In other words, they make these choices either to impress their peers or to gratify their ego, or under the mistaken belief that the amount of weight used (alone) determines muscle load.

Many people (mostly men) are overly concerned with presenting the appearance of being in "beast mode" (seeming very strong). It's much more sensible to focus on training with maximum efficiency—loading your muscles more, while using less weight. This, however, requires a person to have enough knowledge, confidence, and rational thinking to disregard the tendency to impress observers, and to prioritize a strategy that utilizes maximum efficiency.

What's needed is an understanding of the biomechanical principles that apply to resistance exercise, which allows you to select exercises that are most efficient, most productive, and are least likely to cause unnecessary strain to the spine and joints.

## The Influence of Fitness Magazines

For better, or for worse, the health/fitness magazine industry is extremely influential in shaping people's beliefs about exercise. On the other hand, this is often the primary cause of people's confusion about exercise. Figures 26-1 through 26-4 highlight actual statements cut directly from the front covers of various fitness and bodybuilding publications. Unfortunately, fitness magazines are often considered a "primary source" of fitness information by many bodybuilders, trainers, and fitness enthusiasts—despite the fact that they are not "scientific journals."

X-PLOSIVE GUNS
HUGE ARMS IN 6 WEEKS
SCIENTIFICALLY PROVEN!
BUILD HARD ABS
at home in just four weeks
ROCK HARD ABS!
CHISEL GREAT ABS WITH 4 EASY MOVES
Figure 26-1

FEEL ENERGISED WITHOUT COFFEE
BLITZ YOUR BELLY
STRIP AWAY FAT IN JUST 12 MINUTES A DAY
THE CHILL
THAT MAKES
BUILD MUSCLE FAST!
FLAT BELLY FIXES!
EASY ABS IN JUST 3 MOVES
Figure 26-2

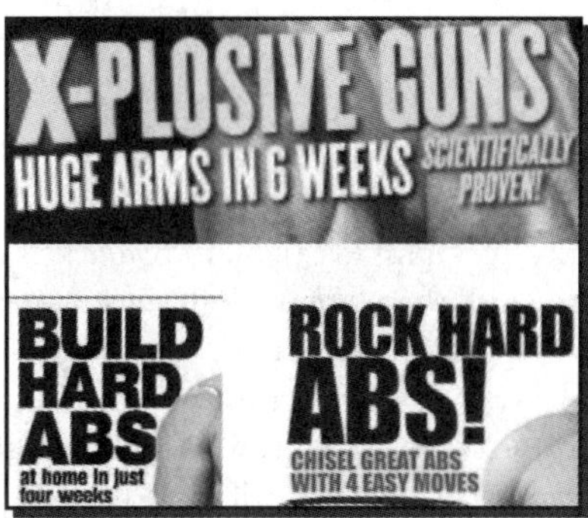

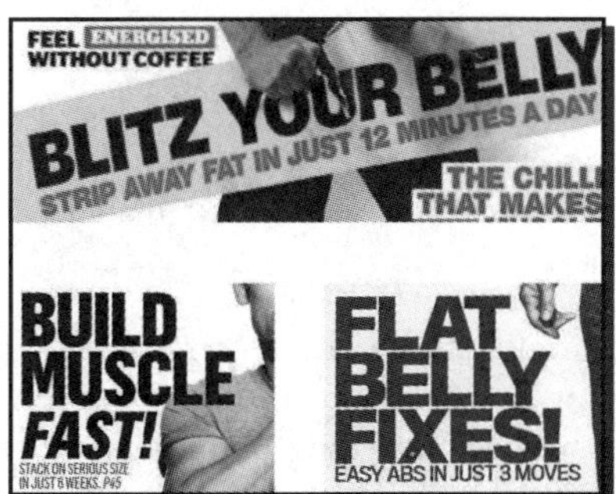

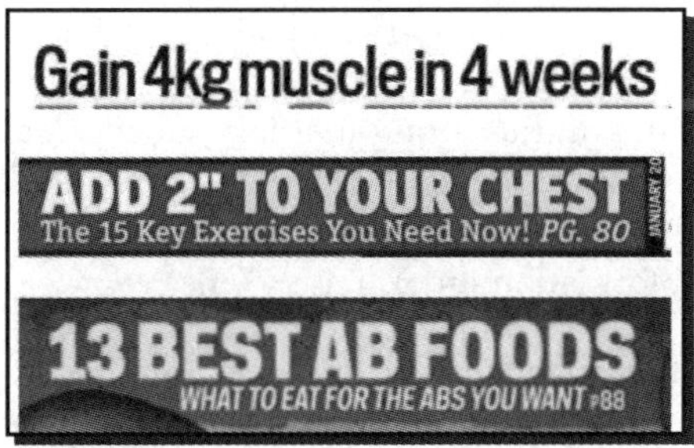

Figure 26-3

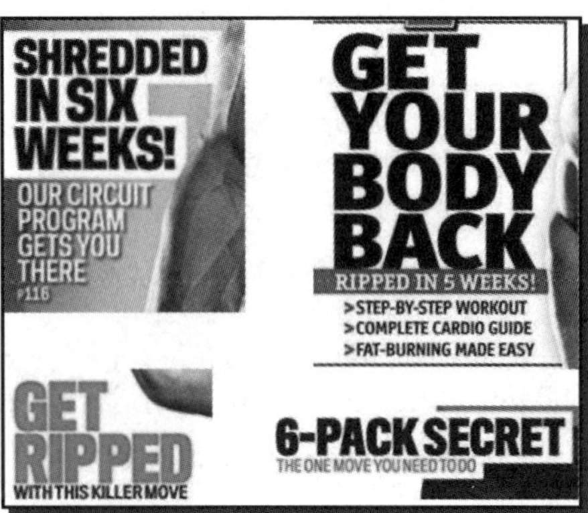

SHREDDED IN SIX WEEKS!
OUR CIRCUIT PROGRAM GETS YOU THERE
GET YOUR BODY BACK
RIPPED IN 5 WEEKS!
>STEP-BY-STEP WORKOUT
>COMPLETE CARDIO GUIDE
>FAT-BURNING MADE EASY
GET RIPPED
WITH THIS KILLER MOVE
6-PACK SECRET
THE ONE MOVE YOU NEED TO DO
Figure 26-4

Every single one of these statements has some degree of falsehood. Either the statement is completely false or unrealistic—physiologically speaking—or it drastically overstates reality. Why are these misleading statements on the front cover of fitness magazines? Obviously, it is because they prompt consumers to buy the magazine.

It should come as no surprise that fitness magazines are not primarily concerned with educating the public. Rather, they are primarily concerned with achieving and maintaining a company's profits, or (at least) their economic survival. They want revenue, and they know that most consumers want "fast," "simple," "easy" guidance ("secret tips") with regard to how to achieve super-hero status (i.e., more muscle, less fat, and more impressive physical prowess). As a result, publishers of these magazines seem very willing to mislead consumers by featuring an array of undocumented, unsubstantiated, unrealistic claims—because doing so increases their sales.

If magazine publishers were truly interested in educating the public, they could do it in about 24 issues (e.g., two years' worth of monthly editions). At that point, however, they'd have nothing more to provide to their readers, so they might have to go out of business.

Unfortunately, there is a large percentage of the population that lacks the intelligence, or perhaps the open-mindedness, to grasp anything other than dogmatic beliefs or simplistic, grandiose claims. Those people would likely be overwhelmed or annoyed by scientifically sound information that challenges their traditional beliefs. Thus, grandiose claims on magazine covers will always have a receptive audience. Furthermore, in the scarcity of better options (more truthful and accurate journals), intellectually curious and open-minded individuals are likely to be fooled into believing that mainstream fitness magazines might be a good source of information on exercise science.

Unfortunately, there is no such thing as a regulatory agency for the fitness industry—a type of fitness industry police—which might serve to prevent "bad" fitness information from being disseminated. As such, all sorts of outrageously inaccurate "information" can be sold to consumers, as well as to trainers—with no consequence, whatsoever.

The U.S. Food and Drug Administration (FDA) has strict guidelines for the "food" and "drug" industries, and a relatively strict set of guidelines for the nutrition supplement industry, under the "Dietary Supplement Health Education Act" (DSHEA) of 1984. As such, supplement manufacturers are not allowed to make "medical" claims on their packaging, or in their advertising, which might cause consumers to have unrealistic expectations with regard to a nutrition product.

No such regulation exists for the fitness/exercise industry, however. As a result, magazines are able to make claims like, "*This exercise will improve your mobility, increase your strength by 20%, and pack on slabs of muscle*"—when, in fact, nothing could be farther from the truth. In this regard, the fitness industry is entirely unregulated—consumers beware.

On a particular day in the 1980s, back when I owned a gym in the town of Pasadena (California), Cory Everson—a well-known champion female bodybuilder at the time—came into my facility with a prominent photographer named Robert Reiff (Figure 26-5). They had scheduled to come to my gym, to do a photo shoot for one of the women's fitness magazines. During that assignment, Cory was photographed doing a variety of exercises that were meant to accompany an upcoming article.

As someone who knows bodybuilding very well, it was obvious to me that the exercises she was demonstrating were not part of her normal workout routine. Some people might refer to the exercises she demonstrated as "fluff" exercises—exercises that are certainly not part of a serious bodybuilding workout, let alone that of a world class champion.*

**Note: Cory Everson won the Ms. Olympia competition—considered by some as the highest level of bodybuilding competition—a historic six times. She also won numerous other competitions during her nine-year career.*

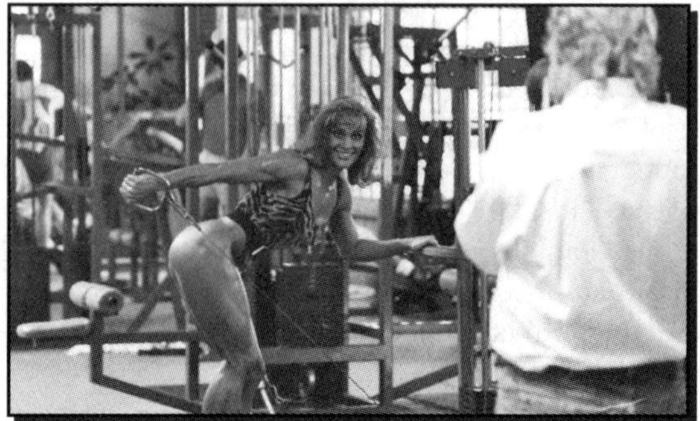

Figure 26-5

It would be natural for most lay people reading the magazine in which that article was to appear, to assume that the exercises Cory Everson was demonstrating were the actual exercises that she used to develop her amazing body. That assumption, however, would be incorrect. In reality, Cory Everson did exercises which were much more demanding than the ones she was shown depicting during this photo shoot.

As someone who has also been photographed for magazine articles, I concede that when bodybuilders/models agree to do a photo shoot, they are usually thrilled to get the exposure, and focused on the fact that their career success has allowed them to have that opportunity. Those images will be regarded as a historical record of that athlete's career path. What is overlooked, however, is that those images will mislead many readers, who will believe that those exercises are key to developing that type of musculature.

A magazine would not hire models who are not impressive to look at—especially for the cover—given that a primary reason people purchase fitness magazines is for inspiration. The publisher also knows the magazine must show something different in every issue, in order to keep readers interested. As a result, publishers (editors) often tell the bodybuilders/models which exercises they would like to show them doing, regardless of whether or not that bodybuilder actually performs those exercises during their workouts.

What matters most, from a publisher's point of view, is what will make the magazine more popular, and thus more profitable. What sells more magazines, will always take precedence over completely truthful and accurate content.

## Dubious Endorsement by Trusted Authorities

From the 1930s through the 1950s, a number of physicians recommended and endorsed the smoking of cigarettes. Needless to say, there is nothing healthful about smoking cigarettes. Some cigarette smokers might be fortunate enough to avoid an early death, cardiac disease or lung cancer, but the vast majority of people who smoke cigarettes suffer severe health consequences as a direct result of this nefarious habit. In fact, at the present time, most doctors state that the single most health-improving thing that a person can do (if they smoke cigarettes) is to STOP smoking.

Figures 26-6 to 26-9 feature a number of ads from the 1930s and 40s, showing the kind of medically endorsed "encouragement" that was aimed at consumers, with regard to smoking cigarettes. Fast forward to November 24, 2017. A *New York Times* article announced that four "Big Tobacco" companies (Altria, and R. J. Reynolds Tobacco, and Lorillard, and Philip Morris USA) were federally court-ordered to begin airing advertisements on prime-time television, as well as in national newspapers, that stated they have known for the past 20 years that smoking was extremely detrimental to a person's health—yet, they knowingly misled the public about it.

"I'm going to grow a hundred years old!"
...and possibly she may—for the amazing strides of medical science have added years to life expectancy
• It's a fact—a warm, wonderful fact—that this five-year-old child, or your own child, has a life expectancy almost a whole decade longer than was her mother's, and a good 15 to 20 years longer than that of her grandmother. Not only the expectation of a longer life, but of a life by far healthier.
Thank medical science for that. Thank your doctor and thousands like him... toiling ceaselessly... that you and yours may enjoy a longer, better life.
According to a recent Nationwide survey:
More Doctors smoke Camels than any other cigarette!
NOT ONE but three outstanding independent research organizations conducted this survey. And they asked not just a few thousand, but 113,597, doctors from coast to coast to name the cigarette they themselves preferred to smoke.
Answers came in by the thousands... from general physicians, diagnosticians, surgeons, nose and throat specialists too. The most-named brand was Camel.
If you are not now smoking Camels, try them. Let your "T-Zone" tell you (see right).
CAMELS Costlier Tobaccos
THE "T-ZONE" TEST WILL TELL YOU
CAMEL
Noted throat specialists report on 30-day test of Camel smokers...
NOT ONE SINGLE CASE OF THROAT IRRITATION due to smoking CAMELS!
Yes, these were the findings of noted throat specialists after a total of 2,470 weekly examinations of the throats of hundreds of men and women who smoked Camels—and only Camels—for 30 consecutive days.
THE TEST WAS REALLY FUN! EVERY CAMEL TASTED SO GOOD! AND I DIDN'T NEED MY DOCTOR'S REPORT TO KNOW CAMELS ARE MILD!
...AND THOUSANDS MORE AGREE!
Start your own 30-Day Camel MILDNESS Test Today!

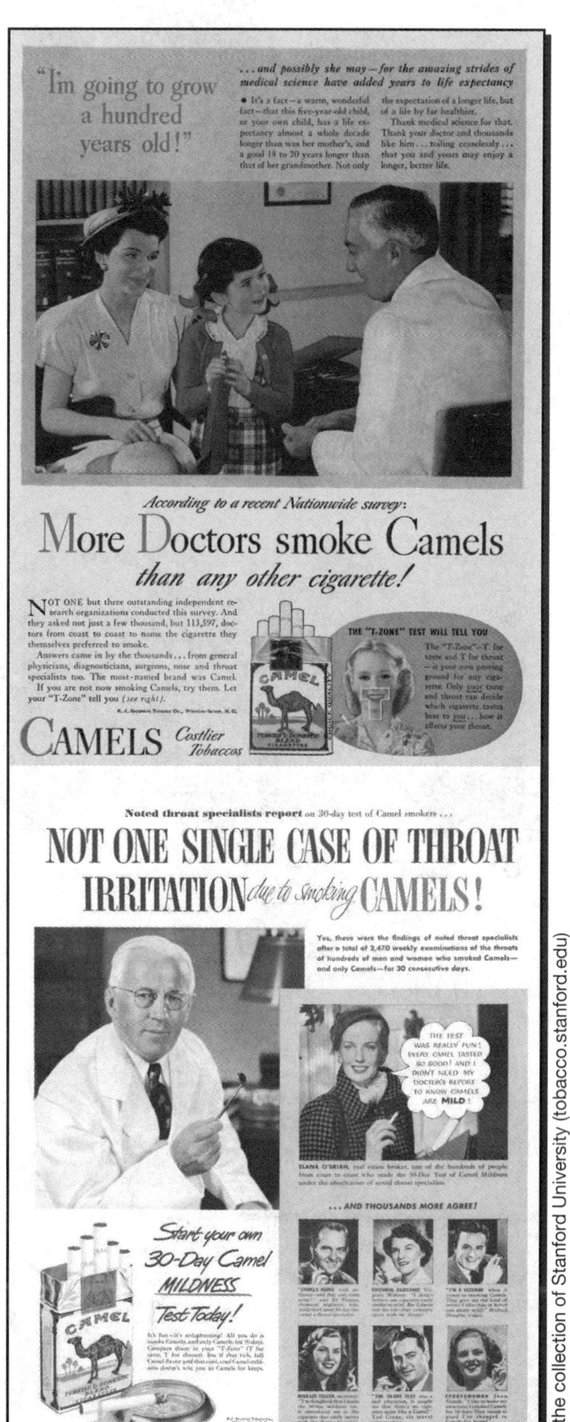

From the collection of Stanford University (tobacco.stanford.edu)

Figure 26-6

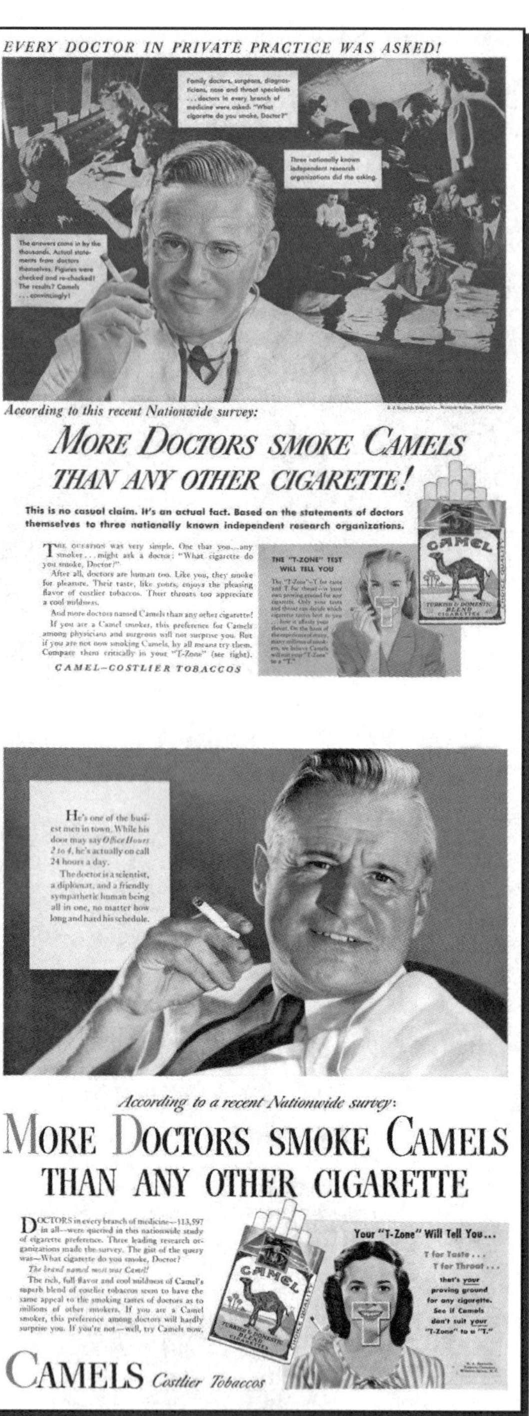


Figure 26-7

From the collection of Stanford University (tobacco.stanford.edu)

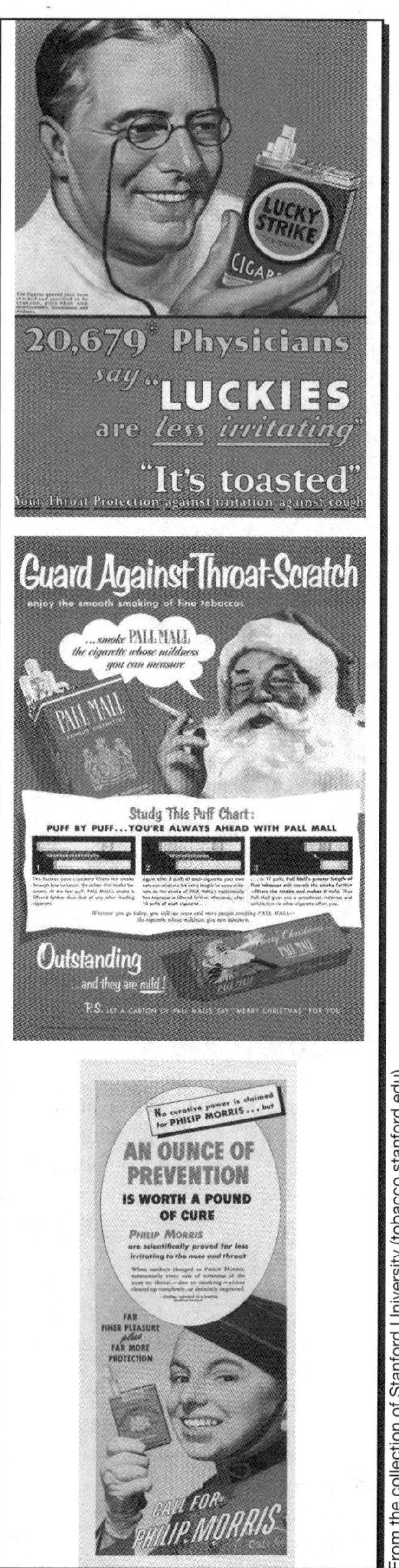


Figure 26-8

From the collection of Stanford University (tobacco.stanford.edu)

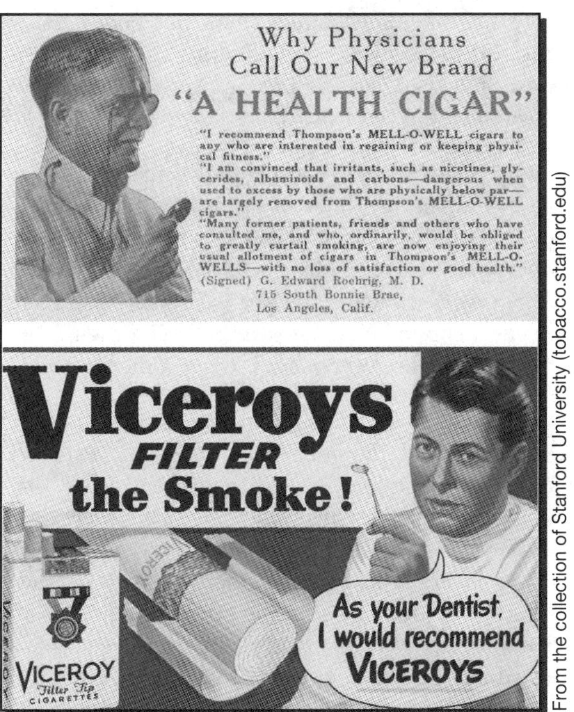

Why Physicians
Call Our New Brand
"A HEALTH CIGAR"
"I recommend Thompson's MELL-O-WELL cigars to any who are interested in regaining or keeping physical fitness."
"I am convinced that irritants, such as nicotines, glycerides, albuminoids and carbons—dangerous when used to excess by those who are physically below par—are largely removed from Thompson's MELL-O-WELL cigars."
"Many former patients, friends and others who have consulted me, and who, ordinarily, would be obliged to greatly curtail smoking, are now enjoying their usual allotment of cigars in Thompson's MELL-O-WELLS—with no loss of satisfaction or good health."
(Signed) G. Edward Roehrig, M. D.
715 South Bonnie Brae,
Los Angeles, Calif.
Viceroys
FILTER
the Smoke!
As your Dentist, I would recommend VICEROYS
VICEROY
Filter Tip
CIGARETTES
From the collection of Stanford University (tobacco.stanford.edu)
Figure 26-9

One of the court-ordered advertisements, created by the tobacco companies, stated that, "*More people die every year from smoking than murder, AIDS, suicide, drugs, car crashes, and alcohol—combined.*" Another read, "*Cigarette companies intentionally designed cigarettes with enough nicotine to create and sustain addiction.*"

This deadly and poisonous product is the same one that was endorsed by physicians—individuals who are regarded as "health experts." Certainly, there has never been any research which has demonstrated health improvements from smoking cigarettes. Did the endorsing physicians base their decision to promote cigarette-smoking on the absence of evidence demonstrating its toxicity? Were those physicians aware of the dangers of cigarette-smoking, but were more influenced by the money they were paid by the cigarette companies, than by their pledge to the Hippocratic Oath—"first, do no harm?" We can only speculate what their rationale was, but this situation is further proof that you cannot always believe those whom you think are knowledgeable and trustworthy—especially when corporate profits are involved.

## Misinformed "Experts"

In the documentary film entitled, "Blackfish," a number of former trainers of SeaWorld, reveal what they were "taught" by their employer about the lives of orcas (killer whales). During the live orca shows, audience members would ask those orca trainers questions about the lives of killer whales. The trainers would respond with answers they believed were correct. Yet, those answers were false, according to marine biologists. For example, one of the questions was, "Why do many of the orcas in the show have a collapsed dorsal fin?" The answer the trainers gave to audiences, which was told to them by SeaWorld management, was that "it's normal for about 25 percent of all orcas to have their dorsal fins collapse" (Figure 26-10, upper and lower images).

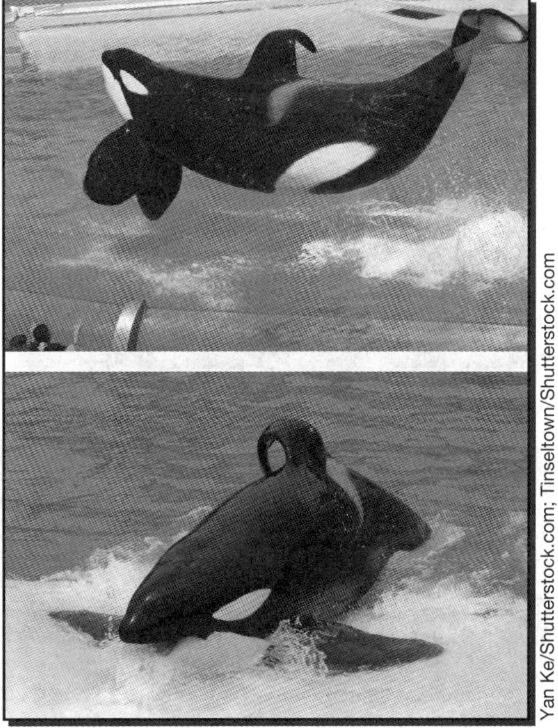

Yan Ke/Shutterstock.com; Tinseltown/Shutterstock.com
Figure 26-10

According to marine biologists, dorsal fin collapse rarely happens in the wild. "It occurs in less than 1 percent of all wild orcas," say marine biologists. The rate of incidence found in captivity—25 percent of orcas—is believed to be due to the limited swim space. According to Debbie Giles, Ph.D. (a marine biologist), orcas in the wild swim hundreds of miles, at speeds between 8 and 29 miles per hour, for which they need an upright dorsal fin (Figures 26-11 and 26-12). In captivity, they mostly just "float," never reaching even a fraction of the speed they could achieve in the open ocean, and certainly not nearly the distance.

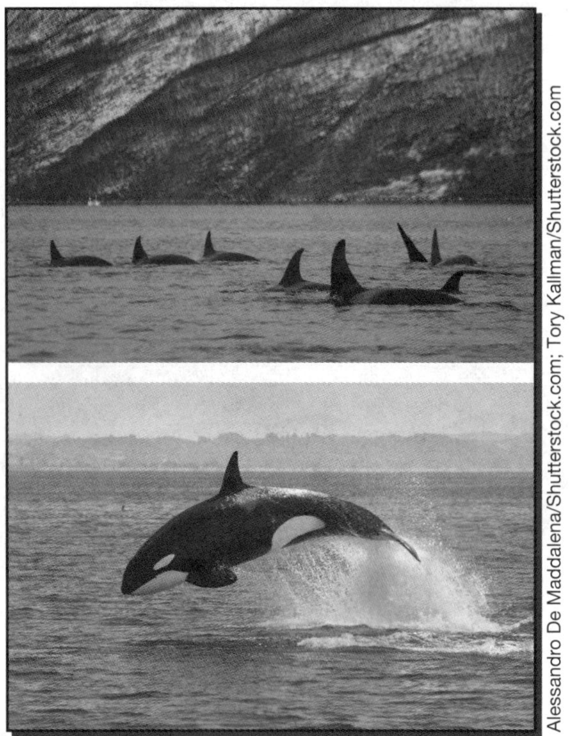

Alessandro De Maddalena/Shutterstock.com; Tory Kallman/Shutterstock.com

Figure 26-11

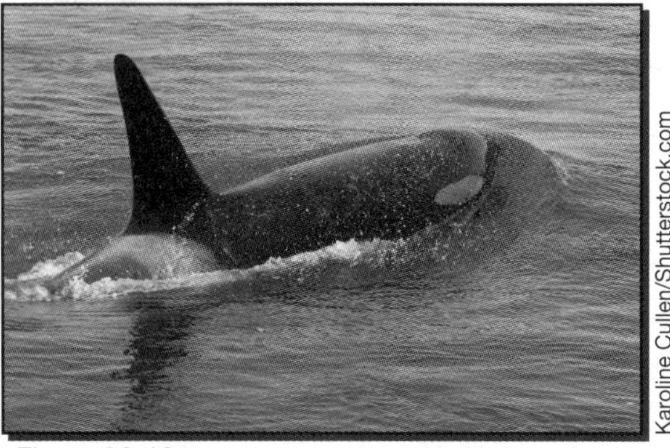

Karoline Cullen/Shutterstock.com

Figure 26-12

Another question that was asked by audience members at SeaWorld events was, "How long do killer whales live?" Again, with complete confidence and an attitude suggesting an advanced education in marine biology (though these trainers did not have that kind of education), the trainers would say that "orcas in captivity live twice as long as they do in the wild." According to independent marine biologists, however, orcas live much longer in the wild, than they do in captivity. "Most orcas in captivity only live about 20 years. In the wild, the average life span of a male orca is 30 years, and for females it's 50 years."

The SeaWorld trainers answered this question (regarding the lifespan of orcas being longer in captivity, than in the wild), believing they answered it accurately and honestly. It was not their intention to mislead the audience—though they did mislead the audience. At the time, they were completely unaware that they had been misinformed by their own their employer (i.e., the "industry").

Why were the SeaWorld trainers misinformed by their employer, about the lives of orcas? A logical explanation might be that it was meant to prevent the sympathy audience members would feel, if they believed that keeping orcas in captivity was detrimental to their well-being. In other words, there was a commercial benefit in avoiding the truth—and a potential economic consequence in revealing the truth.

What's most interesting, perhaps, is that the SeaWorld trainers answered the audience's questions with complete sincerity and confidence, believing that they had been accurately informed by their employer. They were completely unaware that they had been deliberately misinformed by their employer. The same scenario occurs in the fitness industry. Some trainers, with the same misguided confidence as demonstrated by the SeaWorld employees, make false claims about exercise—because that's what's being told to them by their industry "leaders."

This is yet another example of how it is that consumers (as well as those who are "educating" consumers—i.e., trainers) are frequently misled—often by the very same people whom they trust to properly inform them of the truth. Whether it's physicians recommending cigarettes, or trainers recommending exercises that are less than optimally productive and safe, individuals must always question the accuracy of the information they are given. Unfortunately—because of economic conflicts of interest—the information that is given to individuals is often what is most economically advantageous to the employer or the "industry"—even if it's incorrect.

## Knowledge vs. Beliefs

Prior to 9th Century BC, it was believed that the sun rotated around the Earth. It certainly appeared that way, and still does, from the perspective of someone standing on Earth. Even now, people say, "the sun rises in the east, and sets in the west," even though they know that's not technically accurate. In fact, the Sun does not move at all, although that was not known in those years.

Then, in 9th Century BC, an Indian philosopher named Yajnavalkya (Figure 26-13, uppermost image), using mathematics and geometric calculations, concluded that it's actually the Earth that rotates around the Sun. In 270 BC, a Greek mathematician named "Aristarchus" (Figure 26-13, middle-left image) arrived at the same conclusion. Although this finding was announced to the public, no one accepted it. People continued believing that the Sun revolved around the Earth.

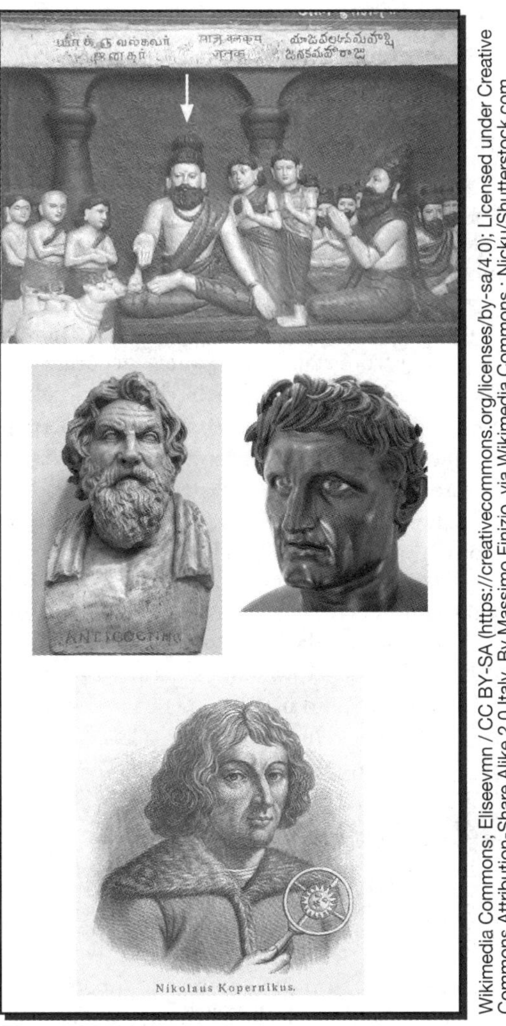


Figure 26-13

Wikimedia Commons; Eliseevmn / CC BY-SA (https://creativecommons.org/licenses/by-sa/4.0); Licensed under Creative Commons Attribution-Share Alike 2.0 Italy. By Massimo Finizio, via Wikimedia Commons.; Nicku/Shutterstock.com

In 190 BC, a Greek philosopher and astronomer named "Seleucus of Selecia" (Figure 26-13, middle-right image) also came to that same conclusion—that the Earth revolved around the Sun. Other scientists, mathematicians and philosophers began realizing the truth as well, and they also declared it publicly. Still, the vast majority of people refused to accept it.

Finally, when German mathematician and astronomer, Nicolaus Copernicus (Figure 26-14, lowermost image) made that same claim in the 16th Century AD, individuals finally began believing the Earth actually rotates around the Sun. That public acceptance, however, was more than 3000 years after the truth was first proposed.

Prior to people embracing the notion that the Earth rotates around the Sun, people claimed to "know" that the Sun rotated around the Earth. They considered it "knowledge," but it was actually a mistaken "belief," based on conjecture, and the absence of better information.

In 1916, Albert Einstein predicted "gravitational waves," as part of his general theory of relativity. Gravitational waves are "ripples in space time" that are caused by objects moving through the universe. At the time, Albert Einstein's prediction was criticized and ridiculed by individuals who refused to accept the possibility of it being correct, even though he gave a rational explanation in support of his theory.

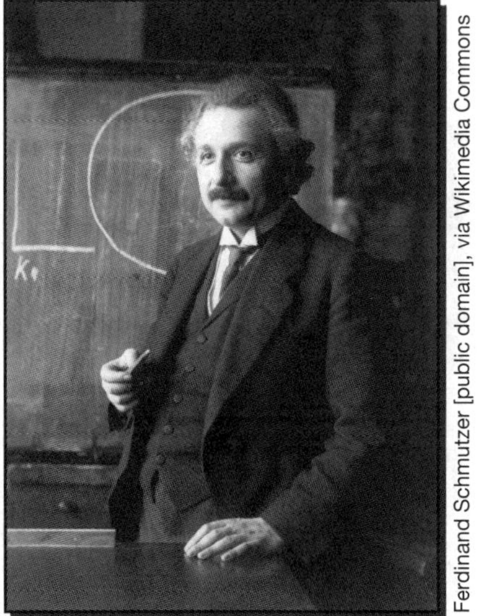

Figure 26-14

Ferdinand Schmutzer [public domain], via Wikimedia Commons

Einstein's theory was eventually proven to be correct on September 14, 2015, by a group of researchers known as "The Laser Interferometer Gravitational-Wave Observatory" (LIGO). As such, the existence of gravitational waves is now considered "knowledge," whereas before it was considered a "crack pot" belief.

As these scenarios demonstrate, there is a long history of people refusing to accept new evidence, or to embrace a more logical approach to a pre-existing belief. The reason for this human tendency is that people typically identify with their beliefs. In other words, the things that people think are true become part of their identity.

If a person's belief about something is demonstrated to be false, it often makes them feel as if their identity is threatened (subconsciously). The longer that belief has been held by a person and the more "invested" they are in that belief, the more difficult it is for them to accept that that belief is false. As a result, people sometimes feel an impulsive need to defend that which they have believed to be true. People who spend many years in a particular field often develop a certain level of confidence—perhaps even arrogance—about their "knowledge" in that particular subject. Sometimes, however, that confidence is misguided.

For example, on occasion, you may see a veteran "weightlifter" (60+ years old) walk into a gym, with a high level of confidence—an attitude suggesting, "*These young kids today don't know a damn thing about weight lifting ... I've spent more years in gyms than they've been alive ... I know my way around a gym.*" That person then proceeds to perform exercises, which are clearly explained in this book as being inefficient, unproductive, or dangerous.

Spending years studying the science of a particular subject can indeed make a person very knowledgeable about that subject. On the other hand, spending years entrenched in the mythology and the "conventional wisdom" of a subject (close to it, but not actually studying the science of it) will only make an individual "knowledgeable" about the way that subject has been practiced—even if it's wrong. As world-renowned physicist, cosmologist, and Lucasian professor of mathematics Stephen Hawking once said, "*The greatest enemy of knowledge is not ignorance. It is the illusion of knowledge.*"

In fact, it can be much worse to have an incorrect understanding of a particular subject, than it is to have no knowledge at all about that subject. As a rule, individuals with no knowledge about a subject tend to be more receptive to new information, than are people with a pre-existing (but incorrect) "knowledge" about that subject. In that regard, "Osho" (Indian spiritual guru and philosopher) once said, "*One of the greatest misfortunes in the world is that the foolish are absolutely certain, and the wise are hesitant.*"

## Psychological Barriers to New (Better) Information

In reality, people who are certain that they fully understand a subject, are often closed-minded about considering new (perhaps more logical) information. A wiser approach might be to take the position that "*We may believe something is true and correct, based on the information we have at this time. If new and better information is made available, however, we are open to the possibility of adjusting our understanding of that subject.*"

For hundreds of years, psychologists have been aware of a phenomenon referred to as "The Einstellung effect," which is a tendency for people to cling to the most familiar solution to a problem (i.e., method of doing something), while stubbornly ignoring alternative solutions (i.e, methods). As such, Francis Bacon—an English philosopher, scientist, and essayist—called it "one of the most common forms of cognitive bias" in his 1620 book entitled, "*Novum Organum.*" ("*Novum Organum*"—Latin for "New Instrument" or "true direction"—is a treatise about the interpretation of science and nature.)

Harvard University professor Steven Jay Gould also addressed this phenomenon in his 1981 book entitled, "*The Mismeasure of Man.*" Gould noted that humans tend to not only preferentially seek and embrace information that supports their already existing beliefs, even when those beliefs are wrong, they often aggressively condemn information that may disprove their belief. In addition, they may also attempt to belittle the person making the claim or who is providing the new information.

As if this type of closed-minded attitude is not enough to block a person from considering more accurate information, there is yet another human behavioral trait that tends to interfere with the learning of truth, and further perpetuates false or inaccurate beliefs. Psychologists refer to this characteristic as "the backfire effect," which is the tendency many people have to defend their belief more aggressively, when more evidence is presented that refutes their belief.

Apparently, the more evidence that is provided, the more it "backfires." Rather than increasing the likelihood that additional evidence will change a person's belief, it often causes that individual to more aggressively defend their belief. A person will either refuse to listen at all, or will use irrational arguments to oppose the new information. This response is very similar to what occurs when a person's character is being assaulted—they become "defensive."

Of course, a person is free to believe whatever they choose to believe, whether it's accurate or not. In general, people have all sorts of beliefs, many of which are not the least bit reasonable. On the other hand, people who are wise tend to thoughtfully and rationally evaluate and consider new information. If they find it sensible, they incorporate that new information into their belief system. The new information is not viewed as an assault on their character, whether it has merit or not.

As you have discovered in this book, many exercises that you may have thought were "good," are actually not so good, when they are examined more closely. Meanwhile, other exercises, which you may have never seen before, are actually very good, when viewed through the lens of sound logic and biomechanics (physics and anatomy).

This "new" information is likely to be unsettling for many people—possibly even you. At the very least, hopefully, it is cause for you to rethink your previous understanding about resistance exercise—intended for the purpose of physique development or for general physical fitness. This new perspective is very logical and sensible, and is perfectly accurate from an engineering (physics) perspective—hence, the endorsement of physics experts, orthopedic physicians, and an evolutionary biologist. Ideally, you'll be more skeptical of the "advice" you hear, when it violates the universal physics principles outlined in this book—even if it comes from people who wear the cloak of authority and of "knowledge."

In fact, the best way to distinguish between good advice about an exercise, and bad advice, is to understand the principles that apply to all things that are mechanical (physics), as well as to understand basic human musculoskeletal facts. These 13 physics and musculoskeletal factors are outlined at the beginning of this chapter.

Resistance exercise is a mechanical event, because the human body is made up of levers, pivots, and "pulleys"—i.e., muscles that pull on their corresponding levers. In reality, no debate should exist about which exercises are "better" or "worse" than other exercises. It's all determined by what constitutes "natural" human anatomical movement and physics (math). It's as black and white as is the engineering of an architectural structure—a bridge or a crane. It's all quantifiable, once you understand the basic principles of biomechanics—explained in this book.

After reading this book, you should no longer be fooled by the plethora of misinformation and the endless trends peddled to the world by commercial enterprises, who are more focused on maximizing their profits than they are in providing individuals with truthful and sensible information for optimal fitness improvements. As such, knowing the truth (about biomechanics) can set you free from being duped or conned into believing unreasonable claims about exercise, ever again.

I am grateful for the opportunity to share with you what I've learned throughout the four decades that I've devoted to exploring and studying the mechanics of resistance exercise. Hopefully, this information will allow you to improve your physical condition beyond what you could have imagined; that it will allow you to stay injury-free; that it will spare you from needlessly wasting time and energy on inefficient exercises; and that (if you are a personal trainer) it will help make you be a better resource of information for the clients you serve.

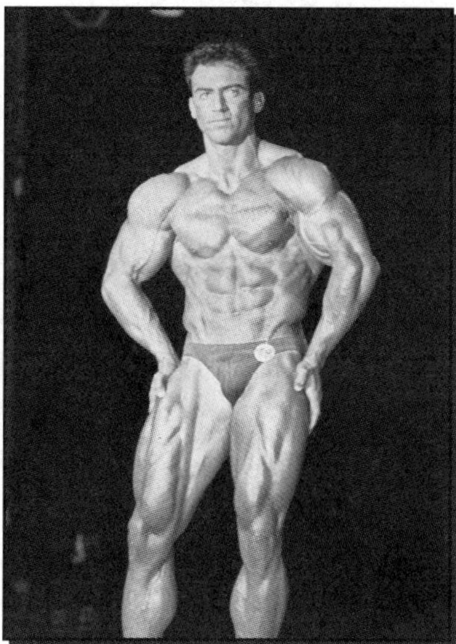

Figure 26-15

# About the Author

Doug Brignole is a bodybuilding champion, author, personal trainer, and public speaker. Certified by both ACE and ACSM, he has dedicated his life to the study of exercise science, particularly the field of biomechanics. In the process, he has written articles for numerous fitness publications, authored or co-authored two well-received books, and conducted seminars on addressing "how fitness actually works" to audiences around the world.

Doug's extensive bodybuilding career has enabled him to put into practice the biomechanics principles he strongly advocates. Starting with weight training at age 14, he began his bodybuilding career at age 16—a mission he continued until the age of 59. Along the way, he won a number of titles and awards, including the Mr. California title in 1982, the 1986 Mr. America competition (medium-tall division), the Mr. Universe competition (medium-tall division) also in 1986, and the 2019 Mr. Universe competition—open division/overall—at the age of 59.

In addition to his renowned expertise in biomechanics, Doug is known for his ability to articulate mechanically complex concepts in layman's terms. In that regard, he is one of the very few individuals who is able to accurately identify and explain the mechanical and musculoskeletal factors by which all resistance exercises can be appropriately evaluated, with respect to efficiency, productivity, and safety.